TRANSLATIONAL IMMUNOLOGY

TRANSLATIONAL IMMUNOLOGY

Mechanisms and Pharmacologic Approaches

Edited by
SENG-LAI TAN, Ph.D.

ELSEVIER

AMSTERDAM • BOSTON • HEIDELBERG • LONDON
NEW YORK • OXFORD • PARIS • SAN DIEGO
SAN FRANCISCO • SINGAPORE • SYDNEY • TOKYO
Academic Press is an imprint of Elsevier

Academic Press is an imprint of Elsevier
225 Wyman Street, Waltham, MA 02451, USA
525 B Street, Suite 1800, San Diego, CA 92101–4495, USA
125 London Wall, London, EC2Y 5AS, UK
The Boulevard, Langford Lane, Kidlington, Oxford OX5 1GB, UK

British Library Cataloguing in Publication Data
A catalogue record for this book is available from the British Library

Library of Congress Cataloging-in-Publication Data
A catalog record for this book is available from the Library of Congress

For information on all Academic Press publications
visit our website at http://store.elsevier.com/

ISBN: 978-0-12-801577-3

Publisher: Janice Audet
Acquisition Editor: Linda Versteeg-Buschman
Editorial Project Manager: Halima Williams
Production Project Manager: Lucía Pérez
Designer: Greg Harris

Typeset by SPi

CONTENTS

CONTRIBUTORS

A. Agua-Doce
Instituto de Medicina Molecular, University of Lisbon, Lisbon, Portugal

O. Awe
Herman B Wells Center for Pediatric Research, and
Indiana University School of Medicine, Indianapolis, IN, United States

R.I. Azevedo
Instituto de Medicina Molecular, University of Lisbon, Lisbon, Portugal

R. Bacchetta
Stanford Medical School, Stanford, CA, United States

R. Bortell
University of Massachusetts Medical School, Diabetes Center of Excellence, Worcester, MA, United States

M.A. Brehm
University of Massachusetts Medical School, Diabetes Center of Excellence, Worcester, MA, United States

A.N. Burska
University of Leeds, Leeds, United Kingdom

K. Csomos
Harvard Medical School, Boston, MA, United States

J.C. Denny
Vanderbilt University, Nashville, TN, United States

J.T. Dudley
Icahn School of Medicine at Mount Sinai, New York, NY, United States

J. Farmer
Harvard Medical School, Boston, MA, United States

D.R. Getts
Department of Microbiology-Immunology and Interdepartmental Immunobiology Center, Feinberg School of Medicine, Northwestern University, Chicago, IL, United States

L. Graca
Instituto de Medicina Molecular, University of Lisbon, Lisbon, Portugal

D.L. Greiner
University of Massachusetts Medical School, Diabetes Center of Excellence, Worcester, MA, United States

S.R. Harrison
University of Leeds, Leeds, United Kingdom

S. Hillion
Université de Brest, and LabEx IGO, and Laboratory of Immunology, Brest University Medical School Hospital, Brest, France

M.H. Kaplan
Herman B Wells Center for Pediatric Research, and
Indiana University School of Medicine, Indianapolis, IN, United States

B.A. Kidd
Icahn School of Medicine at Mount Sinai, New York, NY, United States

J.F. Lacerda
Instituto de Medicina Molecular, University of Lisbon, and Hospital de Santa Maria, Lisbon, Portugal

Y.N. Lee
Division of Immunology, Children's Hospital, Harvard Medical School, Boston, MA, United States

S.D. Miller
Department of Microbiology-Immunology and Interdepartmental Immunobiology Center, Feinberg School of Medicine, Northwestern University, Chicago, IL, United States

M. Monteiro
Instituto de Medicina Molecular, University of Lisbon, Lisbon, Portugal

F. Ponchel
University of Leeds, Leeds, United Kingdom

L.D. Shultz
The Jackson Laboratory, Bar Harbor, ME, United States

Q. Simon
Université de Brest, and LabEx IGO, and Laboratory of Immunology, Brest University Medical School Hospital, Brest, France

C.B. Smarr
Department of Microbiology-Immunology and Interdepartmental Immunobiology Center, Feinberg School of Medicine, Northwestern University, Chicago, IL, United States

H. Ueno
Baylor Institute for Immunology Research, Dallas, TX, United States

M. Verma
The Jackson Laboratory, Bar Harbor, ME, United States

J.E. Walter
Harvard Medical School, Boston, MA, United States

J.L. Warner
Vanderbilt University, Nashville, TN, United States

Jianfei Yang
GlaxoSmithKline, Cambridge, MA, United States

PREFACE

Human disease is complex and is intricately intertwined with some level of deregulation of the immune system. Improved understanding of how our immune system functions to fend off foreign invaders and remove cancerous cells while maintaining immunological tolerance to self and promoting tissue homeostasis is central to the development of more effective therapies for combating a wide variety of human illnesses. This book was prepared to summarize and highlight some of the most important advances in human immunology, examples of clinical translations, new tools to analyze therapeutic targets, and new pharmacological approaches for the treatment of immune disorders. To that end, we have assembled a diverse group of highly regarded experts, as well as emerging thought leaders in the field, who have prepared 12 chapters covering different concepts, which could fundamentally change how we target the immune system for disease therapy.

This monograph is organized into three sections: Human Immunology, Emerging Pharmacological Targets, and New Approaches. In the first section, Kidd and Dudley emphasize the need to understand human immunology at the systems level. Also, they review how recent advances in high-throughput "omics" technologies and computational analysis techniques are improving disease understanding, and accelerating the discovery of better diagnostic markers and therapies (Chapter 1). Next, Walter and colleagues review our current understanding of monogenic primary immunodeficiency disease and its implications for mechanism-based targeted therapies (Chapter 2). Indeed, the advent of electronic personal health records is enabling our ability to phenotype large human populations. In Chapter 3, Warner and Denny discuss how an important translational bioinformatics tool known as phenome-wide association study (PheWAS) can be applied to link diseases or traits to a given genetic variant or biomarker. Not to be outdone, single-cell analysis has the power uncover the complexity inherent in heterogeneous populations of cells and reveal important functional insights. This is showcased in Chapter 4, wherein Lee discusses the application of RNA sequencing in a high-throughput manner to study the T cell receptor repertoire.

Immune cells have the ability to differentiate into functionally distinct effector and regulatory cell subsets, depending on the cytokines present within the microenvironment during an active immune response. Each specialized immune cell subset plays a critical role in fine-tuning our immune responses. This is perhaps best studied in the T lymphocyte population, which is covered in the second section of the book. In Chapter 5, Yang summarizes our current understanding of the T-helper 17 cells (Th17) as key effectors of autoimmune inflammatory diseases, and outlines strategies targeting the lineage of Th17 cells. The growing evidence of Th9 cells' role in contributing to human disease, thus another emerging target for drug development, is discussed by Awe and Kaplan (Chapter 6). Ueno reviews the critical role of T follicular helper cells (Tfh) in providing help to B cells, allowing for the production of high affinity antibodies (Chapter 7). Graca and colleagues summarize our current understanding of the role of regulatory T cell subsets (Treg) play in maintaining peripheral tolerance while preventing autoimmune diseases and limiting chronic inflammation (Chapter 8). In the same vein, a subset of B cells with regulatory functions (Breg) is also gaining traction in their own right as a potential target for therapeutic manipulation. Simon and Hillion cover this topic in Chapter 9.

In the final section of the book, readers are treated to state-of-the-art approaches for interventional immunology. Induction of antigen-specific immune tolerance is the desired goal for the treatment of autoimmune and allergic diseases, and protection of transplanted cells and tissues. Miller and colleagues review recent alternative methods of inducing tolerance for the treatment of allergic diseases (Chapter 10). Humanized mice are increasingly being utilized as a preclinical bridge between mouse studies and clinical trials. Greiner and colleagues discuss advances in the development of mice engrafted with functional human immune systems, and the utility of humanized mice for translating the next generation of cell based and immunomodulatory therapies into the clinic (Chapter 11). Finally, personalized or stratified medicine is recognized as a high priority goal for healthcare providers, pharmaceutical industries, and patients. Ponchel and colleagues discuss the role of immunological biomarkers in stratified medicine, as well as the challenges that needed to be overcome in order to establish their utility in routine clinical practice (Chapter 12).

While this book is not meant to be exhaustive, we hope it will provide readers an understanding of the rationale and mechanisms underlying some of the current and emerging pharmacologic approaches for translational immunology, as well as the gaps therein, and new ideas for better and safer therapeutic approaches.

Seng-Lai Tan, PhD
Editor

SECTION A

Human Immunology

CHAPTER 1

Systems Immunology

B.A. Kidd, J.T. Dudley
Icahn School of Medicine at Mount Sinai, New York, NY, United States

Contents

Translational Immunology
http://dx.doi.org/10.1016/B978-0-12-801577-3.00001-0

1. INTRODUCTION

From the earliest to the latest moments in life, the immune system stands ready to recognize and respond to threats that arise from external (eg, infectious agents) and internal (eg, malignant cells) sources. Potential threats are processed and then acted upon by molecules and cells organized in a distributed network that covers every organ system. The molecular and cellular agents of the immune system coordinate their interactions in time to protect the organism. In the process, the immune system evolves and adapts to an ever-changing environment, forming a complex system that shapes an individual's health.

Throughout the twentieth century, researchers identified the building blocks that comprise the immune system and teased apart the molecular regulatory pathways that govern immunity. These findings led to advances in vaccines and the development of targeted therapeutics like monoclonal antibodies. By contrast, the twenty-first century has ushered in a transition where we are now moving from cataloging the immunological parts list to integrating these components into a whole. In connecting the dots between the elements in this complex system, we are constructing a more complete picture of how these myriad parts coordinate to protect the organism from danger, damage, and disease.

In this chapter, we describe the burgeoning field of systems immunology, which is a discipline that connects the dots between how cells and molecules interact to create functions that are greater than the sum of their parts. We discuss how the confluence of high-throughput technologies and large-scale data generation are providing new insights into disease mechanisms and offering new opportunities for better treatment and prevention of immune-mediated diseases.

2. IMMUNE SYSTEM IS A DISTRIBUTED AND DECENTRALIZED NETWORK THAT PROTECTS AGAINST DISEASE AND PROVIDES A READOUT ON HEALTH

The immune system comprises a complex network of molecules and cells that coordinate their actions to protect against disease and maintain health. Individuals are protected from disease *via* numerous regulatory pathways and mechanisms that are both distributed (ie, found in almost every anatomical location) and work by acting on multiple levels (eg, genes, proteins, cells, tissues, and organ systems). Health is maintained through repair mechanisms that remove infected or dead cells and supervise rebuilding damaged tissue. Both maintenance and protection are ongoing operations that the immune system performs throughout the course of an organism's lifetime. In this section, we examine the interactions among immunological agents—molecules and cells of the immune system—as well as the interface between the immune system and its environment to explore some of the exciting opportunities for new therapies.

2.1 Immune cells are distributed and specialized

The immune system comprises numerous molecular and cellular agents that are distributed throughout the body in a decentralized network. Some agents, eg, antibodies, granulocytes, lymphocytes, and monocytes, circulate throughout the blood and lymphatic systems, the immunological superhighways. Other agents, eg, cytokines, dendritic cells, and macrophages, are found in specific tissues, taking up residence to serve as sentinels against potential threats. All cellular agents of the immune system originate from hematopoietic stem cells in the bone marrow, which differentiate into specialized cells based on environmental cues that activate a particular genetic programming. Once activated, these genetic circuits refine and restrict the molecular arsenal of each leukocyte, turning pluripotent progenitors into distinct cell types that fulfill a specific functional niche (eg, dendritic cells process and present antigens, whereas CD8 + T cells recognize antigens and secrete cytotoxic enzymes). These diverse cell types form a network that together build an immunological wall to protect the host against innumerable threats.

Immune cells have two special properties that make them particularly good at sensing health and preventing disease. First, immune cells can recognize a vast repertoire of molecules and molecular patterns in their environment. In specialized cells, these patterns are encoded and stored in immunological memory so the system can mount a more rapid and vigorous response upon subsequent encounters. This mechanism for creating and storing immunological memories means the immune system can learn from and adapt to its environment. Second, immune cells integrate numerous environmental signals and decide on the most appropriate response based on the contextual cues. These responses setup complex intercellular signaling patterns and feedback loops that can convey a broad array of information between immune cells and their environment. Remarkably, this communication is robust and allows the immune system to disseminate information with high fidelity so cellular actions are coordinated and regulated.

Immune cell signaling is an area where systems approaches have become essential for capturing the full complexity of all the molecular interactions between immune cells and decoding how they influence immune system states. To date, 456 cell-signaling proteins (cytokines, chemokines, growth factors, and hormones) have been identified that can influence the immune system. These molecular messengers interact with one or more of the 306 distinct receptors present on the surface of the more than 450 different immune cell types that have been characterized. This large pool of signaling molecules, receptors, and cell types form a decentralized and distributed communication network that relays information amongst immune cells and regulates their function. To capture and organize the full set of possible interactions between cells and signaling proteins, researchers have applied systematic approaches that mine the scientific knowledge base to connect the dots between cells, cytokines, and function (Shen-Orr et al., 2009; Patil et al., 2010). These text-mining methods construct inter-cellular interaction maps, which can be linked with other systems approaches to connect up to the internal signaling networks responsible for controlling cellular states (Linding et al., 2007; Janes et al., 2008). Using these systematic approaches to analyze and improve our understanding of immune cell-signaling networks is critical because these networks bind the immune system together and connect it to other systems. This more complete picture of how the full communication system operates will help uncover the mechanisms underlying many different diseases (Osborn and Olefsky, 2012; O'Sullivan et al., 2007; O'Shea et al., 2011; Neurath, 2014; Griffin, 2013) and suggest strategies for better treatments (Cosgrove et al., 2010; O'Shea and Plenge, 2012; O'Shea et al., 2013; Feldmann, 2002).

2.2 Immune system connects to all aspects of health and disease

The features that make the immune system effective at recognizing, repelling, and removing danger also establish the immune system as a master integrator of information about health and disease. Moreover, the immune system connects to every other organ system and interfaces with the environment to provide protection and help maintain health (Fig. 1). The immune system plays a central role in allergy, autoimmunity, and infectious disease. Immune surveillance is key for recognizing and removing abnormal cells and many cancerous cells emerge and flourish by finding mechanisms to evade this surveillance. The immune system is highly active and requires continual renewal and regeneration of its cells. Many cancers arise from genetic abnormalities in immune cells that originate during growth and differentiation. Furthermore, dysregulation of inflammatory mechanisms and other immune-mediated processes have been associated with cardiovascular disease, metabolic disorders, and neurodegenerative diseases. This

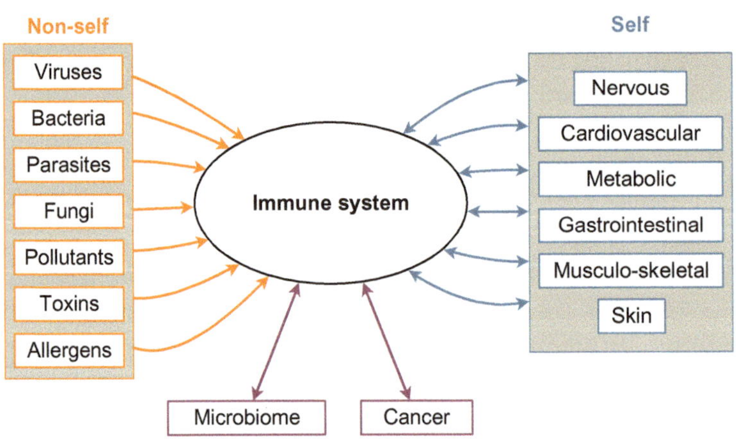

Figure 1 Immune system is a master integrator of information about health and disease. The immune system is a complex network of cells and molecules that integrate information from multiple sources to provide immunity and maintain health.

entrenched connection to every organ system is significant because it implies that immune system health is strongly tied to overall health. Maintaining proper immune function may be the best course of action for preserving health. As we will see later, immune monitoring provides a readout of an individual's well-being and offers more precise feedback on therapeutic interventions.

2.3 Commensal organisms

Investigations into the human microbiome are uncovering complex microbial ecosystems that engage with the immune system and altering how we think about health and disease (Human Microbiome Project, C, 2012a,b; Brown et al., 2013). For example, commensal bacteria play a critical role in both the development, education, and maintenance of proper immune function (Shen et al., 2014; Ahern et al., 2014).This area of research is developing rapidly and in tandem with systems immunology so much remains to be done. However, what's become clear is the microbiome shapes the immune system's response to the environment—diet, infection, and allergy—and influences how the immune system contributes to both the development and treatment of disease (eg, diabetes, cancer, and autoimmunity).

Recent investigations into this immune-microbiome interface are revealing novel regulatory interactions and control that will have implications for clinical medicine. Preliminary findings suggest the microbiome can affect both the development of cancer, as well as the immune response to cancer therapy (Iida et al., 2013; Zitvogel et al., 2015; Viaud et al., 2013). Other studies have shown that the microbiome plays a role in nutritional uptake and influences metabolic control over the immune system in ways that have interesting implications for understanding and treating metabolic disorders including type 2 diabetes (Henao-Mejia et al., 2012; Kau et al., 2011; Dastani et al., 2012). Collectively, these findings have interesting implications for immune homeostasis, allergy, and autoimmunity. These findings clearly need additional follow-up and consideration to determine what role they will play in the clinic. Given the complexity of the interactions between the immune system and the microbiome, systems approaches will be required to identify therapies that restore control from microbe–immune system imbalances.

2.4 Infectious diseases

The main cause of morbidity and mortality for most of human existence has been disease-causing microorganisms. Pathogens exploit transient openings in the immunological wall to invade their host and co-opt cellular machinery or resources for survival. This process causes havoc on the host and results in acute, or sometimes chronic, disease. Not surprisingly, every tissue in the body is susceptible to infection by some microorganism. Fortunately, the immune system's influence extends to every tissue in the body, and the immune system uses its molecular and cellular arsenal to counter pathogens by engaging and fending off these infectious agents wherever they are found. Thus, the immune system and infectious agents remain locked in perpetual battle for survival. While some microorganisms can be challenging to isolate, assaying the immune system yields clues about whether an infection has happened, what type of response was mounted, and whether the host will recover.

All infectious agents interact with the immune system and leave a mark that can be used help track their origin. These agents elicit specific immune responses, which can be helpful in predicting their virulence and identifying therapeutic options for treating the disease. For example, antibodies present in serum signal that the immune system encountered a pathogen at some point in the past. A recent study harnessed this property and showed how to comprehensively characterize the complete history of pathogen encounters by profiling human sera on microarrays displaying viral epitopes (Xu et al., 2015). The abundance of antibodies indicates how well protected an individual will be to future infections and whether that individual might need an immune boost to raise the circulating levels of a particular antibody. The presence of antigen-specific T cells signifies cellular immunity against a particular infectious agent. Further functional and phenotypic characterization of these T cells provides a readout on the strength of immunity. While systems approaches currently offer information on how the immune system responds to, or determines the components of protection against infection, later sections will explore real-time monitoring for immediate feedback on host response.

2.5 Allergic diseases

Asthma, atopy, and allergic diseases are common across all age groups, affecting around 8% of the population in the United States (17 million adults and 7 million children). These conditions are clinically characterized by inflammation of either the airways or skin, brought about by exposure to an allergen or other environmental trigger. In many cases, the environmental triggers of allergic diseases can be difficult to determine. Moreover, the immune response is complex as multiple cellular and molecular players can drive inflammation and allergic reactions. Systems immunology offers tools for building more accurate models of this complexity and suggesting novel treatments.

The primary treatment for atopic diseases is immune and inflammatory suppression with corticosteroids. While effective in the short-term, long-term topical glucocorticoid use leads to cutaneous atrophy, thus making the skin susceptible to damage and infection. One example of how systems immunology approaches can identify novel treatment options comes from a recent study to characterize the transcriptional response to topical glucocorticoids. This study found that combination therapy with steroids and the mTOR inhibitor that regulates development and damage responses (REDD1) could eliminate the adverse side effects while maintaining the therapeutic benefit of steroids (Baida et al., 2014).

Asthma is a complex condition where multiple therapeutic options are employed. These options include fast-acting bronchodilators that relieve airway constriction and enzyme inhibitors that target leukotrienes, inflammatory mediators produced by immune cells. The complex tissue architecture of the airways plus the myriad immune cells contributing to disease and range of therapeutic responses suggest that integrative approaches are needed to identify novel treatments for asthma (Bunyavanich and Schadt, 2015). These approaches have been useful for identifying some of the key pathways that drive allergic responses at the genetic and cellular levels (Sharma et al., 2014; Bunyavanich et al., 2015). The combination of systematic analyses (Bonnelykke et al., 2013) and well-characterized preclinical models (Kelada et al., 2014) provide platforms for discovery and testing that can take advantage of the highly connected nature of the immune system.

2.6 Autoimmune diseases

Autoimmunity represents a clinical condition where the immune system fails to discriminate between self and nonself. The occasional failure to distinguish friend from foe results in a coordinated attack by immunological agents on self-antigens. At a biochemical level, no structural difference exists between self and foreign antigens. In fact, the recognition of self-antigens plays an important part in the development, maintenance, and survival of B cells and T cells. Autoreactive immune cells can, and do, arise against any tissue, yet the prevalence of autoimmunity remains low because additional molecular, cellular, and contextual cues control immune responses to self-antigens. In order to capture and analyze the complex set of regulatory interactions that control autoimmunity, systems approaches offer a natural approach that can integrate high-throughput data collected from environmental, genetic, molecular, cellular, and microbiome measurements into models that can both explain various mechanisms by which autoimmunity arises and predict control points for treating these conditions.

The combination of genetic, environmental, and lifestyle factors that contribute to autoimmunity make these disorders complex diseases. Multiple genomic studies have identified hundreds of genetic loci that are associated with one or more autoimmune diseases (Visscher et al., 2012). While alleles in the human leukocyte antigen (HLA) genes contribute the most to disease susceptibility, a number of immune-related, but non-HLA genes have been linked to autoimmunity (Welter et al., 2014). Although genome-wide association studies (GWAS) permit an unbiased scan of the entire genome and provide strong association with particular regions to disease, understanding the causal drivers require fine mapping of genetic loci or functional studies that link the underlying genotypic variation with a phenotypic trait (Chen et al., 2014; Schadt et al., 2005). Functional data for these studies are often provided from high-throughput scans of all transcripts expressed in a particular sample. Transcriptional profiling of leukocytes collected from peripheral blood has been successfully applied to determine the molecular networks of many autoimmune diseases (Pascual et al., 2010), and the systems approaches have shown promise for characterizing autoimmune and autoinflammatory disorders (Banchereau et al., 2013). More work is required, yet these methods reveal the potential of systems immunology to advance our understanding of disease, identify better biomarkers, and improve drug development.

2.7 Inflammatory diseases

The inflammatory response represents a mechanism employed by the immune system to respond to infection or injury, and to orchestrate repair. The inflammatory response triggers multiple signaling processes and encourages cross talk among multiple cells and tissues. Multiple biomarkers can serve as surrogates for an inflammatory response (eg, C-reactive protein, IL-6, and TNF-alpha) and these molecules are measured clinically to assess whether an individual has chronic inflammation, which implies immune dysregulation and can indicate inflammatory disease. Almost all immune-mediated diseases contain an inflammatory component (McGonagle and McDermott, 2006) and inflammation is a major component of many noncanonical immunological diseases (eg, cardiovascular, obesity, type 2 diabetes, neurodegenerative, cancer). Whether inflammation is causal, or a by-product of other disease processes is not clear. Tracking inflammatory dysregulation and understanding the processes that might shift inflammation from a transient to chronic condition should be a top priority for systems immunology because of the problem's complexity and the societal benefit in identifying new therapies.

Inflammation is a protective response that causes collateral damage to normal healthy tissue in the process of preserving the host from injury and infection. From an evolutionary perspective, the trade-off between host damage and preservation has been optimized over a long timescale across multiple environments. Our current environment provides many immune stimuli that may be misaligned with the immune response traits evolution selected (Okin and Medzhitov, 2012). This suggested mismatch has been proposed as an explanation for why the inflammatory response is associated with so many modern diseases. To explore this evolutionary hypothesis further, one line of inquiry is to examine genetic conditions that lead to autoinflammatory disorders. Although monogenic autoinflammatory conditions are rare, they do shed light on mechanisms for immune dysregulation that influence inflammation and underlie common illnesses. In particular, the discovery of the proinflammatory molecule IL-1b, and its role in both autoinflammatory diseases and inflammasome activation, has made IL-1b antagonists potent therapies for inflammation, sepsis, and immunological disorders (Goldbach-Mansky and Kastner, 2009). However, more studies and follow-up are needed that utilize systems approaches to understand the broader therapeutic consequences and side effects, as well as to connect antiinflammatory therapies to other disorders associated with inflammation.

A strong argument for using systems approaches that consider evolution comes from the fact that the transcriptional response pattern of inflammation is shared across multiple disease models from mouse and rat (Wang et al., 2012b). The conserved immunological features reflect subcomponents of the inflammatory response involved in leukocyte activation, cytokine production, chemotaxis, and toll-like receptor (TLR) signaling. The gene expression profiles show similarity across diseases and the patterns are conserved across tissues and species. The shared biological subnetworks found in the different species and diseases tie together seemingly disparate processes, unifying them into a framework that helps explain molecular mechanisms of disease and identify potential therapies. This inflammatory signature also shows significant overlap with a macrophage-enriched metabolic network that has been found in both humans and mice.

As we've seen, systems approaches to immunological conditions can be applied across diseases to find common regulatory pathways or gene expression signatures that unify diverse conditions at the molecular, cellular, or phenotypic level. These approaches are also suited to focus on a single disease to understand how the different biological levels contribute to a complex disorder. As an example, we highlight a recent study that examined a complex inflammatory condition, inflammatory bowel disease (IBD) (Jostins et al., 2012). This study collected more than 75,000 cases and controls to develop quantitative models that linked genetics, gene expression profiling, evolutionary traits, and host–microbe interactions into the most comprehensive picture to date of inflammatory bowl disease. By combining these data, the authors showed what genetic elements are shared between the two major types of IBD (Crohn's disease and ulcerative colitis), as well as potential links to other inflammatory conditions and responses to infectious agents. Moreover, this type of comprehensive model can be combined with clinical trials data (Colombel et al., 2014; Sandborn et al., 2012) to better understand the connection between molecular profiles and clinical phenotypes in inflammatory diseases. More studies are needed; however, the initial findings from systems immunology approaches to study IBD, as well as the application to better understand other inflammatory diseases (International Multiple Sclerosis Genetics, 2013; International Multiple Sclerosis Genetics et al., 2013; Okada et al., 2014) show promise for stratifying patient cohorts and identifying new therapeutic targets or biomarkers.

2.8 Cancer

The paradigm of cancer is that normal cell processes are disrupted—through somatic mutation or environmental insults—such that cancerous cells are endowed with uncontrolled growth and the ability to invade and damage normal tissues. While certain cells are more or less susceptible to this transformation, cancer covers around 200 diseases that have been associated with almost every cell and tissue type in the human body. Although leukemias and lymphomas account for only ~10% of the estimated annual cancer deaths in adults,[1] the immune system plays a major role in cancer suppression and promotion

[1] US Cancer Statistics Working Group. United States Cancer Statistics: 1999–2011 Incidence and Mortality Web-based Report. Atlanta: US Department of Health and Human Services, Centers for Disease Control and Prevention and National Cancer Institute; 2014.

through the mechanisms of immunosurveillance and immunoediting (Schreiber et al., 2011), as well as protection against viruses associated with an increased risk of cancer (eg, human papillomavirus, Epstein–Barr virus, and Hepatitis C virus). While the intersection between cancer and immunology was postulated more than 100 years ago, evidence over the last decade has shown that infiltrating lymphocytes shape the tumor microenvironment and are associated with favorable prognosis in a variety of cancers (Gajewski et al., 2013; deLeeuw et al., 2012; Odunsi and Old, 2007; Shankaran et al., 2001; Dunn et al., 2002). Furthermore, these connections are revealing promising therapeutic avenues that leverage the immune system to identify and eliminate tumors through immunotherapy (Cancer Target et al., 2010; Gubin et al., 2014; Steinman and Mellman, 2004; Maude et al., 2014). An exciting extension of these approaches is to combine immunotherapy with small molecules to extend survival times even further and potentially drive remission to the point where we have effectively cured certain cancers (Vanneman and Dranoff, 2012). These intersections are where systems approaches can be effective for helping to advance our knowledge about the overlapping boundaries between cancer and immunology and use these connections to identify successful treatment strategies.

2.9 Metabolic diseases

Metabolic diseases such as obesity, insulin resistance, type 2 diabetes, and atherosclerosis have all been associated with a persistent state of inflammation. This chronic inflammatory state appears to be driven by aberrant signaling between the immune system and metabolic processes, both within immune cells and between immune cells and cells in adipose or other metabolic tissues (brain, liver, muscle, and pancreas). Uncovering these connections and how inflammatory processes mediate metabolic diseases is revealing exciting possibilities for targeting the immune system to treat many conditions that are related to obesity, metabolism, and inflammation.

All metabolic tissues contain resident immune cell populations that respond to molecular signals (eg, nutrients, cytokines, and hormones) and help maintain metabolic homeostasis (Lumeng and Saltiel, 2011). For example, macrophages interact with adipocytes to control lipid storage and release (Kosteli et al., 2010). Lipid metabolism and inflammation have been linked through multiple immune cells, signaling molecules, and receptors (Jin et al., 2013). Multiple proinflammatory inputs and pathways converge on genes that ultimately regulate nutrient sensing and metabolism. Drugs that target inflammation aim to interfere with the dysregulation that contributes to metabolic disease. For example, randomized trials on diabetic patients who were overweight or obese showed that modulating NKF-kB activity with salsalate improved glycemic control (Goldfine et al., 2008; Goldfine et al., 2010). In a separate study of obese individuals, blocking TNF-a with etanercept improved insulin sensitivity (Dominguez et al., 2005; Stanley et al., 2011). These examples are just the beginning of therapeutic applications to diseases associated with obesity.

Systems approaches that integrate genotypic, gene expression, and clinical data from human populations with an array of different metabolic diseases are revealing an underlying molecular network that not only is shared among these diverse disorders, but also appears to be causal for these diseases (Schadt, 2009). This molecular network highlights the power of how systems approaches can scan across multiple tissues, cell types, and diseases to identify genes that are significantly enriched in disease-specific transcriptional signatures. This network is highly enriched for genes associated with macrophages, which ties into one of the dominant immune cell types driving these metabolic diseases. Given the macrophage-specific nature of this network and its causal association to a diversity of metabolic traits, we refer to it as the macrophage-enriched metabolic network.

2.10 Neurological diseases

The nervous and immune systems are tightly connected through multiple cells, cytokines, and hormones that each system uses to regulate the other (Steinman, 2004). These complex interactions shape the development of each system, help maintain homeostasis, and when disrupted can contribute to disease pathogenesis (Boulanger and Shatz, 2004). As an example of these regulatory interactions, both autonomic and peripheral neurons are known to regulate inflammatory processes (Andersson and Tracey, 2012; Chiu et al., 2012) and recent evidence suggests that peripheral pain receptors are necessary for an IL-23-mediated inflammatory response in a mouse model of psoriasis (Riol-Blanco et al., 2014). This neural–immune connection is certainly more integrated than previously appreciated as indicated by other studies showing neurons sense and respond to bacterial products by influencing the immune response, even before immune cells respond to the pathogen (Chiu et al., 2013).

Taken together, the early observational studies that viral or bacterial infection (eg, rabies, syphilis, influenza) trigger inflammatory responses in both the periphery and within the central nervous system, along with the recent attempts to tease out whether neural pathology is caused by the infectious agent or host response (Steinman, 2014) and the direct influence of sensory neurons on inflammation, the connections between the nervous and immune systems are clearly more complex and intertwined than we currently understand. Indeed, many neurological diseases have strong genetic components that can be linked to immune genes (Tan et al., 2014) or inflammatory processes (Zhang et al., 2013; Lucin and Wyss-Coray, 2009; Doty et al., 2014; Gonzalez et al., 2014). Determining how these processes are connected and can regulate one another is a perfect challenge for systems immunology.

2.11 Connections between the immune system and other organ systems

Clear cellular communication is essential in order for cells of the immune system to coordinate an appropriate and effective response. These responses require recruitment of the correct cells to the proper place at the right time. To achieve this level of orchestration immune cells secrete soluble factors known as cytokines and chemokines that can act on the secreting cells and other cells within their environment. In addition, immune cells must home to specific locations and adhere to the right tissues, both of which are achieved by surface markers and adhesion molecules. Together this collection of immune molecules make distributed communication amongst immune and nonimmune cells possible.

The HLA provides a striking example of a major molecular player in this distributed communication network. HLA molecules are derived from a family of genes that encode for a set of cell surface molecules that immune cells use to discriminate between self and nonself. Every cell in the human body expresses an HLA molecule, which provides one of the molecular signals immune cells rely on to determine whether another cell is foreign. HLA genes are among the most polymorphic in the genome. Given the thousands of allelic variants and the exquisite specificity of antigen recognition, one could argue the immune system has its own genome. These genes regulate development, perform surveillance, and respond to internal and external threats. The HLA genes, also known as our compatibility genes, resolve many puzzles about how the immune system distinguishes between self and nonself, explaining the molecular similarity needed for a successful organ transplantation, mechanisms for how the adaptive immune system recognizes viral and bacterial products, and how a related family of cell surface proteins found on NK cells (so-called killer cell immunoglobulin-like receptors (KIRs)) can recognize tumors. More importantly, these genes have provided a wellspring for some of the most important scientific questions in medicine and have played a critical role in helping scientists understand and treat disease.

The immune system sits at the boundaries between multiple organ systems, and between genetics and the environment. While immune cells are the quanta of the complex network, the system is multiscale in nature. Thousands of immune-related genes control cellular function, which in turn secrete proteins to control other cells, tissues, or organs. These different levels of organization are tightly regulated to perform critical tasks that are essential for survival. All of these interactions are dynamic and happen over multiple time lines. Reframing the immune system as a master integrator for understanding health permits new approaches to discover biological mechanisms that drive disease and identify therapeutic options that can restore balance to the immune system, and thus restore health.

3. HIGH-THROUGHPUT TECHNOLOGIES AND TECHNIQUES FOR SYSTEMS IMMUNOLOGY

The modern day origins of systems immunology can be traced back to technological innovations stemming from genomic sequencing projects that began in the 1990s. These projects articulated ambitious, yet clear goals for biology, which resulted in large-scale efforts amongst academia, industry, and government. Together, these ventures ushered in the era of high-throughput science where comprehensive sets of molecular interactions can now be examined in parallel from a single experiment and research questions are no longer limited to interrogating specific molecular interactions. The ability to collect comprehensive data on genomes initially, and then ultimately many "omes," has empowered researchers to construct a systems-view of immunology.

The ~3 billion nucleotide sequences in humans presented a challenge that was economically and temporally impractical for the technological capabilities at the Human Genome Project's onset. Thus, new technologies and techniques were invented and developed to address the experimental and computational needs for collecting and analyzing the orders-of-magnitude increase in information waiting to be unlocked in a complete genome. One consequence of these innovations is that high-throughput technologies now exist to probe multiple aspects of the immune system at unprecedented precision and scale. More importantly, high-throughput technologies have enabled the field of systems immunology by providing the data sets needed to synthesize how individual immune components coordinate their actions into a working system (Fig. 2). Below we discuss how various high-throughput technologies and complimentary computational techniques are driving systems immunology and permitting the transplantation of knowledge from immunology into clinical applications.

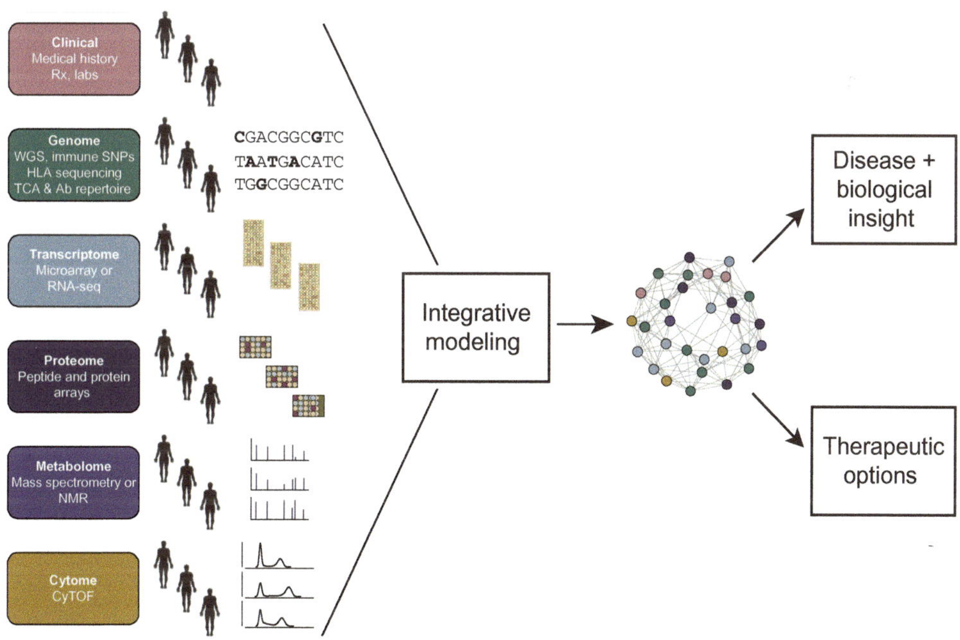

Figure 2 High-throughput technologies generate massive data that form the inputs for detailed and comprehensive models of immune system processes to guide insight into disease and suggest treatment options.

3.1 Genomic profiling of immune system genes

Large-scale sequencing efforts such as the 1000 Genomes Project (Genomes Project et al., 2012) have provided a complete annotation set for the ~6000 noncoding RNA (ncRNA) and the ~19,000 protein-coding genes in the human genome (Gray et al., 2015). Based on these annotations, the number of genetic elements that control immune function turns out to be larger than expected. Conservative estimates suggest that at least 10% of protein-coding genes regulate the immune system in some form, whereas less restrictive definitions of immune function increase this proportion to 40%. This allocation of genomic resources has implications for how we assess genetic control over the immune system, how we evaluate the immune system's contribution to disease, and what transcriptional products provide the best targets for therapies that modulate the immune system and immune-mediated diseases.

Humans harbor natural variation in their genetic code that confers protection and susceptibility to disease. However, most diseases lack a single causative variant. Systematic efforts to understand the specific gene variants that are more likely to be linked with disease conditions (eg, rheumatoid arthritis (RA) or IBD) or phenotypic traits (eg, longevity, lipid levels, or CD4+ to CD8+ ratios) take advantage of high-throughput screens that can interrogate > 100,000 single nucleotide polymorphisms (SNPs) in a single experiment. To connect genotype with phenotype, GWAS aim to identify SNPs in a gene or other regulatory element containing a causal variant that contributes to the disease or trait. GWAS are systematic approaches that take advantage of the natural genetic variation in large cohorts (eg, tens or hundreds of thousands of individuals). Since the introduction of GWAS in the middle of the last decade, the National Human Genome Research Institute (NHGRI) has compiled a catalog of published GWAS that as of this writing includes >1750 curated publications and over 11,900 SNPs that associate with disease, drug response, and phenotypic traits (Welter et al., 2014).

The immune system is shaped by genetic and environmental control. In the era prior to GWAS, clinical genetics identified a number of rare inherited disorders that increased susceptibility to multiple infectious agents. These primary immunodeficiencies gave rise to the dominant paradigm that alteration of a single immune gene increased susceptibility for a specific infectious disease (Picard et al., 2006). For example, individuals with mutations in the molecular circuit for IL-12/23 and IFN-g signaling have increased risk of mycobacterial disease, whereas those with inherited interleukin-1 receptor-associated kinase-4 (IRAK-4) deficiency are prone to pneumococcal disease (Casanova and Abel, 2007). While rare, these genetic alterations have provided insight into the genetic circuits that control immune response to infection.

The variation in an outbred population provides a natural experiment to determine the links between genotype and phenotype. Population studies in humans have revealed hundreds of genetic variants that control immune system function (Casanova et al., 2013;

Xavier and Rioux, 2008). For example, 23 SNPs have been found to regulate immune cell frequencies (Orru et al., 2013). At the time of publication, more than 300 genetic loci have been linked to one or more of the 80 autoimmune diseases (Visscher et al., 2012; Welter et al., 2014). A number of these loci can be mapped to shared biological pathways, indicating some sort of shared mechanism driving autoimmunity (Cho and Gregersen, 2011; Cotsapas et al., 2011; Voight and Cotsapas, 2012; Goris and Liston, 2012). By implementing a combination of systems approaches with whole-genome sequencing and high-resolution mapping on the loci described, we can tease apart the causal links and find the similarities that unify diseases processes.

Next-generation sequencing technologies are finding many applications to problems in immunology. One challenge is sorting out the tremendous repertoire diversity that provides exquisite antigen specificity. High-throughput technologies are revealing the breadth of both the T cell antigen receptor (TCR) (Robins et al., 2010) and antibody repertoires (Boyd et al., 2009), which have multiple applications for medicine in diagnosis and monitoring of clinical care (Boyd, 2013). These methodologies have also successfully been applied to identify immunogenetic risk factors for disease (Trowsdale, 2011), examine HLA polymorphism across population and pathogenic diversity (Prugnolle et al., 2005), and select immunodominant HLA-restricted T cell epitopes, eg, for vaccine or tetramer design (Newell et al., 2013). As these techniques are combined with other methodologies, they provide a more complete picture that connects receptor sequence and cell function (Han et al., 2014).

3.2 Transcriptional profiling of immune cells

Transcriptional profiling measures the functional and dynamic landscape of gene regulation and the cell-specific programming that drives immune cell function. When performed at a whole-genome level, these approaches provide an unbiased examination of how transcript changes correlate with diverse states of the immune system. For example, immune cell subsets have specific transcriptional signatures, and systems immunology approaches have associated these expression patterns with a range of immunological conditions such as autoimmunity (Boisson et al., 2012; Chaussabel et al., 2008; Pascual et al., 2010), response to vaccination (Nakaya et al., 2011; Querec et al., 2009; Furman et al., 2013; Banchereau et al., 2014; Obermoser et al., 2013), and infectious disease (Berry et al., 2010; Cliff et al., 2013; Bloom et al., 2012; Law et al., 2013). Moreover, these molecular signatures have identified therapeutic strategies that might be helpful for patients with rheumatological diseases (Chiche et al., 2013) and lymphomas (Hummel et al., 2006). Although critics of high-throughput biology have suggested that little has come from an approach that measures everything and figures it out later, two clear facts have surfaced that would not have been identified from other means. The first is that multiple pathways drive immune cell responses, and these pathways offer new understanding of disease as well as therapeutic targets. The second is that comprehensive and unbiased profiling of the entire transcriptional landscape has provided data to generate complete regulatory networks, which serve as wiring diagrams for explaining the immune response to a diverse range of immune perturbations. However, the real power of these networks is they are (i) hypothesis-generating tools that lead to verifiable experimental designs and (ii) predictive models for exploring our knowledge of biology and testing out multiple therapeutic leads prior to moving toward more costly experimental validations.

Studies on genome-wide patterns of mRNA expression in immune cells have identified drivers of the immune response to antigens, cytokines, small molecules, and other environmental perturbations. For example, high-throughput technologies have identified cell-specific signatures and the genetic regulatory programs that govern lineage differentiation and pathogen response (Fairfax et al., 2012; Zhang et al., 2012; Shalek et al., 2013; Yosef et al., 2013). To understand the complex and adaptive nature of the immune system, these transcriptional profiles can be connected to SNP data to determine immune regulatory networks and causal drivers of disease. This approach has been recently demonstrated for complex diseases such as IBD, lupus, and type 1 diabetes (T1D) (Jostins et al., 2012; Westra et al., 2013).

3.3 High-throughput technologies to profile immune cells

Immune cells are the functional building blocks of the immune system and they offer readouts for the organism's state of health. High-throughput techniques provide the capability to examine millions of cells at the resolution of the single-cell level. New technologies such as mass cytometry have more than doubled the number of molecular probes that can be used to interrogate a single cell. This technological advance has vastly expanded the number of distinct cell types and functional states that can be examined in an experiment. This scale of experimental inquiry is unprecedented in the history of immunology and has great promise to answer many long-standing questions in immunology such as: what is the diversity of the immune repertoire, how many different cell types does the immune system need, and what are the functional states for different immune cells. The frontiers for systems immunology will be to examine time series data from various immune responses to construct the interaction maps associated with different states and how these states evolve. One key question that needs to be addressed is what immune cell subsets associate with different physiological states so the cells can serve as immunological indicators of health and disease states.

Over the past 40 years, cytometric measurements by flow have progressed by probing a steadily increasing number of cell surface proteins. Currently, single-cell mass cytometry (CyTOF) technology can measure >40 surface markers or intracellular proteins simultaneously, providing an unprecedented number of possible parameters to characterize distinct cell types (Bendall et al., 2011, 2012). Given the large number of markers, automated strategies are now required to process the high-dimensional information and identify cell types based on the extent of similarity among a specified set of markers.

These data-driven approaches select the combinations of markers that identify distinct cell types and can be used to classify differences between cohorts (Amir el et al., 2013; Bruggner et al., 2014), profile drug perturbation responses (Bodenmiller et al., 2012), or map lineage development (Bendall et al., 2014). The computational tools for these advanced cytometric technologies are rapidly evolving, yet areas for which there are unmet needs include (i) techniques to integrate cytometric with other high-throughput data (eg, proteomic, genome-wide profiling, or genetic data), (ii) automated annotation calls for cell subsets based on the complete marker sets, and (iii) statistical methods for data transformation and normalization amongst large numbers of samples.

4. CONTROLLING THE IMMUNE SYSTEM TO TREAT DISEASE

4.1 Vaccination to control infectious disease

The field of immunology has made unparalleled contributions to human health through vaccination. In the United States, vaccination has decreased the annual morbidity, as compared to figures from the twentieth century, by orders of magnitude, driving the numbers to zero for smallpox, diphtheria, and polio (Roush et al., 2007; Centers for Disease Control and Prevention, 2011). Global numbers in developed countries follow similar trends. To date, global vaccination efforts have resulted in the eradication of smallpox, with realistic estimates to eradicate polio by 2018. Despite these vaccine successes, humans are still plagued by many viruses (eg, HIV, hepatitis C), bacteria (eg, mycobacterium tuberculosis (TB)), and parasites (eg, malaria) for which we have poor or nonexistent vaccines. These pathogens are responsible for more than five million deaths per year and continue to challenge effective vaccine efforts because of their complex interplay with the immune system. Thus, multiple opportunities exist for applying systems immunology to direct the development of biologics or cellular therapies that can be used as prophylactic vaccines.

Systems immunology offers an entirely new approach to investigate how the immune system interacts with pathogens. Instead of simply scaling-up targeted approaches, high-throughput technologies, and by extension the system-wide analytical approaches they enable, augment what's possible. For example, data from whole-genome transcriptional profiling permit the construction of regulatory networks that can be used to infer the activities of transcription factors, RNA-binding proteins, and micro-RNAs from the transcriptome patterns. Such inferences are critical for identifying and understanding links between molecular responses induced by vaccine perturbations and physiological or phenotypic responses that correspond to protection.

One uncertainty in vaccine development is whether a new vaccine will provoke a protective immune response. To reduce this uncertainty, systems analyses can identify the molecular signatures associated with immune responses to vaccines, and then apply supervised learning algorithms to determine what molecular features in the signature can be used to predict high- versus low-antibody titers to the pathogen, which is a clinical surrogate for protection and vaccine efficacy. This approach has been applied to a number of different vaccines including yellow fever (Querec et al., 2009), influenza (Nakaya et al., 2011), meningococcus (Li et al., 2014), and pneumococcal (Obermoser et al., 2013).

The results from these initial studies in systems vaccinology highlight three important points. First, distinct immune response pathways are responsible for protection against different vaccines (Li et al., 2014). This result might not be surprising given that divergent microbial stimulation (eg, viral versus bacterial) activate different molecular elements or various vaccine formulations (eg, inactivated versus live-attenuated) trigger separate cell types. However, this study was the first concrete molecular demonstration in humans and these signatures provide guidance on how to tailor vaccines to induce an appropriate immune response that will create protection. Second, collecting molecular and cellular data from early time points postvaccination reveals a more picture of the interaction between innate and adaptive immune responses. In addition, these data permit a better understanding of the role and predictive power that each immunological component has in accurately classifying individual vaccine responders and nonresponders (Tsang et al., 2014). Third, multiple components of the immune system contribute to an effective vaccine response (Furman et al., 2013). Future studies that apply systems immunology to understand vaccine efficacy and help direct its development will need to embrace high-resolution time sampling along with collection of additional immunological features to capture the full complexity of immune responses to vaccination.

4.2 Immunotherapy to manipulate surveillance and control cancer

Cancer can arise when there's a breakdown in the normal cellular regulatory mechanisms that control cell growth, repair, and death. Cancerous cells survive and thrive by passive and active evasion of immune surveillance mechanisms that would otherwise remove abnormal host cells. Although multiple treatment options often exist for a particular cancer, selecting the right drug from among the various alternatives can be a challenge because (i) its usually not clear what molecular mechanism to modulate so as to knock out the main drivers of the cancerous cells and (ii) tumors can adapt by developing resistant to a particular treatment. Systems approaches capture the complexity of immunity and offer guidance for (i) determining key drivers of disease, (ii) matching the treatment to the individual, and (iii) identifying novel therapeutic approaches, all of which aim to better harness the immune system's natural capacity for surveillance and control.

Cancer immunotherapy aims to upgrade immune surveillance by training immune cells to recognize and remove tumors. The concept is simple in theory. Combine immune cells with tumor-specific antigens while providing a stimulus to mimic the process by which effector cells are created so that these newly created effector cells recognize and kill any tumor cell expressing the specific antigen. One practical challenge is determining the best antigen for eliciting a strong antitumor response. Bioinformatics provides computational tools for finding the optimal antigen that is both specific to the cancer cells and representative of tumor composition. To paraphrase Goldilocks, the antigen needs to be just right.

The work of our colleagues Drs. Losic, Rubinsteyn, and Finnigan highlights some of the more recent advancements in bioinformatics approaches that can identify tumor-derived amino acid sequences to help create vaccines for personalized cancer therapy. This process extends current efforts to determine good candidate binding peptides for any combination of HLA alleles (Karosiene et al., 2012) by adding a scoring system that ranks amino acid sequences based on their predicted "immunogenecity," the ability to elicit strong antitumor responses. The scoring algorithm integrates proteomic and genomic information from public repositories with RNA-sequencing data from a tumor sample. Data from the public domain provide a collection of reference sequences to filter out self peptides, and the sequencing data measures the transcriptome to determine preferentially expressed tumor transcripts that allow us to select patient-specific tumor sequences with high statistical confidence. These diverse data inputs are fed into a classification algorithm, in our case a random forest model, to classify and prioritize candidate vaccine peptides that we can synthesize in a clinical-grade facility. This bioinformatics pipeline is currently serving clinical trials designed to evaluate cancer vaccine immunotherapies in both melanoma and pancreatic cancer.

4.3 Biologics to control autoimmune disease

Autoimmune disease results from a blurring of the immunological boundary between self and nonself. As this boundary blurs, the immune system redirects its resources to attack host cells (eg, beta islet cells in T1D), tissues (eg, synovium in RA or myelin in multiple sclerosis (MS)), or organs (eg, skin in psoriasis and systemic lupus erhthematosus (lupus) or intestines in IBD). The most common autoimmune disorders include psoriasis, RA, lupus, T1D, MS, and IBD. However, with more than 80 different autoimmune diseases classified, the prevalence of each disorder is relatively small, but collectively autoimmunity affects 5–10% of the population in Western countries (Cooper et al., 2009).

The dominant paradigm for treating autoimmunity in the twentieth century was to dampen the immune response by administering antiinflammatory and immunosuppressive agents such as corticosteroids or nonsteroidal antiinflammatory drugs (NSAIDs). These therapeutic agents offered some relief but did little to alter the course of disease. Individuals with autoimmunity began to receive real benefit when disease-modifying antirheumatic drugs (DMARDs) such as the small molecule methotrexate or the more recent biologics (eg, monoclonal antibodies) were introduced and used to target rapidly dividing immune cells or specific proinflammatory cytokines and receptors present on immune cells. However, in the autoimmune diseases where therapies exist, patients exhibit a full spectrum of response that ranges from none to complete. For example, even though TNF blockade has been one of most effective therapies for RA, psoriasis, and IBD, around one-third of patients do not respond to treatment even though their clinical presentation is indistinguishable from complete responders. This puzzle persists because for most autoimmune diseases, the underlying pathogenesis, which includes the complete set of antigens targeted by the immune system (eg, antibodies or T cells), as well as other immune cell players, remains unknown.

System-wide approaches in autoimmune disorders offer opportunities to discover antigenic drivers of disease, diagnose disease severity, and monitor disease course to potentially alter treatment. One approach for discovery involves creating ordered microarrays of overlapping peptide fragments based on proteins from targeted tissue, and then probing the arrays with antibodies from patient sera. Based on this systematic look at hundreds of potential molecular targets, novel antigens have been found for RA, MS, and lupus (Hueber et al., 2005; Price et al., 2013; Van Haren et al., 2013). Diagnosing autoimmunity can be a challenge due to the fact that the episodic nature of disease and symptoms are often nonspecific. Molecular profiling and systems analysis provides more precise diagnostic and prognostic markers (Hueber et al., 2002, 2003, 2007; Maecker et al., 2012a). Moreover, monitoring changes in the patterns of targeted epitopes correlates with disease severity and can guide therapy (Kidd et al., 2008; Van Haren et al., 2013).

4.4 Drugs or other therapeutics to control asthma and allergy

There is a pressing need for novel biomedical insights and innovative solutions for addressing open clinical challenges in diagnosis, treatment, control, and prevention of asthma. Asthma is a major public health concern affecting an estimated 300 million individuals worldwide, and accounting for approximately 1 in every 250 deaths globally (Masoli et al., 2004). Current estimates suggest the prevalence of asthma in the United States is 8% (~25 million individuals) with great disparities in susceptibility and disease characteristics observed among individuals in different age, ethnic, and socioeconomic categories (Akinbami et al., 2012). Individuals affected by asthma often experience reduced quality of life due to manifest disease symptoms and associated psychosocial factors. Additionally, expenditures associated with clinical management of asthma contribute substantially to both personal and national health care costs (Akinbami et al., 2012; Sullivan et al., 2011), which is mainly attributable to poor long-term control of disease through therapeutic and lifestyle interventions.

Incomplete understanding of the complex molecular pathophysiology underlying asthma and the long path of the traditional drug development pipeline are two main challenges impeding the development of safer and more effective asthma therapies. A profoundly complex system of interactions between numerous genetic, immune, cellular, metabolic, and environmental factors underlie and give rise to a broad range of asthma clinical phenotypes. Genetic association studies conducted so far implicate hundreds of genes as having a role in the etiology and pathophysiology of asthma, and also highlight several differences in the genetic architecture of asthma traits among ethnic populations. The complexity of asthma does not lend itself well to reductionist approaches and it is important to have a better understanding of the complete system of molecular interactions that underlie asthma to ensure that therapies can target disease more precisely while minimizing nonspecific biological activity that gives risk of side effects. Even when a novel asthma target is discovered, it can take up to 13 years and cost close to $2 billion to develop and deliver a novel therapeutic to the clinic (Paul et al., 2010).

Recent advances in high-throughput molecular profiling technologies and computational analysis techniques offer novel opportunities to improve disease understanding and accelerate discovery of novel therapeutic strategies for asthma. High-throughput molecular profiling technologies such as microarrays and next-generation genomic sequencing technologies enable efficient, unbiased methods for measuring system-wide molecular "snapshots" or signatures that capture the broad molecular activity in a biological system (eg, cell or tissue). Bioinformatics provides computational techniques for comparing (eg, disease vs. health), interrogating, and integrating molecular profiling data to identify patterns and relationships that inform on the molecular basis of disease and drug response. There is now a wealth of molecular profiling data for asthma and hundreds of other diseases available from public data repositories such as the NCBI Gene Expression Omnibus (GEO). We were amongst the first to demonstrate that collecting and integrating molecular disease profiles from the public domain can identify novel molecular connections and shared drug targets between diseases (Suthram et al., 2010). We were also amongst the first to demonstrate that a systematic computational approach can identify novel opportunities to repurpose drugs for novel disease indications based on similarities in genome-wide molecular profiles (Dudley et al., 2011; Sirota et al., 2011).

4.5 Drugs or other therapeutics to aid transplantation and resist rejection

A central and defining feature of the immune system is the ability to distinguish between self and nonself. While this characteristic is essential for protecting the host against potential threats to survival, it creates a major barrier for organ transplantation. In fact, although more than 60 years have passed since the first successful organ transplant in 1954 (Guild et al., 1955), the central issue for transplantation is still preventing allograft rejection. To prevent rejection, standard clinical care is to employ immunosuppressive measures that deplete reactive immunological agents (eg, lymphocytes or antibodies) or block the immune response (Halloran, 2004). Beside general immunosuppressive drugs (eg, glucocorticoids or azathioprine) or antibody depletion with intravenous immunoglobulin (IVIG), current immunosuppressive therapies target B or T cell activation and proliferation. Treatment protocols have focussed managing different stages posttransplantation through careful monitoring of immunological markers. High-throughput approaches are beginning to advance our understanding and procedures for organ transplantation. Systems approaches that integrate these high-throughput measurements offer promise for better diagnostic markers to monitor transplant stages (Li et al., 2012), superior molecular matching between donors and recipients (Spellman et al., 2012; Wang et al., 2012a), and improved therapeutic strategies (Khatri et al., 2011, 2013).

4.6 Drug repurposing

Drug repurposing can minimize the costs and risks associated with drug development programs. While examples exist for drug repurposing, eg, sildenafil for erectile dysfunction and pulmonary hypertension, thalidomide for severe erythema nodosum leprosum and multiple myeloma, and retinoic acid for acute promyelocytic leukemia (Aronson, 2007), most successful cases where new indications were found for approved compounds resulted from serendipitous association rather than systematic examination. To remedy this situation, systematic approaches have been developed based on high-throughput screening (Ashburn and Thor, 2004) or computational approaches. One of us (J.T.D.) developed a computational drug repurposing approach that matches transcriptional profiles from drug perturbations with disease signatures (Sirota et al., 2011). Experimental validation of several novel drug indications identified by this computational drug repurposing system supports the broad biological relevance of the approach for systems immunology.

When we applied the drug repurposing approach to transcriptional profiles of IBD measured from human surgical specimens, we identified and experimentally validated a novel IBD indication predicted for the anticonvulsant agent topiramate (Dudley et al., 2011). Topiramate, which has primary indications for seizure disorders, has no history of efficacious use for IBD or other inflammatory diseases. There are no established therapeutic targets for IBD or other inflammatory diseases among the canonical targets of topiramate, which is known to enhance the activity of GABA-A receptors, antagonize AMPA/kinate glutamate receptor subtypes, and serve as a weak inhibitor of carbonic anhydrase isozymes II and IV (Knox et al., 2011). We used a chemically induced (2,4,6-trinitrobenzenesulfonic acid) rodent model of IBD to evaluate the activity of topiramate administered in the presence of an IBD phenotype. The experimental results demonstrated statistically significant reductions in gross pathophysiological and histopathological measures of severity of the induced IBD phenotype in the population of animals receiving topiramate compared to untreated controls. Furthermore, topiramate exhibited more pronounced amelioration of the IBD phenotype than was observed for the prednisolone corticosteroid positive control.

In a separate study (Jahchan et al., 2013), we applied our computational drug repurposing approach to transcriptional profiles of tumor versus adjacent normal tissue to identify novel drug repurposing candidates for small cell lung cancer (SCLC). This study identified a number of pharmacologically diverse compounds as novel drug repurposing candidates for SCLC, including imipramine; a tricyclic antidepressant (TCA), bepridil; a calcium channel blocker' and promethazine, a phenothiazine antihistamine. Anti-SCLC or other antineoplastic effects were not previously established for these drugs, or for other drugs from the same pharmacological class. We experimentally validated the anti-SCLC of these compounds across a number of *in vitro* and *in vivo* experiments using human and animal model systems.

Drugs of all therapeutic classes influence the immune system but the mechanisms through which these treatments alter the immune system are seldom understood. Characterizing the connections between immune cells and drugs provides multiple opportunities for determining immune-mediated side effects and identifying new therapeutic avenues. To better grasp the connections between immune cells and drugs, we developed a method to quantify the likely effect of a drug on an immune cell based on the similarity between molecular profiles of drug perturbations (treated vs. untreated) and immunological state changes (eg, activated vs. inactivated T cell). This systematic analysis of interactions between molecular perturbations induced by pharmaceutical compounds and immune response allowed us to construct an immunepharmacology map that provides a framework for developing novel approaches for direct manipulation of immune activity through integrative systems pharmacology.

4.7 Cellular therapies

Immune cells naturally remove, repair, and rebuild diseased or damaged tissue, making them ideal candidates for cellular therapies to maintain health and treat human disease. Capitalizing on this potential requires a better understanding of the molecular programs that drive immune cell responses in healthy and diseased conditions. Cellular therapies are showing great potential for treating diseases that can evolve such as cancer, infection, and autoimmunity. Some recent and exciting examples demonstrate that the immune system can be programmed to treat cancer using cell-based therapies.

Adaptive immune cells possess an inherent recognition and response mechanism that, if properly harnessed, could be a more effective treatment for a cancer. Evidence from tumor-infiltrating lymphocytes shows that the immune system does respond to and kill tumor cells; however, sometimes T cells require an extra boost to eliminate the tumor. Such boosts are being made possible by better methods that identify tumor-specific antigens and use this information to reprogram T cells *ex vivo* before being introduced as a more effective therapeutic (Restifo et al., 2012). In a more radical reengineering approach, tumor-specific antigen receptors are expressed in T cells to express a chimeric antigen receptor (CAR) that becomes a more effective tumor targeting therapeutic (Zhang et al., 2005, 2006; Urba and Longo, 2011). This novel cellular therapy is showing promise in treating a range of B cell malignancies (Haso et al., 2013; Kochenderfer and Rosenberg, 2013; Davila et al., 2014; Kochenderfer et al., 2015) and phase 1 clinical trials are underway as of this writing (Sentman and Meehan, 2014). More futuristic and speculative reprogramming efforts have even been suggested by leveraging principles from synthetic biology and systems immunology (Fischbach et al., 2013). In the not-to-distant future, perhaps we will be able to use whole-cell programming (Karr et al., 2012) to create cells that the body has never seen before. These designs will be liberated from the constraints that biological systems currently operate under and will take systems immunology to a completely new realm.

5. IMMUNE MONITORING

The immune system is a complex network of dozens of different cell types and molecules that interact to orchestrate essential defense mechanisms. These defense mechanisms protect against pathogens and disease, and are critical for maintaining health. Despite decades of productive research on the immune system and numerous immunomodulatory therapies, no robust set of metrics currently exists for human immune health. Over the past couple decades, a number of technological advances in high-throughput assays (see Section 2) have made it possible to measure thousands of immunological parameters from the peripheral blood of individuals. At the same time, progress in consumer electronics has resulted in low-cost, wearable devices that can collect data on our physiology and environment in real time (Fig. 3). In this section, we discuss efforts to develop human immune monitoring by integrating longitudinal measurements obtained from multiple modalities to quantify, track, diagnose, predict, and promote immunological health.

5.1 Understanding global health challenges

Global health challenges for the upcoming decades remain focussed on the global burden of disease. The leading preventable contributions to disease burden are infectious disease (eg, HIV, malaria, diarrheal disease, and pneumonia) and malnutrition, both of which disproportionality affect children. To provide financial and scientific incentives for addressing these global health challenges, the Bill and Melinda Gates Foundations has created a number of Grand Challenges in Global Health (http://gcgh.grandchallenges.org/) that are aimed at new interventions for global health and integrated solutions for healthy birth, growth, and development. These programs intend to develop new vaccines or therapeutics, and to monitor health status and diagnostics for point-of-care solutions in resource-limited settings, thus providing an opportunity for systems immunology approaches.

The decreasing cost of high-throughput technologies provides many opportunities to capture a comprehensive set of immunological factors that contribute to disease burden in a global health setting. Furthermore, low sample volumes required for these technologies permit studies in children. Both advances have been key for examining questions about

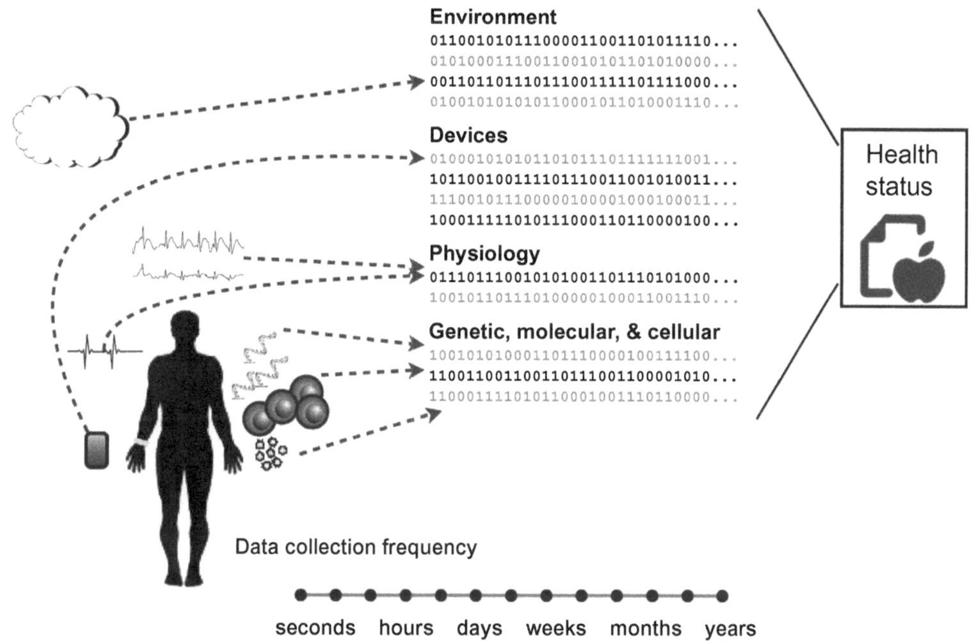

Figure 3 Technological advances in multiple fronts (eg, consumer electronics, devices, medical, and research equipment) have made it possible to collect longitudinal measurements on individuals and perform predictive modeling that provide more precise health reports ("scorecards") for personalized medicine.

host–gene–environment interactions in children who have increased risk of infection. Recent studies are revealing that the microbiome composition plays a role in host response and recovery from *V. cholera*, a causative agent of severe diarrheal disease (Hsiao et al., 2014). The time series data collected from this study indicate how immune monitoring can be used to understand infection dynamics and identify intervention strategies.

Another aspect of host–gene–environment interactions that hasn't been well appreciated is the influence of malnutrition on the immune system and disease susceptibility. Two recent studies have shown how the complex interplay between host microbes, genetics, the immune system, and infectious burden contribute to disease and can alter developmental trajectories. Children with severe acute malnutrition have a markedly different composition of bacterial species in their intestines. These studies have provided the first evidence for how nutrients influence the host's microbial composition and determined that particular species influence growth (Subramanian et al., 2014; Smith et al., 2013). Mapping the comprehensive set of host–environment factors that contribute to infection susceptibility and childhood development, and how other factors such as malnutrition alter this balance, is the first step toward developing new diagnostics and evaluating therapeutic interventions.

5.2 Predicting, tracking, and preventing emerging epidemics

The influenza pandemic that followed World War I spurred public health agencies to improve disease tracking and forecasting to forestall future pandemics. Since the initial 1918–19 pandemic, three other pandemics have occurred, with the most recent happening between April 2009 and April 2010 (http://www.flu.gov/). Our interconnected world of the internet, mobile technologies, and social media can now aid in monitoring and even predicting potential outbreaks. In 2008, Google implemented an influenza surveillance and tracking program (http://www.google.org/flutrends/). This application, labeled flu trends, was created by using hundreds of billions of individual searches to predict influenza-like illness physician visits from query terms over a 5 year period, and this simple model was highly correlated with the weekly reports from the US Centers for Disease Control and Prevention (CDC) over the same time frame, yet at higher temporal resolution than the CDC reports (Ginsberg et al., 2009).

While the flu trends model is overly simplistic and produced inaccurate reports in 2013 (Ginsberg et al., 2009), the approach demonstrated how large-scale data streams can be used to improve forecasting and tracking of both epidemics and emerging infectious diseases. Other web-scale data mining platforms such as HealthMap (http://www.healthmap.org/) (Freifeld et al., 2008) and BioCaster (http://biocaster.org/) (Collier et al., 2008) monitor public health emergencies in near real time by aggregating information from news and social media, rich site summary (RSS) news feeds, government reports, and other web outlets. These types of automated algorithms provide high-resolution spatial and temporal information on disease dynamics that complement official data reports from an outbreak, thus arming officials, aid workers, and citizens with important information to better manage epidemics.

Emerging infections can create confusion and panic about a disease's origin as well as its incidence, distribution, mortality, and how best to control its spread. Tapping into the vast ecosystem of electronic information sources offers many promising new approaches to monitor emerging infections in near real time. High-throughput technologies have improved in speed and accuracy so they can provide important biological information on infectious disease. In the past few years, rapid sequencing technology has identified the origins of the cholera strain that contributed to the Haitian cholera outbreak and the *E. coli* strain that caused an outbreak of hemolytic-uremic syndrome in Germany (Chin et al., 2011; Rasko et al., 2011). More recently, sequencing efforts helped determine virus origin and transmission patterns of the ebola outbreak (Gire et al., 2014). Although infectious diseases will continue to challenge humanity, the combined use of electronic and biologic information will greatly improve disease monitoring and forecasting. By connecting these advancements to smart cities and learning healthcare systems, we can move toward better treatments and possibly even prevention.

5.3 Identifying baseline states

Immunology has followed a trend over the past 50 years where findings from basic research are moving into clinical practice. Stem cell therapies, organ transplants, and monoclonal antibody treatments are just some of the examples of discoveries in immunology that have been translated from bench to bedside. While translational efforts in immunology have shined in the therapeutic domain, immune monitoring and metrics of immune health have lagged behind. Unlike medical specialties such as endocrinology, cardiology, or nephrology that have lab panels that provide quantitative measures of metabolic, cardiovascular, or renal health respectively, clinical immunology lacks definitive metrics for immune health.

The main immunological test used in routine clinical care is the complete blood count (CBC). The CBC measures the proportions of five white blood cell types (granulocytes, lymphocytes, monocytes, basophils, and eosinophils) in the blood, and is based on technology developed in the 1950s. The lymphocyte proportion includes many dozens of immune cell subsets that are drivers for specific immunological diseases and associated with many other diseases. However, with the exception of a few specific conditions (eg, HIV and blood cancers), cell subset frequency and function are not factored into standard medical care. The massive gains in our knowledge of the immune system, its contribution to disease, and advances in immune profiling have not resulted in corresponding changes in how the immune system is evaluated in the clinic. Moreover, healthy ranges for almost all immunological parameters are unknown. Thus, it's not surprising that individuals lack information on whether their immune system is healthy. Fortunately, large-scale collaborative efforts are changing this situation.

The Human Immunology Project Consortium (HIPC; http://www.immuneprofiling.org/) is a large-scale initiative by the US National Institute of Allergy and Infectious Diseases to create a public repository of immunological data based on the latest technologies for immune profiling (as of February 1, 2015, more than 20,000 subjects from 115 studies and over 300,000 results across multiple data types such as enzyme-linked immunosorbent assay, enzyme-linked immunospot, flow cytometry, and gene expression). The data feeding this repository has been collected using standardized protocols that measure the immune system in relevant clinical states (eg, following infection or pre- and postvaccination). In addition to holding these data in a publicly accessible warehouse, the initiative has created a computational interface for all researchers to take advantage of this valuable resource (https://immport.niaid.nih.gov/). Similar to other public repositories, the value of these data increases as more researchers use them to address their specific hypotheses or construct models that aim to solve the biggest challenges facing clinical and basic immunology (Kidd et al., 2014).

Advances in immune profiling methods and high-throughput technologies now provide a suite of tools for characterizing the immune system in a diverse array of states (eg, disease, infection, and following vaccination). These new tools offer powerful ways to identify biomarkers that can be used to monitor health and help manage disease (Maecker et al., 2012a; Chang et al., 2014). To make these tools useful for clinical measurements, we need to standardize the protocols for how immunological parameters are collected, processed, and analyzed, such as what has been proposed for immunophenotyping (Maecker et al., 2012b; Finak et al., 2014; Aghaeepour et al., 2013).

A critical component of immune monitoring is collecting periodic measurements to establish baseline values and normal reference ranges that can be applied on both individuals and populations. At the individual level, combining technology with integrative analysis permits frequent monitoring of thousands of immunological parameters for applications in personalized medicine (Chen et al., 2012; Yao et al., 2014). At the population level, systems approaches provide reference ranges for immunological parameters that can improve diagnosis and disease classification (Brodin et al., 2015; Mei et al., 2015). A clever twist on collecting reference ranges for immune monitoring is the recent effort to map the micriobial landscape of New York City (Afshinnekoo et al., 2015) (http://www.pathomap.org). While microorganisms undoubtedly play a role in human health, the diversity and abundance of any citywide microbiome has remained a mystery. More importantly, its unclear how this landscape contributes to disease. The PathoMap presents a baseline of the microbial ecosystem and has clear applications for disease surveillance that could be coordinated with individual immune health data to guide both personal and public health management.

5.4 Monitoring for healthy aging and longevity

Individuals born in developed countries after the latter half of the twentieth century are expected to enjoy a longer lifespan than our ancestors. With increased longevity, society faces new medical challenges for how to maintain immune system vitality beyond the reproductive years. Immune system function declines with age, a phenomenon known as immunosenescence, and these impairments place elderly individuals at increased risk for infectious disease, cancer, and inflammatory disorders (Hakim and Gress, 2007). In addition, the decreased production of naïve lymphocytes and the altered competence of the adaptive immune response diminish vaccine effectiveness in older adults (Goronzy and Weyand, 2013). Given the complexity of the immune system and the multiple components that can contribute to immunosenescence, systems immunology can be used to address multiple questions:

- What molecular and cellular markers should be monitored for healthy aging and to help prevent age-related diseases?
- How do individual immune systems differ between centenarians—winning the so-called immunological lottery—and younger cohorts with chronic inflammatory conditions?

- How can we bolster, or even augment, the immune system so it responds appropriately to diseases at every age?
- What are the best ways to treat an immune system that evolved to protect against threats that limited reproductive success?

5.5 Monitoring for critical care situations

There's a strong need to identify immune markers that correlate with different recovery trajectories during critical care situations such as following organ transplantation. Unlike the other situations we've described, posttransplantation monitoring is performed in a hospital and the outcomes encompass a broad spectrum. Multiple factors influence recovery following the procedure (eg, drug response, immune response, infection) and the list of biomarkers is far from complete. Thus, multiplexed immunological assays could be leveraged to identify biomarkers that correlate with various aspects of recovery. In combination, validation studies based on systems approaches could alleviate some of the confusion surrounding best practices for successful transplantation (Cravedi and Heeger, 2012; Sawitzki et al., 2011). In the past, complicated protocols and lengthy assays times might have limited the use of advanced technologies such as sequencing and multiplex immunological assays. However, recent demonstrations have shown that sequencing pipelines and sophisticated assays can be completed in near real time, thus making them useful for clinical monitoring and decision making (Wilson et al., 2014; Chang et al., 2014). While more studies are needed in the specific area of transplantation, these examples highlight how powerful monitoring tools can be used in critical care situations, which will further our understanding of host–graft tolerance and improve patient outcomes for some of the most vulnerable medical situations.

6. CONCLUSION

All roads to health and wellness seem to pass through the immune system. Systems immunology is about connecting the dots between all the interacting parts, which make up a whole that is greater than the sum of its parts. By interrogating the immune system with high-throughput technologies, we aim to collect comprehensive sets of immunological parameters that feed into integrative mathematical models to determine the relationships amongst all the parameters and link these measurements of immune and overall health. Such models can be used to determine the complex associations and causal interactions that drive immunological states in health and disease. More importantly, these models can be used to identify new therapeutic targets and predict how immune states will respond to perturbation.

Just as blood pressure and heart rate serve as metrics of cardiovascular health, immune cells and cytokines provide potential metrics of immune health. Collecting these immunological measures under various conditions will help define the range of these parameters and their connection to health. Powerful new multiplexed assays and wearable devices provide great promise for identifying clinically actionable biomarkers. Some examples in this chapter highlight the state of the art for systems immunology, whereas others were slightly more speculative. The future of systems immunology holds great potential for generating better models for how the immune system works, identifying new therapies for disease, and helping usher in personalized medicine.

REFERENCES

Afshinnekoo, E., Meydan, C., Chowdhury, S., Jaroudi, D., Boyer, C., Bernstein, N., Martiz, J.M., Reeves, D., Gandara, J., Chhangawala, S., Ahsanuddin, S., Simmons, A., Nessel, T., Sundaresh, B., Pereira, E., Jorgensen, E., Kolokotronis, S.-O., Kirchberger, N., Garcia, I., Gandara, D., Dhanraj, S., Nawrin, T., Saletore, Y., Alexander, N., Vijay, P., Hénaff, E.M., Zumbo, P., Walsh, M., O'Mullan, G.D., Tighe, S., Dudley, J.T., Dunaif, A., Ennis, S., O'Halloran, E.R., Magalhaes, T., Boone, B., Jones, A.L., Muth, T.R., Paolantonio, K.S., Alter, E., Schadt, E.E., Garbarino, J., Prill, R.J., Carlton, J.M., Levy, S., Mason, C.M., 2015. Geospatial resolution of human and bacterial diversity with city-scale metagenomics. Cell Systems 1, 1–15.

Aghaeepour, N., Finak, G., Flow, C.A.P.C., Consortium, D., Hoos, H., Mosmann, T.R., Brinkman, R., Gottardo, R., Scheuermann, R.H., 2013. Critical assessment of automated flow cytometry data analysis techniques. Nat. Methods 10, 228–238.

Ahern, P.P., Faith, J.J., Gordon, J.I., 2014. Mining the human gut microbiota for effector strains that shape the immune system. Immunity 40, 815–823.

Akinbami, L.J., Morroman, J.E., Bailey, C., Zahran, H.S., King, M., Johnson, C.A., Liu, X., 2012. Trends in asthma prevalence, health care use, and mortality in the United States, 2001–2010. NCHS Data Brief 94, 1–8.

Amir El, A.D., Davis, K.L., Tadmor, M.D., Simonds, E.F., Levine, J.H., Bendall, S.C., Shenfeld, D.K., Krishnaswamy, S., Nolan, G.P., Pe'er, D., 2013. viSNE enables visualization of high dimensional single-cell data and reveals phenotypic heterogeneity of leukemia. Nat. Biotechnol. 31, 545–552.

Andersson, U., Tracey, K.J., 2012. Reflex principles of immunological homeostasis. Annu. Rev. Immunol. 30, 313–335.

Aronson, J.K., 2007. Old drugs–new uses. Br. J. Clin. Pharmacol. 64, 563–565.

Ashburn, T.T., Thor, K.B., 2004. Drug repositioning: identifying and developing new uses for existing drugs. Nat. Rev. Drug Discov. 3, 673–683.

Baida, G., Bhalla, P., Kirsanov, K., Lesovaya, E., Yakubovskaya, M., Yuen, K., Guo, S., Lavker, R.M., Readhead, B., Dudley, J.T., Budunova, I., 2014. REDD1 functions at the crossroads between the therapeutic and adverse effects of topical glucocorticoids. EMBO Mol. Med. 7, 42–58.

Banchereau, R., Cepika, A.M., Pascual, V., 2013. Systems approaches to human autoimmune diseases. Curr. Opin. Immunol. 25, 598–605.

Banchereau, R., Baldwin, N., Cepika, A.M., Athale, S., Xue, Y., Yu, C.I., Metang, P., Cheruku, A., Berthier, I., Gayet, I., Wang, Y., Ohouo, M., Snipes, L., Xu, H., Obermoser, G., Blankenship, D., Oh, S., Ramilo, O., Chaussabel, D., Banchereau, J., Palucka, K., Pascual, V., 2014. Transcriptional specialization of human dendritic cell subsets in response to microbial vaccines. Nat. Commun. 5, 5283.

Bendall, S.C., Simonds, E.F., Qiu, P., Amir El, A.D., Krutzik, P.O., Finck, R., Bruggner, R.V., Melamed, R., Trejo, A., Ornatsky, O.I., Balderas, R.S., Plevritis, S.K., Sachs, K., Pe'er, D., Tanner, S.D., Nolan, G.P., 2011. Single-cell mass cytometry of differential immune and drug responses across a human hematopoietic continuum. Science 332, 687–696.

Bendall, S., Nolan, G., Roederer, M., Chattopadhyay, P., 2012. A deep profiler's guide to cytometry. Trends Immunol. 33, 323–332.

Bendall, S.C., Davis, K.L., Amir El, A.D., Tadmor, M.D., Simonds, E.F., Chen, T.J., Shenfeld, D.K., Nolan, G.P., Pe'er, D., 2014. Single-cell trajectory detection uncovers progression and regulatory coordination in human B cell development. Cell 157, 714–725.

Berry, M.P., Graham, C.M., Mcnab, F.W., Xu, Z., Bloch, S.A., Oni, T., Wilkinson, K.A., Banchereau, R., Skinner, J., Wilkinson, R.J., Quinn, C., Blankenship, D., Dhawan, R., Cush, J.J., Mejias, A., Ramilo, O., Kon, O.M., Pascual, V., Banchereau, J., Chaussabel, D., O'Garra, A., 2010. An interferon-inducible neutrophil-driven blood transcriptional signature in human tuberculosis. Nature 466, 973–977.

Bloom, C.I., Graham, C.M., Berry, M.P., Wilkinson, K.A., Oni, T., Rozakeas, F., Xu, Z., Rossello-Urgell, J., Chaussabel, D., Banchereau, J., Pascual, V., Lipman, M., Wilkinson, R.J., O'Garra, A., 2012. Detectable changes in the blood transcriptome are present after two weeks of antituberculosis therapy. PLoS One 7, e46191.

Bodenmiller, B., Zunder, E., Finck, R., Chen, T., Savig, E., Bruggner, R., Simonds, E., Bendall, S., Sachs, K., Krutzik, P., Nolan, G., 2012. Multiplexed mass cytometry profiling of cellular states perturbed by small-molecule regulators. Nat. Biotechnol. 30, 858–867.

Boisson, B., Laplantine, E., Prando, C., Giliani, S., Israelsson, E., Xu, Z., Abhyankar, A., Israel, L., Trevejo-Nunez, G., Bogunovic, D., Cepika, A.M., MacDuff, D., Chrabieh, M., Hubeau, M., Bajolle, F., Debre, M., Mazzolari, E., Vairo, D., Agou, F., Virgin, H.W., Bossuyt, X., Rambaud, C., Facchetti, F., Bonnet, D., Quartier, P., Fournet, J.C., Pascual, V., Chaussabel, D., Notarangelo, L.D., Puel, A., Israel, A., Casanova, J.L., Picard, C., 2012. Immunodeficiency, autoinflammation and amylopectinosis in humans with inherited HOIL-1 and LUBAC deficiency. Nat. Immunol. 13, 1178–1186.

Bonnelykke, K., Matheson, M.C., Pers, T.H., Granell, R., Strachan, D.P., Alves, A.C., Linneberg, A., Curtin, J.A., Warrington, N.M., Standl, M., Kerkhof, M., Jonsdottir, I., Bukvic, B.K., Kaakinen, M., Sleimann, P., Thorleifsson, G., Thorsteinsdottir, U., Schramm, K., Baltic, S., Kreiner-Moller, E., Simpson, A., St Pourcain, B., Coin, L., Hui, J., Walters, E.H., Tiesler, C.M., Duffy, D.L., Jones, G., Ring, S.M., Mcardle, W.L., Price, L., Robertson, C.F., Pekkanen, J., Tang, C.S., Thiering, E., Montgomery, G.W., Hartikainen, A.L., Dharmage, S.C., Husemoen, L.L., Herder, C., Kemp, J.P., Elliot, P., James, A., Waldenberger, M., Abramson, M.J., Fairfax, B.P., Knight, J.C., Gupta, R., Thompson, P.J., Holt, P., Sly, P., Hirschhorn, J.N., Blekic, M., Weidinger, S., Hakonarsson, H., Stefansson, K., Heinrich, J., Postma, D.S., Custovic, A., Pennell, C.E., Jarvelin, M.R., Koppelman, G.H., Timpson, N., Ferreira, M.A., Bisgaard, H., Henderson, A.J., Australian Asthma Genetics C, Genetics E. A., Lifecourse Epidemiology C., 2013. Meta-analysis of genome-wide association studies identifies ten loci influencing allergic sensitization. Nat. Genet. 45, 902–906.

Boulanger, L.M., Shatz, C.J., 2004. Immune signalling in neural development, synaptic plasticity and disease. Nat. Rev. Neurosci. 5, 521–531.

Boyd, S.D., 2013. Diagnostic applications of high-throughput DNA sequencing. Annu. Rev. Pathol. 8, 381–410.

Boyd, S.D., Marshall, E.L., Merker, J.D., Maniar, J.M., Zhang, L.N., Sahaf, B., Jones, C.D., Simen, B.B., Hanczaruk, B., Nguyen, K.D., Nadeau, K.C., Egholm, M., Miklos, D.B., Zehnder, J.L., Fire, A.Z., 2009. Measurement and clinical monitoring of human lymphocyte clonality by massively parallel VDJ pyrosequencing. Sci. Transl. Med. 1, 12ra23.

Brodin, P., Jojic, V., Gao, T., Bhattacharya, S., Angel, C.J., Furman, D., Shen-Orr, S., Dekker, C.L., Swan, G.E., Butte, A.J., Maecker, H.T., Davis, M.M., 2015. Variation in the human immune system is largely driven by non-heritable influences. Cell 160, 37–47.

Brown, J., De Vos, W.M., Distefano, P.S., Dore, J., Huttenhower, C., Knight, R., Lawley, T.D., Raes, J., Turnbaugh, P., 2013. Translating the human microbiome. Nat. Biotechnol. 31, 304–308.

Bruggner, R.V., Bodenmiller, B., Dill, D.L., Tibshirani, R.J., Nolan, G.P., 2014. Automated identification of stratifying signatures in cellular subpopulations. Proc. Natl. Acad. Sci. U. S. A. 111, E2770–E2777.

Bunyavanich, S., Schadt, E.E., 2015. Systems biology of asthma and allergic diseases: A multiscale approach. J. Allergy Clin. Immunol. 135 (1), 31–42.

Bunyavanich, S., Schadt, E.E., Himes, B.E., Lasky-Su, J., Qiu, W., Lazarus, R., Ziniti, J.P., Cohain, A., Linderman, M., Torgerson, D.G., Eng, C.S., Pino-Yanes, M., Padhukasahasram, B., Yang, J.J., Mathias, R.A., Beaty, T.H., Li, X., Graves, P., Romieu, I., Navarro Bdel, R., Salam, M.T., Vora, H., Nicolae, D.L., Ober, C., Martinez, F.D., Bleecker, E.R., Meyers, D.A., Gauderman, W.J., Gilliland, F., Burchard, E.G., Barnes, K.C., Williams, L.K., London, S.J., Zhang, B., Raby, B.A.,

Weiss, S.T., 2014. Integrated genome-wide association, coexpression network, and expression single nucleotide polymorphism analysis identifies novel pathway in allergic rhinitis. BMC Med. Genet. 7, 48.

Cancer Target, D., Development, N., Schreiber, S.L., Shamji, A.F., Clemons, P.A., Hon, C., Koehler, A.N., Munoz, B., Palmer, M., Stern, A.M., Wagner, B.K., Powers, S., Lowe, S.W., Guo, X., Krasnitz, A., Sawey, E.T., Sordella, R., Stein, L., Trotman, L.C., Califano, A., Dalla-Favera, R., Ferrando, A., Iavarone, A., Pasqualucci, L., Silva, J., Stockwell, B.R., Hahn, W.C., Chin, L., Depinho, R.A., Boehm, J.S., Gopal, S., Huang, A., Root, D.E., Weir, B.A., Gerhard, D.S., Zenklusen, J.C., Roth, M.G., White, M.A., Minna, J.D., MacMillan, J.B., Posner, B.A., 2010. Towards patient-based cancer therapeutics. Nat. Biotechnol. 28, 904–906.

Casanova, J.L., Abel, L., 2007. Human genetics of infectious diseases: a unified theory. EMBO J. 26, 915–922.

Casanova, J.L., Abel, L., Quintana-Murci, L., 2013. Immunology taught by human genetics. Cold Spring Harb. Symp. Quant. Biol. 78, 157–172.

Centers for Disease, Control & Prevention, 2011. Notifiable diseases and mortality tables. MMWR Morb. Mortal. Wkly Rep. 59, 1704–1717.

Chang, S., Kohrt, H., Maecker, H.T., 2014. Monitoring the immune competence of cancer patients to predict outcome. Cancer Immunol. Immunother. 63, 713–719.

Chaussabel, D., Quinn, C., Shen, J., Patel, P., Glaser, C., Baldwin, N., Stichweh, D., Blankenship, D., Li, L., Munagala, I., Bennett, L., Allantaz, F., Mejias, A., Ardura, M., Kaizer, E., Monnet, L., Allman, W., Randall, H., Johnson, D., Lanier, A., Punaro, M., Wittkowski, K.M., White, P., Fay, J., Klintmalm, G., Ramilo, O., Palucka, A.K., Banchereau, J., Pascual, V., 2008. A modular analysis framework for blood genomics studies: application to systemic lupus erythematosus. Immunity 29, 150–164.

Chen, R., Mias, G.I., Li-Pook-Than, J., Jiang, L., Lam, H.Y., Chen, R., Miriami, E., Karczewski, K.J., Hariharan, M., Dewey, F.E., Cheng, Y., Clark, M.J., Im, H., Habegger, L., Balasubramanian, S., O'Huallachain, M., Dudley, J.T., Hillenmeyer, S., Haraksingh, R., Sharon, D., Euskirchen, G., Lacroute, P., Bettinger, K., Boyle, A.P., Kasowski, M., Grubert, F., Seki, S., Garcia, M., Whirl-Carrillo, M., Gallardo, M., Blasco, M.A., Greenberg, P.L., Snyder, P., Klein, T.E., Altman, R.B., Butte, A.J., Ashley, E.A., Gerstein, M., Nadeau, K.C., Tang, H., Snyder, M., 2012. Personal omics profiling reveals dynamic molecular and medical phenotypes. Cell 148, 1293–1307.

Chen, J.C., Alvarez, M.J., Talos, F., Dhruv, H., Rieckhof, G.E., Iyer, A., Diefes, K.L., Aldape, K., Berens, M., Shen, M.M., Califano, A., 2014. Identification of causal genetic drivers of human disease through systems-level analysis of regulatory networks. Cell 159, 402–414.

Chiche, L., Jourde-Chiche, N., Pascual, V., Chaussabel, D., 2013. Current perspectives on systems immunology approaches to rheumatic diseases. Arthritis Rheum. 65, 1407–1417.

Chin, C.S., Sorenson, J., Harris, J.B., Robins, W.P., Charles, R.C., Jean-Charles, R.R., Bullard, J., Webster, D.R., Kasarskis, A., Peluso, P., Paxinos, E.E., Yamaichi, Y., Calderwood, S.B., Mekalanos, J.J., Schadt, E.E., Waldor, M.K., 2011. The origin of the Haitian cholera outbreak strain. N. Engl. J. Med. 364, 33–42.

Chiu, I.M., Von Hehn, C.A., Woolf, C.J., 2012. Neurogenic inflammation and the peripheral nervous system in host defense and immunopathology. Nat. Neurosci. 15, 1063–1067.

Chiu, I.M., Heesters, B.A., Ghasemlou, N., Von Hehn, C.A., Zhao, F., Tran, J., Wainger, B., Strominger, A., Muralidharan, S., Horswill, A.R., Bubeck Wardenburg, J., Hwang, S.W., Carroll, M.C., Woolf, C.J., 2013. Bacteria activate sensory neurons that modulate pain and inflammation. Nature 501, 52–57.

Cho, J.H., Gregersen, P.K., 2011. Genomics and the multifactorial nature of human autoimmune disease. N. Engl. J. Med. 365, 1612–1623.

Cliff, J.M., Lee, J.S., Constantinou, N., Cho, J.E., Clark, T.G., Ronacher, K., King, E.C., Lukey, P.T., Duncan, K., Van Helden, P.D., Walzl, G., Dockrell, H.M., 2013. Distinct phases of blood gene expression pattern through tuberculosis treatment reflect modulation of the humoral immune response. J. Infect. Dis. 207, 18–29.

Collier, N., Doan, S., Kawazoe, A., Goodwin, R.M., Conway, M., Tateno, Y., Ngo, Q.H., Dien, D., Kawtrakul, A., Takeuchi, K., Shigematsu, M., Taniguchi, K., 2008. BioCaster: detecting public health rumors with a Web-based text mining system. Bioinformatics 24, 2940–2941.

Colombel, J.F., Rutgeerts, P.J., Sandborn, W.J., Yang, M., Camez, A., Pollack, P.F., Thakkar, R.B., Robinson, A.M., Chen, N., Mulani, P.M., Chao, J., 2014. Adalimumab induces deep remission in patients with Crohn's disease. Clin. Gastroenterol. Hepatol. 12 (3), 414-22.e5.

Cooper, G.S., Bynum, M.L., Somers, E.C., 2009. Recent insights in the epidemiology of autoimmune diseases: improved prevalence estimates and understanding of clustering of diseases. J. Autoimmun. 33, 197–207.

Cosgrove, B.D., Alexopoulos, L.G., Hang, T.C., Hendriks, B.S., Sorger, P.K., Griffith, L.G., Lauffenburger, D.A., 2010. Cytokine-associated drug toxicity in human hepatocytes is associated with signaling network dysregulation. Mol. BioSyst. 6, 1195–1206.

Cotsapas, C., Voight, B.F., Rossin, E., Lage, K., Neale, B.M., Wallace, C., Abecasis, G.R., Barrett, J.C., Behrens, T., Cho, J., De Jager, P.L., Elder, J.T., Graham, R.R., Gregersen, P., Klareskog, L., Siminovitch, K.A., Van Heel, D.A., Wijmenga, C., Worthington, J., Todd, J.A., Hafler, D.A., Rich, S.S., Daly, M.J., F.O.N.O. Consortia, 2011. Pervasive sharing of genetic effects in autoimmune disease. PLoS Genet. 7, e1002254.

Cravedi, P., Heeger, P.S., 2012. Immunologic monitoring in transplantation revisited. Curr. Opin. Organ Transplant. 17, 26–32.

Dastani, Z., Hivert, M.F., Timpson, N., Perry, J.R., Yuan, X., Scott, R.A., Henneman, P., Heid, I.M., Kizer, J.R., Lyytikainen, L.P., Fuchsberger, C., Tanaka, T., Morris, A.P., Small, K., Isaacs, A., Beekman, M., Coassin, S., Lohman, K., Qi, L., Kanoni, S., Pankow, J.S., Uh, H.W., Wu, Y., Bidulescu, A., Rasmussen-Torvik, L.J., Greenwood, C.M., Ladouceur, M., Grimsby, J., Manning, A.K., Liu, C.T., Kooner, J., Mooser, V.E., Vollenweider, P., Kapur, K.A., Chambers, J., Wareham, N.J., Langenberg, C., Frants, R., Willems-Vandijk, K., Oostra, B.A., Willems, S.M., Lamina, C., Winkler, T.W., Psaty, B.M., Tracy, R.P., Brody, J., Chen, I., Viikari, J., Kahonen, M., Pramstaller, P.P., Evans, D.M., St Pourcain, B., Sattar, N., Wood, A.R., Bandinelli, S., Carlson, O.D., Egan, J.M., Bohringer, S., Van Heemst, D., Kedenko, L., Kristiansson, K., Nuotio, M.L., Loo, B.M., Harris, T., Garcia, M., Kanaya, A., Haun, M., Klopp, N., Wichmann, H.E., Deloukas, P., Katsareli, E., Couper, D.J., Duncan, B.B., Kloppenburg, M., Adair, L.S., Borja, J.B., Consortium, D., Consortium, M., Investigators, G., Mu, T.C., Wilson, J.G., Musani, S., Guo, X., Johnson, T., Semple, R., Teslovich, T.M., Allison, M.A., Redline, S., Buxbaum, S.G., Mohlke, K.L., Meulenbelt, I., Ballantyne, C.M., Dedoussis, G.V., Hu, F.B., Liu, Y., Paulweber, B., Spector, T.D., Slagboom, P.E., Ferrucci, L., Jula, A., et al., 2012. Novel loci for adiponectin levels and their influence on type 2 diabetes and metabolic traits: a multi-ethnic meta-analysis of 45,891 individuals. PLoS Genet. 8, e1002607.

Davila, M.L., Riviere, I., Wang, X., Bartido, S., Park, J., Curran, K., Chung, S.S., Stefanski, J., Borquez-Ojeda, O., Olszewska, M., Qu, J., Wasielewska, T., He, Q., Fink, M., Shinglot, H., Youssif, M., Satter, M., Wang, Y., Hosey, J., Quintanilla, H., Halton, E., Bernal, Y., Bouhassira, D.C., Arcila, M.E., Gonen, M., Roboz, G.J., Maslak, P., Douer, D., Frattini, M.G., Giralt, S., Sadelain, M., Brentjens, R., 2014. Efficacy and toxicity management of 19-28z CAR T cell therapy in B cell acute lymphoblastic leukemia. Sci. Transl. Med. 6, 224ra25.

Deleeuw, R.J., Kost, S.E., Kakal, J.A., Nelson, B.H., 2012. The prognostic value of FoxP3+ tumor-infiltrating lymphocytes in cancer: a critical review of the literature. Clin. Cancer Res. 18, 3022–3029.

Dominguez, H., Storgaard, H., Rask-Madsen, C., Steffen Hermann, T., Ihlemann, N., Baunbjerg Nielsen, D., Spohr, C., Kober, L., Vaag, A., Torp-Pedersen, C., 2005. Metabolic and vascular effects of tumor necrosis factor-alpha blockade with etanercept in obese patients with type 2 diabetes. J. Vasc. Res. 42, 517–525.

Doty, K.R., Guillot-Sestier, M.V., Town, T., 2014. The role of the immune system in neurodegenerative disorders: adaptive or maladaptive? Brain Res. 1617, 155–173

Dudley, J.T., Sirota, M., Shenoy, M., Pai, R.K., Roedder, S., Chiang, A.P., Morgan, A.A., Sarwal, M.M., Pasricha, P.J., Butte, A.J., 2011. Computational repositioning of the anticonvulsant topiramate for inflammatory bowel disease. Sci. Transl. Med. 3, 96ra76.

Dunn, G.P., Bruce, A.T., Ikeda, H., Old, L.J., Schreiber, R.D., 2002. Cancer immunoediting: from immunosurveillance to tumor escape. Nat. Immunol. 3, 991–998.

Fairfax, B.P., Makino, S., Radhakrishnan, J., Plant, K., Leslie, S., Dilthey, A., Ellis, P., Langford, C., Vannberg, F.O., Knight, J.C., 2012. Genetics of gene expression in primary immune cells identifies cell type-specific master regulators and roles of HLA alleles. Nat. Genet. 44, 502–510.
Feldmann, M., 2002. Development of anti-TNF therapy for rheumatoid arthritis. Nat. Rev. Immunol. 2, 364–371.
Finak, G., Frelinger, J., Jiang, W., Newell, E.W., Ramey, J., Davis, M.M., Kalams, S.A., De Rosa, S.C., Gottardo, R., 2014. OpenCyto: an open source infrastructure for scalable, robust, reproducible, and automated, end-to-end flow cytometry data analysis. PLoS Comput. Biol. 10, e1003806.
Fischbach, M.A., Bluestone, J.A., Lim, W.A., 2013. Cell-based therapeutics: the next pillar of medicine. Sci. Transl. Med. 5, 179ps7.
Freifeld, C.C., Mandl, K.D., Reis, B.Y., Brownstein, J.S., 2008. HealthMap: global infectious disease monitoring through automated classification and visualization of Internet media reports. J. Am. Med. Inform. Assoc. 15, 150–157.
Furman, D., Jojic, V., Kidd, B., Shen-Orr, S., Price, J., Jarrell, J., Tse, T., Huang, H., Lund, P., Maecker, H.T., Utz, P.J., Dekker, C.L., Koller, D., Davis, M.M., 2013. Apoptosis and other immune biomarkers predict influenza vaccine responsiveness. Mol. Syst. Biol. 9, 659.
Gajewski, T.F., Schreiber, H., Fu, Y.X., 2013. Innate and adaptive immune cells in the tumor microenvironment. Nat. Immunol. 14, 1014–1022.
Genomes Project, C., Abecasis, G.R., Auton, A., Brooks, L.D., Depristo, M.A., Durbin, R.M., Handsaker, R.E., Kang, H.M., Marth, G.T., Mcvean, G.A., 2012. An integrated map of genetic variation from 1,092 human genomes. Nature 491, 56–65.
Ginsberg, J., Mohebbi, M.H., Patel, R.S., Brammer, L., Smolinski, M.S., Brilliant, L., 2009. Detecting influenza epidemics using search engine query data. Nature 457, 1012–1014.
Gire, S.K., Goba, A., Andersen, K.G., Sealfon, R.S., Park, D.J., Kanneh, L., Jalloh, S., Momoh, M., Fullah, M., Dudas, G., Wohl, S., Moses, L.M., Yozwiak, N.L., Winnicki, S., Matranga, C.B., Malboeuf, C.M., Qu, J., Gladden, A.D., Schaffner, S.F., Yang, X., Jiang, P.P., Nekoui, M., Colubri, A., Coomber, M.R., Fonnie, M., Moigboi, A., Gbakie, M., Kamara, F.K., Tucker, V., Konuwa, E., Saffa, S., Sellu, J., Jalloh, A.A., Kovoma, A., Koninga, J., Mustapha, I., Kargbo, K., Foday, M., Yillah, M., Kanneh, F., Robert, W., Massally, J.L., Chapman, S.B., Bochicchio, J., Murphy, C., Nusbaum, C., Young, S., Birren, B.W., Grant, D.S., Scheiffelin, J.S., Lander, E.S., Happi, C., Gevao, S.M., Gnirke, A., Rambaut, A., Garry, R.F., Khan, S.H., Sabeti, P.C., 2014. Genomic surveillance elucidates Ebola virus origin and transmission during the 2014 outbreak. Science 345, 1369–1372.
Goldbach-Mansky, R., Kastner, D.L., 2009. Autoinflammation: the prominent role of IL-1 in monogenic autoinflammatory diseases and implications for common illnesses. J. Allergy Clin. Immunol. 124, 1141–1149. quiz 1150–1.
Goldfine, A.B., Silver, R., Aldhahi, W., Cai, D., Tatro, E., Lee, J., Shoelson, S.E., 2008. Use of salsalate to target inflammation in the treatment of insulin resistance and type 2 diabetes. Clin. Transl. Sci. 1, 36–43.
Goldfine, A.B., Fonseca, V., Jablonski, K.A., Pyle, L., Staten, M.A., Shoelson, S.E., T.-T.D.S. Team, 2010. The effects of salsalate on glycemic control in patients with type 2 diabetes: a randomized trial. Ann. Intern. Med. 152, 346–357.
Gonzalez, H., Elgueta, D., Montoya, A., Pacheco, R., 2014. Neuroimmune regulation of microglial activity involved in neuroinflammation and neurodegenerative diseases. J. Neuroimmunol. 274, 1–13.
Goris, A., Liston, A., 2012. The immunogenetic architecture of autoimmune disease. Cold Spring Harbor Perspect. Biol. 4, a007260.
Goronzy, J.J., Weyand, C.M., 2013. Understanding immunosenescence to improve responses to vaccines. Nat. Immunol. 14, 428–436.
Gray, K.A., Yates, B., Seal, R.L., Wright, M.W., Bruford, E.A., 2015. Genenames.org: the HGNC resources in 2015. Nucleic Acids Res. 43, D1079–D1085.
Griffin, W.S., 2013. Neuroinflammatory cytokine signaling and Alzheimer's disease. N. Engl. J. Med. 368, 770–771.
Gubin, M.M., Zhang, X., Schuster, H., Caron, E., Ward, J.P., Noguchi, T., Ivanova, Y., Hundal, J., Arthur, C.D., Krebber, W.J., Mulder, G.E., Toebes, M., Vesely, M.D., Lam, S.S., Korman, A.J.,

Allison, J.P., Freeman, G.J., Sharpe, A.H., Pearce, E.L., Schumacher, T.N., Aebersold, R., Rammensee, H.G., Melief, C.J., Mardis, E.R., Gillanders, W.E., Artyomov, M.N., Schreiber, R.D., 2014. Checkpoint blockade cancer immunotherapy targets tumour-specific mutant antigens. Nature 515, 577–581.

Guild, W.R., Harrison, J.H., Merrill, J.P., Murray, J., 1955. Successful homotransplantation of the kidney in an identical twin. Trans. Am. Clin. Climatol. Assoc. 67, 167–173.

Hakim, F.T., Gress, R.E., 2007. Immunosenescence: deficits in adaptive immunity in the elderly. Tissue Antigens 70, 179–189.

Halloran, P.F., 2004. Immunosuppressive drugs for kidney transplantation. N. Engl. J. Med. 351, 2715–2729.

Han, A., Glanville, J., Hansmann, L., Davis, M.M., 2014. Linking T-cell receptor sequence to functional phenotype at the single-cell level. Nat. Biotechnol. 32, 684–692.

Haso, W., Lee, D.W., Shah, N.N., Stetler-Stevenson, M., Yuan, C.M., Pastan, I.H., Dimitrov, D.S., Morgan, R.A., Fitzgerald, D.J., Barrett, D.M., Wayne, A.S., Mackall, C.L., Orentas, R.J., 2013. Anti-CD22-chimeric antigen receptors targeting B-cell precursor acute lymphoblastic leukemia. Blood 121, 1165–1174.

Henao-Mejia, J., Elinav, E., Jin, C., Hao, L., Mehal, W.Z., Strowig, T., Thaiss, C.A., Kau, A.L., Eisenbarth, S.C., Jurczak, M.J., Camporez, J.P., Shulman, G.I., Gordon, J.I., Hoffman, H.M., Flavell, R.A., 2012. Inflammasome-mediated dysbiosis regulates progression of NAFLD and obesity. Nature 482, 179–185.

Hsiao, A., Ahmed, A.M., Subramanian, S., Griffin, N.W., Drewry, L.L., Petri, W.A.J.R., Haque, R., Ahmed, T., Gordon, J.I., 2014. Members of the human gut microbiota involved in recovery from Vibrio cholerae infection. Nature 515, 423–426.

Hueber, W., Utz, P.J., Steinman, L., Robinson, W.H., 2002. Autoantibody profiling for the study and treatment of autoimmune disease. Arthritis Res. 4, 290–295.

Hueber, W., Utz, P.J., Robinson, W.H., 2003. Autoantibodies in early arthritis: advances in diagnosis and prognostication. Clin. Exp. Rheumatol. 21, S59–S64.

Hueber, W., Kidd, B.A., Tomooka, B.H., Lee, B.J., Bruce, B., Fries, J.F., Sonderstrup, G., Monach, P., Drijfhout, J.W., Van Venrooij, W.J., Utz, P.J., Genovese, M.C., Robinson, W.H., 2005. Antigen microarray profiling of autoantibodies in rheumatoid arthritis. Arthritis Rheum. 52, 2645–2655.

Hueber, W., Tomooka, B.H., Zhao, X.Y., Kidd, B.A., Drijfhout, J.W., Fries, J.F., Van Venrooij, W.J., Metzger, A.L., Genovese, M.C., Robinson, W.H., 2007. Proteomic analysis of secreted proteins in early rheumatoid arthritis: anti-citrulline autoreactivity is associated with up regulation of proinflammatory cytokines. Ann. Rheum. Dis. 66, 712–719.

Human Microbiome Project, C, 2012a. A framework for human microbiome research. Nature 486, 215–221.

Human Microbiome Project, C, 2012b. Structure, function and diversity of the healthy human microbiome. Nature 486, 207–214.

Hummel, M., Bentink, S., Berger, H., Klapper, W., Wessendorf, S., Barth, T.F., Bernd, H.W., Cogliatti, S.B., Dierlamm, J., Feller, A.C., Hansmann, M.L., Hummel, M., Bentink, S., Berger, H., Klapper, W., Wessendorf, S., Barth, T.F., Bernd, H.W., Cogliatti, S.B., Dierlamm, J., Feller, A.C., Hansmann, M.L., Haralambieva, E., Harder, L., Hasenclever, D., Kuhn, M., Lenze, D., Lichter, P., Martin-Subero, J.I., Moller, P., Muller-Hermelink, H.K., Ott, G., Parwaresch, R.M., Pott, C., Rosenwald, A., Rosolowski, M., Schwaenen, C., Sturzenhofecker, B., Szczepanowski, M., Trautmann, H., Wacker, H.H., Spang, R., Loeffler, M., Trumper, L., Stein, H., Siebert, R., Molecular Mechanisms In Malignant Lymphomas Network Project Of The Deutsche K, 2006. A biologic definition of Burkitt's lymphoma from transcriptional and genomic profiling. N. Engl. J. Med. 354, 2419–2430.

Iida, N., Dzutsev, A., Stewart, C.A., Smith, L., Bouladoux, N., Weingarten, R.A., Molina, D.A., Salcedo, R., Back, T., Cramer, S., Dai, R.M., Kiu, H., Cardone, M., Naik, S., Patri, A.K., Wang, E., Marincola, F.M., Frank, K.M., Belkaid, Y., Trinchieri, G., Goldszmid, R.S., 2013. Commensal bacteria control cancer response to therapy by modulating the tumor microenvironment. Science 342, 967–970.

International Multiple Sclerosis Genetics, C., 2013. Network-based multiple sclerosis pathway analysis with GWAS data from 15,000 cases and 30,000 controls. Am. J. Hum. Genet. 92, 854–865.

International Multiple Sclerosis Genetics, C., Beecham, A.H., Patsopoulos, N.A., Xifara, D.K., Davis, M.F., Kemppinen, A., Cotsapas, C., Shah, T.S., Spencer, C., Booth, D., Goris, A., Oturai, A., Saarela, J., Fontaine, B., Hemmer, B., Martin, C., Zipp, F., D'Alfonso, S., Martinelli-Boneschi, F., Taylor, B., Harbo, H.F., Kockum, I., Hillert, J., Olsson, T., Ban, M., Oksenberg, J.R., Hintzen, R., Barcellos, L.F., Wellcome Trust Case Control C., International I. B. D. G. C., Agliardi, C., Alfredsson, L., Alizadeh, M., Anderson, C., Andrews, R., Sondergaard, H.B., Baker, A., Band, G., Baranzini, S.E., Barizzone, N., Barrett, J., Bellenguez, C., Bergamaschi, L., Bernardinelli, L., Berthele, A., Biberacher, V., Binder, T.M., Blackburn, H., Bomfim, I.L., Brambilla, P., Broadley, S., Brochet, B., Brundin, L., Buck, D., Butzkueven, H., Caillier, S.J., Camu, W., Carpentier, W., Cavalla, P., Celius, E.G., Coman, I., Comi, G., Corrado, L., Cosemans, L., Cournu-Rebeix, I., Cree, B.A., Cusi, D., Damotte, V., Defer, G., Delgado, S.R., Deloukas, P., Di Sapio, A., Dilthey, A.T., Donnelly, P., Dubois, B., Duddy, M., Edkins, S., Elovaara, I., Esposito, F., Evangelou, N., Fiddes, B., Field, J., Franke, A., Freeman, C., Frohlich, I.Y., Galimberti, D., Gieger, C., Gourraud, P.A., Graetz, C., Graham, A., Grummel, V., Guaschino, C., Hadjixenofontos, A., Hakonarson, H., Halfpenny, C., Hall, G., Hall, P., Hamsten, A., Harley, J., Harrower, T., et al., 2013. Analysis of immune-related loci identifies 48 new susceptibility variants for multiple sclerosis. Nat. Genet. 45, 1353–1360.

Jahchan, N.S., Dudley, J.T., Mazur, P.K., Flores, N., Yang, D., Palmerton, A., Zmoos, A.F., Vaka, D., Tran, K.Q., Zhou, M., Krasinska, K., Riess, J.W., Neal, J.W., Khatri, P., Park, K.S., Butte, A.J., Sage, J., 2013. A drug repositioning approach identifies tricyclic antidepressants as inhibitors of small cell lung cancer and other neuroendocrine tumors. Cancer Discovery 3, 1364–1377.

Janes, K.A., Reinhardt, H.C., Yaffe, M.B., 2008. Cytokine-induced signaling networks prioritize dynamic range over signal strength. Cell 135, 343–354.

Jin, C., Henao-Mejia, J., Flavell, R.A., 2013. Innate immune receptors: key regulators of metabolic disease progression. Cell Metab. 17, 873–882.

Jostins, L., Ripke, S., Weersma, R.K., Duerr, R.H., Mcgovern, D.P., Hui, K.Y., Lee, J.C., Schumm, L.P., Sharma, Y., Anderson, C.A., Essers, J., Mitrovic, M., Ning, K., Cleynen, I., Theatre, E., Spain, S.L., Raychaudhuri, S., Goyette, P., Wei, Z., Abraham, C., Achkar, J.P., Ahmad, T., Amininejad, L., Ananthakrishnan, A.N., Andersen, V., Andrews, J.M., Baidoo, L., Balschun, T., Bampton, P.A., Bitton, A., Boucher, G., Brand, S., Buning, C., Cohain, A., Cichon, S., D'Amato, M., De Jong, D., Devaney, K.L., Dubinsky, M., Edwards, C., Ellinghaus, D., Ferguson, L.R., Franchimont, D., Fransen, K., Gearry, R., Georges, M., Gieger, C., Glas, J., Haritunians, T., Hart, A., Hawkey, C., Hedl, M., Hu, X., Karlsen, T.H., Kupcinskas, L., Kugathasan, S., Latiano, A., Laukens, D., Lawrance, I.C., Lees, C.W., Louis, E., Mahy, G., Mansfield, J., Morgan, A.R., Mowat, C., Newman, W., Palmieri, O., Ponsioen, C.Y., Potocnik, U., Prescott, N.J., Regueiro, M., Rotter, J.I., Russell, R.K., Sanderson, J.D., Sans, M., Satsangi, J., Schreiber, S., Simms, L.A., Sventoraityte, J., Targan, S.R., Taylor, K.D., Tremelling, M., Verspaget, H.W., De Vos, M., Wijmenga, C., Wilson, D.C., Winkelmann, J., Xavier, R.J., Zeissig, S., Zhang, B., Zhang, C.K., Zhao, H., International, I.B.D.G.C., Silverberg, M.S., Annese, V., Hakonarson, H., Brant, S.R., Radford-Smith, G., Mathew, C.G., Rioux, J.D., et al., 2012. Host-microbe interactions have shaped the genetic architecture of inflammatory bowel disease. Nature 491, 119–124.

Karosiene, E., Lundegaard, C., Lund, O., Nielsen, M., 2012. NetMHCcons: a consensus method for the major histocompatibility complex class I predictions. Immunogenetics 64, 177–186.

Karr, J.R., Sanghvi, J.C., Macklin, D.N., Gutschow, M.V., Jacobs, J.M., Bolival Jr., B., Assad-Garcia, N., Glass, J.I., Covert, M.W., 2012. A whole-cell computational model predicts phenotype from genotype. Cell 150, 389–401.

Kau, A.L., Ahern, P.P., Griffin, N.W., Goodman, A.L., Gordon, J.I., 2011. Human nutrition, the gut microbiome and the immune system. Nature 474, 327–336.

Kelada, S.N., Carpenter, D.E., Aylor, D.L., Chines, P., Rutledge, H., Chesler, E.J., Churchill, G.A., Pardo-Manuel De Villena, F., Schwartz, D.A., Collins, F.S., 2014. Integrative genetic analysis of allergic inflammation in the murine lung. Am. J. Respir. Cell Mol. Biol. 51, 436–445.

Khatri, P., Sarwal, M.M., Butte, A.J., 2011. Applications of translational bioinformatics in transplantation. Clin. Pharmacol. Ther. 90, 323–327.

Khatri, P., Roedder, S., Kimura, N., De Vusser, K., Morgan, A.A., Gong, Y., Fischbein, M.P., Robbins, R.C., Naesens, M., Butte, A.J., Sarwal, M.M., 2013. A common rejection module (CRM) for acute rejection across multiple organs identifies novel therapeutics for organ transplantation. J. Exp. Med. 210, 2205–2221.

Kidd, B.A., Ho, P.P., Sharpe, O., Zhao, X., Tomooka, B.H., Kanter, J.L., Steinman, L., Robinson, W.H., 2008. Epitope spreading to citrullinated antigens in mouse models of autoimmune arthritis and demyelination. Arthritis Res. Ther. 10, R119.

Kidd, B.A., Peters, L.A., Schadt, E.E., Dudley, J.T., 2014. Unifying immunology with informatics and multiscale biology. Nat. Immunol. 15, 118–127.

Knox, C., Law, V., Jewison, T., Liu, P., Ly, S., Frolkis, A., Pon, A., Banco, K., Mak, C., Neveu, V., Djoumbou, Y., Eisner, R., Guo, A.C., Wishart, D.S., 2011. DrugBank 3.0: a comprehensive resource for 'omics' research on drugs. Nucleic Acids Res. 39, D1035–D1041.

Kochenderfer, J.N., Rosenberg, S.A., 2013. Treating B-cell cancer with T cells expressing anti-CD19 chimeric antigen receptors. Nat. Rev. Clin. Oncol. 10, 267–276.

Kochenderfer, J.N., Dudley, M.E., Kassim, S.H., Somerville, R.P., Carpenter, R.O., Stetler-Stevenson, M., Yang, J.C., Phan, G.Q., Hughes, M.S., Sherry, R.M., Raffeld, M., Feldman, S., Lu, L., Li, Y.F., Ngo, L.T., Goy, A., Feldman, T., Spaner, D.E., Wang, M.L., Chen, C.C., Kranick, S.M., Nath, A., Nathan, D.A., Morton, K.E., Toomey, M.A., Rosenberg, S.A., 2015. Chemotherapy-refractory diffuse large B-Cell lymphoma and indolent B-Cell malignancies can be effectively treated with autologous T cells expressing an Anti-CD19 chimeric antigen receptor. J. Clin. Oncol. 33, 540–549.

Kosteli, A., Sugaru, E., Haemmerle, G., Martin, J.F., Lei, J., Zechner, R., Ferrante Jr., A.W., 2010. Weight loss and lipolysis promote a dynamic immune response in murine adipose tissue. J. Clin. Invest. 120, 3466–3479.

Law, G.L., Korth, M.J., Benecke, A.G., Katze, M.G., 2013. Systems virology: host-directed approaches to viral pathogenesis and drug targeting. Nat. Rev. Microbiol. 11, 455–466.

Li, L., Khatri, P., Sigdel, T.K., Tran, T., Ying, L., Vitalone, M.J., Chen, A., Hsieh, S., Dai, H., Zhang, M., Naesens, M., Zarkhin, V., Sansanwal, P., Chen, R., Mindrinos, M., Xiao, W., Benfield, M., Ettenger, R.B., Dharnidharka, V., Mathias, R., Portale, A., McDonald, R., Harmon, W., Kershaw, D., Vehaskari, V.M., Kamil, E., Baluarte, H.J., Warady, B., Davis, R., Butte, A.J., Salvatierra, O., Sarwal, M.M., 2012. A peripheral blood diagnostic test for acute rejection in renal transplantation. Am. J. Transplant. 12, 2710–2718.

Li, S., Rouphael, N., Duraisingham, S., Romero-Steiner, S., Presnell, S., Davis, C., Schmidt, D.S., Johnson, S.E., Milton, A., Rajam, G., Kasturi, S., Carlone, G.M., Quinn, C., Chaussabel, D., Palucka, A.K., Mulligan, M.J., Ahmed, R., Stephens, D.S., Nakaya, H.I., Pulendran, B., 2014. Molecular signatures of antibody responses derived from a systems biology study of five human vaccines. Nat. Immunol. 15, 195–204.

Linding, R., Jensen, L.J., Ostheimer, G.J., Van Vugt, M.A., Jorgensen, C., Miron, I.M., Diella, F., Colwill, K., Taylor, L., Elder, K., Metalnikov, P., Nguyen, V., Pasculescu, A., Jin, J., Park, J.G., Samson, L.D., Woodgett, J.R., Russell, R.B., Bork, P., Yaffe, M.B., Pawson, T., 2007. Systematic discovery of in vivo phosphorylation networks. Cell 129, 1415–1426.

Lucin, K.M., Wyss-Coray, T., 2009. Immune activation in brain aging and neurodegeneration: too much or too little? Neuron 64, 110–122.

Lumeng, C.N., Saltiel, A.R., 2011. Inflammatory links between obesity and metabolic disease. J. Clin. Invest. 121, 2111–2117.

Maecker, H.T., Lindstrom, T.M., Robinson, W.H., Utz, P.J., Hale, M., Boyd, S.D., Shen-Orr, S.S., Fathman, C.G., 2012a. New tools for classification and monitoring of autoimmune diseases. Nat. Rev. Rheumatol. 8, 317–328.

Maecker, H.T., McCoy, J.P., Nussenblatt, R., 2012b. Standardizing immunophenotyping for the human immunology project. Nat. Rev. Immunol. 12, 191–200.

Masoli, M., Fabian, D., Holt, S., Beasley, R., Global Initiative For Asthma Patients, 2004. The global burden of asthma: executive summary of the GINA Dissemination Committee report. Allergy 59, 469–478.

Maude, S.L., Frey, N., Shaw, P.A., Aplenc, R., Barrett, D.M., Bunin, N.J., Chew, A., Gonzalez, V.E., Zheng, Z., Lacey, S.F., Mahnke, Y.D., Melenhorst, J.J., Rheingold, S.R., Shen, A., Teachey, D.T., Levine, B.L., June, C.H., Porter, D.L., Grupp, S.A., 2014. Chimeric antigen receptor T cells for sustained remissions in leukemia. N. Engl. J. Med. 371, 1507–1517.

Mcgonagle, D., McDermott, M.F., 2006. A proposed classification of the immunological diseases. PLoS Med. 3, e297.

Mei, H.E., Leipold, M.D., Schulz, A.R., Chester, C., Maecker, H.T., 2015. Barcoding of live human peripheral blood mononuclear cells for multiplexed mass cytometry. J. Immunol. 194, 2022–2031.

Nakaya, H.I., Wrammert, J., Lee, E.K., Racioppi, L., Marie-Kunze, S., Haining, W.N., Means, A.R., Kasturi, S.P., Khan, N., Li, G.M., McCausland, M., Kanchan, V., Kokko, K.E., Li, S., Elbein, R., Mehta, A.K., Aderem, A., Subbarao, K., Ahmed, R., Pulendran, B., 2011. Systems biology of vaccination for seasonal influenza in humans. Nat. Immunol. 12, 786–795.

Neurath, M.F., 2014. Cytokines in inflammatory bowel disease. Nat. Rev. Immunol. 14, 329–342.

Newell, E.W., Sigal, N., Nair, N., Kidd, B.A., Greenberg, H.B., Davis, M.M., 2013. Combinatorial tetramer staining and mass cytometry analysis facilitate T-cell epitope mapping and characterization. Nat. Biotechnol. 31, 623–629.

Obermoser, G., Presnell, S., Domico, K., Xu, H., Wang, Y., Anguiano, E., Thompson-Snipes, L., Ranganathan, R., Zeitner, B., Bjork, A., Anderson, D., Speake, C., Ruchaud, E., Skinner, J., Alsina, L., Sharma, M., Dutartre, H., Cepika, A., Israelsson, E., Nguyen, P., Nguyen, Q.A., Harrod, A.C., Zurawski, S.M., Pascual, V., Ueno, H., Nepom, G.T., Quinn, C., Blankenship, D., Palucka, K., Banchereau, J., Chaussabel, D., 2013. Systems scale interactive exploration reveals quantitative and qualitative differences in response to influenza and pneumococcal vaccines. Immunity 38, 831–844.

Odunsi, K., Old, L.J., 2007. Tumor infiltrating lymphocytes: indicators of tumor-related immune responses. Cancer Immun. 7, 3.

Okada, Y., Wu, D., Trynka, G., Raj, T., Terao, C., Ikari, K., Kochi, Y., Ohmura, K., Suzuki, A., Yoshida, S., Graham, R.R., Manoharan, A., Ortmann, W., Bhangale, T., Denny, J.C., Carroll, R.J., Eyler, A.E., Greenberg, J.D., Kremer, J.M., Pappas, D.A., Jiang, L., Yin, J., Ye, L., Su, D.F., Yang, J., Xie, G., Keystone, E., Westra, H.J., Esko, T., Metspalu, A., Zhou, X., Gupta, N., Mirel, D., Stahl, E.A., Diogo, D., Cui, J., Liao, K., Guo, M.H., Myouzen, K., Kawaguchi, T., Coenen, M.J., Van Riel, P.L., Van De Laar, M.A., Guchelaar, H.J., Huizinga, T.W., Dieude, P., Mariette, X., Bridges, S.L.J.R., Zhernakova, A., Toes, R.E., Tak, P.P., Miceli-Richard, C., Bang, S.Y., Lee, H.S., Martin, J., Gonzalez-Gay, M.A., Rodriguez-Rodriguez, L., Rantapaa-Dahlqvist, S., Arlestig, L., Choi, H.K., Kamatani, Y., Galan, P., Lathrop, M., Consortium, R., Consortium, G., Eyre, S., Bowes, J., Barton, A., De Vries, N., Moreland, L.W., Criswell, L.A., Karlson, E.W., Taniguchi, A., Yamada, R., Kubo, M., Liu, J.S., Bae, S.C., Worthington, J., Padyukov, L., Klareskog, L., Gregersen, P.K., Raychaudhuri, S., Stranger, B.E., De Jager, P.L., Franke, L., Visscher, P.M., Brown, M.A., Yamanaka, H., Mimori, T., Takahashi, A., Xu, H., Behrens, T.W., Siminovitch, K.A., Momohara, S., Matsuda, F., Yamamoto, K., Plenge, R.M., 2014. Genetics of rheumatoid arthritis contributes to biology and drug discovery. Nature 506, 376–381.

Okin, D., Medzhitov, R., 2012. Evolution of inflammatory diseases. Curr. Biol. 22, R733–R740.

Orru, V., Steri, M., Sole, G., Sidore, C., Virdis, F., Dei, M., Lai, S., Zoledziewska, M., Busonero, F., Mulas, A., Floris, M., Mentzen, W.I., Urru, S.A., Olla, S., Marongiu, M., Piras, M.G., Lobina, M., Maschio, A., Pitzalis, M., Urru, M.F., Marcelli, M., Cusano, R., Deidda, F., Serra, V., Oppo, M., Pilu, R., Reinier, F., Berutti, R., Pireddu, L., Zara, I., Porcu, E., Kwong, A., Brennan, C., Tarrier, B., Lyons, R., Kang, H.M., Uzzau, S., Atzeni, R., Valentini, M., Firinu, D., Leoni, L., Rotta, G., Naitza, S., Angius, A., Congia, M., Whalen, M.B., Jones, C.M., Schlessinger, D., Abecasis, G.R., Fiorillo, E., Sanna, S., Cucca, F., 2013. Genetic variants regulating immune cell levels in health and disease. Cell 155, 242–256.

Osborn, O., Olefsky, J.M., 2012. The cellular and signaling networks linking the immune system and metabolism in disease. Nat. Med. 18, 363–374.

O'Shea, J.J., Plenge, R., 2012. JAK and STAT signaling molecules in immunoregulation and immune-mediated disease. Immunity 36, 542–550.

O'Shea, J.J., Gadina, M., Kanno, Y., 2011. Cytokine signaling: birth of a pathway. J. Immunol. 187, 5475–5478.

O'Shea, J.J., Holland, S.M., Staudt, L.M., 2013. JAKs and STATs in immunity, immunodeficiency, and cancer. N. Engl. J. Med. 368, 161–170.

O'Sullivan, L.A., Liongue, C., Lewis, R.S., Stephenson, S.E., Ward, A.C., 2007. Cytokine receptor signaling through the Jak-Stat-Socs pathway in disease. Mol. Immunol. 44, 2497–2506.

Pascual, V., Chaussabel, D., Banchereau, J., 2010. A genomic approach to human autoimmune diseases. Annu. Rev. Immunol. 28, 535–571.

Patil, S., Pincas, H., Seto, J., Nudelman, G., Nudelman, I., Sealfon, S.C., 2010. Signaling network of dendritic cells in response to pathogens: a community-input supported knowledgebase. BMC Syst. Biol. 4, 137.

Paul, S.M., Mytelka, D.S., Dunwiddie, C.T., Persinger, C.C., Munos, B.H., Lindborg, S.R., Schacht, A.L., 2010. How to improve R&D productivity: the pharmaceutical industry's grand challenge. Nat. Rev. Drug Discov. 9, 203–214.

Picard, C., Casanova, J.L., Abel, L., 2006. Mendelian traits that confer predisposition or resistance to specific infections in humans. Curr. Opin. Immunol. 18, 383–390.

Price, J.V., Haddon, D.J., Kemmer, D., Delepine, G., Mandelbaum, G., Jarrell, J.A., Gupta, R., Balboni, I., Chakravarty, E.F., Sokolove, J., Shum, A.K., Anderson, M.S., Cheng, M.H., Robinson, W.H., Browne, S.K., Holland, S.M., Baechler, E.C., Utz, P.J., 2013. Protein microarray analysis reveals BAFF-binding autoantibodies in systemic lupus erythematosus. J. Clin. Invest. 123, 5135–5145.

Prugnolle, F., Manica, A., Charpentier, M., Guegan, J.F., Guernier, V., Balloux, F., 2005. Pathogen-driven selection and worldwide HLA class I diversity. Curr. Biol. 15, 1022–1027.

Querec, T.D., Akondy, R.S., Lee, E.K., Cao, W., Nakaya, H.I., Teuwen, D., Pirani, A., Gernert, K., Deng, J., Marzolf, B., Kennedy, K., Wu, H., Bennouna, S., Oluoch, H., Miller, J., Vencio, R.Z., Mulligan, M., Aderem, A., Ahmed, R., Pulendran, B., 2009. Systems biology approach predicts immunogenicity of the yellow fever vaccine in humans. Nat. Immunol. 10, 116–125.

Rasko, D.A., Webster, D.R., Sahl, J.W., Bashir, A., Boisen, N., Scheutz, F., Paxinos, E.E., Sebra, R., Chin, C.S., Iliopoulos, D., Klammer, A., Peluso, P., Lee, L., Kislyuk, A.O., Bullard, J., Kasarskis, A., Wang, S., Eid, J., Rank, D., Redman, J.C., Steyert, S.R., Frimodt-Moller, J., Struve, C., Petersen, A.M., Krogfelt, K.A., Nataro, J.P., Schadt, E.E., Waldor, M.K., 2011. Origins of the E. coli strain causing an outbreak of hemolytic-uremic syndrome in Germany. N. Engl. J. Med. 365, 709–717.

Restifo, N.P., Dudley, M.E., Rosenberg, S.A., 2012. Adoptive immunotherapy for cancer: harnessing the T cell response. Nat. Rev. Immunol. 12, 269–281.

Riol-Blanco, L., Ordovas-Montanes, J., Perro, M., Naval, E., Thiriot, A., Alvarez, D., Paust, S., Wood, J.N., Von Andrian, U.H., 2014. Nociceptive sensory neurons drive interleukin-23-mediated psoriasiform skin inflammation. Nature 510, 157–161.

Robins, H.S., Srivastava, S.K., Campregher, P.V., Turtle, C.J., Andriesen, J., Riddell, S.R., Carlson, C.S., Warren, E.H., 2010. Overlap and effective size of the human CD8+ T cell receptor repertoire. Sci. Transl. Med. 2, 47ra64.

Roush, S.W., Murphy, T.V., Vaccine-Preventable Disease Table Working Group, 2007. Historical comparisons of morbidity and mortality for vaccine-preventable diseases in the United States. JAMA 298, 2155–2163.

Sandborn, W.J., Gasink, C., Gao, L.L., Blank, M.A., Johanns, J., Guzzo, C., Sands, B.E., Hanauer, S.B., Targan, S., Rutgeerts, P., Ghosh, S., De Villiers, W.J., Panaccione, R., Greenberg, G., Schreiber, S., Lichtiger, S., Feagan, B.G., Group C. S., 2012. Ustekinumab induction and maintenance therapy in refractory Crohn's disease. N. Engl. J. Med. 367, 1519–1528.

Sawitzki, B., Schlickeiser, S., Reinke, P., Volk, H.D., 2011. Monitoring tolerance and rejection in organ transplant recipients. Biomarkers 16 (Suppl 1), S42–S50.

Schadt, E.E., Lamb, J., Yang, X., Zhu, J., Edwards, S., Guhathakurta, D., Sieberts, S.K., Monks, S., Reitman, M., Zhang, C., Lum, P.Y., Leonardson, A., Thieringer, R., Metzger, J.M., Yang, L., Castle, J., Zhu, H., Kash, S.F., Drake, T.A., Sachs, A., Lusis, A.J., 2005. An integrative genomics approach to infer causal associations between gene expression and disease. Nat. Genet. 37, 710–717.

Schadt, E.E., 2009. Molecular networks as sensors and drivers of common human diseases. Nature 461, 218–223.

Schreiber, R.D., Old, L.J., Smyth, M.J., 2011. Cancer immunoediting: integrating immunity's roles in cancer suppression and promotion. Science 331, 1565–1570.

Sentman, C.L., Meehan, K.R., 2014. NKG2D CARs as cell therapy for cancer. Cancer J. 20, 156–159.

Shalek, A., Satija, R., Adiconis, X., Gertner, R., Gaublomme, J., Raychowdhury, R., Schwartz, S., Yosef, N., Malboeuf, C., Lu, D., Trombetta, J., Gennert, D., Gnirke, A., Goren, A., Hacohen, N., Levin, J., Park, H., Regev, A., 2013. Single-cell transcriptomics reveals bimodality in expression and splicing in immune cells. Nature 498, 236–240.

Shankaran, V., Ikeda, H., Bruce, A.T., White, J.M., Swanson, P.E., Old, L.J., Schreiber, R.D., 2001. IFNgamma and lymphocytes prevent primary tumour development and shape tumour immunogenicity. Nature 410, 1107–1111.

Sharma, S., Zhou, X., Thibault, D.M., Himes, B.E., Liu, A., Szefler, S.J., Strunk, R., Castro, M., Hansel, N.N., Diette, G.B., Vonakis, B.M., Adkinson, N.F.J.R., Avila, L., Soto-Quiros, M., Barraza-Villareal, A., Lemanske, R.F.J.R., Solway, J., Krishnan, J., White, S.R., Cheadle, C., Berger, A.E., Fan, J., Boorgula, M.P., Nicolae, D., Gilliland, F., Barnes, K., London, S.J., Martinez, F., Ober, C., Celedon, J.C., Carey, V.J., Weiss, S.T., Raby, B.A., 2014. A genome-wide survey of CD4(+) lymphocyte regulatory genetic variants identifies novel asthma genes. J. Allergy Clin. Immunol. 134, 1153–1162.

Shen, P., Roch, T., Lampropoulou, V., O'Connor, R.A., Stervbo, U., Hilgenberg, E., Ries, S., Dang, V.D., Jaimes, Y., Daridon, C., Li, R., Jouneau, L., Boudinot, P., Wilantri, S., Sakwa, I., Miyazaki, Y., Leech, M.D., Mcpherson, R.C., Wirtz, S., Neurath, M., Hoehlig, K., Meinl, E., Grutzkau, A., Grun, J.R., Horn, K., Kuhl, A.A., Dorner, T., Bar-Or, A., Kaufmann, S.H., Anderton, S.M., Fillatreau, S., 2014. IL-35-producing B cells are critical regulators of immunity during autoimmune and infectious diseases. Nature 507, 366–370.

Shen-Orr, S.S., Goldberger, O., Garten, Y., Rosenberg-Hasson, Y., Lovelace, P.A., Hirschberg, D.L., Altman, R.B., Davis, M.M., Butte, A.J., 2009. Towards a cytokine-cell interaction knowledgebase of the adaptive immune system. Pac. Symp. Biocomput. 14, 439–450.

Sirota, M., Dudley, J.T., Kim, J., Chiang, A.P., Morgan, A.A., Sweet-Cordero, A., Sage, J., Butte, A.J., 2011. Discovery and preclinical validation of drug indications using compendia of public gene expression data. Sci. Transl. Med. 3, 96ra77.

Smith, M.I., Yatsunenko, T., Manary, M.J., Trehan, I., Mkakosya, R., Cheng, J., Kau, A.L., Rich, S.S., Concannon, P., Mychaleckyj, J.C., Liu, J., Houpt, E., Li, J.V., Holmes, E., Nicholson, J., Knights, D., Ursell, L.K., Knight, R., Gordon, J.I., 2013. Gut microbiomes of Malawian twin pairs discordant for kwashiorkor. Science 339, 548–554.

Spellman, S.R., Eapen, M., Logan, B.R., Mueller, C., Rubinstein, P., Setterholm, M.I., Woolfrey, A.E., Horowitz, M.M., Confer, D.L., Hurley, C.K., National Marrow Donor P., Center For International B., Marrow Transplant R., 2012. A perspective on the selection of unrelated donors and cord blood units for transplantation. Blood 120, 259–265.

Stanley, T.L., Zanni, M.V., Johnsen, S., Rasheed, S., Makimura, H., Lee, H., Khor, V.K., Ahima, R.S., Grinspoon, S.K., 2011. TNF-alpha antagonism with etanercept decreases glucose and increases the proportion of high molecular weight adiponectin in obese subjects with features of the metabolic syndrome. J. Clin. Endocrinol. Metab. 96, E146–E150.

Steinman, L., 2004. Elaborate interactions between the immune and nervous systems. Nat. Immunol. 5, 575–581.

Steinman, L., 2014. Going viral and the fatal vulnerability of neurons from immunity, not from infection. Proc. Natl. Acad. Sci. U. S. A. 111, 16982–16983.

Steinman, R.M., Mellman, I., 2004. Immunotherapy: bewitched, bothered, and bewildered no more. Science 305, 197–200.

Subramanian, S., Huq, S., Yatsunenko, T., Haque, R., Mahfuz, M., Alam, M.A., Benezra, A., Destefano, J., Meier, M.F., Muegge, B.D., Barratt, M.J., Vanarendonk, L.G., Zhang, Q., Province, M.A., Petri JR., W.A., Ahmed, T., Gordon, J.I., 2014. Persistent gut microbiota immaturity in malnourished Bangladeshi children. Nature 510, 417–421.

Sullivan, P.W., Ghushchyan, V.H., Slejko, J.F., Belozeroff, V., Globe, D.R., Lin, S.L., 2011. The burden of adult asthma in the United States: evidence from the Medical Expenditure Panel Survey. J. Allergy Clin. Immunol. 127 (363–369), e1–e3.

Suthram, S., Dudley, J.T., Chiang, A.P., Chen, R., Hastie, T.J., Butte, A.J., 2010. Network-based elucidation of human disease similarities reveals common functional modules enriched for pluripotent drug targets. PLoS Comput. Biol. 6, e1000662.

Tan, M.S., Jiang, T., Tan, L., Yu, J.T., 2014. Genome-wide association studies in neurology. Ann. Transl. Med. 2, 124.

Trowsdale, J., 2011. The MHC, disease and selection. Immunol. Lett. 137, 1–8.

Tsang, J.S., Schwartzberg, P.L., Kotliarov, Y., Biancotto, A., Xie, Z., Germain, R.N., Wang, E., Olnes, M.J., Narayanan, M., Golding, H., Moir, S., Dickler, H.B., Perl, S., Cheung, F., Baylor, H.C., Consortium, C.H.I., 2014. Global analyses of human immune variation reveal baseline predictors of postvaccination responses. Cell 157, 499–513.

Urba, W.J., Longo, D.L., 2011. Redirecting T cells. N. Engl. J. Med. 365, 754–757.

Van Haren, K., Tomooka, B.H., Kidd, B.A.B.A.N.W.E.L.L.B., Bar-Or, A., Chitnis, T., Tenembaum, S.N., Pohl, D., Rostasy, K., Dale, R.C., O'Connor, K.C., Hafler, D.A., Steinman, L., Robinson, W.H., 2013. Serum autoantibodies to myelin peptides distinguish acute disseminated encephalomyelitis from relapsing-remitting multiple sclerosis. Mult. Scler. 19, 1726–1733.

Vanneman, M., Dranoff, G., 2012. Combining immunotherapy and targeted therapies in cancer treatment. Nat. Rev. Cancer 12, 237–251.

Viaud, S., Saccheri, F., Mignot, G., Yamazaki, T., Daillere, R., Hannani, D., Enot, D.P., Pfirschke, C., Engblom, C., Pittet, M.J., Schlitzer, A., Ginhoux, F., Apetoh, L., Chachaty, E., Woerther, P.L., Eberl, G., Berard, M., Ecobichon, C., Clermont, D., Bizet, C., Gaboriau-Routhiau, V., Cerf-Bensussan, N., Opolon, P., Yessaad, N., Vivier, E., Ryffel, B., Elson, C.O., Dore, J., Kroemer, G., Lepage, P., Boneca, I.G., Ghiringhelli, F., Zitvogel, L., 2013. The intestinal microbiota modulates the anticancer immune effects of cyclophosphamide. Science 342, 971–976.

Visscher, P.M., Brown, M.A., McCarthy, M.I., Yang, J., 2012. Five years of GWAS discovery. Am. J. Hum. Genet. 90, 7–24.

Voight, B.F., Cotsapas, C., 2012. Human genetics offers an emerging picture of common pathways and mechanisms in autoimmunity. Curr. Opin. Immunol. 24, 552–557.

Wang, C., Krishnakumar, S., Wilhelmy, J., Babrzadeh, F., Stepanyan, L., Su, L.F., Levinson, D., Fernandez-Vina, M.A., Davis, R.W., Davis, M.M., Mindrinos, M., 2012a. High-throughput, high-fidelity HLA genotyping with deep sequencing. Proc. Natl. Acad. Sci. U. S. A. 109, 8676–8681.

Wang, I.M., Zhang, B., Yang, X., Zhu, J., Stepaniants, S., Zhang, C., Meng, Q., Peters, M., He, Y., Ni, C., Slipetz, D., Crackower, M.A., Houshyar, H., Tan, C.M., Asante-Appiah, E., O'Neill, G., Luo, M.J., Thieringer, R., Yuan, J., Chiu, C.S., Lum, P.Y., Lamb, J., Boie, Y., Wilkinson, H.A., Schadt, E.E., Dai, H., Roberts, C., 2012b. Systems analysis of eleven rodent disease models reveals an inflammatome signature and key drivers. Mol. Syst. Biol. 8, 594.

Welter, D., Macarthur, J., Morales, J., Burdett, T., Hall, P., Junkins, H., Klemm, A., Flicek, P., Manolio, T., Hindorff, L., Parkinson, H., 2014. The NHGRI GWAS catalog, a curated resource of SNP-trait associations. Nucleic Acids Res. 42, D1001–D1006.

Westra, H.J., Peters, M.J., Esko, T., Yaghootkar, H., Schurmann, C., Kettunen, J., Christiansen, M.W., Fairfax, B.P., Schramm, K., Powell, J.E., Zhernakova, A., Zhernakova, D.V., Veldink, J.H., Van Den Berg, L.H., Karjalainen, J., Withoff, S., Uitterlinden, A.G., Hofman, A., Rivadeneira, F., 't Hoen, P.A., Reinmaa, E., Fischer, K., Nelis, M., Milani, L., Melzer, D., Ferrucci, L., Singleton, A.B., Hernandez, D.G., Nalls, M.A., Homuth, G., Nauck, M., Radke, D., Volker, U., Perola, M., Salomaa, V., Brody, J., Suchy-Dicey, A., Gharib, S.A., Enquobahrie, D.A., Lumley, T., Montgomery, G.W., Makino, S., Prokisch, H., Herder, C., Roden, M., Grallert, H., Meitinger, T., Strauch, K., Li, Y., Jansen, R.C., Visscher, P.M., Knight, J.C., Psaty, B.M., Ripatti, S., Teumer, A., Frayling, T.M., Metspalu, A., Van Meurs, J.B., Franke, L., 2013. Systematic identification of trans eQTLs as putative drivers of known disease associations. Nat. Genet. 45, 1238–1243.

Wilson, M.R., Naccache, S.N., Samayoa, E., Biagtan, M., Bashir, H., Yu, G., Salamat, S.M., Somasekar, S., Federman, S., Miller, S., Sokolic, R., Garabedian, E., Candotti, F., Buckley, R.H., Reed, K.D., Meyer, T.L., Seroogy, C.M., Galloway, R., Henderson, S.L., Gern, J.E., Derisi, J.L., Chiu, C.Y., 2014. Actionable diagnosis of neuroleptospirosis by next-generation sequencing. N. Engl. J. Med. 370, 2408–2417.

Xavier, R.J., Rioux, J.D., 2008. Genome-wide association studies: a new window into immune-mediated diseases. Nat. Rev. Immunol. 8, 631–643.
Xu, G.J., Kula, T., Xu, Q., Li, M.Z., Vernon, S.D., Ndung'u, T., Ruxrungtham, K., Sanchez, J., Brander, C., Chung, R.T., O'connor, K.C., Walker, B., Larman, H.B., Elledge, S.J., 2015. Viral immunology. Comprehensive serological profiling of human populations using a synthetic human virome. Science. 348, aaa0698.
Yao, Y., Liu, R., Shin, M.S., Trentalange, M., Allore, H., Nassar, A., Kang, I., Pober, J.S., Montgomery, R.R., 2014. CyTOF supports efficient detection of immune cell subsets from small samples. J. Immunol. Methods 415, 1–5.
Yosef, N., Shalek, A.K., Gaublomme, J.T., Jin, H., Lee, Y., Awasthi, A., Wu, C., Karwacz, K., Xiao, S., Jorgolli, M., Gennert, D., Satija, R., Shakya, A., Lu, D.Y., Trombetta, J.J., Pillai, M.R., Ratcliffe, P.J., Coleman, M.L., Bix, M., Tantin, D., Park, H., Kuchroo, V.K., Regev, A., 2013. Dynamic regulatory network controlling TH17 cell differentiation. Nature 496, 461–468.
Zhang, T., Lemoi, B.A., Sentman, C.L., 2005. Chimeric NK-receptor-bearing T cells mediate antitumor immunotherapy. Blood 106, 1544–1551.
Zhang, T., Barber, A., Sentman, C.L., 2006. Generation of antitumor responses by genetic modification of primary human T cells with a chimeric NKG2D receptor. Cancer Res. 66, 5927–5933.
Zhang, J.A., Mortazavi, A., Williams, B.A., Wold, B.J., Rothenberg, E.V., 2012. Dynamic transformations of genome-wide epigenetic marking and transcriptional control establish T cell identity. Cell 149, 467–482.
Zhang, B., Gaiteri, C., Bodea, L.G., Wang, Z., Mcelwee, J., Podtelezhnikov, A.A., Zhang, C., Xie, T., Tran, L., Dobrin, R., Fluder, E., Clurman, B., Melquist, S., Narayanan, M., Suver, C., Shah, H., Mahajan, M., Gillis, T., Mysore, J., MacDonald, M.E., Lamb, J.R., Bennett, D.A., Molony, C., Stone, D.J., Gudnason, V., Myers, A.J., Schadt, E.E., Neumann, H., Zhu, J., Emilsson, V., 2013. Integrated systems approach identifies genetic nodes and networks in late-onset Alzheimer's disease. Cell 153, 707–720.
Zitvogel, L., Galluzzi, L., Viaud, S., Vetizou, M., Daillere, R., Merad, M., Kroemer, G., 2015. Cancer and the gut microbiota: an unexpected link. Sci. Transl. Med. 7, 271ps1.

CHAPTER 2

Congenital Immunodeficiency Diseases: Crossroad of Infection, Autoimmunity, and Hyperinflammation

J. Farmer[1], K. Csomos[1], R. Bacchetta[2], J.E. Walter[1]
[1]Harvard Medical School, Boston, MA, United States
[2]Stanford Medical School, Stanford, CA, United States

Contents

1. INTRODUCTION

Primary immunodeficiency diseases (PIDs) are inherent disorders of immune system function. Today the term encompasses over 200 known hereditary disorders (Al-Herz et al., 2014). Initially the causative genetic mutations were identified using

Translational Immunology
http://dx.doi.org/10.1016/B978-0-12-801577-3.00002-2

time-intensive laboratory techniques including Sanger sequencing, fluorescent *in situ* hybridization (FISH), linkage mapping, positional cloning, and animal modeling of candidate genes. Such approaches led to notable discoveries in the field that include the role of recombination-activating gene 1 and 2 (*RAG1* and *RAG2*) in severe combined immunodeficiency disease (SCID) (Shinkai et al., 1992; Mombaerts et al., 1992; Schwarz et al., 1996), the role of Bruton's tyrosine kinase (BTK) in X-linked agammaglobulinemia (Vetrie et al., 1993), and the causative 22q11 deletion in DiGeorge Syndrome (de la Chapelle et al., 1981). Since the development of next generation sequencing, the field of PID genetics has been expanding exponentially, empowering the clinical immunologist to efficiently whole-exome or whole-genome sequence a single patient or family (Picard and Fischer, 2014). Classical PID genes are now identified in association with unexpected disease phenotypes. Unlike in early pediatric onset severe disease, where most PIDs are caused by a single genetic mutation or "monogenic" in origin, there is now an evolving spectrum of cases with mild to moderate severity where the clinical phenotype is likely driven by other susceptibility genes or epigenetic modifiers. The interpretation of whole-genome and whole-exome sequencing in these cases may be challenging, and functional testing for evidence of causative role is essential.

PIDs are still subclassified according to etiology of the underlying immune defect. The 2014 International Consensus (ICON) document recently described the following groups: innate immunodeficiencies including toll-like receptor (TLR) pathway defects in addition to phagocytic and complement deficiencies (group 1), disorders of T cells and B cells known as combined immunodeficiencies (CIDs) (group 2), isolated antibody deficiencies (group 3), and immunodeficiencies associated with syndromes (group 4) (Routes et al., 2014). In this chapter, we will focus on specific disease etiologies that best represent the gamut of PID with an emphasis on noninfectious clinical features and mechanisms that lead to autoimmunity and hyperinflammation. From group 1, we will discuss chronic granulomatous disease (CGD), a disease of impaired phagocytosis, and isolated complement deficiencies. From group 2, we will focus on SCID, Omenn syndrome, and late-onset CIDs secondary to a selection of genetic defects (*IL7RA, IL7RG, RAG1/2, Ligase IV, DCLRE1C, RMRP, CHD7, AK2, DOCK8*, and *STAT5b*). From group 3, we will discuss common variable immune deficiency (CVID), a deficiency of total IgG in combination with a deficiency of IgA or IgM. From group 4, we will discuss immunodeficiencies associated with syndromes including Wiskott-Aldrich syndrome, autoimmune polyendocrinopathy candidiasis and ectodermal dystrophy (APECED), autoimmune lymphoproliferative syndrome (ALPS), immune dysregulation polyendocrinopathy enteropathy X-linked (IPEX) syndrome, and mutations of the LPS-responsive beige-like anchor (*LRBA*) and cytotoxic T cell antigen-4 (*CTLA-4*) genes. Finally, we will review the emerging group or PIDs due to gain-of-function (GOF) alleles. Remarkably immunodeficiency has been described with *STAT1*, *STAT3*, and *PIK3R1* heterozygous GOF alleles that result in autoinflammation and/or autoimmunity with a wide range of immunological and clinical forms.

In 2013 epidemiologic modeling for PIDs estimated a worldwide prevalence of 6 million people, which is far less than the actual 27,000–60,000 individuals who report a diagnosis (Bousfiha et al., 2013). These data suggest that many patients with pathogenic PID genes go undiagnosed, either symptomatic or asymptomatic. With increasing knowledge that hypomorphic and hypermorphic mutations in PID genes may result in less severe and narrow spectrum infections in combination with increasing dominance of noninfectious complications (autoimmunity, malignancy, and inflammatory bowel disease (IBD) for example), many of the patients may be initially seen by other specialties such as hematology/oncology, rheumatology, or gastroenterology. The field of PID epidemiology is further complicated by incidence and prevalence rates that vary widely by specific disease etiology and geographic location. Within the United States and Europe, prevalence of all PIDs has been estimated at 1:1,200–1:500,000 (Gathmann et al., 2009; Boyle and Buckley, 2007). CVID is the most common symptomatic PID with an estimated incidence of 1:10,000–1:50,000 (Al-Herz et al., 2014; IUIS, 1999; Park et al., 2008).

The clinical presentation of PID is also varied. In the case of SCID, patients present with life-threatening infections at around 4–6 months of age, once maternal antibodies are no longer available to protect the infant. The high mortality related to a missed or delayed SCID diagnosis prompted the development of rapid T cell receptor excision circle (TREC) testing as part of the initial newborn screening process, which has now been implemented as mandatory in several states throughout the United States (Kwan et al., 2014). The early detection of SCID at birth, even in the asymptomatic phase under the protection of maternal antibodies, has not only prepared the patient for a more successful hematopoietic stem cell transplantation but has been proven to be cost effective as well (Chan et al., 2011; Kubiak et al., 2014). In contrast, the presentation of isolated antibody deficiency can be subtle, masked as recurrent sinopulmonary infections that may go unrecognized for years by the outpatient primary care physician. Data now demonstrate that a delayed PID diagnosis incurs significant morbidity to the patient (Resnick et al., 2012; Joshi et al., 2009). Too often a thorough diagnostic immune workup is not initiated and temporizing organ-based therapies, such as short courses of antibiotics or bronchodilators in the case of an acute pulmonary infection, take the place of preventive mechanism-based therapies, such as immunoglobulin replacement in the case of a patient with an underlying antibody deficiency or targeted treatment for autoimmune complications in CVID.

The long-term consequences of a missed or delayed PID diagnosis have been best characterized for CVID due to its often insidious onset and relative frequency in the general population. Both in Europe (Edgar et al., 2014; Gathmann et al., 2014) and in the United States (Resnick et al., 2012) these data demonstrate a significant risk for recurrent infections, transition to malignancy, and development of autoimmune pathology including cytopenias, end-organ granulomatous disease, and systemic autoinflammation such as rheumatoid arthritis and lupus. The mechanism behind how tolerance is disrupted and impaired immune defense can progress to autoimmunity has been a topic of much interest in the PID field. Not only do we gain insight into how better to manage our PID patients, but there is also the potential to use these rare monogenic diseases to elucidate basic immune mechanisms that drive hyperinflammation, loss of self-tolerance, and ultimately autoimmune disease. These fundamental concepts have implications on a much broader patient population spanning the disciplines of rheumatology, hematology/oncology, and even pulmonology, nephrology, gastroenterology, and neurology.

In this chapter we will review monogenic PIDs with a specific focus on the clinical spectrum of autoimmunity and hyperinflammation. We will discuss known mechanisms leading to these complications and contrast current commonly used approaches with mechanism-based investigational treatment strategies. At the end of the chapter, we will reflect on how early detection of PID patients prone to autoimmunity can alter disease course and prevent the onset or escalation of autoimmune complications.

2. CLINICAL FEATURES OF AUTOIMMUNE AND INFLAMMATORY MANIFESTATIONS IN PID

Development of autoimmune disease in patients with PID is much more common than previously recognized. In a population of Canadian pediatric patients with chronic rheumatologic disease, 15% tested positive for an underlying and previously undiagnosed PID (Barsalou et al., 2011). Analysis of the US Immunodeficiency Network (USIDNET) data bank additionally uncovered autoimmune disease in 1–10% of PID patients with the most frequent disease etiologies being autoimmune hemolytic anemia (AIHA), idiopathic thrombocytopenia purpura (ITP), and IBD (Maggadottir and Sullivan, 2014). Beyond the patients who carry an official diagnosis, many more may suffer from hyperinflammation, as demonstrated by a recent survey of patients with X-linked agammaglobulinemia, which identified at least one inflammatory symptom in 69% of respondents (Hernandez-Trujillo et al., 2014). Moreover, development of autoimmune disease pathology incurs significant morbidity and mortality to the PID patient. Four decades of outcomes analysis in US patients with CVID recently demonstrated an 11-fold higher risk of death in patients who developed noninfectious disease complications (Resnick et al., 2012), which correlates with previous analysis of the European Common Variable Immunodeficiency Disorders registry, demonstrating increased mortality in patients with CVID-associated autoimmune disease specifically (Chapel et al., 2008). Together these data highlight the need to for improved clinical screening and treatment regimens aimed specifically at addressing autoimmune disease pathology in PID.

Autoimmune cytopenias are some of the most common noninfectious disease complications seen in PID and can include AIHA, ITP, and autoimmune neutropenia (AIN). Autoimmune cytopenias are frequently observed in CVID and ALPS, which share prominent autoantibody production (Seidel, 2014). In a retrospective chart review of 326 patients with CVID, 11% had a history of autoimmune cytopenias, 54% of which predated the patient's diagnosis of CVID (Wang and Cunningham-Rundles, 2005). Perhaps most strikingly, the prevalence of autoimmune cytopenias in patients with CVID has been estimated at 100- to 1000-fold higher than that of the general population (Notarangelo, 2009). ALPS can also present with autoimmune cytopenias as the first clinical sign. AIHA and ITP are most frequently observed (23–51% of patients), although AIN is also common (19–27% of patients), and 80% of ALPS patients test positive for autoantibodies, most often Coombs and anticardiolipin (Notarangelo, 2009). While counterintuitive, autoimmune cytopenias can also be observed in CID on account of hypomorphic genetic defects supporting low levels of autoreactive T and B cell populations (Milner et al., 2008; Hillion et al., 2005; Walter et al., 2015). Finally, autoimmune cytopenias are a prominent feature of multiple PIDs associated with syndromes including Wiskott-Aldrich syndrome and IPEX with AIHA estimated in 15–36% and 30% of patients, respectively (Arason et al., 2010).

Systemic autoimmunity as a complication of PID can also develop, including inflammatory arthritis, sarcoidosis, Sjögren's syndrome, and even systemic lupus erythematous (SLE) and antiphospholipid syndrome in severe cases. Most notable among these associations is the development of SLE in patients with classical complement cascade deficiencies, which approaches 93% in patients with C1q deficiency and is observed to a lesser extent in patients with C1r, C1s, C4, and C2 deficiencies (Arason et al., 2010). The etiology of this was initially linked to defective clearance of immune complexes and apoptotic material, which exposes the immune system to nuclear debris and drives the production of nuclear autoantibodies. However, more recently dynamic interactions between the complement cascade and the adaptive arm of the immune system have been described (Leffler et al., 2014). To a lesser degree, CVID has also been linked to the development of systemic autoimmunity. Analysis of the USIDNET data bank recently demonstrated progression to rheumatoid arthritis in 3.2% of CVID patients and progression to severe systemic autoimmune disease including SLE and antiphospholipid syndrome in < 1% of CVID patients (Resnick et al., 2012). While it would be of great clinical yield to identify the subset of CVID patients who will progress to severe autoimmunity in order to initiate early treatment and prevent permanent end-organ damage, such methods have yet to be routinely implemented (Chapel et al., 2008). In addition, clinical management of systemic autoimmune disease in PID can be particularly challenging on account of delayed diagnosis, additional requirement for immune replacement therapy to avoid tendency for infections, and coordination between multiple providers (Swierkot et al., 2006).

One of the most striking and complex pathologies in PID is the development of granulomas, which has been well described for both CVID and CGD. In the two largest CVID cohorts to date, granulomas were identified in 8–9.7% of patients with common sites being the lungs, lymph nodes, liver, skin, and spleen (Resnick et al., 2012; Chapel et al., 2008). In addition, 7 of the 46 patients who developed granulomas in the US cohort had hyperinflammatory disease in more than one location (Resnick et al., 2012). In a recent single center cohort analysis of CGD, granuloma formation was histologically confirmed in 50% of patients with inflammatory disease localizing to the gastrointestinal tract (88.2%), lungs (26.4%), urogenital tract (17.6%), eyes (8.8%), and other sites including the skin (19.1%) (Magnani et al., 2014). While recurrent infection is one plausible explanation for granuloma formation in the PID patient, data in the CGD model suggest a prominent component of aseptic hyperinflammatory disease. First, in many instances no pathogens can be cultured from the inflammatory nodules. Second, the inflammatory nodules respond to immune modulators such as steroids but not to antibiotics. Third, IBD can be induced in a mouse model of CGD using only sterile preparations of branched beta-glucan proteins (reviewed in Schappi et al., 2008). Increased understanding of the pathogenesis of granulomatous disease in PID is a critical first step toward improving clinical management. Currently, IBD accounts for significant morbidity in CGD with 11–71% of patients progressing to failure to thrive (Marciano et al., 2004; Schappi et al., 2001). Furthermore, CVID patients who demonstrate a polyclonal lymphocytic infiltrative phenotype that includes granuloma formation are in one of the highest risk cohorts for PID-related death (Chapel et al., 2008).

Finally, end-organ specific autoimmune disease can occur in PID. Diffuse organ involvement has been described, including autoinflammatory disease of the endocrine system, lungs, gastrointestinal tract, skin, and even central nervous system. APECED derives its name from the autoimmune polyendocrinopathy that develops, most frequently adrenal cortical failure and hypoparathyroidism; however, type 1 diabetes mellitus (T1DM) and autoimmune thyroid disease have also been described (Arason et al., 2010). In contrast, IPEX is characterized by severe and early onset T1DM in the vast majority of patients (Barzaghi et al., 2012). Autoimmune endocrinopathy has been described to a lesser extent for CVID with autoimmune thyroid disease being most common (Resnick et al., 2012). Recently, the clinical spectrum of APECED has been expanding to include chronic lung disease, gastrointestinal dysfunction, and chronic inflammatory demyelinating polyneuropathy correlating with the discovery of new end-organ specific autoantibodies (Valenzise et al., 2014). However, autoimmune enteropathy is still most pronounced for IPEX, where life-threatening malabsorption often requiring parenteral nutrition is a feared complication. Specific autoantibodies against autoimmune enteropathy-related 75 kDa antigen (AIE-75) (Kobayashi et al., 1998) and villin (Kobayashi et al., 2011) are hypothesized to mediate the subtotal villous atrophy observed in IPEX patients (Patey-Mariaud de Serre et al., 2009). Finally, IPEX pathology extends to the skin where eczematous dermatitis and psoriasis have been well described, and more recently direct evidence of autoreactivity against keratin has been confirmed (Huter et al., 2010). On the other hand, anti-tryptophan hydroxylase-1 (TPH-1) antibodies are detected in APECED, a central tolerance defect, especially when complicated with gastrointestinal dysfunction. In a recent study, the presence of anti-AIE-75, anti-villin antibodies, and anti-TPH-1 antibodies were compared in APECED and IPEX syndrome and confirmed the disease specificity of both anti-AIE-75 and anti-TPH-1, although anti-villin antibodies were detected in some patients with APECED. The authors suggest that immune tolerance to AIE-75 and TPH-1 depends on the peripheral versus central tolerance mechanism, respectively (Chida et al., 2015).

3. MECHANISMS LEADING TO AUTOIMMUNITY AND HYPERINFLAMMATION IN PID

The clinical spectrum of autoimmune pathology undoubtedly relates to the underlying immune dysregulation at play. In the subsequent section, we will review in detail our up-to-date understanding of the development of autoimmunity and hyperinflammation in PID.

3.1 Increased apoptosis and decreased clearance

3.1.1 Complement defects

The association of complement defects with autoimmune diseases is well known. The complement system is a complex network with an important role in immediate defense of the host, controlling or promoting inflammation and clearance of apoptotic cells. Genetic deficiencies in early components of the classical complement pathway (C2, C4, C1q) or autoantibodies targeting C1q are associated with an increased risk for the development of SLE (Atkinson, 1986; Day et al., 1973; Meyer et al., 1985). In fact, there is a strong and frequent association with immune complex disease in 93% of C1q, 60–66% of C1s/r, and 90% of C4 deficient patients (Pickering et al., 2000; Sullivan, 1998). As the complement system is responsible for safe elimination of immune complexes and apoptotic cells, if deficient there is the potential for increased release of cellular antigens including DNA and RNA. In accordance with this mechanism, macrophages from individuals deficient in C1q, C4, C2, or C3 have been shown to have a reduced ability to uptake apoptotic material (Gullstrand et al., 2009).

As a further safety mechanism, opsonization of apoptotic cells by the complement system suppresses IL-12 and mitigates the proinflammatory activation of macrophages and dendritic cells (Ricklin et al., 2010). While controlled complement activation is therefore critical for effective removal of apoptotic material and maintenance of self-tolerance, unregulated and grossly amplified complement activation can alternatively promote autoinflammatory disease. First, uncontrolled complement activation can lead to direct end-organ tissue damage and exposure of autoantigens. Second, complement activation can have dynamic effects on the innate and adaptive arms of the immune system. Prominent mechanisms include the potential for complement activation to synergistically enhance TLR-dependent proinflammatory cytokine production (Zhang et al., 2007) as well as the potential for complement activation to lower the threshold for Fcγ receptor activation, which has been implicated in the pathogenesis of AIHA (Kumar et al., 2006). Finally, recurrent stimulation of the complement cascade may play a pathologic role in a variety of other inflammatory diseases including age-related macular degeneration (Anderson et al., 2010) and Alzheimer's disease (Alexander et al., 2008).

3.1.2 Chronic granulomatous disease (CGD)

Apoptosis is a form of programmed cellular death that results in controlled removal of damaged or terminal cells from the system. It occurs as a cascade of events that begins with cellular stress and ends with externalization of phosphatidylserine at the cellular surface as a signal for phagocytosis. Phosphatidylserine is recognized by counterpart receptors on the cellular surface of phagocytes, primarily macrophages. The ultimate result is efficient uptake of the apoptotic cell, an act that prevents further inflammation in the surrounding tissue by several mechanisms. First, effective uptake of the apoptotic cell inhibits toxic components, such as reactive oxygen species, from interacting with the surrounding tissue and causing damage. Second, effective uptake by the macrophage results in downstream production of inhibitory cytokines, mainly TGFβ, which suppresses an inflammatory response in the surrounding tissue. In CGD, impaired apoptosis promoting autoantibody generation has been described (Sanford et al., 2006). Patients with CGD as well as a mouse model of gp91 deficiency have been shown to have defective expression of phosphatidylserine at the neutrophil cell surface (Frasch et al., 2008; Hampton et al., 2002).

In addition, macrophages in CGD patients have been shown to be ineffectively programmed and thus unable to effectively phagocytose apoptotic material (Ricklin et al., 2010). Together, this neutrophil-macrophage dysfunction has been hypothesized to promote hyperinflammatory disease pathology in CGD. The macrophage dysfunction can be rescued in part by phosphatidylserine-dependent IL-4 production (Fernandez-Boyanapalli et al., 2009) or alternatively by IFNγ treatment, which promotes NO production and endogenous TNFα and Rac activation (Fernandez-Boyanapalli et al., 2010).

3.2 Tendency for hyperinflammation

3.2.1 Chronic granulomatous disease (CGD)

Patients with CGD have a primary defect in nicotinamide adenine dinucleotide phosphate (NADPH) oxidase activity. This oxidase response is essential to forming a functional defense mechanism against various bacterial and fungal pathogens, and thus patients with CGD are at significant risk for infection starting at birth (Marciano et al., 2015).

A functional oxidative defense mechanism requires formation of the phox complex, which consists of cell membrane integrated gp91-phox (CYBB) and p22-phox (CYBA) subunits in combination with cytosolic p47-phox (NCF1), p67-phox (NCF2), and p40-phox (NCF4) subunits. Mutations in all components of the NADPH oxidative complex can result in a CGD phenotype; however, two-thirds of CGD patients carry an X-linked recessive mutation in gp91-phox (Holland, 2013). Patients with CGD develop early-onset hyperinflammation in multiple sites including the gastrointestinal, urogenital, pulmonary, ocular system, and systemic autoimmune complications (Magnani et al., 2014). Autoimmune complications may include SLE, antiphospholipid syndrome, Kawasaki disease, arthritis, IgA nephropathy, and granulomatous pulmonary disease (De Ravin et al., 2008). Recently, the etiology of an underlying hyperinflammation in these patients was connected to hyperactivation of the type I interferon pathway (Kelkka et al., 2014). Patients with CGD demonstrated increased expression of type I IFN-responsive genes (most notably *STAT1*). They additionally were found to have increased production of lupus autoantibodies. These findings were confirmed in a Ncf1m1J-mutated mouse model of CGD and were reproducible in a germ-free setting, suggesting that hyperactivation of the type I IFN pathway in patients with CGD is native and not pathogen-driven. Even in heterozygous form, if NADPH oxidative complex activity is decreased to a certain threshold, clinical symptoms of lupus appear in female carriers. Occasionally, with decreased inactivation and skewing toward the diseased X chromosome, female carriers can develop profound CGD-like disease (Anderson-Cohen et al., 2003).

3.2.2 Omenn syndrome

In Omenn syndrome, autoimmune pathology is alternatively driven by expansion and activation of an oligoclonal population of autoreactive T and B cells. One of the clinical hallmarks of Omenn syndrome is scaly exudative erythroderma very early in life with highly elevated IgE levels and eosinophilia that distinguish this syndrome from SCID (Villa et al., 2008). Against the overall lymphopenia, autoreactive oligoclonal T cells infiltrate into lymph nodes, spleen, liver, and gastrointestinal tract to cause diffuse end-organ disease, which is fatal within months unless managed with complete immune reconstitution (de Saint-Basile et al., 1991; Signorini et al., 1999). Omenn syndrome was initially linked to partial ablation of recombinase function in V(D)J rearrangement secondary to pathogenic mutations in the *RAG1/RAG2* genes (Villa et al., 1998). Recently, individual case reports describe a similar phenotype with partial defects in other SCID-associated genes such as *IL2RG* (Shibata et al., 2007), *LIG4* (Grunebaum et al., 2008), *IL7RA* (Giliani et al., 2006), *ADA* (Roifman et al., 2008), *DCLRE1C* (Ege et al., 2005), *AK2* (Henderson et al., 2013a), *RMRP* (Roifman et al., 2006), *ZAP70* (Turul et al., 2009), and *CHD7* (Gennery et al., 2008). Most of the inflammatory pathology is attributable to a dysregulated T cell compartment secondary to partial defects in SCID-associated genes (Notarangelo, 2014), although recent investigation of the molecular and cellular basis of immune dysregulation in patients and animal models has revealed impaired tolerance mechanisms in both T and B cell development (Cassani et al., 2010a; Cavadini et al., 2005; Marrella et al., 2007; Poliani et al., 2009; Walter et al., 2010).

3.3 Impaired B or T cell tolerance checkpoints

There are numerous checkpoints in both T and B cell development that attempt to reduce the generation and/or survival of autoreactive cells. These mechanisms can be selectively impaired in certain PIDs. Hereby we briefly review the importance of central and peripheral B and T cell tolerance checkpoints and their impairment in specific PIDs.

3.3.1 Defects in B cell tolerance that induce autoimmunity in PID

Normally, two important processes accompany the maturation of B cells. By positive selection B cells acquire the ability to recognize foreign antigens and respond to them (immune competence), and by negative selection they develop tolerance against self-antigens preventing autoimmunity (immune tolerance). B cells arise in the bone marrow from the common myeloid progenitor and through pro-B and pre-B cell stages progress to immature B cells that express a functional B cell receptor (BCR). A large fraction of the B cells in the bone marrow is autoreactive even in a normal host (Wardemann et al., 2003). Deletion of cells with increased BCR binding to self and repeated rearrangement of the BCR (RAG-dependent receptor editing) allow for elimination of a subset of autoreactive cells (Gay et al., 1993; Tiegs et al., 1993). In addition, centrally the strength of BCR signaling can strongly influence selective survival of non-autoreactive B cells. Underlying the importance of BCR signaling in the establishment of tolerance, patients with *BTK* mutation and impaired B cell signaling (X-linked agammaglobulinemia) have a small fraction of immature B cells in the peripheral blood with high frequency of self-reactivity although bearing no mature B cells (Ng et al., 2004).

B cells then migrate into the red pulp of the spleen through the bloodstream. In the spleen they continue their maturation through transitional stages. Depending on the specificity of the newly formed BCR, they either become marginal zone B cells and short-lived plasma cells, or evolve into the follicular B cell compartment and progress to memory B cells or long-lived plasma cells in a T helper (Th) cell-dependent manner and enter into the circulation. The establishment of immune competence is furthered by somatic hypermutation (SHM), affinity maturation, and class-switch recombination (CSR) in the periphery, which result in a high-affinity BCR on the surface of the mature B cells with different isotypes of antibodies. Loss of CD40 on the surface of B cells (or CD40L on T cells) precludes immunoglobulin class switch recombination and leads to the accumulation of IgM-type immunoglobulins and the lack of other isotypes (hyper IgM syndrome). Similarly, mutation in other genes contributing to the class-switch and SHM (activation-induced cytidine deaminase (*AID*) or uracil-DNA glycosylase

(*UNG*)) provoke hyper IgM syndrome (Qamar and Fuleihan, 2014). During this maturation process in the periphery, a fraction of B cells still exists with autoreactive properties. Mechanisms of elimination include anergy and decreased survival signals of the autoreactive cells secondary to low B cell activation factor (BAFF) receptor expression (Pillai et al., 2011).

In summary, tolerance mechanisms can be divided into central and peripheral steps. Central B cell tolerance includes pre-BCR censoring, deletion, anergy, and receptor editing, while peripheral B cell tolerance includes clonal deletion and anergy. Understandably, defects in genes involved in B cell maturation and establishment of immune competence could not only make patients prone to immune deficiency but also generation and survival of autoreactive cells and ultimately autoimmunity.

Regarding specific PIDs with an impaired B cell tolerance mechanism, defects in the generation of B and T cell receptors and receptor editing such as leaky SCID or Omenn syndrome and defects in B cell receptor signaling such as *BTK* or B cell linker protein (*BLNK*) mutations can result in the generation of a small fraction of immature B cells that are inadequately censored, giving rise to an increased number of autoreactive B cells leaving to the periphery (Cassani et al., 2010a; Walter et al., 2010; Ng et al., 2004). In addition, TLRs expressed on B cells can play a role in the establishment of central and peripheral tolerance. TLR7, TLR8, and TLR9 operate with interleukin-1 receptor-associated kinase 4 (IRAK4) and myeloid differentiation factor 88 (MyD88) to transduce signal into the nucleus. In both IRAK4- and MyD88-deficient patients, significantly increased frequency of autoreactive newly emigrant/transitional B cells have been observed. As autoreactive antibodies in patients' sera have not been detected to date, likely peripheral tolerance mechanisms compensate for central dysregulation (Isnardi et al., 2008).

Beyond Omenn syndrome and leaky SCID, a CID phenotype with distinct features of granuloma and/or autoimmunity (CID-G/AI) secondary to *RAG* mutations was recently described in the literature (De Ravin et al., 2010; Schuetz et al., 2008). Similar to Omenn syndrome, patients with CID-G/AI secondary to hypomorphic *RAG1/2* mutations have residual V(D)J activity leading to a compromised immature B cell repertoire with autoreactive clones that are likely due to impaired receptor editing as part of dysregulated central tolerance. Unlike Omenn syndrome, however, these patients present later in life with fewer infections but more autoimmune manifestations including the presence of vast autoantibodies (warm IgG agglutinin to red blood cells, lupus anticoagulant, anti-neutrophil, anti-myeloperoxidase, anti-thyroglobulin, anti-thyroid peroxidase, anti-neutrophil cytoplasmic antibody (ANCA) in addition to recently detected anti–IFN-α), clinical evidence of autoimmunity (autoimmune cytopenias, vitiligo, psoriasis, Guillain-Barré syndrome, myasthenia gravis), and granuloma formation (De Ravin et al., 2010; Avila et al., 2010; Buchbinder et al., 2015; Chen et al., 2014; Walter et al., 2015).

Rescue of autoreactive immature B cells from the bone marrow has also been demonstrated in hyper IgM syndrome caused by AID deficiency. Indeed, AID deficient patients often display autoimmune diseases such as AIHA, thrombocytopenia, and/or autoimmune hepatitis. Higher frequency of autoreactive newly emigrant/transitional B cells in the circulation of these patients suggests that AID may be involved in a process contributing to the central tolerance (Durandy et al., 2013; Cantaert et al., 2015).

In the periphery, PID genes associated with B cell tolerance mechanisms are less clear. Autoantibodies and autoimmunity are generated in Wiskott-Aldrich syndrome likely secondary to peripheral B cell dysregulation (Castiello et al., 2014). Additionally, increased BAFF levels in B cell lymphopenia with elevated BAFF levels in the case of partial RAG deficiency was shown to be associated with autoantibody production in the periphery of patients and a mouse model of Omenn syndrome (Walter et al., 2010; Walter et al., 2015).

3.3.2 Defects in T cell tolerance that induce autoimmunity in PID

The maturation process of a T lineage progenitor from a bone marrow hematopoietic stem cell includes somatic gene rearrangement with positive and negative selection steps. T cell development occurs in the thymus in three phases. In the first phase, CD4 and CD8 negative (double negative) pre-T cells colonize thymic cortex and gradually become committed to the T cell lineage. In the second phase, cells migrate deeper in the thymic cortex and induce the expression of CD4 and CD8 (double positive) and RAG1/2 that assemble and diversify the T cell receptor (TCR). Depending on the TCR-gene usage, cells proceed to either $\alpha\beta$ or $\gamma\delta$ lineages (Krangel, 2009). In the third phase, maturing T cells complete their final differentiation and mature thymocytes are released back into the circulation. The T cell maturation process heavily depends on a cross talk between the naïve T cells and a three-dimensional thymic stromal cell network including thymic epithelial cells (TECs), dendritic cells (DCs), and macrophages. In the cortical region of the thymus, positive selection of functional TCR carrying T cells is mediated by the DCs and macrophages presenting MHC-bound self-peptides. In addition, exposure to medullary TECs presenting autoimmune regulator (AIRE)-driven expression of tissue-specific antigens allows selection of T cells with high self-antigen specificity. These T cells will either be deleted by apoptosis or converted into regulatory T cells (Tregs) (Watanabe et al., 2005).

Similar to B cells, the elimination of autoreactive T cells (negative selection) consists of central and peripheral mechanisms. The central tolerance occurs in the medullary region of the thymus. Presentation of self-antigens in this specialized microenvironment depends on the transcription factor AIRE that mediates thymic expression of thousands of peripheral tissue-specific antigens and therefore is a key player in central T cell tolerance (Heino et al., 1999). Strong recognition of self-peptide–MHC complexes displayed on medullary TECs by the TCR leads to the induction of apoptosis and the consequent deletion of autoreactive T cell clones. Therefore, defects in AIRE expression are associated with decreased filtering of autoreactive T cells and consequent break in T cell tolerance. Leaking to the periphery, autoreactive T cells can induce organ-specific autoimmunity. In the absence of AIRE, impaired thymic presentation of tissue-specific antigens results in the survival of autoreactive T cells and leads to a clinical presentation of autoimmunity known as APECED, which is notable for a wide spectrum of autoimmune-mediated conditions including hypoparathyroidism, thyroiditis, adrenocortical failure, hepatitis, primary biliary cirrhosis (PBC), hypogonadism, AIHA, pernicious anemia, T1DM, vitiligo, alopecia, keratoconjunctivitis, and ectodermal dysplasia (Bussone and Mouthon, 2009; Lehman and Ballow, 2008; Ahonen et al., 1990). As a part of B cell dysregulation in APECED, antibodies to cytokines (IL-17) have been found and are associated with candidiasis (Kisand et al., 2010).

As previously mentioned, there is a fundamental cross talk between early T cells and medullary TECs, where T cell development depends on the proper function and presence of mTECs, but medullary T cells also promote the maturation of mTECs through LTβ-receptor signaling. This cross talk is an essential part of central T cell tolerance as mTECs are the main source of AIRE-dependent tissue-specific antigen presentation (Zuklys et al., 2000; Boehm et al., 2003). PIDs characterized by decreased T cell development preclude the development of normal thymic architecture and, thereby, lead to a secondary defect in central T cell tolerance as observed in Omenn or DiGeorge syndromes (Arason et al., 2010; Coutinho and Carneiro-Sampaio, 2008; Todoric et al., 2013). DiGeorge syndrome is an autosomal dominant disorder resulting in partial or complete failure of T cell development due to defective thymic development caused by a deletion on chromosome 22q11. Besides the series of nonimmune complications (facial dysmorphisms, cardiac and parathyroid abnormalities, deafness), clonal expansion of autoreactive T cells and consequent autoimmune manifestations occur in 5–30% of patients that include cytopenias, AIHA, hepatitis, IBD, arthritis, psoriasis, vitiligo, and thyroiditis (Gennery, 2012; Gennery, 2013; Gennery et al., 2002; McLean-Tooke et al., 2007; Tison et al., 2011; Davies et al., 2003). Similarly, thymic dysplasia was noted among patients with *FoxN1* mutations, which is required for thymic epithelial differentiation and development of mTECs for cross talk with the lymphoid compartment (Palamaro et al., 2014). Autoimmune manifestations have not been reported in large cohorts, but there is a recent case report of autoimmunity post-thymus transplant in a patient with FoxN1 deficiency (Levy et al., 2012).

Autoreactive T cells that escape central checkpoint could be suppressed by natural regulatory T cells (nTregs) as a part of the peripheral T cell tolerance. These nTregs originate from the thymus via conversion of subsets of T cells with high-affinity, potentially autoreactive TCR selected by mTEC cells (Watanabe et al., 2005; Apostolou et al., 2002; Aschenbrenner et al., 2007). Peripheral development and function of nTregs depend on the transcription factor FOXP3 with coexpression of the IL-2 receptor (CD25) and CD4. nTregs exert their suppressive activity mainly by cell contact–dependent mechanisms or by the secretion of immunosuppressive cytokines including IL-10,

TGF-β, and IL-35 (Vignali, 2008; Vignali et al., 2008; Shevach, 2009). nTregs are able to suppress autoimmune responses executed not only by the T cell compartment but also those of B cells, therefore constituting an essential part of the peripheral tolerance checkpoint.

Genetic defects affecting nTreg development are accompanied by the disruption of peripheral T cell tolerance. Development of functional nTregs essentially depends upon the expression of FOXP3, and the lack of this critical transcription factor results in a clinical syndrome known as immune dysregulation polyendocrinopathy enteropathy X-linked (IPEX). IPEX is associated with early-onset diffuse autoimmune manifestations and can be fatal in males if unrecognized at infancy. The clinical picture is marked by severe autoimmune enteropathy and T1DM at birth to within weeks of life, often worsening to include dermatitis within months of life. In subsets of patients, autoimmune-mediated thyroiditis, cytopenias, nephritis, and arthritis have also been described (Barzaghi et al., 2012). Serologically IPEX is notable for a rapid accumulation of autoantibodies, which correlates with end-organ disease development (i.e. Coombs antibodies, anti-platelet antibodies, and anti-neutrophil antibodies in patients who progress to autoimmune cytopenias). More recently, specific anti-enterocyte antibodies (villin and autoimmune enteropathy-related 75 kDa, named harmonin protein) were described (Kobayashi et al., 1998; Lampasona et al., 2013). These brush border autoantibodies are predicted to mediate significant gastrointestinal inflammation, which ultimately drives the histologic loss of gastrointestinal villa and results in gross protein-wasting enteropathy and failure to thrive in IPEX patients. Less commonly, patients may develop hepatitis, vasculitis, sarcoidosis, vitiligo, and adrenal failure (Chida et al., 2015; Bussone and Mouthon, 2009; Lehman and Ballow, 2008; Moraes-Vasconcelos et al., 2008; Pessach et al., 2009). Furthermore, because nTreg maintenance strongly depends on IL-2 signaling, mutations in *STAT5b* and/or in the α chain of the IL-2 receptor (CD25) lead to the development of an IPEX-like PID similar to FOXP3 deficiency (Goudy et al., 2013; Caudy et al., 2007; Hwa et al., 2011).

Regulatory T cell dysfunction has also been linked to a novel gene known as LPS-responsive beige-like anchor (*LRBA*) (Charbonnier et al., 2015). LRBA is implicated in the regulation of endosomal vesicle trafficking, particularly those vesicles containing immune effector molecules. Patients with LRBA deficiency were noted to have increased apoptosis and marked Treg cell depletion with decreased suppression function. In addition, detailed immune phenotyping revealed decreased expression of canonical Treg cell markers (FOXP3, CD25, Helios, and CTLA-4) (Charbonnier et al., 2015). Patients with *LRBA* mutations may present with a wide selection of phenotypes ranging from ALPS features (autoimmune cytopenias) to CVID and IBD (Charbonnier et al., 2015; Serwas et al., 2015; Seidel et al., 2014; Lopez-Herrera et al., 2012; Burns et al., 2012; Alangari et al., 2012).

Furthermore, germline heterozygous *STAT1* mutations were identified among patients with IPEX-like disease with the triad of polyendocrinopathy, enteropathy, and dermatitis (Uzel et al., 2013) and *STAT3* gain-of-function mutations have been recently linked to clinical presentations of autoimmune cytopenias and multiorgan autoimmunity and regulatory T cell dysfunction. (Milner et al., 2015; Haapaniemi et al., 2015).

Finally, IL-10 is a potent immunosuppressive cytokine that plays a major role in the homeostasis of the gut. In the case of defects in IL-10 signaling (with genetic mutations in *IL10RA, IL10RB,* or *IL10*), patients present with the hyperinflammatory clinical phenotype of bloody diarrhea, abscesses, colitis, perianal fistulas and folliculitis, oral aphthous lesions, arthritis, and gastrointestinal symptoms within the first 3 months of life. As part of the pathogenic process, Tregs cannot exert control of inflammation via IL-10 (Glocker et al., 2010; Glocker et al., 2009; Kotlarz et al., 2012).

3.3.3 Defects in multiple tolerance checkpoints that induce autoimmunity in PID

Combined dysfunction of central and peripheral tolerance is noted among patients where mutations affect the signaling pathway of the apoptotic program. In ALPS, mutations in *Fas, FasL,* or less commonly in caspase 8 (*CASP8*) and 10 (*CASP10*), result in the production of autoreactive T cells that cannot undergo clonal deletion via apoptosis and thus persist in the periphery. Autoimmune consequences are reported in approximately 50–80% of individuals and can include autoimmune cytopenias, Guillain-Barré syndrome, glomerulonephritis, hepatitis, arthritis, optic neuritis, cutaneous vasculitis, blistering dermatosis, and acquired factor VIII deficiency (Arason et al., 2010; Bussone and Mouthon, 2009; Coutinho and Carneiro-Sampaio, 2008; Campagnoli et al., 2006).

T and B cell tolerance mechanisms intersect on many levels, as demonstrated by a single genetic defect disrupting multiple T and B cell tolerance checkpoints in patients and mouse models of RAG deficiency. In detail, decreased AIRE expression occurs (disruption of central T cell tolerance) (Poliani et al., 2009), Tregs are decreased (disruption of peripheral T cell tolerance) (Cassani et al., 2010b), receptor editing is impaired in the bone marrow (disruption of central B cell tolerance) (Walter et al., 2010), and increased BAFF levels enable survival of autoreactive B cells (disruption of peripheral B cell tolerance) (Cassani et al., 2010a; Walter et al., 2010). The relative importance of central versus peripheral tolerance has been extensively examined in multiple primary immunodeficiencies for B cells (Ng et al., 2004; Isnardi et al., 2008; Durandy et al., 2013; Castiello et al., 2014; Janssen et al., 2014; Menard et al., 2014; Meyers et al., 2011). In contrast, the description of autoreactive T cells in humans has been much more limited to date, primarily due to a lack of definitive laboratory markers.

Finally, combined dysfunction in peripheral B and T cell tolerance has been described in DOCK8 deficiency, the autosomal recessive variant of hyper IgE syndrome, where Treg cells are decreased in number and suppressor function and autoreactive B cells are increased in peripheral compartments (Janssen et al., 2014). In contrast, Wiskott-Aldrich syndrome is characterized by eczema, thrombocytopenia, and susceptibility to infection, and may present with autoimmune complications such has AIHA, neutropenia, arthritis, and vasculitis (Catucci et al., 2012). Studies in B cell tolerance in patients with Wiskott-Aldrich syndrome have revealed unusual expansion of CD21(low) B cell populations and increased plasma BAFF levels, suggesting an impaired B cell tolerance checkpoint (Castiello et al., 2014).

4. CURRENT TREATMENT STRATEGIES FOR AUTOIMMUNITY IN PID

Treatment of autoimmune disease pathology in PID is an actively emerging and often controversial field. For the most common complication of autoimmune cytopenias, treatment historically consisted of immune suppression with corticosteroids. More recently, corticosteroid-sparing agents have become increasingly popular in treating a spectrum of PID-driven autoimmune complications, including rituximab (a chimeric monoclonal antibody directed against CD20 and targeting B cells), mycophenolate mofetil (MMF) (a purine synthesis inhibitor targeting the development of T and B cells), methotrexate (a competitive inhibitor of dihydrofolate reductase that has a number of distinct regulatory effects on T and B cells), and even tumor necrosis factor-alpha (TNF-α) inhibitors such as etanercept. Alternative treatment options include the use of high-dose (1.5–2 g/kg) intravenous immunoglobulin (IVIG) (purified monomeric IgG that is pooled from the plasma of healthy donors) (Podjasek and Abraham, 2012), and hematopoietic stem cell transplantation (HSCT) in the case of severe PID with autoimmunity where the underlying genetic defect is clear, such as in IPEX syndrome (Seidel et al., 2014; Mazzolari et al., 2005).

While the development of steroid-sparing immunosuppression has revolutionized the treatment of isolated autoimmune diseases including rheumatoid arthritis and IBD, its use in treating PID-driven autoimmune disease has been complicated by fear of predisposition toward infection. Use of IVIG continues to be popular among immunologists due to the fact that it is well tolerated and targets both the underlying immune deficiency as well as the complicating autoimmunity; however, there is a lack of consensus regarding appropriate dosing schedules. Finally, while allogeneic HSCT is preferred in severe PID in order to reconstitute a functional immune system with the added potential to reset peripheral and central tolerance, autologous stem cell transplantation is increasingly the standard of care in refractory cases of isolated autoimmune disease due to the decreased risk of graft-versus-host disease and severe infectious complications. In 1997, the first consensus guidelines for HSCT in autoimmune diseases were published, while an international coordinated clinical program was launched and served as data collection. Recently the guidelines were revised and updated for both the current application and future development (Snowden et al., 2012). Autologous HSCT, however, would not correct an underlying immunodeficiency and could make the patient prone to recurrence of autoimmune complications in the future. Therapeutic management of autoimmune disease in a background of PID is therefore frequently challenging and continues to be an area of active academic research.

CVID is distinct among PIDs due to its relative frequency in the general population. Therefore, clinical guidelines are best characterized for the treatment of autoimmune cytopenias in patients with CVID (Podjasek and Abraham, 2012). First, an adult patient must progress to the threshold for treatment, platelets below $30 \times 10^9/L$ in the case of ITP or neutrophils below $500/mm^3$ without a history of severe or recurrent infections in the case of AIN. First-line therapy for ITP, AIHA, and AIN is steroids (typically 1 mg/kg for at least 3 weeks) with an appropriate alternative or cotreatment being IVIG (typically dosed at 1 g/kg with repeat dosing pending an appropriate initial response). For ITP and AIHA, Rho(D) immune globulin can be utilized in Rh-positive individuals who have not undergone a splenectomy and are unable to tolerate steroid treatment. Splenectomy is recommended only in patients who fail steroid therapy. In a recent retrospective study, the outcome of splenectomy was examined in 45 CVID patients over a 40-year period. Autoimmune cytopenias resolved in 75% of the patients, even in some cases that were refractory to rituximab treatment. It is encouraging that splenectomy did not worsen mortality among patients with CVID, likely protected from overwhelming postsplenectomy infections by proper immunoglobulin replacement therapy (Wong et al., 2013).

For AIN, G-CSF can be utilized in patients with a limited bone marrow reserve, and splenectomy is not recommended given the often-transient improvement in cell counts and increased risk for infection. In patients who fail these initial therapies, progression to steroid-sparing immunosuppressive agents including rituximab (Gobert et al., 2011), alone or in combination with alemtuzumab (a monoclonal antibody directed against CD52 (Gomez-Almaguer et al., 2010)) and MMF (Kotb et al., 2005; Rao et al., 2005), has been described. To date these studies report excellent response rates in severe cases of autoimmune cytopenias that have failed first-line therapy for both rituximab alone (84%) and MMF (78–92%). While there was initial concern over high rates of infectious complications in patients receiving steroid-sparing immunosuppression, infectious complication rates were in fact comparable to standard of care autoimmune cytopenia treatment in CVID (Michel et al., 2004), and autoimmune cytopenia episodes mainly occurred for subjects not on immunoglobulin replacement therapy (Wang and Cunningham-Rundles, 2005).

Outside of CVID, IVIG has been shown to be effective in the treatment of primary autoimmune diseases including ITP, Kawasaki disease, Guillain-Barré syndrome, myasthenia gravis, and others (Kerr et al., 2014; Hartung et al., 2009). However, the delivered concentration of IVIG differs depending on these two distinct clinical scenarios, from a peak level of 12–14 mg/mL for "replacement therapy" to 25–35 mg/mL for "high-dose" immunomodulatory therapy (Kaveri et al., 2011). These data bring about several questions in the use of IVIG to treat PID. First, what is the mechanism of clinical benefit? Second, has IVIG been historically underdosed in PID in terms of preventing the development of autoimmune disease complications? The clinical benefit of IVIG has been shown to outlast its half-life in the serum, suggesting that IVIG has both direct antiinfective and immunomodulatory effects in addition to long-lasting effects on cellular immunity. A variety of underlying mechanisms have been proposed including Fc receptor modulation, interaction with the complement cascade, modulation of cytokine profiles, and finally long-lasting cellular effects including promotion of T cell-independent B cell proliferation (thus stimulating Ig production) as well as dendritic cell rescue from a proinflammatory default state of differentiation (thus decreasing hyperinflammation) (Kaveri et al., 2011). Unfortunately, clinical guidelines for the use of IVIG in the treatment of autoimmune disease are based on empiric dosing schedules for ITP (Imbach et al., 1981; Blanchette et al., 1994) and Kawasaki disease (Furusho et al., 1984; Newburger et al., 1991). We currently lack a systematic approach to more accurately guide our use of IVIG therapy. Ideally, future dosing schedules for IVIG in PID will be informed both by infectious complication rates as well as rates of autoimmune disease progression.

Treatment of autoimmune cytopenias is more of an evolving field in ALPS. Some patients can be controlled with corticosteroids alone. In contrast to CVID, however, the benefit of IVIG is variable and limited to patients with severe AIHA (Rao and Oliveira, 2011), and splenectomy carries a significant risk for life-threatening sepsis (Bleesing et al., 2000). Thus, escalation to steroid-sparing immunosuppression is often required. MMF has been best studied in ALPS, notable for limited toxicity and a remarkable 80% reduction in autoimmune disease pathology (Rao et al., 2005; Kossiva et al., 2006). However, an exciting and emerging new therapy in ALPS is sirolimus (rapamycin), inhibiting mTORs (mammalian target of rapamycin). Sirolimus has been demonstrated to resolve autoimmune disease pathology in MMF-refractory ALPS patients with novel normalization of the double negative T cell count (Janic et al., 2009; Teachey et al., 2009). The proposed mechanism of clinical benefit stems from the ability of sirolimus to both preserve and enhance T regulatory cells and induce apoptosis in dysfunctional lymphocytes. Related to this latter mechanism, while a feared complication of classical immunosupression in ALPS has been increased risk of malignant transformation, sirolimus may in fact reduce this risk. Proof of principle was demonstrated in a population of renal transplant recipients who developed Kaposi's sarcoma on MMF or cyclosporine therapy that subsequently resolved upon transition to sirolimus for ongoing immunosuppression (Stallone et al., 2005). Given these distinct benefits of sirolimus, a recent algorithm for the treatment of autoimmune cytopenias in ALPS highlights the use of MMF in patients who fail steroid therapy alone in cases of moderate disease versus immediate progression to sirolimus in cases of severe disease (Teachey et al., 2010). HSCT for the treatment of ALPS-related autoimmune disease is effective (Cohen et al., 2007; Kahwash et al., 2007; Sleight et al., 1998); however, it is often not preferred given that the majority of ALPS patients can be managed successfully on single agent regimens.

The clinical benefit of steroid-sparing immunosuppression in treating PID-driven autoimmune pathology extends well beyond the confines of autoimmune cytopenias. In a recent case series on CGD, the authors demonstrate failure of corticosteroid therapy alone to control autoimmune disease pathology in several distinct cases: CGD complicated by antiphospholipid syndrome that ultimately required methotrexate therapy, four cases of CGD complicated by noninfectious pulmonary interstitial granulomatous inflammation and lymphocytic infiltrates that also required escalation to methotrexate therapy, and finally one case of CGD complicated by juvenile idiopathic arthritis that was managed with etanercept (De Ravin et al., 2008). Transition to a steroid-sparing immunosuppressive agent in these cases reduced long-term exposure to steroids, achieved improved control of autoimmune pathology as compared to steroids alone, and was not reported to increase the propensity of infectious complications in these patients.

In contrast to CVID, ALPS, and CGD, HSCT has been more readily utilized in patients with SCID or SCID–gene-associated CIDs, both from the perspective of immune reconstitution and also from the perspective of autoimmune disease prevention. Recently an unfortunate family with compound heterozygous *RAG1* mutations was described (Chen et al., 2014). The initial clinical presentation of two siblings was autoimmune cytopenias, lymphopenia, and moderate-to-severe infections. The diagnosis and subsequent HSCT of the older sibling (Patient 1) was delayed until the patient was 8 years old. In contrast, the younger sibling (Patient 2) was screened at disease onset, which allowed for HSCT at the age of 29 months. In addition to conventional autoantibodies, both patients carried a specific panel of anticytokine autoantibodies targeting IFN-α and IFN-ω that may serve as biomarkers for larger cohorts to identify individual cases of RAG deficiency/CID phenotype and prompt early HSCT if clinically indicated. Similar case reports are available in the literature for RAG-associated CIDs (De Ravin et al., 2010; Schuetz et al., 2008; Patiroglu et al., 2014; Walter et al., 2015). These data highlight the importance of early screening for CID in patients with a primary presentation of autoimmune disease and a background of lymphopenias and recurrent infections to facilitate early HSCT and reduce the risk for autoimmune disease progression. As an extreme example, a child was reported to undergo HSCT at 3 months of age after diagnosed with naive T cell lymphopenia as reflected by low T cell receptor excision circles (TRECs). Additional immune phenotyping confirmed poor T cell proliferation. Her sister died early in life and had a complex history of autoimmune disease (cytopenias, vasculitis, Raynaud's disease) and infections (RSV bronchiolitis, urinary tract infections, and a fatal *Enterobacter*-related central line infection). Genetic testing revealed a compound heterozygous pathogenic mutation in the *RAG1* gene. In the context of the family history and current immunological phenotype, the younger sibling underwent HSCT and has been healthy since with no autoimmune or infectious complications (Henderson et al., 2013b).

HSCT has yet to be routinely adopted for other PIDs, including LRBA deficiency. Treatment of LRBA deficiency has been challenging to date given the limited and often temporary response to immune suppression. However, the first case report of HSCT for the treatment of LBRA deficiency was recently described (Seidel et al., 2014). The authors demonstrate significant reduction in recurrent infectious and autoimmune disease pathology at 9 years posttransplantation from an HLA-identical mother. The patient's posttransplantation course has been complicated by a relapse of ITP, which required a short course of high-dose IVIG; however, since then the patient is clinically stable on romiplostim therapy alone. The relapse of autoimmune disease in this case is confounded by a heterozygous *LRBA* donor, the patient's mother. Though additional data on HSCT in the context of LRBA deficiency is required, this isolated case report raises the intriguing possibility of early HSCT as a potential treatment for LRBA deficiency-mediated autoimmune disease.

Case series on IPEX have brought into question patients who are too ill, on account of PID-related comorbidities, to undergo traditional HSCT transplantation (Wildin et al., 2002). While proof of principle was first demonstrated in 2001 that HSCT could reconstitute partial immune system function in IPEX and significantly reduce autoimmune disease pathology, these patients ultimately passed away from hypothesized transplantation-related toxicity (Baud et al., 2001). More recently, a modified protocol was attempted in two patients with IPEX who received HLA-matched related bone marrow or peripheral blood stem cell grafts following low-intensity nonmyeloablative conditioning (Burroughs et al., 2010). Long-term clinical recovery with regards to enteropathy and autoimmune-mediated cytopenias was observed in both patients, whereas diabetes and thyroid disease persisted, likely due to already permanent end-organ damage. Most importantly, the two patients were alive and functional at the 1- and 4-year follow-ups, respectively.

5. INVESTIGATIONAL TREATMENT STRATEGIES FOR AUTOIMMUNITY IN PID

While steroids, steroid-sparing immunosuppression, IVIG, and HSCT continue to be the major treatment modalities for autoimmune disease in PID, our growing understanding of underlying immune mechanisms that drive hyperinflammation and loss of self-tolerance have led to multiple new therapeutic targets.

5.1 Small molecule inhibitors

T cell coreceptor cytotoxic T cell antigen-4 (CTLA-4) is a critical coinhibitor of T cell proliferation that has implications both in autoimmune disease pathology and cancer. Its negative regulatory effect on autoinflammation was first described using knockout mouse models (Tivol et al., 1995; Waterhouse et al., 1995). Subsequently, CTLA-4 was implicated as a susceptibility gene in autoimmune diseases, such as AIHA (Pavkovic et al., 2003).

Finally, patients with PID and severe immune dysregulation were identified with germline heterozygous *CTLA-4* mutations that resulted in haploinsufficiency (Kuehn et al., 2014; Kristiansen et al., 2000; Ueda et al., 2003). The majority of CTLA-4 is located intracellularly, and surface levels are carefully regulated by endocytosis, recycling, and newly synthesized CTLA-4 (Schneider and Rudd, 2014). Inhibitory control of T cells can be lost with even subtle changes in surface expression, promoting self-recognition of low-affinity antigens. Thus, biologic agents that target CTLA-4 can have dramatic effects on cellular immunity. Ipilimumab is a checkpoint-blocking antibody directed against CTLA-4, which is known to have antitumor properties (Hodi et al., 2010; Robert et al., 2011). More recently, ipilimumab was shown to be effective in treating autoimmune disease pathology in two patients with melanoma; specifically, seronegative rheumatoid arthritis and multiple sclerosis (Kyi et al., 2014). Just this year abatacept, a CTLA-4-immunoglobulin fusion protein that inhibits T cell responses by competing for costimulatory ligands, was trialed in nine patients with LRBA deficiency (Lo et al., 2015). Of great interest, the LRBA deficient patients were shown to have substantially lower CTLA-4 T regulatory cell levels. Furthermore, treatment of the LRBA deficient patients with abatercept was shown to improve autoimmune disease pathology, including marked reduction in inflammatory interstitial lung disease in particular. These data highlight the intimate connection between LRBA and CTLA-4, which are known to display similar clinical phenotypes when deficient. Also of interest, chloroquine was shown to prevent CTLA-4 loss in LRBA deficient cells via inhibition of lysosomal degradation, which raises the intriguing question of whether this old medication acts through a novel CTLA-4 mechanism to induce its anti-inflammatory effects. Given the complex nature of CTLA-4 cell surface expression, there is great potential for the development of additional CTLA-4-targeted therapies that could be efficacious in multiple clinical arenas including malignancy, autoimmune disease, and PID.

Proteasome inhibitors are also gaining momentum as novel therapeutics for refractory autoimmune disease. Bortezomib was the first proteasome inhibitor to be tested in humans (Adams and Elliott, 2000). Initially approved for the treatment of refractory and relapsed multiple myeloma, it is now a cornerstone of multiple myeloma combination therapy (Moreau et al., 2012), and its use extends to other malignancies including mantle cell lymphoma (Kane et al., 2007). Bortezomib can promote cellular apoptosis *via* p53-dependent and p53-independent mechanisms by increasing the accumulation of cell cycle inhibitors (Skrott and Cvek, 2014). However, bortezomib was first described as an antiinflammatory molecule (Palombella et al., 1998) and a prominent mechanism of action includes the suppression of NF-κB pathway activation (Palombella et al., 1994). Moreover, cellular response to bortezomib may be in part driven by degree of macromolecular processing (Powers et al., 2009), which is notably increased in plasma cells due to Ig processing and production. In line with this mechanism, bortezomib has now been trialed as a direct therapeutic for autoimmune disease. To date, clinical efficacy has been best described for autoimmune cytopenias. A recent case report of seven pediatric patients with severe and refractory autoimmune disease demonstrated initial clinical response to bortezomib in six patients and sustained clinical response in four patients. Toxicity included thrombocytopenia (two patients) and infectious complications (three patients with infections as follows: colitis, cellulitis, and febrile neutropenia) (Khandelwal et al., 2014). Bortezomib may be clinically efficacious in other diseases of prominent autoantibody production as well. Early research shows promise in myasthenia gravis (Gomez et al., 2014), primary Sjögren's syndrome (Jakez-Ocampo et al., 2015), lupus nephritis (Neubert et al., 2008), and even autoimmune uveitis (Hsu et al., 2015).

5.2 Gene therapy

As monogenic diseases have by definition a causative genetic target of disease pathology, gene-based therapy and in essence a complete cure has long been the Holy Grail in PID. However, the practical application of gene therapy has been notoriously complex. The first studies in humans were accomplished in patients with SCID in the 1990s and early 2000s (Bordignon et al., 1993; Cavazzana-Calvo et al., 2000; Gaspar et al., 2004). Both X-linked SCID (accounting for the majority of cases and caused by a mutation in *IL2GR*, a prominent cytokine receptor required for lymphocyte lineage production and differentiation) and ADA SCID (accounting for 15–20% of cases and caused by a mutation in adenosine deaminase (*ADA*), resulting in metabolite accumulation and lymphocyte toxicity when deficient) were excellent initial clinical targets. Patients received autologous infusions of CD34+ cells that had been transduced *ex vivo* with γ-retroviral vectors containing the intact gene. While immune reconstitution was demonstrated in the majority of X-linked SCID patients initially trialed (improved thymopoesis and production of diverse T cell repertoires with intact functional response to pathogen (Hacein-Bey-Abina et al., 2010; Gaspar et al., 2011)), T cell leukemia was an unfortunate consequence in 5 out of the 20 patients first studied, most often on account of retroviral integration adjacent to a known oncogene (Howe et al., 2008; Hacein-Bey-Abina et al., 2008). In contrast, gene therapy for ADA SCID was much more promising from onset. Long-term outcomes were recently described in a cohort of 10 patients who received nonmyeloablative conditioning followed by infusion of autologous CD34+ cells from bone marrow that had been transduced with a viral vector carrying the *ADA* gene. Remarkably, 9 of 10 patients had sustained immune reconstitution with normalization of their T cell function, 8 patients no longer required enzyme-replacement therapy, 5 patients could mount immunoglobulin responses to antigen, and all patients were alive at the median 4 year follow-up with serious complications limited to infections (EBV reactivation in one patient and catheter-associated infections in two patients), autoimmune disease (autoimmune hepatitis in one patient), cytopenias (neutropenia in one patient), and hypertension (one patient) (Aiuti et al., 2009). Given the initial risk for malignant transformation associated with the use of γ-retroviral vectors for the treatment of X-linked SCID, more recent clinical trials are evolving toward the use of self-inactivating lentiviral vectors (Cicalese and Aiuti, 2015). Self-inactivating lentiviral vectors appear to be safe and less oncogenic than their retroviral ancestors (Naldini, 2011). Finally, HIV-1-based vectors are also promising due to their robust transduction potential, broad cellular tropism, and ability to integrate through transcription, which limits dependence on promoter regions.

Retroviral gene transfer was also trialed in patients with Wiskott-Aldrich syndrome. The first clinical trial of two patients demonstrated improved platelet counts, restored NK, T, and B cell functions, and resolved clinical symptoms of bleeding, eczema, autoimmunity, and recurrent infections at the 3 year follow-up (Boztug et al., 2010). Similar to the X-linked SCID trials, however, progression to leukemia was ultimately found to be a significant and limiting long-term complication (Braun et al., 2014). However, the lentiviral vector delivery system has been more recently trialed in Wiskott-Aldrich syndrome with early clinical promise (Aiuti et al., 2013). To date, the authors demonstrate functional immune reconstitution in all three patients treated, without early gene integration near oncogenes, and with clinical stability at the 20–32 month follow-up. Long-term clinical outcomes in this cohort will be critical to establish safety and efficacy for the use of gene therapy in Wiskott-Aldrich syndrome going forward.

Gene therapy in CGD has perhaps proven most challenging with failed long-term clinical benefit to date (Kaufmann et al., 2014). Unlike SCID and Wiskott-Aldrich syndrome, CGD is confounded by a terminal lineage cellular defect and a pathogenic inclination toward myeloid hyperplasia, neither of which favor a selective advantage for the transduced HSC (Grez et al., 2011). Furthermore, gene therapy in CGD has also been complicated by genotoxicity; specifically, transformation to myelodysplastic syndrome (Stein et al., 2010).

Gene therapy is now on the horizon for several other PIDs, including IPEX. The severe autoimmune pathology in IPEX is driven by FOXP3 deficiency, which in turn leads to loss of function of circulating T regulatory cells in favor of lineage differentiation toward T effector cells (Passerini et al., 2011). Recently, CD4+ T cells isolated from the peripheral blood of IPEX patients were successfully converted into T regulatory cells *via* lentiviral-mediated *FOXP3* gene transfer. These genetically modified *FOXP3*-mutated CD4+ T cells acquired T regulatory cell phenotype and function both *in vitro* and in an *in vivo* mouse model of xenograft versus host disease. While not yet trialed in patients, these data suggest potentials to restore immune regulation and inhibit severe lymphoproliferation (Passerini et al., 2013; Passerini et al., 2014).

5.3 Cell-based therapy

5.3.1 T regulatory Type 1 (Tr1) cells

Our growing understanding of immune cell dynamics and increasing awareness of unique T cell subsets has diversified our potential for treatment of PID and autoimmune disease. T regulatory Type 1 (Tr1) cells were first identified in the peripheral blood of SCID patients who developed tolerance after HLA-mismatched HSCT, highlighting their potential as immunomodulators (Bacchetta et al., 1994). Tr1 cells are now known to produce abundant IL-10 and TGF-β and to play a prominent role in suppressing T cell-mediated hyperinflammation and maintaining immunologic homeostasis (Roncarolo et al., 2014). Their preventative role in autoimmune disease pathology has been demonstrated for a variety of clinical entities including colitis (Groux et al., 1997), neuroinflammation (Kleinewietfeld and Hafler, 2014), and rheumatoid arthritis (Gol-Ara et al., 2012). Potential use of Tr1 as a targeted therapy in humans was first described in 2014. Twelve patients with high-risk hematologic malignancy were selected to receive T cell-depleted haploidentical-HSCT in combination with IL-10-anergized donor T cells, which were enriched in Tr1 specific to host alloantigens. Remarkably, four of these patients demonstrated full normalization of the immune repertoire and complete disease remission off of all immunosuppression at an average of 7.2 years follow-up posttransplantation (Bacchetta et al., 2014). Further evidence for the clinical application of Tr1 to modify self-tolerance has been demonstrated using animal models. Tr1 cell infusion was shown to decrease incidence and clinical symptoms in two distinct mouse models of arthritis (Asnagli et al., 2014). Additionally, Tr1 induction *in vivo* has been shown to suppress autoinflammation in mouse models of EAE (Zohar et al., 2014; Meiron et al., 2008) and diabetes (Battaglia et al., 2006). Progress toward elucidating exact mechanisms of Tr1 induction and downstream signaling will only further these therapeutic opportunities (Pot et al., 2011). The generation or enrichment of antigen-specific Tr1 cells show great promise to be used as cell therapy for known antigens.

5.3.2 Virus-specific T cells

Patients with PID, particularly those with underlying defects in cytotoxic T cell immunity, are at chronic risk for viral infection or reactivation. Among the most morbid of these are EBV and CMV, which have been implicated in significant end-organ inflammatory disease and even progression to malignancy (Sankaran-Walters et al., 2011; Ok et al., 2015). Virus-specific T cell reconstitution was first trialed against EBV in HSCT recipients. These data demonstrated significant reduction in EBV-driven lymphoma in patients who received the donor-derived EBV-specific T lymphocytes (Rooney et al., 1998). The principle of cellular-based antiviral therapy has now been extended to PID. Recently, infusion of autologous CMV-specific cytotoxic T cells was trialed in two patients with life-threatening CMV-mediated enteritis refractory to conventional antiviral therapy. This intervention was shown to promote intestinal healing and decrease mucosa-specific viral load (Ciccocioppo et al., 2014). Curiously, partial HLA match is sufficient for the donor T cells currently banked at few academic centers. Longer-term follow-up will be necessary to observe for a sustained clinical response.

However, these initial studies demonstrate proof of principle for virus-specific cellular-based therapy in patients with PID.

6. SUMMARY STATEMENT

PIDs complicated by noninfectious clinical features are at a disadvantage as currently treatment strategies are often empirical. As our knowledge grows, mechanism-based targeted therapy will become more feasible to treat autoimmunity and hyperinflammation in PID and ultimately opens the era of precision medicine in the field of congenital immunodeficiencies.

REFERENCES

Adams, J., Elliott, P.J., 2000. New agents in cancer clinical trials. Oncogene 19 (56), 6687–6692.

Ahonen, P., Myllarniemi, S., Sipila, I., Perheentupa, J., 1990. Clinical variation of autoimmune polyendocrinopathy-candidiasis-ectodermal dystrophy (APECED) in a series of 68 patients. N. Engl. J. Med. 322 (26), 1829–1836.

Aiuti, A., Cattaneo, F., Galimberti, S., Benninghoff, U., Cassani, B., Callegaro, L., Scaramuzza, S., Andolfi, G., Mirolo, M., Brigida, I., et al., 2009. Gene therapy for immunodeficiency due to adenosine deaminase deficiency. N. Engl. J. Med. 360 (5), 447–458.

Aiuti, A., Biasco, L., Scaramuzza, S., Ferrua, F., Cicalese, M.P., Baricordi, C., Dionisio, F., Calabria, A., Giannelli, S., Castiello, M.C., et al., 2013. Lentiviral hematopoietic stem cell gene therapy in patients with Wiskott-Aldrich syndrome. Science 341 (6148), 1233151.

Alangari, A., Alsultan, A., Adly, N., Massaad, M.J., Kiani, I.S., Aljebreen, A., Raddaoui, E., Almomen, A.K., Al-Muhsen, S., Geha, R.S., et al., 2012. LPS-responsive beige-like anchor (LRBA) gene mutation in a family with inflammatory bowel disease and combined immunodeficiency. J. Allergy Clin. Immunol. 130 (2), 481–488, 2.

Alexander, J.J., Anderson, A.J., Barnum, S.R., Stevens, B., Tenner, A.J., 2008. The complement cascade: Yin-Yang in neuroinflammation–neuro-protection and -degeneration. J. Neurochem. 107 (5), 1169–1187.

Al-Herz, W., Bousfiha, A., Casanova, J.L., Chatila, T., Conley, M.E., Cunningham-Rundles, C., Etzioni, A., Franco, J.L., Gaspar, H.B., Holland, S.M., et al., 2014. Primary immunodeficiency diseases: an update on the classification from the international union of immunological societies expert committee for primary immunodeficiency. Front. Immunol. 5, 162.

Anderson, D.H., Radeke, M.J., Gallo, N.B., Chapin, E.A., Johnson, P.T., Curletti, C.R., Hancox, L.S., Hu, J., Ebright, J.N., Malek, G., et al., 2010. The pivotal role of the complement system in aging and age-related macular degeneration: hypothesis re-visited. Prog. Retin. Eye Res. 29 (2), 95–112.

Anderson-Cohen, M., Holland, S.M., Kuhns, D.B., Fleisher, T.A., Ding, L., Brenner, S., Malech, H.L., Roesler, J., 2003. Severe phenotype of chronic granulomatous disease presenting in a female with a de novo mutation in gp91-phox and a non familial, extremely skewed X chromosome inactivation. Clin. Immunol. 109 (3), 308–317.

Apostolou, I., Sarukhan, A., Klein, L., von Boehmer, H., 2002. Origin of regulatory T cells with known specificity for antigen. Nat. Immunol. 3 (8), 756–763.

Arason, G.J., Jorgensen, G.H., Ludviksson, B.R., 2010. Primary immunodeficiency and autoimmunity: lessons from human diseases. Scand. J. Immunol. 71 (5), 317–328.

Aschenbrenner, K., D'Cruz, L.M., Vollmann, E.H., Hinterberger, M., Emmerich, J., Swee, L.K., Rolink, A., Klein, L., 2007. Selection of Foxp3+ regulatory T cells specific for self antigen expressed and presented by Aire+ medullary thymic epithelial cells. Nat. Immunol. 8 (4), 351–358.

Asnagli, H., Martire, D., Belmonte, N., Quentin, J., Bastian, H., Boucard-Jourdin, M., Fall, P.B., Mausset-Bonnefont, A.L., Mantello-Moreau, A., Rouquier, S., et al., 2014. Type 1 regulatory T cells specific for collagen type II as an efficient cell-based therapy in arthritis. Arthritis Res. Ther. 16 (3), R115.

Atkinson, J.P., 1986. Complement activation and complement receptors in systemic lupus erythematosus. Springer Semin. Immunopathol. 9 (2–3), 179–194.

Avila, E.M., Uzel, G., Hsu, A., Milner, J.D., Turner, M.L., Pittaluga, S., Freeman, A.F., Holland, S.M., 2010. Highly variable clinical phenotypes of hypomorphic RAG1 mutations. Pediatrics 126 (5), e1248–e1252.

Bacchetta, R., Bigler, M., Touraine, J.L., Parkman, R., Tovo, P.A., Abrams, J., de Waal Malefyt, R., de Vries, J.E., Roncarolo, M.G., 1994. High levels of interleukin 10 production in vivo are associated with tolerance in SCID patients transplanted with HLA mismatched hematopoietic stem cells. J. Exp. Med. 179 (2), 493–502.

Bacchetta, R., Lucarelli, B., Sartirana, C., Gregori, S., Lupo Stanghellini, M.T., Miqueu, P., Tomiuk, S., Hernandez-Fuentes, M., Gianolini, M.E., Greco, R., et al., 2014. Immunological Outcome in Haploidentical-HSC Transplanted Patients Treated with IL-10-Anergized Donor T Cells. Front. Immunol. 5, 16.

Barsalou, J., Saint-Cyr, C., Drouin, E., Le Deist, F., Haddad, E., 2011. High prevalence of primary immune deficiencies in children with autoimmune disorders. Clin. Exp. Rheumatol. 29 (1), 125–130.

Barzaghi, F., Passerini, L., Bacchetta, R., 2012. Immune dysregulation, polyendocrinopathy, enteropathy, x-linked syndrome: a paradigm of immunodeficiency with autoimmunity. Front. Immunol. 3, 211.

Battaglia, M., Stabilini, A., Draghici, E., Migliavacca, B., Gregori, S., Bonifacio, E., Roncarolo, M.G., 2006. Induction of tolerance in type 1 diabetes via both CD4+CD25+ T regulatory cells and T regulatory type 1 cells. Diabetes 55 (6), 1571–1580.

Baud, O., Goulet, O., Canioni, D., Le Deist, F., Radford, I., Rieu, D., Dupuis-Girod, S., Cerf-Bensussan, N., Cavazzana-Calvo, M., Brousse, N., et al., 2001. Treatment of the immune dysregulation, polyendocrinopathy, enteropathy, X-linked syndrome (IPEX) by allogeneic bone marrow transplantation. N. Engl. J. Med. 344 (23), 1758–1762.

Blanchette, V., Imbach, P., Andrew, M., Adams, M., McMillan, J., Wang, E., Milner, R., Ali, K., Barnard, D., Bernstein, M., et al., 1994. Randomised trial of intravenous immunoglobulin G, intravenous anti-D, and oral prednisone in childhood acute immune thrombocytopenic purpura. Lancet 344 (8924), 703–707.

Bleesing, J.J., Straus, S.E., Fleisher, T.A., 2000. Autoimmune lymphoproliferative syndrome. A human disorder of abnormal lymphocyte survival. Pediatr. Clin. N. Am. 47 (6), 1291–1310.

Boehm, T., Scheu, S., Pfeffer, K., Bleul, C.C., 2003. Thymic medullary epithelial cell differentiation, thymocyte emigration, and the control of autoimmunity require lympho-epithelial cross talk via LTbetaR. J. Exp. Med. 198 (5), 757–769.

Bordignon, C., Mavilio, F., Ferrari, G., Servida, P., Ugazio, A.G., Notarangelo, L.D., Gilboa, E., Rossini, S., O'Reilly, R.J., Smith, C.A., et al., 1993. Transfer of the ADA gene into bone marrow cells and peripheral blood lymphocytes for the treatment of patients affected by ADA-deficient SCID. Hum. Gene Ther. 4 (4), 513–520.

Bousfiha, A.A., Jeddane, L., Ailal, F., Benhsaien, I., Mahlaoui, N., Casanova, J.L., Abel, L., 2013. Primary immunodeficiency diseases worldwide: more common than generally thought. J. Clin. Immunol. 33 (1), 1–7.

Boyle, J.M., Buckley, R.H., 2007. Population prevalence of diagnosed primary immunodeficiency diseases in the United States. J. Clin. Immunol. 27 (5), 497–502.

Boztug, K., Schmidt, M., Schwarzer, A., Banerjee, P.P., Diez, I.A., Dewey, R.A., Bohm, M., Nowrouzi, A., Ball, C.R., Glimm, H., et al., 2010. Stem-cell gene therapy for the Wiskott-Aldrich syndrome. N. Engl. J. Med. 363 (20), 1918–1927.

Braun, C.J., Boztug, K., Paruzynski, A., Witzel, M., Schwarzer, A., Rothe, M., Modlich, U., Beier, R., Gohring, G., Steinemann, D., et al., 2014. Gene therapy for Wiskott-Aldrich syndrome–long-term efficacy and genotoxicity. Sci. Transl. Med. 6 (227), 227ra33.

Buchbinder, D., Baker, R., Lee, Y.N., Ravell, J., Zhang, Y., McElwee, J., Nugent, D., Coonrod, E.M., Durtschi, J.D., Augustine, N.H., et al., 2015. Identification of patients with RAG mutations previously diagnosed with common variable immunodeficiency disorders. J. Clin. Immunol. 35 (2), 119–124.

Burns, S.O., Zenner, H.L., Plagnol, V., Curtis, J., Mok, K., Eisenhut, M., Kumararatne, D., Doffinger, R., Thrasher, A.J., Nejentsev, S., 2012. LRBA gene deletion in a patient presenting with autoimmunity without hypogammaglobulinemia. J. Allergy Clin. Immunol. 130 (6), 1428–1432.

Burroughs, L.M., Torgerson, T.R., Storb, R., Carpenter, P.A., Rawlings, D.J., Sanders, J., Scharenberg, A.M., Skoda-Smith, S., Englund, J., Ochs, H.D., et al., 2010. Stable hematopoietic cell engraftment after low-intensity nonmyeloablative conditioning in patients with immune dysregulation, polyendocrinopathy, enteropathy, X-linked syndrome. J. Allergy Clin. Immunol. 126 (5), 1000–1005.

Bussone, G., Mouthon, L., 2009. Autoimmune manifestations in primary immune deficiencies. Autoimmun. Rev. 8 (4), 332–336.

Campagnoli, M.F., Garbarini, L., Quarello, P., Garelli, E., Carando, A., Baravalle, V., Doria, A., Biava, A., Chiocchetti, A., Rosolen, A., et al., 2006. The broad spectrum of autoimmune lymphoproliferative disease: molecular bases, clinical features and long-term follow-up in 31 patients. Haematologica 91 (4), 538–541.

Cantaert, T., Schickel, J.N., Bannock, J.M., Ng, Y.S., Massad, C., Oe, T., Wu, R., Lavoie, A., Walter, J.E., Notarangelo, L.D., et al., AID expression in human B-cell precursors is essential for central B-cell tolerance. Immunity, in press.

Cassani, B., Poliani, P.L., Marrella, V., Schena, F., Sauer, A.V., Ravanini, M., Strina, D., Busse, C.E., Regenass, S., Wardemann, H., et al., 2010a. Homeostatic expansion of autoreactive immunoglobulin-secreting cells in the Rag2 mouse model of Omenn syndrome. J. Exp. Med. 207 (7), 1525–1540.

Cassani, B., Poliani, P.L., Moratto, D., Sobacchi, C., Marrella, V., Imperatori, L., Vairo, D., Plebani, A., Giliani, S., Vezzoni, P., et al., 2010b. Defect of regulatory T cells in patients with Omenn syndrome. J. Allergy Clin. Immunol. 125 (1), 209–216.

Castiello, M.C., Bosticardo, M., Pala, F., Catucci, M., Chamberlain, N., van Zelm, M.C., Driessen, G.J., Pac, M., Bernatowska, E., Scaramuzza, S., et al., 2014. Wiskott-Aldrich Syndrome protein deficiency perturbs the homeostasis of B-cell compartment in humans. J. Autoimmun. 50, 42–50.

Catucci, M., Castiello, M.C., Pala, F., Bosticardo, M., Villa, A., 2012. Autoimmunity in wiskott-Aldrich syndrome: an unsolved enigma. Front. Immunol. 3, 209.

Caudy, A.A., Reddy, S.T., Chatila, T., Atkinson, J.P., Verbsky, J.W., 2007. CD25 deficiency causes an immune dysregulation, polyendocrinopathy, enteropathy, X-linked-like syndrome, and defective IL-10 expression from CD4 lymphocytes. J. Allergy Clin. Immunol. 119 (2), 482–487.

Cavadini, P., Vermi, W., Facchetti, F., Fontana, S., Nagafuchi, S., Mazzolari, E., Sediva, A., Marrella, V., Villa, A., Fischer, A., et al., 2005. AIRE deficiency in thymus of 2 patients with Omenn syndrome. J. Clin. Invest. 115 (3), 728–732.

Cavazzana-Calvo, M., Hacein-Bey, S., de Saint, Basile G., Gross, F., Yvon, E., Nusbaum, P., Selz, F., Hue, C., Certain, S., Casanova, J.L., et al., 2000. Gene therapy of human severe combined immunodeficiency (SCID)-X1 disease. Science 288 (5466), 669–672.

Chan, K., Davis, J., Pai, S.Y., Bonilla, F.A., Puck, J.M., Apkon, M., 2011. A Markov model to analyze cost-effectiveness of screening for severe combined immunodeficiency (SCID). Mol. Genet. Metab. 104 (3), 383–389.

Chapel, H., Lucas, M., Lee, M., Bjorkander, J., Webster, D., Grimbacher, B., Fieschi, C., Thon, V., Abedi, M.R., Hammarstrom, L., 2008. Common variable immunodeficiency disorders: division into distinct clinical phenotypes. Blood 112 (2), 277–286.

Charbonnier, L.M., Janssen, E., Chou, J., Ohsumi, T.K., Keles, S., Hsu, J.T., Massaad, M.J., Garcia-Lloret, M., Hanna-Wakim, R., Dbaibo, G., et al., 2015. Regulatory T-cell deficiency and immune dysregulation, polyendocrinopathy, enteropathy, X-linked-like disorder caused by loss-of-function mutations in LRBA. J. Allergy Clin. Immunol. 135 (1), 217–227.

Chen, K., Wu, W., Mathew, D., Zhang, Y., Browne, S.K., Rosen, L.B., McManus, M.P., Pulsipher, M.A., Yandell, M., Bohnsack, J.F., et al., 2014. Autoimmunity due to RAG deficiency and estimated disease incidence in RAG1/2 mutations. J. Allergy Clin. Immunol. 133 (3), 880–882, 3.

Chida, N., Kobayashi, I., Takezaki, S., Ueki, M., Yamazaki, Y., Garelli, S., Scarpa, R., Horikawa, R., Yamada, M., Betterle, C., et al., 2015. Disease specificity of anti-tryptophan hydroxylase-1 and anti-AIE-75 autoantibodies in APECED and IPEX syndrome. Clin. Immunol. 156 (1), 36–42.

Cicalese, M.P., Aiuti, A., 2015. Clinical applications of gene therapy for primary immunodeficiencies. Hum. Gene Ther. 26 (4), 210–219.

Ciccocioppo, R., Comoli, P., Gallia, A., Basso, S., Baldanti, F., Corazza, G.R., 2014. Autologous human cytomegalovirus-specific cytotoxic T cells as rescue therapy for ulcerative enteritis in primary immunodeficiency. J. Clin. Immunol. 34 (6), 681–685.
Cohen, J.M., Sebire, N.J., Harvey, J., Gaspar, H.B., Cathy, C., Jones, A., Rao, K., Cubitt, D., Amrolia, P.J., Davies, E.G., et al., 2007. Successful treatment of lymphoproliferative disease complicating primary immunodeficiency/immunodysregulatory disorders with reduced-intensity allogeneic stem-cell transplantation. Blood 110 (6), 2209–2214.
Coutinho, A., Carneiro-Sampaio, M., 2008. Primary immunodeficiencies unravel critical aspects of the pathophysiology of autoimmunity and of the genetics of autoimmune disease. J. Clin. Immunol. 28 (Suppl 1), S4–S10.
Davies, J.K., Telfer, P., Cavenagh, J.D., Foot, N., Neat, M., 2003. Autoimmune cytopenias in the 22q11.2 deletion syndrome. Clin. Lab. Haematol. 25 (3), 195–197.
Day, N.K., Geiger, H., McLean, R., Michael, A., Good, R.A., 1973. C2 deficiency. Development of lupus erythematosus. J. Clin. Invest. 52 (7), 1601–1607.
de la Chapelle, A., Herva, R., Koivisto, M., Aula, P., 1981. A deletion in chromosome 22 can cause DiGeorge syndrome. Hum. Genet. 57 (3), 253–256.
De Ravin, S.S., Naumann, N., Cowen, E.W., Friend, J., Hilligoss, D., Marquesen, M., Balow, J.E., Barron, K.S., Turner, M.L., Gallin, J.I., et al., 2008. Chronic granulomatous disease as a risk factor for autoimmune disease. J. Allergy Clin. Immunol. 122 (6), 1097–1103.
De Ravin, S.S., Cowen, E.W., Zarember, K.A., Whiting-Theobald, N.L., Kuhns, D.B., Sandler, N.G., Douek, D.C., Pittaluga, S., Poliani, P.L., Lee, Y.N., et al., 2010. Hypomorphic Rag mutations can cause destructive midline granulomatous disease. Blood 116 (8), 1263–1271.
de Saint-Basile, G., Le Deist, F., de Villartay, J.P., Cerf-Bensussan, N., Journet, O., Brousse, N., Griscelli, C., Fischer, A., 1991. Restricted heterogeneity of T lymphocytes in combined immunodeficiency with hypereosinophilia (Omenn's syndrome). J. Clin. Invest. 87 (4), 1352–1359.
Durandy, A., Cantaert, T., Kracker, S., Meffre, E., 2013. Potential roles of activation-induced cytidine deaminase in promotion or prevention of autoimmunity in humans. Autoimmunity 46 (2), 148–156.
Edgar, J.D., Buckland, M., Guzman, D., Conlon, N.P., Knerr, V., Bangs, C., Reiser, V., Panahloo, Z., Workman, S., Slatter, M., et al., 2014. The United Kingdom Primary Immune Deficiency (UKPID) Registry: report of the first 4 years' activity 2008–2012. Clin. Exp. Immunol. 175 (1), 68–78.
Ege, M., Ma, Y., Manfras, B., Kalwak, K., Lu, H., Lieber, M.R., Schwarz, K., Pannicke, U., 2005. Omenn syndrome due to ARTEMIS mutations. Blood 105 (11), 4179–4186.
Fernandez-Boyanapalli, R.F., Frasch, S.C., McPhillips, K., Vandivier, R.W., Harry, B.L., Riches, D.W., Henson, P.M., Bratton, D.L., 2009. Impaired apoptotic cell clearance in CGD due to altered macrophage programming is reversed by phosphatidylserine-dependent production of IL-4. Blood 113 (9), 2047–2055.
Fernandez-Boyanapalli, R., McPhillips, K.A., Frasch, S.C., Janssen, W.J., Dinauer, M.C., Riches, D.W., Henson, P.M., Byrne, A., Bratton, D.L., 2010. Impaired phagocytosis of apoptotic cells by macrophages in chronic granulomatous disease is reversed by IFN-gamma in a nitric oxide-dependent manner. J. Immunol. 185 (7), 4030–4041.
Frasch, S.C., Berry, K.Z., Fernandez-Boyanapalli, R., Jin, H.S., Leslie, C., Henson, P.M., Murphy, R.C., Bratton, D.L., 2008. NADPH oxidase-dependent generation of lysophosphatidylserine enhances clearance of activated and dying neutrophils via G2A. J. Biol. Chem. 283 (48), 33736–33749.
Furusho, K., Kamiya, T., Nakano, H., Kiyosawa, N., Shinomiya, K., Hayashidera, T., Tamura, T., Hirose, O., Manabe, Y., Yokoyama, T., et al., 1984. High-dose intravenous gammaglobulin for Kawasaki disease. Lancet 2 (8411), 1055–1058.
Gaspar, H.B., Parsley, K.L., Howe, S., King, D., Gilmour, K.C., Sinclair, J., Brouns, G., Schmidt, M., Von Kalle, C., Barington, T., et al., 2004. Gene therapy of X-linked severe combined immunodeficiency by use of a pseudotyped gammaretroviral vector. Lancet 364 (9452), 2181–2187.
Gaspar, H.B., Cooray, S., Gilmour, K.C., Parsley, K.L., Adams, S., Howe, S.J., Al Ghonaium, A., Bayford, J., Brown, L., Davies, E.G., et al., 2011. Long-term persistence of a polyclonal T cell repertoire after gene therapy for X-linked severe combined immunodeficiency. Sci. Transl. Med. 3 (97), 97ra79.

Gathmann, B., Grimbacher, B., Beaute, J., Dudoit, Y., Mahlaoui, N., Fischer, A., Knerr, V., Kindle, G., Party, E.R.W., 2009. The European internet-based patient and research database for primary immunodeficiencies: results 2006–2008. Clin. Exp. Immunol. 157 (Suppl 1), 3–11.

Gathmann, B., Mahlaoui, N., CEREDIH, Gerard, L., Oksenhendler, E., Warnatz, K., Schulze, I., Kindle, G., Kuijpers, T.W., Dutch, W.I.D., et al., 2014. Clinical picture and treatment of 2212 patients with common variable immunodeficiency. J. Allergy Clin. Immunol. 134 (1), 116–126.

Gay, D., Saunders, T., Camper, S., Weigert, M., 1993. Receptor editing: an approach by autoreactive B cells to escape tolerance. J. Exp. Med. 177 (4), 999–1008.

Gennery, A.R., 2012. Immunological aspects of 22q11.2 deletion syndrome. Cell. Mol. Life Sci. 69 (1), 17–27.

Gennery, A.R., 2013. Immunological features of 22q11 deletion syndrome. Curr. Opin. Pediatr. 25 (6), 730–735.

Gennery, A.R., Barge, D., O'Sullivan, J.J., Flood, T.J., Abinun, M., Cant, A.J., 2002. Antibody deficiency and autoimmunity in 22q11.2 deletion syndrome. Arch. Dis. Child. 86 (6), 422–425.

Gennery, A.R., Slatter, M.A., Rice, J., Hoefsloot, L.H., Barge, D., McLean-Tooke, A., Montgomery, T., Goodship, J.A., Burt, A.D., Flood, T.J., et al., 2008. Mutations in CHD7 in patients with CHARGE syndrome cause T-B + natural killer cell + severe combined immune deficiency and may cause Omenn-like syndrome. Clin. Exp. Immunol. 153 (1), 75–80.

Giliani, S., Bonfim, C., de Saint, Basile G., Lanzi, G., Brousse, N., Koliski, A., Malvezzi, M., Fischer, A., Notarangelo, L.D., Le Deist, F., 2006. Omenn syndrome in an infant with IL7RA gene mutation. J. Pediatr. 148 (2), 272–274.

Glocker, E.O., Kotlarz, D., Boztug, K., Gertz, E.M., Schaffer, A.A., Noyan, F., Perro, M., Diestelhorst, J., Allroth, A., Murugan, D., et al., 2009. Inflammatory bowel disease and mutations affecting the interleukin-10 receptor. N. Engl. J. Med. 361 (21), 2033–2045.

Glocker, E.O., Frede, N., Perro, M., Sebire, N., Elawad, M., Shah, N., Grimbacher, B., 2010. Infant colitis–it's in the genes. Lancet 376 (9748), 1272.

Gobert, D., Bussel, J.B., Cunningham-Rundles, C., Galicier, L., Dechartres, A., Berezne, A., Bonnotte, B., DeRevel, T., Auzary, C., Jaussaud, R., et al., 2011. Efficacy and safety of rituximab in common variable immunodeficiency-associated immune cytopenias: a retrospective multicentre study on 33 patients. Br. J. Haematol. 155 (4), 498–508.

Gol-Ara, M., Jadidi-Niaragh, F., Sadria, R., Azizi, G., Mirshafiey, A., 2012. The role of different subsets of regulatory T cells in immunopathogenesis of rheumatoid arthritis. Arthritis 2012, 805875.

Gomez, A.M., Willcox, N., Vrolix, K., Hummel, J., Nogales-Gadea, G., Saxena, A., Duimel, H., Verheyen, F., Molenaar, P.C., Buurman, W.A., et al., 2014. Proteasome inhibition with bortezomib depletes plasma cells and specific autoantibody production in primary thymic cell cultures from early-onset myasthenia gravis patients. J. Immunol. 193 (3), 1055–1063.

Gomez-Almaguer, D., Solano-Genesta, M., Tarin-Arzaga, L., Herrera-Garza, J.L., Cantu-Rodriguez, O.G., Gutierrez-Aguirre, C.H., Jaime-Perez, J.C., 2010. Low-dose rituximab and alemtuzumab combination therapy for patients with steroid-refractory autoimmune cytopenias. Blood 116 (23), 4783–4785.

Goudy, K., Aydin, D., Barzaghi, F., Gambineri, E., Vignoli, M., Ciullini Mannurita, S., Doglioni, C., Ponzoni, M., Cicalese, M.P., Assanelli, A., Tommasini, A., Brigida, I., Dellepiane, R.M., Martino, S., Olek, S., Aiuti, A., Ciceri, F., Roncarolo, M.G., Bacchetta, R., 2013. Human IL2RA null mutation mediates immunodeficiency with lymphoproliferation and autoimmunity. Clin. Immunol. 146 (3), 248–261.

Grez, M., Reichenbach, J., Schwable, J., Seger, R., Dinauer, M.C., Thrasher, A.J., 2011. Gene therapy of chronic granulomatous disease: the engraftment dilemma. Mol. Ther. 19 (1), 28–35.

Groux, H., O'Garra, A., Bigler, M., Rouleau, M., Antonenko, S., de Vries, J.E., Roncarolo, M.G., 1997. A CD4+ T-cell subset inhibits antigen-specific T-cell responses and prevents colitis. Nature 389 (6652), 737–742.

Grunebaum, E., Bates, A., Roifman, C.M., 2008. Omenn syndrome is associated with mutations in DNA ligase IV. J. Allergy Clin. Immunol. 122 (6), 1219–1220.

Gullstrand, B., Martensson, U., Sturfelt, G., Bengtsson, A.A., Truedsson, L., 2009. Complement classical pathway components are all important in clearance of apoptotic and secondary necrotic cells. Clin. Exp. Immunol. 156 (2), 303–311.

Haapaniemi, E.M., Kaustio, M., Rajala, H.L., van Adrichem, A.J., Kainulainen, L., Glumoff, V., Doffinger, R., Kuusanmaki, H., Heiskanen-Kosma, T., Trotta, L., et al., 2015. Autoimmunity, hypogammaglobulinemia, lymphoproliferation, and mycobacterial disease in patients with activating mutations in STAT3. Blood 125 (4), 639–648.

Hacein-Bey-Abina, S., Garrigue, A., Wang, G.P., Soulier, J., Lim, A., Morillon, E., Clappier, E., Caccavelli, L., Delabesse, E., Beldjord, K., et al., 2008. Insertional oncogenesis in 4 patients after retrovirus-mediated gene therapy of SCID-X1. J. Clin. Invest. 118 (9), 3132–3142.

Hacein-Bey-Abina, S., Hauer, J., Lim, A., Picard, C., Wang, G.P., Berry, C.C., Martinache, C., Rieux-Laucat, F., Latour, S., Belohradsky, B.H., et al., 2010. Efficacy of gene therapy for X-linked severe combined immunodeficiency. N. Engl. J. Med. 363 (4), 355–364.

Hampton, M.B., Vissers, M.C., Keenan, J.I., Winterbourn, C.C., 2002. Oxidant-mediated phosphatidylserine exposure and macrophage uptake of activated neutrophils: possible impairment in chronic granulomatous disease. J. Leukoc. Biol. 71 (5), 775–781.

Hartung, H.P., Mouthon, L., Ahmed, R., Jordan, S., Laupland, K.B., Jolles, S., 2009. Clinical applications of intravenous immunoglobulins (IVIg)–beyond immunodeficiencies and neurology. Clin. Exp. Immunol. 158 (Suppl 1), 23–33.

Heino, M., Peterson, P., Kudoh, J., Nagamine, K., Lagerstedt, A., Ovod, V., Ranki, A., Rantala, I., Nieminen, M., Tuukkanen, J., et al., 1999. Autoimmune regulator is expressed in the cells regulating immune tolerance in thymus medulla. Biochem. Biophys. Res. Commun. 257 (3), 821–825.

Henderson, L.A., Frugoni, F., Hopkins, G., Al-Herz, W., Weinacht, K., Comeau, A.M., Bonilla, F.A., Notarangelo, L.D., Pai, S.Y., 2013a. First reported case of Omenn syndrome in a patient with reticular dysgenesis. J. Allergy Clin. Immunol. 131 (4), 1227–1230, 30 e1-3.

Henderson, L.A., Frugoni, F., Hopkins, G., de Boer, H., Pai, S.Y., Lee, Y.N., Walter, J.E., Hazen, M.M., Notarangelo, L.D., 2013b. Expanding the spectrum of recombination-activating gene 1 deficiency: a family with early-onset autoimmunity. J. Allergy Clin. Immunol. 132 (4), 969–971, e1-2.

Hernandez-Trujillo, V.P., Scalchunes, C., Cunningham-Rundles, C., Ochs, H.D., Bonilla, F.A., Paris, K., Yel, L., Sullivan, K.E., 2014. Autoimmunity and inflammation in X-linked agammaglobulinemia. J. Clin. Immunol. 34 (6), 627–632.

Hillion, S., Rochas, C., Youinou, P., Jamin, C., 2005. Expression and reexpression of recombination activating genes: relevance to the development of autoimmune states. Ann. N. Y. Acad. Sci. 1050, 10–18.

Hodi, F.S., O'Day, S.J., McDermott, D.F., Weber, R.W., Sosman, J.A., Haanen, J.B., Gonzalez, R., Robert, C., Schadendorf, D., Hassel, J.C., et al., 2010. Improved survival with ipilimumab in patients with metastatic melanoma. N. Engl. J. Med. 363 (8), 711–723.

Holland, S.M., 2013. Chronic granulomatous disease. Hematol. Oncol. Clin. North Am. 27 (1), 89–99, 1.

Howe, S.J., Mansour, M.R., Schwarzwaelder, K., Bartholomae, C., Hubank, M., Kempski, H., Brugman, M.H., Pike-Overzet, K., Chatters, S.J., de Ridder, D., et al., 2008. Insertional mutagenesis combined with acquired somatic mutations causes leukemogenesis following gene therapy of SCID-X1 patients. J. Clin. Invest. 118 (9), 3143–3150.

Hsu, S.M., Yang, C.H., Shen, F.H., Chen, S.H., Lin, C.J., Shieh, C.C., 2015. Proteasome inhibitor bortezomib suppresses nuclear factor-kappa B activation and ameliorates eye inflammation in experimental autoimmune uveitis. Mediat. Inflamm. 2015, 847373.

Huter, E.N., Natarajan, K., Torgerson, T.R., Glass, D.D., Shevach, E.M., 2010. Autoantibodies in scurfy mice and IPEX patients recognize keratin 14. J. Invest. Dermatol. 130 (5), 1391–1399.

Hwa, V., Nadeau, K., Wit, J.M., Rosenfeld, R.G., 2011. STAT5b deficiency: lessons from STAT5b gene mutations. Best Pract. Res. Clin. Endocrinol. Metab. 25 (1), 61–75.

Imbach, P., Barandun, S., d'Apuzzo, V., Baumgartner, C., Hirt, A., Morell, A., Rossi, E., Schoni, M., Vest, M., Wagner, H.P., 1981. High-dose intravenous gammaglobulin for idiopathic thrombocytopenic purpura in childhood. Lancet 1 (8232), 1228–1231.

Isnardi, I., Ng, Y.S., Srdanovic, I., Motaghedi, R., Rudchenko, S., von Bernuth, H., Zhang, S.Y., Puel, A., Jouanguy, E., Picard, C., et al., 2008. IRAK-4- and MyD88-dependent pathways are essential for the removal of developing autoreactive B cells in humans. Immunity 29 (5), 746–757.

Primary immunodeficiency diseases. Report of an IUIS Scientific Committee. 1999. International Union of Immunological Societies. Clin. Exp. Immunol. 118 (Suppl 1), 1–28.
Jakez-Ocampo, J., Atisha-Fregoso, Y., Llorente, L., 2015. Refractory primary Sjögren syndrome successfully treated with bortezomib. Int. J. Clin. Rheumatol. 21 (1), 31–32.
Janic, M.D., Brasanac, C.D., Jankovic, J.S., Dokmanovic, B.L., Krstovski, R.N., Kraguljac Kurtovic, J.N., 2009. Rapid regression of lymphadenopathy upon rapamycin treatment in a child with autoimmune lymphoproliferative syndrome. Pediatr. Blood Cancer 53 (6), 1117–1119.
Janssen, E., Morbach, H., Ullas, S., Bannock, J.M., Massad, C., Menard, L., Barlan, I., Lefranc, G., Su, H., Dasouki, M., et al., 2014. Dedicator of cytokinesis 8-deficient patients have a breakdown in peripheral B-cell tolerance and defective regulatory T cells. J. Allergy Clin. Immunol. 134 (6), 1365–1374.
Joshi, A.Y., Iyer, V.N., Hagan, J.B., St Sauver, J.L., Boyce, T.G., 2009. Incidence and temporal trends of primary immunodeficiency: a population-based cohort study. Mayo Clin. Proc. 84 (1), 16–22.
Kahwash, S.B., Fung, B., Savelli, S., Bleesing, J.J., Qualman, S.J., 2007. Autoimmune lymphoproliferative syndrome (ALPS): a case with congenital onset. Pediatr. Dev. Pathol. 10 (4), 315–319.
Kane, R.C., Dagher, R., Farrell, A., Ko, C.W., Sridhara, R., Justice, R., Pazdur, R., 2007. Bortezomib for the treatment of mantle cell lymphoma. Clin. Cancer Res. 13 (18 Pt 1), 5291–5294.
Kaufmann, K.B., Chiriaco, M., Siler, U., Finocchi, A., Reichenbach, J., Stein, S., Grez, M., 2014. Gene therapy for chronic granulomatous disease: current status and future perspectives. Curr. Gene Ther. 14 (6), 447–460.
Kaveri, S.V., Maddur, M.S., Hegde, P., Lacroix-Desmazes, S., Bayry, J., 2011. Intravenous immunoglobulins in immunodeficiencies: more than mere replacement therapy. Clin. Exp. Immunol. 164 (Suppl 2), 2–5.
Kelkka, T., Kienhofer, D., Hoffmann, M., Linja, M., Wing, K., Sareila, O., Hultqvist, M., Laajala, E., Chen, Z., Vasconcelos, J., et al., 2014. Reactive oxygen species deficiency induces autoimmunity with type 1 interferon signature. Antioxid. Redox Signal. 21 (16), 2231–2245.
Kerr, J., Quinti, I., Eibl, M., Chapel, H., Spath, P.J., Sewell, W.A., Salama, A., van Schaik, I.N., Kuijpers, T.W., Peter, H.H., 2014. Is dosing of therapeutic immunoglobulins optimal? A review of a three-decade long debate in europe. Front. Immunol. 5, 629.
Khandelwal, P., Davies, S.M., Grimley, M.S., Jordan, M.B., Curtis, B.R., Jodele, S., Marsh, R., Filipovich, A.J., 2014. Bortezomib for refractory autoimmunity in pediatrics. Biol. Blood Marrow Transplant. 20 (10), 1654–1659.
Kisand, K., Boe Wolff, A.S., Podkrajsek, K.T., Tserel, L., Link, M., Kisand, K.V., Ersvaer, E., Perheentupa, J., Erichsen, M.M., Bratanic, N., et al., 2010. Chronic mucocutaneous candidiasis in APECED or thymoma patients correlates with autoimmunity to Th17-associated cytokines. J. Exp. Med. 207 (2), 299–308.
Kleinewietfeld, M., Hafler, D.A., 2014. Regulatory T cells in autoimmune neuroinflammation. Immunol. Rev. 259 (1), 231–244.
Kobayashi, I., Imamura, K., Yamada, M., Okano, M., Yara, A., Ikema, S., Ishikawa, N., 1998. A 75-kD autoantigen recognized by sera from patients with X-linked autoimmune enteropathy associated with nephropathy. Clin. Exp. Immunol. 111 (3), 527–531.
Kobayashi, I., Kubota, M., Yamada, M., Tanaka, H., Itoh, S., Sasahara, Y., Whitesell, L., Ariga, T., 2011. Autoantibodies to villin occur frequently in IPEX, a severe immune dysregulation, syndrome caused by mutation of FOXP3. Clin. Immunol. 141 (1), 83–89.
Kossiva, L., Theodoridou, M., Mostrou, G., Vrachnou, E., Le Deist, F., Rieux-Laucat, F., Kanariou, M.G., 2006. Mycophenolate mofetil as an alternate immunosuppressor for autoimmune lymphoproliferative syndrome. J. Pediatr. Hematol. Oncol. 28 (12), 824–826.
Kotb, R., Pinganaud, C., Trichet, C., Lambotte, O., Dreyfus, M., Delfraissy, J.F., Tchernia, G., Goujard, C., 2005. Efficacy of mycophenolate mofetil in adult refractory auto-immune cytopenias: a single center preliminary study. Eur. J. Haematol. 75 (1), 60–64.
Kotlarz, D., Beier, R., Murugan, D., Diestelhorst, J., Jensen, O., Boztug, K., Pfeifer, D., Kreipe, H., Pfister, E.D., Baumann, U., et al., 2012. Loss of interleukin-10 signaling and infantile inflammatory bowel disease: implications for diagnosis and therapy. Gastroenterology 143 (2), 347–355.

Krangel, M.S., 2009. Mechanics of T cell receptor gene rearrangement. Curr. Opin. Immunol. 21 (2), 133–139.
Kristiansen, O.P., Larsen, Z.M., Pociot, F., 2000. CTLA-4 in autoimmune diseases–a general susceptibility gene to autoimmunity? Genes Immun. 1 (3), 170–184.
Kubiak, C., Jyonouchi, S., Kuo, C., Garcia-Lloret, M., Dorsey, M.J., Sleasman, J., Zbrozek, A.S., Perez, E.E., 2014. Fiscal implications of newborn screening in the diagnosis of severe combined immunodeficiency. J. Allergy Clin. Immunol. 2 (6), 697–702.
Kuehn, H.S., Ouyang, W., Lo, B., Deenick, E.K., Niemela, J.E., Avery, D.T., Schickel, J.N., Tran, D.Q., Stoddard, J., Zhang, Y., et al., 2014. Immune dysregulation in human subjects with heterozygous germline mutations in CTLA4. Science 345 (6204), 1623–1627.
Kumar, V., Ali, S.R., Konrad, S., Zwirner, J., Verbeek, J.S., Schmidt, R.E., Gessner, J.E., 2006. Cell-derived anaphylatoxins as key mediators of antibody-dependent type II autoimmunity in mice. J. Clin. Invest. 116 (2), 512–520.
Kwan, A., Abraham, R.S., Currier, R., Brower, A., Andruszewski, K., Abbott, J.K., Baker, M., Ballow, M., Bartoshesky, L.E., Bonilla, F.A., et al., 2014. Newborn screening for severe combined immunodeficiency in 11 screening programs in the United States. JAMA 312 (7), 729–738.
Kyi, C., Carvajal, R.D., Wolchok, J.D., Postow, M.A., 2014. Ipilimumab in patients with melanoma and autoimmune disease. J. Immunother. Cancer 2 (1), 35.
Lampasona, V., Passerini, L., Barzaghi, F., Lombardoni, C., Bazzigaluppi, E., Brigatti, C., Bacchetta, R., Bosi, E., 2013. Autoantibodies to harmonin and villin are diagnostic markers in children with IPEX syndrome. Plos One 8 (11), e78664.
Leffler, J., Bengtsson, A.A., Blom, A.M., 2014. The complement system in systemic lupus erythematosus: an update. Ann. Rheum. Dis. 73 (9), 1601–1606.
Lehman, H.K., Ballow, M., 2008. Immune deficiency disorders with autoimmunity and abnormalities in immune regulation-monogenic autoimmune diseases. Clin. Rev. Allergy Immunol. 34 (2), 141–145.
Levy, E., Neven, B., Entz-Werle, N., Cribier, B., Lipsker, D., 2012. Post-thymus transplant vitiligo in a child with Foxn1 deficiency. Ann. Dermatol. Venereol. 139 (6–7), 468–471.
Lo, B., Zhang, K., Lu, W., Zheng, L., Zhang, Q., Kanellopoulou, C., Zhang, Y., Liu, Z., Fritz, J.M., et al., 2015. Patients with LRBA deficiency show CTLA4 loss and immune dysregulation responsive to abatacept therapy. Science 349 (6246), 436–440.
Lopez-Herrera, G., Tampella, G., Pan-Hammarstrom, Q., Herholz, P., Trujillo-Vargas, C.M., Phadwal, K., Simon, A.K., Moutschen, M., Etzioni, A., Mory, A., et al., 2012. Deleterious mutations in LRBA are associated with a syndrome of immune deficiency and autoimmunity. Am. J. Hum. Genet. 90 (6), 986–1001.
Maggadottir, S.M., Sullivan, K.E., 2014. The intersection of immune deficiency and autoimmunity. Curr. Opin. Rheumatol. 26 (5), 570–578.
Magnani, A., Brosselin, P., Beaute, J., de Vergnes, N., Mouy, R., Debre, M., Suarez, F., Hermine, O., Lortholary, O., Blanche, S., et al., 2014. Inflammatory manifestations in a single-center cohort of patients with chronic granulomatous disease. J. Allergy Clin. Immunol. 134 (3), 655–662, e8.
Marciano, B.E., Rosenzweig, S.D., Kleiner, D.E., Anderson, V.L., Darnell, D.N., Anaya-O'Brien, S., Hilligoss, D.M., Malech, H.L., Gallin, J.I., Holland, S.M., 2004. Gastrointestinal involvement in chronic granulomatous disease. Pediatrics 114 (2), 462–468.
Marciano, B.E., Spalding, C., Fitzgerald, A., Mann, D., Brown, T., Osgood, S., Yockey, L., Darnell, D.N., Barnhart, L., Daub, J., et al., 2015. Common severe infections in chronic granulomatous disease. Clin. Infect. Dis. 60, 1176–1183.
Marrella, V., Poliani, P.L., Casati, A., Rucci, F., Frascoli, L., Gougeon, M.L., Lemercier, B., Bosticardo, M., Ravanini, M., Battaglia, M., et al., 2007. A hypomorphic R229Q Rag2 mouse mutant recapitulates human Omenn syndrome. J. Clin. Invest. 117 (5), 1260–1269.
Mazzolari, E., Forino, C., Fontana, M., D'Ippolito, C., Lanfranchi, A., Gambineri, E., Ochs, H., Badolato, R., Notarangelo, L.D., 2005. A new case of IPEX receiving bone marrow transplantation. Bone Marrow Transplant. 35 (10), 1033–1034.
McLean-Tooke, A., Spickett, G.P., Gennery, A.R., 2007. Immunodeficiency and autoimmunity in 22q11.2 deletion syndrome. Scand. J. Immunol. 66 (1), 1–7.
Meiron, M., Zohar, Y., Anunu, R., Wildbaum, G., Karin, N., 2008. CXCL12 (SDF-1alpha) suppresses ongoing experimental autoimmune encephalomyelitis by selecting antigen-specific regulatory T cells. J. Exp. Med. 205 (11), 2643–2655.

Menard, L., Cantaert, T., Chamberlain, N., Tangye, S.G., Riminton, S., Church, J.A., Klion, A., Cunningham-Rundles, C., Nichols, K.E., Meffre, E., 2014. Signaling lymphocytic activation molecule (SLAM)/SLAM-associated protein pathway regulates human B-cell tolerance. J. Allergy Clin. Immunol. 133 (4), 1149–1161.

Meyer, O., Hauptmann, G., Tappeiner, G., Ochs, H.D., Mascart-Lemone, F., 1985. Genetic deficiency of C4, C2 or C1q and lupus syndromes. Association with anti-Ro (SS-A) antibodies. Clin. Exp. Immunol. 62 (3), 678–684.

Meyers, G., Ng, Y.S., Bannock, J.M., Lavoie, A., Walter, J.E., Notarangelo, L.D., Kilic, S.S., Aksu, G., Debre, M., Rieux-Laucat, F., et al., 2011. Activation-induced cytidine deaminase (AID) is required for B-cell tolerance in humans. Proc. Natl. Acad. Sci. U. S. A. 108 (28), 11554–11559.

Michel, M., Chanet, V., Galicier, L., Ruivard, M., Levy, Y., Hermine, O., Oksenhendler, E., Schaeffer, A., Bierling, P., Godeau, B., 2004. Autoimmune thrombocytopenic purpura and common variable immunodeficiency: analysis of 21 cases and review of the literature. Medicine 83 (4), 254–263.

Milner, J.D., Fasth, A., Etzioni, A., 2008. Autoimmunity in severe combined immunodeficiency (SCID): lessons from patients and experimental models. J. Clin. Immunol. 28 (Suppl 1), S29–S33.

Milner, J.D., Vogel, T.P., Forbes, L., Ma, C.A., Stray-Pedersen, A., Niemela, J.E., Lyons, J.J., Engelhardt, K.R., Zhang, Y., Topcagic, N., et al., 2015. Early-onset lymphoproliferation and autoimmunity caused by germline STAT3 gain-of-function mutations. Blood 125 (4), 591–599.

Mombaerts, P., Iacomini, J., Johnson, R.S., Herrup, K., Tonegawa, S., Papaioannou, V.E., 1992. RAG-1-deficient mice have no mature B and T lymphocytes. Cell 68 (5), 869–877.

Moraes-Vasconcelos, D., Costa-Carvalho, B.T., Torgerson, T.R., Ochs, H.D., 2008. Primary immune deficiency disorders presenting as autoimmune diseases: IPEX and APECED. J. Clin. Immunol. 28 (Suppl 1), S11–S19.

Moreau, P., Richardson, P.G., Cavo, M., Orlowski, R.Z., San Miguel, J.F., Palumbo, A., Harousseau, J.L., 2012. Proteasome inhibitors in multiple myeloma: 10 years later. Blood 120 (5), 947–959.

Naldini, L., 2011. Ex vivo gene transfer and correction for cell-based therapies. Nat. Rev. Genet. 12 (5), 301–315.

Neubert, K., Meister, S., Moser, K., Weisel, F., Maseda, D., Amann, K., Wiethe, C., Winkler, T.H., Kalden, J.R., Manz, R.A., et al., 2008. The proteasome inhibitor bortezomib depletes plasma cells and protects mice with lupus-like disease from nephritis. Nat. Med. 14 (7), 748–755.

Newburger, J.W., Takahashi, M., Beiser, A.S., Burns, J.C., Bastian, J., Chung, K.J., Colan, S.D., Duffy, C.E., Fulton, D.R., Glode, M.P., et al., 1991. A single intravenous infusion of gamma globulin as compared with four infusions in the treatment of acute Kawasaki syndrome. N. Engl. J. Med. 324 (23), 1633–1639.

Ng, Y.S., Wardemann, H., Chelnis, J., Cunningham-Rundles, C., Meffre, E., 2004. Bruton's tyrosine kinase is essential for human B cell tolerance. J. Exp. Med. 200 (7), 927–934.

Notarangelo, L.D., 2009. Primary immunodeficiencies (PIDs) presenting with cytopenias. Hematol. Am. Soc. Hematol. Educ. Progr. 1, 139–143.

Notarangelo, L.D., 2014. Combined immunodeficiencies with nonfunctional T lymphocytes. Adv. Immunol. 121, 121–190.

Ok, C.Y., Li, L., Young, K.H., 2015. EBV-driven B-cell lymphoproliferative disorders: from biology, classification and differential diagnosis to clinical management. Exp. Mol. Med. 47, e132.

Palamaro, L., Romano, R., Fusco, A., Giardino, G., Gallo, V., Pignata, C., 2014. FOXN1 in organ development and human diseases. Int. Rev. Immunol. 33 (2), 83–93.

Palombella, V.J., Rando, O.J., Goldberg, A.L., Maniatis, T., 1994. The ubiquitin-proteasome pathway is required for processing the NF-kappa B1 precursor protein and the activation of NF-kappa B. Cell 78 (5), 773–785.

Palombella, V.J., Conner, E.M., Fuseler, J.W., Destree, A., Davis, J.M., Laroux, F.S., Wolf, R.E., Huang, J., Brand, S., Elliott, P.J., et al., 1998. Role of the proteasome and NF-kappaB in streptococcal cell wall-induced polyarthritis. Proc. Natl. Acad. Sci. U. S. A. 95 (26), 15671–15676.

Park, M.A., Li, J.T., Hagan, J.B., Maddox, D.E., Abraham, R.S., 2008. Common variable immunodeficiency: a new look at an old disease. Lancet 372 (9637), 489–502.

Passerini, L., Olek, S., Di Nunzio, S., Barzaghi, F., Hambleton, S., Abinun, M., Tommasini, A., Vignola, S., Cipolli, M., Amendola, M., et al., 2011. Forkhead box protein 3 (FOXP3) mutations lead to increased TH17 cell numbers and regulatory T-cell instability. J. Allergy Clin. Immunol. 128 (6), 1376–1379, e1.

Passerini, L., Rossi Mel, E., Sartirana, C., Fousteri, G., Bondanza, A., Naldini, L., Roncarolo, M.G., Bacchetta, R., 2013. CD4(+) T cells from IPEX patients convert into functional and stable regulatory T cells by FOXP3 gene transfer. Sci. Transl. Med. 5 (215), 215ra174.

Passerini, L., Sio, F.R., Porteus, M.H., Bacchetta, R., 2014. Gene/cell therapy approaches for Immune Dysregulation Polyendocrinopathy Enteropathy X-linked syndrome. Curr. Gene Ther. 14 (6), 422–428.

Patey-Mariaud de Serre, N., Canioni, D., Ganousse, S., Rieux-Laucat, F., Goulet, O., Ruemmele, F., Brousse, N., 2009. Digestive histopathological presentation of IPEX syndrome. Mod. Pathol. 22 (1), 95–102.

Patiroglu, T., Akar, H.H., Gilmour, K., Ozdemir, M.A., Bibi, S., Henriquez, F., Burns, S.O., Unal, E., 2014. Atypical severe combined immunodeficiency caused by a novel homozygous mutation in Rag1 gene in a girl who presented with pyoderma gangrenosum: a case report and literature review. J. Clin. Immunol. 34 (7), 792–795.

Pavkovic, M., Georgievski, B., Cevreska, L., Spiroski, M., Efremov, D.G., 2003. CTLA-4 exon 1 polymorphism in patients with autoimmune blood disorders. Am. J. Hematol. 72 (2), 147–149.

Pessach, I., Walter, J., Notarangelo, L.D., 2009. Recent advances in Primary Immunodeficiencies: identification of novel genetic defects and unanticipated phenotypes. Pediatr. Res. 65, 3R–12R.

Picard, C., Fischer, A., 2014. Contribution of high-throughput DNA sequencing to the study of primary immunodeficiencies. Eur. J. Immunol. 44 (10), 2854–2861.

Pickering, M.C., Botto, M., Taylor, P.R., Lachmann, P.J., Walport, M.J., 2000. Systemic lupus erythematosus, complement deficiency, and apoptosis. Adv. Immunol. 76, 227–324.

Pillai, S., Mattoo, H., Cariappa, A., 2011. B cells and autoimmunity. Curr. Opin. Immunol. 23 (6), 721–731.

Podjasek, J.C., Abraham, R.S., 2012. Autoimmune cytopenias in common variable immunodeficiency. Front. Immunol. 3, 189.

Poliani, P.L., Facchetti, F., Ravanini, M., Gennery, A.R., Villa, A., Roifman, C.M., Notarangelo, L.D., 2009. Early defects in human T-cell development severely affect distribution and maturation of thymic stromal cells: possible implications for the pathophysiology of Omenn syndrome. Blood 114 (1), 105–108.

Pot, C., Apetoh, L., Kuchroo, V.K., 2011. Type 1 regulatory T cells (Tr1) in autoimmunity. Semin. Immunol. 23 (3), 202–208.

Powers, E.T., Morimoto, R.I., Dillin, A., Kelly, J.W., Balch, W.E., 2009. Biological and chemical approaches to diseases of proteostasis deficiency. Annu. Rev. Biochem. 78, 959–991.

Qamar, N., Fuleihan, R.L., 2014. The hyper IgM syndromes. Clin. Rev. Allergy Immunol. 46 (2), 120–130.

Rao, V.K., Oliveira, J.B., 2011. How I treat autoimmune lymphoproliferative syndrome. Blood 118 (22), 5741–5751.

Rao, V.K., Dugan, F., Dale, J.K., Davis, J., Tretler, J., Hurley, J.K., Fleisher, T., Puck, J., Straus, S.E., 2005. Use of mycophenolate mofetil for chronic, refractory immune cytopenias in children with autoimmune lymphoproliferative syndrome. Br. J. Haematol. 129 (4), 534–538.

Resnick, E.S., Moshier, E.L., Godbold, J.H., Cunningham-Rundles, C., 2012. Morbidity and mortality in common variable immune deficiency over 4 decades. Blood 119 (7), 1650–1657.

Ricklin, D., Hajishengallis, G., Yang, K., Lambris, J.D., 2010. Complement: a key system for immune surveillance and homeostasis. Nat. Immunol. 11 (9), 785–797.

Robert, C., Thomas, L., Bondarenko, I., O'Day, S., Weber, J., Garbe, C., Lebbe, C., Baurain, J.F., Testori, A., Grob, J.J., et al., 2011. Ipilimumab plus dacarbazine for previously untreated metastatic melanoma. N. Engl. J. Med. 364 (26), 2517–2526.

Roifman, C.M., Gu, Y., Cohen, A., 2006. Mutations in the RNA component of RNase mitochondrial RNA processing might cause Omenn syndrome. J. Allergy Clin. Immunol. 117 (4), 897–903.

Roifman, C.M., Zhang, J., Atkinson, A., Grunebaum, E., Mandel, K., 2008. Adenosine deaminase deficiency can present with features of Omenn syndrome. J. Allergy Clin. Immunol. 121 (4), 1056–1058.

Roncarolo, M.G., Gregori, S., Bacchetta, R., Battaglia, M., 2014. Tr1 cells and the counter-regulation of immunity: natural mechanisms and therapeutic applications. Curr. Top. Microbiol. Immunol. 380, 39–68.

Rooney, C.M., Smith, C.A., Ng, C.Y., Loftin, S.K., Sixbey, J.W., Gan, Y., Srivastava, D.K., Bowman, L.C., Krance, R.A., Brenner, M.K., et al., 1998. Infusion of cytotoxic T cells for the prevention and treatment of Epstein-Barr virus-induced lymphoma in allogeneic transplant recipients. Blood 92 (5), 1549–1555.

Routes, J., Abinun, M., Al-Herz, W., Bustamante, J., Condino-Neto, A., De La Morena, M.T., Etzioni, A., Gambineri, E., Haddad, E., Kobrynski, L., et al., 2014. ICON: the early diagnosis of congenital immunodeficiencies. J. Clin. Immunol. 34 (4), 398–424.
Sanford, A.N., Suriano, A.R., Herche, D., Dietzmann, K., Sullivan, K.E., 2006. Abnormal apoptosis in chronic granulomatous disease and autoantibody production characteristic of lupus. Rheumatology 45 (2), 178–181.
Sankaran-Walters, S., Ransibrahmanakul, K., Grishina, I., Hung, J., Martinez, E., Prindiville, T., Dandekar, S., 2011. Epstein-Barr virus replication linked to B cell proliferation in inflamed areas of colonic mucosa of patients with inflammatory bowel disease. J. Clin. Virol. 50 (1), 31–36.
Schappi, M.G., Smith, V.V., Goldblatt, D., Lindley, K.J., Milla, P.J., 2001. Colitis in chronic granulomatous disease. Arch. Dis. Child. 84 (2), 147–151.
Schappi, M.G., Jaquet, V., Belli, D.C., Krause, K.H., 2008. Hyperinflammation in chronic granulomatous disease and anti-inflammatory role of the phagocyte NADPH oxidase. Semin. Immunopathol. 30 (3), 255–271.
Schneider, H., Rudd, C.E., 2014. Diverse mechanisms regulate the surface expression of immunotherapeutic target ctla-4. Front. Immunol. 5, 619.
Schuetz, C., Huck, K., Gudowius, S., Megahed, M., Feyen, O., Hubner, B., Schneider, D.T., Manfras, B., Pannicke, U., Willemze, R., et al., 2008. An immunodeficiency disease with RAG mutations and granulomas. N. Engl. J. Med. 358 (19), 2030–2038.
Schwarz, K., Gauss, G.H., Ludwig, L., Pannicke, U., Li, Z., Lindner, D., Friedrich, W., Seger, R.A., Hansen-Hagge, T.E., Desiderio, S., et al., 1996. RAG mutations in human B cell-negative SCID. Science 274 (5284), 97–99.
Seidel, M.G., 2014. Autoimmune and other cytopenias in primary immunodeficiencies: pathomechanisms, novel differential diagnoses, and treatment. Blood 124 (15), 2337–2344.
Seidel, M.G., Hirschmugl, T., Gamez-Diaz, L., Schwinger, W., Serwas, N., Deutschmann, A., Gorkiewicz, G., Zenz, W., Windpassinger, C., Grimbacher, B., et al., 2014. Long-term remission after allogeneic hematopoietic stem cell transplantation in LPS-responsive beige-like anchor (LRBA) deficiency. J. Allergy Clin. Immunol. 135 (5), 1384–1390.
Serwas, N.K., Kansu, A., Santos-Valente, E., Kuloglu, Z., Demir, A., Yaman, A., Yaneth Gamez Diaz, L., Artan, R., Sayar, E., Ensari, A., et al., 2015. Atypical manifestation of LRBA deficiency with predominant IBD-like phenotype. Inflamm. Bowel Dis. 21 (1), 40–47.
Shevach, E.M., 2009. Mechanisms of foxp3 + T regulatory cell-mediated suppression. Immunity 30 (5), 636–645.
Shibata, H., Tani-ichi, S., Lee, H.C., Maki, K., Ikuta, K., 2007. Induction of the IL-7 receptor alpha chain in mouse peripheral B cells by glucocorticoids. Immunol. Lett. 111 (1), 45–50.
Shinkai, Y., Rathbun, G., Lam, K.P., Oltz, E.M., Stewart, V., Mendelsohn, M., Charron, J., Datta, M., Young, F., Stall, A.M., et al., 1992. RAG-2-deficient mice lack mature lymphocytes owing to inability to initiate V(D)J rearrangement. Cell 68 (5), 855–867.
Signorini, S., Imberti, L., Pirovano, S., Villa, A., Facchetti, F., Ungari, M., Bozzi, F., Albertini, A., Ugazio, A.G., Vezzoni, P., et al., 1999. Intrathymic restriction and peripheral expansion of the T-cell repertoire in Omenn syndrome. Blood 94 (10), 3468–3478.
Skrott, Z., Cvek, B., 2014. Linking the activity of bortezomib in multiple myeloma and autoimmune diseases. Crit. Rev. Oncol. Hematol. 92 (2), 61–70.
Sleight, B.J., Prasad, V.S., DeLaat, C., Steele, P., Ballard, E., Arceci, R.J., Sidman, C.L., 1998. Correction of autoimmune lymphoproliferative syndrome by bone marrow transplantation. Bone Marrow Transplant. 22 (4), 375–380.
Snowden, J.A., Saccardi, R., Allez, M., Ardizzone, S., Arnold, R., Cervera, R., Denton, C., Hawkey, C., Labopin, M., Mancardi, G., et al., 2012. Haematopoietic SCT in severe autoimmune diseases: updated guidelines of the european group for blood and marrow transplantation. Bone Marrow Transplant. 47 (6), 770–790.
Stallone, G., Schena, A., Infante, B., Di Paolo, S., Loverre, A., Maggio, G., Ranieri, E., Gesualdo, L., Schena, F.P., Grandaliano, G., 2005. Sirolimus for Kaposi's sarcoma in renal-transplant recipients. N. Engl. J. Med. 352 (13), 1317–1323.
Stein, S., Ott, M.G., Schultze-Strasser, S., Jauch, A., Burwinkel, B., Kinner, A., Schmidt, M., Kramer, A., Schwable, J., Glimm, H., et al., 2010. Genomic instability and myelodysplasia with monosomy 7 consequent to EVI1 activation after gene therapy for chronic granulomatous disease. Nat. Med. 16 (2), 198–204.

Sullivan, K.E., 1998. Complement deficiency and autoimmunity. Curr. Opin. Pediatr. 10 (6), 600–606.
Swierkot, J., Lewandowicz-Uszynska, A., Chlebicki, A., Szmyrka-Kaczmarek, M., Polanska, B., Jankowski, A., Szechinski, J., 2006. Rheumatoid arthritis in a patient with common variable immunodeficiency: difficulty in diagnosis and therapy. Clin. Rheumatol. 25 (1), 92–94.
Teachey, D.T., Greiner, R., Seif, A., Attiyeh, E., Bleesing, J., Choi, J., Manno, C., Rappaport, E., Schwabe, D., Sheen, C., et al., 2009. Treatment with sirolimus results in complete responses in patients with autoimmune lymphoproliferative syndrome. Br. J. Haematol. 145 (1), 101–106.
Teachey, D.T., Seif, A.E., Grupp, S.A., 2010. Advances in the management and understanding of autoimmune lymphoproliferative syndrome (ALPS). Br. J. Haematol. 148 (2), 205–216.
Tiegs, S.L., Russell, D.M., Nemazee, D., 1993. Receptor editing in self-reactive bone marrow B cells. J. Exp. Med. 177 (4), 1009–1020.
Tison, B.E., Nicholas, S.K., Abramson, S.L., Hanson, I.C., Paul, M.E., Seeborg, F.O., Shearer, W.T., Perez, M.D., Noroski, L.M., Chinen, J., 2011. Autoimmunity in a cohort of 130 pediatric patients with partial DiGeorge syndrome. J. Allergy Clin. Immunol. 128 (5), 1115–1117, e1-3.
Tivol, E.A., Borriello, F., Schweitzer, A.N., Lynch, W.P., Bluestone, J.A., Sharpe, A.H., 1995. Loss of CTLA-4 leads to massive lymphoproliferation and fatal multiorgan tissue destruction, revealing a critical negative regulatory role of CTLA-4. Immunity 3 (5), 541–547.
Todoric, K., Koontz, J.B., Mattox, D., Tarrant, T.K., 2013. Autoimmunity in immunodeficiency. Curr. Allergy Asthma Rep. 13 (4), 361–370.
Turul, T., Tezcan, I., Artac, H., de Bruin-Versteeg, S., Barendregt, B.H., Reisli, I., Sanal, O., van Dongen, J.J., van der Burg, M., 2009. Clinical heterogeneity can hamper the diagnosis of patients with ZAP70 deficiency. Eur. J. Pediatr. 168 (1), 87–93.
Ueda, H., Howson, J.M., Esposito, L., Heward, J., Snook, H., Chamberlain, G., Rainbow, D.B., Hunter, K.M., Smith, A.N., Di Genova, G., et al., 2003. Association of the T-cell regulatory gene CTLA4 with susceptibility to autoimmune disease. Nature 423 (6939), 506–511.
Uzel, G., Sampaio, E.P., Lawrence, M.G., Hsu, A.P., Hackett, M., Dorsey, M.J., Noel, R.J., Verbsky, J.W., Freeman, A.F., Janssen, E., et al., 2013. Dominant gain-of-function STAT1 mutations in FOXP3 wild-type immune dysregulation-polyendocrinopathy-enteropathy-X-linked-like syndrome. J. Allergy Clin. Immunol. 131 (6), 1611–1623.
Valenzise, M., Alessi, L., Bruno, E., Cama, V., Costanzo, D., Genovese, C., Mignosa, C., Scuderi, V., De Luca, F., 2014. APECED syndrome in childhood: clinical spectrum is enlarging. Minerva Pediatr.
Vetrie, D., Vorechovsky, I., Sideras, P., Holland, J., Davies, A., Flinter, F., Hammarstrom, L., Kinnon, C., Levinsky, R., Bobrow, M., et al., 1993. The gene involved in X-linked agammaglobulinaemia is a member of the src family of protein-tyrosine kinases. Nature 361 (6409), 226–233.
Vignali, D., 2008. How many mechanisms do regulatory T cells need? Eur. J. Immunol. 38 (4), 908–911.
Vignali, D.A., Collison, L.W., Workman, C.J., 2008. How regulatory T cells work. Nat. Rev. Immunol. 8 (7), 523–532.
Villa, A., Santagata, S., Bozzi, F., Giliani, S., Frattini, A., Imberti, L., Gatta, L.B., Ochs, H.D., Schwarz, K., Notarangelo, L.D., et al., 1998. Partial V(D)J recombination activity leads to Omenn syndrome. Cell 93 (5), 885–896.
Villa, A., Notarangelo, L.D., Roifman, C.M., 2008. Omenn syndrome: inflammation in leaky severe combined immunodeficiency. J. Allergy Clin. Immunol. 122 (6), 1082–1086.
Walter, J.E., Rucci, F., Patrizi, L., Recher, M., Regenass, S., Paganini, T., Keszei, M., Pessach, I., Lang, P.A., Poliani, P.L., et al., 2010. Expansion of immunoglobulin-secreting cells and defects in B cell tolerance in Rag-dependent immunodeficiency. J. Exp. Med. 207 (7), 1541–1554.
Walter, J.E., Rosen, L.B., Csomos, K., Rosenberg, J.M., Mathew, D., Keszei, M., Ujhazi, B., Chen, K., Lee, Y.N., Tirosh, I., Dobbs, K., Al-Herz, W., Cowan, M., Puck, J., Bleesing, J., Grimley, M.S., Melch, H., De Ravin, S.S., Gennery, A.R., Abraham, R.S., Joshi, A.Y., Boyce, T.G., Butte, M.J., Nadeau, K.C., Balboni, I., Sullivan, K.E., Akhter, J., Adeli, M., El-Feky, R., El-Ghoneimy, D., Dbaibo, G., Wakim, R., Azzari, C., Palma, P., Cancrini, C., Capuder, K., Condino-Neto, A., Costa-Carvalho, B.T., Oliveira, J.B., Roifman, C., Buchbinder, D., Kumanovics, A., Franco, J.L., Niehues, T., Schuetz, C., Kuijpers, T., Yee, C., Chou, J., Masaad, M.M., Geha, R., Uzel, G., Geller, R., Holland, S.M., Recher, M., Utz, P.J., Browne, S.K., Notarangelo, L.D., Broad spectrum antibodies to self-antigens and cytokines in RAG deficiency. J. Clin. Invest., in press.

Wang, J., Cunningham-Rundles, C., 2005. Treatment and outcome of autoimmune hematologic disease in common variable immunodeficiency (CVID). J. Autoimmun. 25 (1), 57–62.
Wardemann, H., Yurasov, S., Schaefer, A., Young, J.W., Meffre, E., Nussenzweig, M.C., 2003. Predominant autoantibody production by early human B cell precursors. Science 301 (5638), 1374–1377.
Watanabe, N., Wang, Y.H., Lee, H.K., Ito, T., Wang, Y.H., Cao, W., Liu, Y.J., 2005. Hassall's corpuscles instruct dendritic cells to induce CD4+CD25+ regulatory T cells in human thymus. Nature 436 (7054), 1181–1185.
Waterhouse, P., Penninger, J.M., Timms, E., Wakeham, A., Shahinian, A., Lee, K.P., Thompson, C.B., Griesser, H., Mak, T.W., 1995. Lymphoproliferative disorders with early lethality in mice deficient in Ctla-4. Science 270 (5238), 985–988.
Wildin, R.S., Smyk-Pearson, S., Filipovich, A.H., 2002. Clinical and molecular features of the immunodysregulation, polyendocrinopathy, enteropathy, X linked (IPEX) syndrome. J. Med. Genet. 39 (8), 537–545.
Wong, G.K., Goldacker, S., Winterhalter, C., Grimbacher, B., Chapel, H., Lucas, M., Alecsandru, D., McEwen, D., Quinti, I., Martini, H., et al., 2013. Outcomes of splenectomy in patients with common variable immunodeficiency (CVID): a survey of 45 patients. Clin. Exp. Immunol. 172 (1), 63–72.
Zhang, X., Kimura, Y., Fang, C., Zhou, L., Sfyroera, G., Lambris, J.D., Wetsel, R.A., Miwa, T., Song, W.C., 2007. Regulation of Toll-like receptor-mediated inflammatory response by complement in vivo. Blood 110 (1), 228–236.
Zohar, Y., Wildbaum, G., Novak, R., Salzman, A.L., Thelen, M., Alon, R., Barsheshet, Y., Karp, C.L., Karin, N., 2014. CXCL11-dependent induction of FOXP3-negative regulatory T cells suppresses autoimmune encephalomyelitis. J. Clin. Invest. 124 (5), 2009–2022.
Zuklys, S., Balciunaite, G., Agarwal, A., Fasler-Kan, E., Palmer, E., Hollander, G.A., 2000. Normal thymic architecture and negative selection are associated with Aire expression, the gene defective in the autoimmune-polyendocrinopathy-candidiasis-ectodermal dystrophy (APECED). J. Immunol. 165 (4), 1976–1983.

CHAPTER 3

Phenome-Wide Association Study

J.L. Warner, J.C. Denny
Vanderbilt University, Nashville, TN, United States

Contents

1. INTRODUCTION

Typically, genetic and biomarker association studies have begun with cases and controls for a well-defined disease phenotype and have asked whether biomarkers or genetic variants are associated with the disease. The standard for genetic studies has become the genome-wide association study (GWAS) and, more recently, whole-exome or genome sequencing

Translational Immunology
http://dx.doi.org/10.1016/B978-0-12-801577-3.00003-4

studies, both of which can assay hundreds of thousands to billions of genetic variants. These large-scale studies have led to the serendipitous discovery of some instances in which genetic variants can be associated with multiple diseases, a condition termed pleiotropy. The purpose of this chapter is to introduce a set of techniques that are collectively referred to as phenotype-wide association studies (PheWAS). PheWAS is essentially the reverse experiment of a GWAS, and provides a systematic method for studying what diseases or traits may be associated with a given genetic variant or biomarker. In essence, the PheWAS concept is simple: perform a series of statistical tests across a human population of varying phenotypes, to discover significant associations with some defining factor of interest (eg, single-nucleotide polymorphisms (SNPs)). PheWAS can also be applied to other biomarkers, such as laboratory test results or even physical exam findings. Due to the nature in which the data of interest are captured in electronic health records (EHRs), the capability to perform large, well-powered PheWAS studies now exists across many institutions—in part thanks to endeavors such as Informatics for Integrating Biology and the Bedside (i2b2) at the national level (Murphy et al., 2010; Kohane, 2011; Kohane et al., 2012) and institutional efforts such as the BioVU project at Vanderbilt (Roden et al., 2008; Danciu et al., 2014). In practice, each step in a PheWAS can be quite challenging: (1) defining and normalizing the independent variable(s); (2) defining the phenotypes; (3) identifying cases and controls; (4) choosing the appropriate statistical test(s); (5) defining thresholds of significance; and (6) interpreting and visualizing the results.

In this chapter, we will first review the history of phenotyping in the medical record, which has been an evolution over centuries, but not approached systematically or comprehensively until relatively recently. We will then introduce the PheWAS concept in some detail, and review some of the published studies to date. Next, we will review PheWAS techniques dealing with noncategorical (eg, continuous) data. Finally, we will focus on some future directions for PheWAS, including the integration of network analytics and of data that reside outside of traditional EHRs.

2. PHENOTYPING FROM THE MEDICAL RECORD

2.1 History of the classification of the human phenome

The idea of classifying, or compartmentalizing, the spectrum of diseases afflicting the human condition dates back centuries and has its roots in public health efforts. Back when human life was considered to be "nasty, brutish, and short" the exact reasons for so much mortality were obscure (Hobbes, 1651). Aside from well-recorded instances of periodic plagues and deaths due to war activities, very little detail was available about causes of death. Spurred by the extreme mortality resulting from plague, some information about causes of death began to be recorded as early as the mid-fifteenth century, in Italy (Moriyama et al., 2011). In the early 1530s, the city of London began to collect detailed weekly records of "Bills of Mortality." These were concatenated and published by John Graunt as the "Natural and Political Observations Made upon the Bills of Mortality," which may be the earliest attempt to define the human phenome (Graunt, 1662). This treatise was updated periodically and also included rudimentary death tables, as shown in Fig. 1. Afflictions recognizable to the contemporary clinician, such as plague, tuberculosis, thrush, scurvy, and rickets, are accompanied by unfamiliar ones, such as "teeth and worms" (death of an infant when

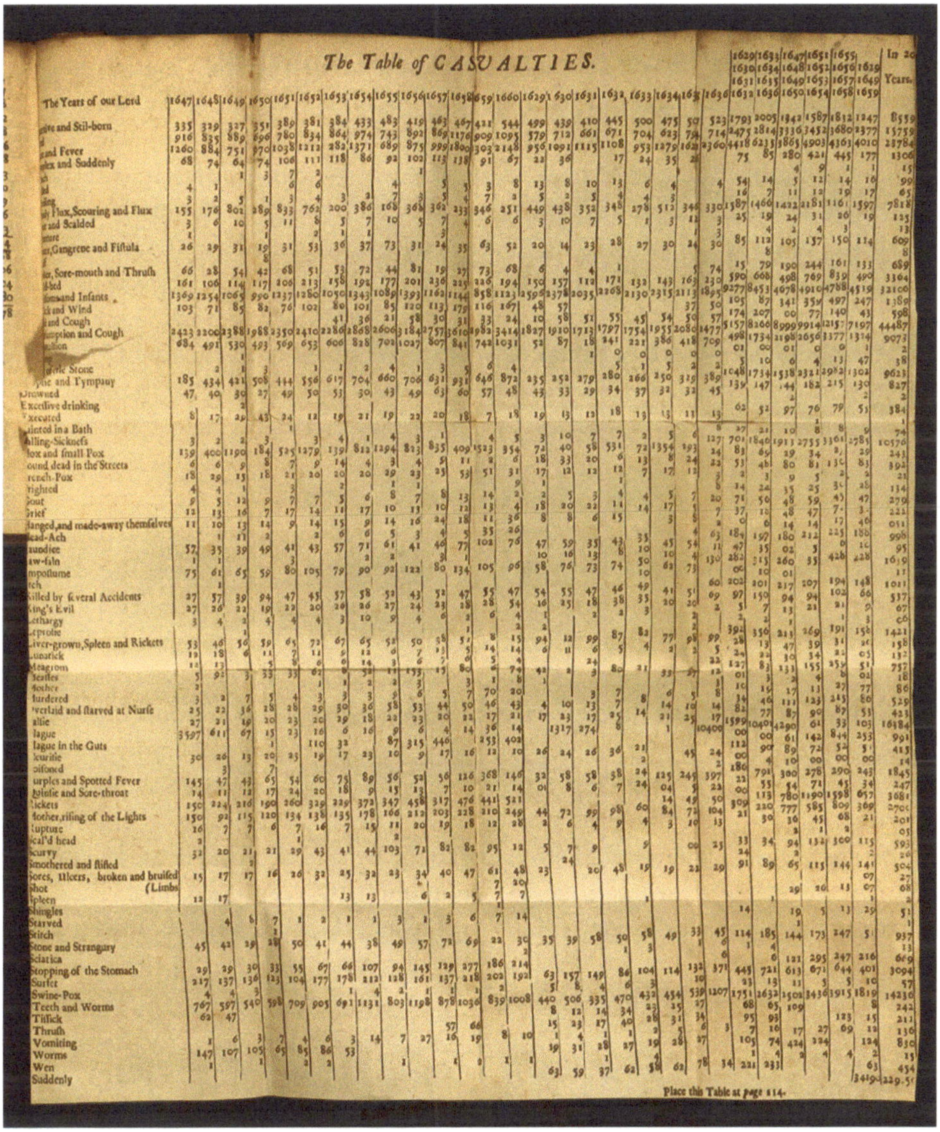
The Table of CASUALTIES.

Place this Table at page 114.

Figure 1 A page from the 5th edition of John Graunt's *Natural and Political Observations Made Upon the Bills of Mortality, 1676. (Reproduced with permission from The Royal Society).*

teething or convulsions associated with teething, worms, elevated temperature, or diarrhea), surfet (vomiting from overeating or gluttony), and "rising of the lights" (generally considered to be croup) (definitions in parentheses from the Glossary of Old Disease Names: http://www.homeoint.org/cazalet/oldnames.htm).

The next serious effort to classify human disease occurred nearly 200 years later, in 1853. This was the year that the First International Statistical Congress was held in Brussels, and amongst other topics, "Causes of Death" was discussed, with a focus on the need for uniformity across countries, for comparison purposes. The task of developing a uniform classification schema fell upon two medical statisticians: Marc-Jacob D'Espine of Geneva, Switzerland and William Farr of England. In a foreshadowing of some of the challenges that still confront medical phenotyping to this day, D'Espine and Farr came up with disparate methods for classification; D'Espine classified diseases by their nature (eg, affecting the joints, the liver, the heart, and so forth) whereas Farr classified diseases by their behavior (eg, general diseases, those affecting specific locations, developmental diseases, etc.). These differences were resolved by committee and led to the formulation of "the 1855 list" of 139 causes of death. This list and subsequent revisions did not really gain much traction until 1860, when Florence Nightingale proposed the systematic collection of hospital data across England. This suggestion was carried out approximately 30 years later for the city of Paris, by a physician named Jacques Bertillon, who introduced the Bertillon Classification of Causes of Death in 1893. This systematized nomenclature was based on the distinction between conditions afflicting the whole organism versus those that were organ-specific, although it initially had only 44 classes of disease. As this volume was translated into other languages, it was also revised and expanded to 161 classes in 5 short years. The American Public Health Association (founded in 1872 and still operating) recommended adoption of the nomenclature in 1898 with an important additional stipulation; that it be revised once per decade "to keep up with the progress of medical science." This recommendation led to the inaugural International Conference for the Revision of the International List of Causes of Death, held in Paris on August 18, 1900. The product of this meeting was the "First Revision": ICD-1. Revisions did occur with regularity, although it was not until the 6th revision (ICD-6) that the classification schema began to resemble its current form. In 1948 this new edition introduced morbidity to the Bertillon nomenclature and the acronym was reconfigured as the International Classification of *Diseases* (also abbreviated ICD). With this important change in focus from mortality to morbidity, the stage was set for electronic phenotyping. For a much more detailed overview, the interested reader is directed to the monograph by Moriyama et al. (2011).

2.2 Phenotyping from ICD data

The current version of ICD being used in the United States is the ICD-9-CM, where the CM stands for "Clinical Modification." Elsewhere around the world, ICD-10 has been adopted; ICD-10-CM is due to be adopted in the United States on October 1, 2015, after several delays. ICD-9-CM has approximately 17,000 descriptive codes covering the gamut of human disease; ICD-10-CM will have nearly 68,000. This breadth, along with the widespread requirement that ICD codes be used to justify the billing of medical encounters, led to the current situation where a patient's phenotype can potentially be well described through the judicious use of billing codes.

Typically, the billing for an outpatient encounter (including doctor's visits, laboratory and radiology testing, etc.) can be justified with up to five ICD codes; inpatient hospitalizations allow for many more. What this means is that, with a longitudinal EHR, a patient with regular contact with the health care system can accumulate hundreds or thousands of individual billing codes, which begin to offer a complex phenotype representation. In typical practice, we have seen that an individual typically has an average of 34 *distinct* ICD-9-CM codes, while cohorts that have been chosen for research have had up to an average of 107 distinct ICD-9-CM codes per person (Denny et al., 2013).

It must be noted that some clinicians do not enthusiastically support the idea of a systematic classification of disease conditions. This is most true for the psychiatric diseases (Meyer-Lindenberg, 2010). While there is an ongoing effort to classify these conditions (the most well-known being the Diagnostic and Statistical Manual of Mental Disorders, currently in its Fifth Edition (American Psychiatric Association, 2013)), some argue that by their nature, psychiatric conditions are unique to the individual afflicted (Jablensky, 1988). Others have shown that psychiatric phenotypes such as treatment-resistant depression can be extracted from EHRs with natural language processing (NLP; see Section 2.4.5) (Perlis et al., 2012).

2.3 Challenges of the current ICD classification

Although the current ICD system of disease nomenclature can be unwieldy, it is also a very useful starting point to approach the analysis of human phenotypes. Nevertheless, there are some significant issues with the ICD system that must be understood before using the system for phenotyping purposes. Some of the notable shortcomings are summarized as follows and then briefly discussed in turn.

- Numeric organization that is not based on clinical or biological knowledge
- Widespread use of the terms "not otherwise specified (NOS)" and "not elsewhere classified (NEC)" for disease names
- Diseases not found in the classification system
- Jumble of subclassifications by anatomy, status, etc.
- Institutional variability

2.3.1 Numeric organization

The original ordinal basis of Bertillon's classification system was by convenience and anatomically based; the ICD revisions loosely followed this system of chapters with the introduction of disease-specific chapters such as Chapter 1: Infectious Diseases and Chapter 2: Neoplasms. Individual diseases are numbered to the fourth or fifth significant digit, with three digits before and one or two after a decimal point. The numbering of diseases across the chapters does not follow logic, however (eg, Chapter 1 ranges from 001.0 to 139.8, whereas Chapter 2 ranges from 140.0 to 239.9). The arbitrariness of an ordinal system is worsened by the fact that, due to mainly historical reasons, the numeric axis is nonlinear. This is perhaps best illustrated by the fact that tuberculosis, a disease with different manifestations but all caused by a single microorganism, occupies the territory of 010.00–018.96 and 137.*, whereas type 1 diabetes mellitus (T1DM) and type 2 diabetes mellitus (T2DM), which have different pathophysiology and are usually treated distinctly differently, are both coded under 250.* (250.00 is T2DM [or unspecified; see below] and 250.01 is T2DM).

2.3.2 Widespread NOS and NEC classifications

Although medical knowledge is admittedly not all-encompassing, the widespread use of these terms, along with derivations such as "unspecified" or "other specified" throughout the ICD classification is useful for billing but problematic for understanding a patient's true disease. Essentially, these definitions rely on other ICD codes to delineate their formal definition. Again, two examples are illustrative of the problem. Consider ICD-9-CM code 189.8: Malignant neoplasm of other specified sites of urinary organs. In order to consider what this code might encompass, one must possess the knowledge that there are specific codes for kidney, renal pelvis, ureter, urethra, and paraurethral glands in ICD-9-CM. As another example, consider the very frequently used ICD-9-CM code 038.9: Unspecified septicemia. What is it that is unspecified? Is it the causative organism (eg, 038.10: Staphylococcal septicemia)? Is it a description of the nature of the bacteria (eg, 038.12: Methicillin resistant *Staphylococcus aureus* septicemia)? Is it a description of the vehicle of the sepsis (eg, 999.39: Sepsis following infusion, injection, transfusion and/or vaccination; 659.3: Septicemia during labor) or of the host (eg, 771.81: Septicemia of newborn)? Note that many of these codes have no numeric relationship to the "unspecified" code, which has been colocated to the codes representing particular causative microorganisms. While this was a choice of the designers of ICD-9-CM, it does not necessarily follow that clinicians or billing coders have used the code in the organism-specific sense. The fact that many NOS/NEC codes such as 038.9 are billable for reimbursement leads to their overrepresentation in ICD-defined phenotypes, as they are often the "path of least resistance." For further reading on the topic of NOS/NEC, we refer the reader to the excellent paper by Cimino, "Desiderata for Controlled Medical Vocabularies in the Twenty-First Century" (Cimino, 1998).

2.3.3 Missing diseases

The ICD system can be quite comprehensive, although this comprehensiveness is not evenly distributed over the span of human diseases. An example was given before, with the many codes covering various facets of human tubercular disease. Another example is from ICD-10-CM, which separately specifies injuries caused by chickens (*W61.33: Pecked by chicken*), turkeys (*W61.43: Pecked by turkey*), ducks (*W61.61: Bitten by duck*), and geese (*W61.51: Bitten by goose*). The coding system even lets a user specify whether the unfortunate victim was struck (*W61.32*), pecked (*W61.33*), or had "other contact" with the chicken (*W61.39*) (another example of the NOS/NEC problem; see above). While this tour de force of domestic fowl incidents might help the phenotyper with an interest in the deleterious effects of animal husbandry, other conditions are left out. For example, disease-specific characteristics with treatment implications, such as the presence of the *BCR:ABL* T315I mutation in chronic myelogenous leukemia, which confers resistance to most available tyrosine kinase inhibitors, is not represented in any ICD system. Additionally, rare diseases are underrepresented. In a recent evaluation, Fung et al. (2014) compared a list of 6519 rare diseases assembled by the Office of Rare Diseases Research to concepts present in ICD-9-CM, ICD-10-CM, and SNOMED-CT (see Section 2.4.1). They found that only 11% of these rare diseases were represented in ICD-9-CM; ICD-10-CM fared little better with 21% coverage; SNOMED-CT had the best performance but still only 44% coverage. This has unfortunate implications for the usefulness of the ICD system for phenotyping of rare diseases and unusual syndromes.

2.3.4 Jumble of subclassifications

ICD is by nature hierarchical. That is, the three digit codes are considered "parents" of the four digit codes, and the four digit codes are "parents" of the five digit codes. For example, 123 is the parent of 123.1, which is the parent of 123.11. While this hierarchical schema makes a great deal of sense, and hierarchies tend to be internally consistent, they are by no means consistent across disease entities. This is well illustrated by two lymphoid malignancies: Hodgkin's disease and multiple myeloma. In Table 1, the parent codes and the first three codes from each of the nested hierarchies are shown. In this case, the Level One hierarchy is consistent across the two disease entities, and is based on histology. However, the Level Two hierarchy differs completely: in the case of Hodgkin's lymphoma, it is an *anatomic* subclassification, whereas in multiple myeloma, it is a *disease status* subclassification. Unfortunately, there are many similar instances across ICD, an echo of the divergent approaches to disease classification in the 1850s.

2.3.5 Institutional variability

With the preceding discussion of some of the challenges of ICD, it should come as no surprise that there might be considerable variability across regions and local institutions. Although some degree of variability would be expected to represent true local variations in the phenotypes of populations, much variability is also due to local coding practices and customs. It bears emphasizing that ICD codes are an abstraction, often several times removed from reality. Consider these two extremes and how the ICD encoding might

Table 1 The left-most column contains the parent ICD-9-CM codes; the middle column contains the first three child codes (in numeric order) of the parent, and the right-most column contains the first three child codes of the first child code in the middle column

Parent code	Level one hierarchy	Level two hierarchy
201: Hodgkin's disease	201.0 Hodgkin's paragranuloma	201.00: Hodgkin's paragranuloma, unspecified site, extranodal and solid organ sites
	201.1 Hodgkin's granuloma	201.01: Hodgkin's paragranuloma, lymph nodes of head, face, and neck
	201.2 Hodgkin's sarcoma	201.02: Hodgkin's paragranuloma, intrathoracic lymph nodes
203: Multiple myeloma and immunoproliferative neoplasms	203.0: Multiple myeloma	203.00: Multiple myeloma, without mention of having achieved remission
	203.1: Plasma cell leukemia	203.01: Multiple myeloma, in remission
	203.8: Other immunoproliferative neoplasms	203.02: Multiple myeloma, in relapse

differ: Patient John Smith has rheumatoid arthritis (RA) and has seen the same specialist for more than a decade, 3–4 times per year. Over that period of time, the specialist has diagnosed several RA-associated conditions, and recorded these while filling out the outpatient billing forms shortly after each visit. Patient Sally Jones has acute leukemia and spends 30 days in the hospital, during which time she is transferred to and from the intensive care unit twice. She sees approximately 50 different medical providers during this period, some of whom may generate distinct but short lists of ICD codes for professional services rendered. When she is discharged, a busy resident who has known her for 2 days is responsible for writing the discharge summary of her entire hospital stay. A nonclinician billing coder then abstracts the information contained within the discharge summary to develop a potentially large list of ICD codes. While John Smith and Sally Jones both will have a complex phenotype, it is more likely that Mr Smith has a "truer" representation of his complex disease process than Ms Jones.

Several studies have sought to compare the accuracy of ICD codes to other sources such as population surveys. For example, Orueta et al. (2012) found considerable variance in the prevalence of chronic diseases in ICD-9-CM billing data compared to the Basque Health Interview Study. Muggah et al. (2013) found poor agreement between administrative data and self-report for stroke, congestive heart failure, and COPD in a population of ~85,000 Canadians. The published data on variability between ICD coding practices at differing institutions are not robust; however, Schildcrout et al.

(2010) demonstrated that patients with similar diseases tend to have similar ICD distributions between sites. In addition, phenotype definitions relying on ICD data across different sites have shown high validity at multiple institutions (Denny et al., 2011; Carroll et al., 2012; Kho et al., 2012).

2.4 Other sources of phenotype data in EHRs

As the complexity and comprehensiveness of EHRs continues to grow, new sources of phenotyping data are becoming available (Pathak et al., 2013). Most of the early EHRs were simply elaborate billing systems, and as such the administrative data such as the ICD billing codes have historically been the most plentiful. Given the numerous limitations described above, there is great interest in utilizing new data sources to increase the richness and accuracy of electronic phenotyping. Here, we briefly discuss some of these alternative data sources.

2.4.1 SNOMED-CT

The Systematized Nomenclature of Medicine (SNOMED) has a more recent pedigree than ICD, having been founded in 1973 by the College of American Pathologists. Unlike ICD, SNOMED was designed with the computer in mind, and the "Clinical Terms" (CT) expansion even more so. SNOMED-CT is a rigorously hierarchical terminology, where all relationships are defined by the "*is a*" concept. Thus, SNOMED-CT can be broad, deep, and expandable. SNOMED-CT does have its limitations, many of which are pragmatic (Ingenerf and Linder, 2009; Schulz et al., 2009), but the coverage of clinical diagnoses, signs, and symptoms can be much more extensive than ICD, as in the case of rare diseases. Many EHR vendors have incorporated SNOMED-CT for varying parts of their products; eg, problem lists that are driven in part by the increased importance of semantic interoperability (Tapuria et al., 2013) and incentive-driven mandates such as the Medicare/Medicaid EHR Incentive Program (Meaningful Use) (Blumenthal, 2010).

2.4.2 PHIN-VADS

The Public Health Information Network Vocabulary Access and Distribution System (PHIN-VADS) was created by the US Centers for Disease Control and Prevention in 2009 to standardize the reporting of conditions of interest to public health. This includes communicable diseases and other reportable conditions such as cancer. Some of the advantages of PHIN-VADS are the ability to rapidly create and disseminate new terminologies. For example, in October 2014 the "Ebola Virus Disease (EVD) Reporting" terminology was released, with seven coded data elements (eg, "Symptoms (EVD Triage)") with eight allowed concepts (abdominal pain, weakness, fever, headache, hemorrhage, muscle pain, vomiting, other) which are standardized to SNOMED-CT. A disadvantage to PHIN-VADS is that many EHR vendors have not yet adopted the system except for rudimentary reporting needs.

2.4.3 "Universal" terminologies

With even the modest number of terminologies that have been introduced thus far, it would not be surprising if the reader were to ask: "Why can't there just be one master terminology for all of medicine?" While this desire is understandable, that situation is unlikely to come to pass, for several reasons. First, many terminologies are based on information models that are incompatible, hearkening back to the original experience of D'Espine and Farr. Second, many terminologies are protected by intellectual property, such as the Common Procedural Terminology (CPT©, American Medical Association). Third, there is a role for purpose-built terminologies of limited scope, such as the ebola virus reporting. To attempt to provide a solution, the Unified Medical Language System (UMLS) was begun in 1986 by the US National Library of Medicine (Humphreys et al., 1998). This remains the most comprehensive source of medical terminologies, with over 150 different terminologies, including SNOMED-CT, ICD-9-CM, ICD-10-CM, and many other vocabularies. The UMLS links like concepts from separate vocabularies together using concept unique identifiers. For instance, "congestive heart failure" in the UMLS has a single identifier of C0018802 that includes ICD-9-CM (428.0), ICD-10-CM (I50.9), and SNOMED-CT (42343007) concepts. The UMLS also includes many synonyms, abbreviations, and multiple languages for concepts. Major limitations of UMLS are that it inherits the advantages and disadvantages of the underlying vocabularies, the mappings are not perfect, and EHR vendors have not necessarily robustly implemented it.

2.4.4 Indirect measures of phenotype

Much of the information captured in structured fashion in EHRs can be used to infer phenotype. Procedural codes can be quite specific to certain diseases. For example, a patient with a CPT code recorded for percutaneous transluminal balloon angioplasty of a renal artery can be fairly assumed to have renal artery stenosis.

Another potentially rich source of inferential phenotyping data is medication information. There are three important structured sources of medication information that are present in most modern EHRs: computerized provider order entry (CPOE), electronic medication administration records (eMARs), and outpatient electronic prescribing "e-prescribing" tools. CPOE best reflects the *intent* of the ordering physician, whereas eMAR is the actual record of medications received (there is of course not a 1:1 correlation, as patients with capacity are free to refuse medications, whether or not this is in their best interest). Because of the closed nature of the environment, inpatient data are usually more complete than outpatient data. While many medications may have multiple indications, many others are quite specific to a particular phenotype or small set of phenotypes. For example, rituximab is essentially prescribed for only two purposes: (1) the treatment of B-lymphocyte malignancies and (2) the treatment of antibody-mediated autoimmune processes, such as rheumatoid arthritis, autoimmune thrombocytopenia, and pemphigus. Compare that to aspirin, which is prescribed in a wide variety of conditions. Phenotype can thus be inferred for a subset of very specific drugs. Even drugs with more than one indication can be used to infer a probabilistic phenotype. It is important to note that many prescriptions, however, may only be noted in the clinical documentation; eg, phone call records from pharmacies or a provider who handwrites a prescription. Expensive medications (eg, biologics) are often routed through specialty pharmacies and not well-traced in the EHR environment. For these, NLP approaches can be used to identify medications prescribed to patients (see the next section).

Laboratory data are another very important indirect measure of phenotype. Analogous to medications, for phenotyping purposes there are two types of laboratory data: the CPOE, which reflects the *intent* of the ordering provider, and the actual laboratory results. It is often possible to make inferences of phenotype when the results are not present or not available, perhaps due to being stored in an inaccessible image format. HLA-B27 testing on a young male patient may enable an inference about the presence of ankylosing spondylitis (AS), whereas hepatitis C viral genotyping would only ever be ordered on a patient with hepatitis C infection. Conversely, the complete blood counts are ordered routinely for almost all patients and thus their presence or absence in the medical record does not correlate with the presence or absence of a phenotype.

2.4.5 Clinical narratives

The bulk of medical documentation continues to reside in prose format. This is due to the simple fact that natural language allows for expressivity that cannot be easily captured in structured formats (Rosenbloom et al., 2011). While there has been a move toward a more structured clinical documentation in some realms, notably synoptic reporting in pathology (Rosenbloom et al., 2004, 2013; Srigley et al., 2009), much of the clinical narrative for the process of documenting a patient's presentation, radiological findings, differential diagnoses, and treatment plan remains in free text. Thus, the narrative clinical record will remain a major potential source for phenotype information. In a comprehensive EHR system, this includes clinical progress notes, hospital documents, letters to patients and providers, informal communications such as telephone calls, interpretations of complex medical tests such as pulmonary function testing, and pathology and radiology reports. Additionally, many EHRs contain a centralized longitudinal problem list, which may be periodically or continuously updated. An example of the information content of structured versus unstructured (narrative) data is shown in Fig. 2.

NLP is a subspecialty of computer science and computational linguistics that seeks to address the problem of transforming prose into machine-computable data. Although the exact date of the birth of the subspecialty is debated, its origins stem from the famous Turing Test (Turing, 1950). Clinical NLP is the subdomain of NLP that focuses specifically on the extraction of clinical concepts, assertions, and relationships (Nadkarni et al., 2011). A review of clinical NLP is beyond the scope of this chapter, but a summary of

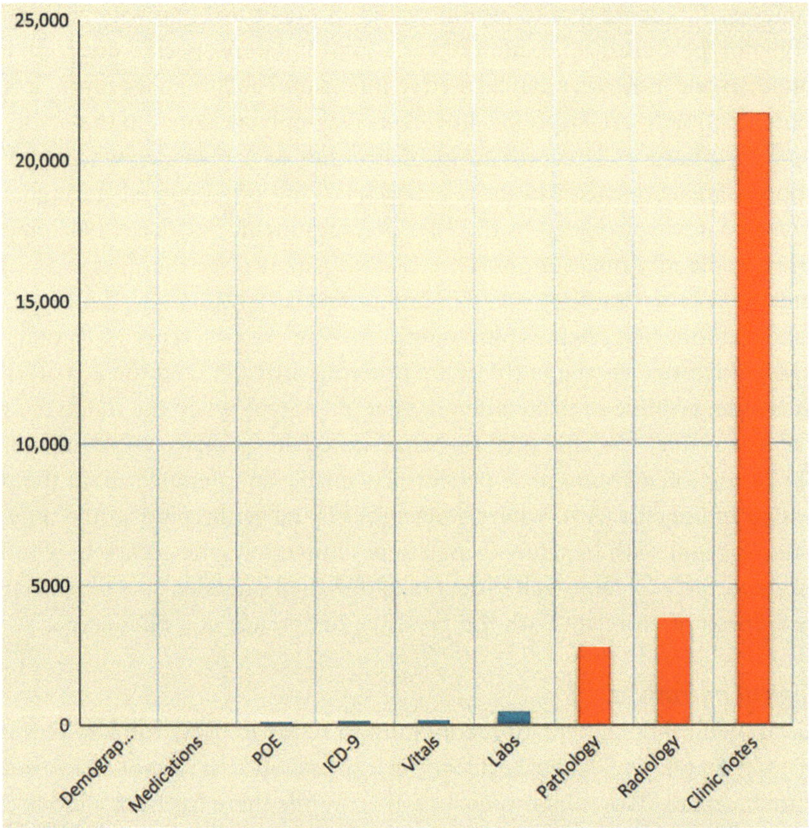

Figure 2 The information content of structured (blue) versus unstructured (red) data for a single patient who has undergone diagnosis, staging, and treatment for diffuse large B-cell lymphoma. This particular patient had, in an approximately 6-month period 21 demographic measurements (eg, gender, ethnicity, age); 34 prescriptions; 106 provider order entry events; 136 ICD-9-CM codes; 167 vital sign measurements; 484 laboratory value measurements; eight pathology reports containing 2779 words; eight radiology reports containing 3803 words; and 26 oncology clinic notes containing 21,702 words. Not shown are 277 pages of scanned PDFs from outside facilities, corresponding to approximately 69,250 words (250 words per page), which are essentially unusable for secondary analysis.

accomplishments include extraction of medication exposure information (Xu et al., 2010); extraction of adverse drug effects (Aramaki et al., 2010); identification of postoperative complications (Murff et al., 2011); and quantification of the degree of redundancy present in EHRs (Wrenn et al., 2010). The interested reader is directed to several recent reviews of the subject (Meystre et al., 2008; Sun et al., 2013).

2.5 Putting it all together

It is obvious from this overview of methods of phenotyping (a.k.a. phenomics) that there is no one "source of truth" in the EHR (Lanktree et al., 2010; Pathak et al., 2013).

Rather, there are many competing imperfect data sources, each with their pros and cons. Due to their ubiquity, ICD codes remain the most common source of phenotyping today, although there are two notable efforts focussed on developing an unambiguous relational definition of phenotype: the Human Phenotype Ontology project (Kohler et al., 2014) and the Human Disease Ontology database (Kibbe et al., 2015). Many investigators have begun to evaluate the accuracy of combining various structured and unstructured data sources (Wright et al., 2011; Boland et al., 2013b; Shivade et al., 2014). Here, we briefly discuss the National Human Genome Research Institute's (NHGRI) Electronic Medical Records and Genomics (eMERGE) network as an example of a consortium using EHR data for genomic investigation.

Started in 2007, the eMERGE network was funded with the goal of using the EHRs linked to DNA biobanks for genomic and pharmacogenomic investigation (Gottesman et al., 2013). eMERGE initially included five sites (McCarty et al., 2011), and expanded to nine sites by 2012 and currently includes in excess of 100,000 patients with GWAS samples linked to EHR data (Gottesman et al., 2013). The primary model of investigation has been into particular phenotypes using algorithms that combine billing codes, medication exposures, laboratory data, and NLP for particular phenotypes, such as cataracts (Peissig et al., 2012), T2DM (Kho et al., 2012), and hypothyroidism (Denny et al., 2011). Importantly, each algorithm includes algorithms to find both cases and controls (because absence of a disease, especially common diseases such as diabetes, cataracts, and hypothyroidism, cannot be assumed). Algorithms are typically validated through manual chart review of randomly selected cases to determine positive predictive values. Often the algorithms are rule-based, but others have utilized machine learning approaches such as trained logistic regression models (Liao et al., 2010) or support vector machines (Lin et al., 2014). Many of these algorithms have been collected for reuse by others at http://PheKB.org.

3. PHENOME-WIDE ASSOCIATION STUDIES

3.1 Introduction to and overview of the PheWAS methodology

The eMERGE phenotyping approaches just described are designed to capture genetic associations with a single disease or trait, such as the typical GWAS. Such analyses by their nature cannot identify pleiotropic associations except by observation from multiple independent studies, and may also miss important confounders in an analysis, such as the correlation between T2DM and obesity, a famous example of "pseudopleiotropy" seen in an early GWAS for T2DM not adjusted for body mass index (Wellcome Trust Case Control Consortium, 2007). PheWAS is an alternative approach, enabled by densely phenotyped records such as those included in the EHR. The first PheWAS (and most subsequently) have focussed on a reverse genetics approach starting with a variant of interest (the independent variable) and studying the effect it has on a wide range of phenotypes. PheWAS investigations require large representative patient populations with definable phenotypic characteristics. The first and majority of PheWAS to date have leveraged EHR billing code data but subsequent PheWAS have also used cohort observational data as well (see Table 3).

The first demonstration of the PheWAS approach used 6005 patients genotyped for five SNPs with seven previously known disease associations (Denny et al., 2010). This PheWAS used ICD-9-CM codes linked to a code-translation table that mapped the ~17,000 ICD-9-CM codes to 776 disease phenotypes, each matched to a control definition. Although the translational table used the three-digit groupings as a guide, the primary mapping were driven by suspected etiology to create new groupings. For example, codes that represented common etiologies were brought together (eg, creating a single "tuberculosis" code group), and diseases with distinct etiologies combined into one three-digit ICD-9-CM code were separated, such as T1DM and T2DM. Finally, ICD-9-CM codes that were unlikely to be useful in a genetic context, such as external injury "E codes" were marked as "ignorable."

In addition, we used the ICD-9-CM coding system to generate comparison groups (controls) for all case groups, which included all patients that did not have a prevalent ICD-9-CM code belonging to a specified list of disease exclusions defined for each case group. Eligibility to the control group required absence of the case disease and related diseases. For example, controls for Crohn's disease excluded patients with Crohn's, ulcerative colitis, and several other related gastrointestinal complaints. In this study, PheWAS methods replicated four of seven previously known associations with $p \leq 0.011$. Fig. 3 shows one illustrative Manhattan plot of phenotype associations with an HLA-DRA

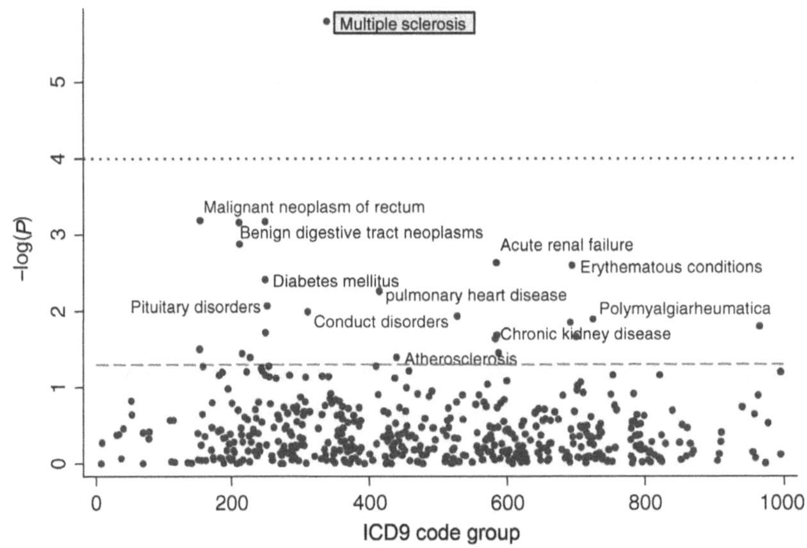

Figure 3 Phenome-wide scan for association with rs3135388. MS is replicated from prior analyses. The dashed line represents $P = 0.05$; the dotted line represents the Bonferroni correction. *(Denny et al. (2010), by permission of Oxford University Press).*

SNP known to be associated with multiple sclerosis. Of note, this PheWAS also highlights other possible associations, such as Type 1 diabetes, acquired hypothyroidism, and "erythematous conditions" (which includes the diagnosis of lupus). This latter possible association was later replicated in another PheWAS by Hebbring et al. (2013), performed with similar ICD-9-CM data from the Marshfield Clinic Personalized Medicine Research Program.

Since that original PheWAS study, the code mapping has been revised and expanded to include 1689 hierarchical phenotypes with 1087 leaf concepts by (1) including V and E billing codes in the PheWAS code mapping, (2) redesigning the code system to include hierarchical relationships such that one phenotype could be a parent of another "subphenotype" (eg, cardiac arrhythmias is a parent of atrial fibrillation, atrial flutter, and other arrhythmias), and (3) including more granular phenotypes into the coding system (eg, "T1DM with ketoacidosis," which has a parent phenotype of "T1DM"). In this model, an individual with "T1DM with ketoacidosis" receives all appropriate hierarchical phenotypes during the mapping: "diabetes mellitus," "T1DM," and "T1DM with ketoacidosis." The development of parent hierarchical phenotypes included creation of new phenotypes not present in the ICD-9-CM billing hierarchy, such as "inflammatory bowel disease" as the parent phenotype for "Crohn's disease" and "ulcerative colitis." In this process, we were guided by the hierarchical organization of the Clinical Classifications Software (CCS) produced by the Agency for Healthcare Research and Quality which contains >700 hierarchical phenotypes designed primarily for epidemiological research (Cowen et al., 1998). An example of the ICD-9-CM to PheWAS mappings and control groups is shown in Table 2.

Table 2 Example ICD-9-CM mappings to PheWAS codes and control groupings

PheWAS code	PheWAS Phenotype	ICD-9-CM codes to be a case	Controls cannot have these ICD-9-CMs
250	Diabetes	250.*	250.* (Diabetes), 249.* (secondary diabetes), 790.2* (abnormal glucose codes), V45.85 (insulin pump), and other insulin pump codes
250.1	Type 1 diabetes	250.01 250.11 250.21	
250.2	Type 2 diabetes	250.00 250.10 250.20	
714	Rheumatoid and other inflammatory arthritis	714.*	714.* (rheumatoid arthritis), 720.* (Ankylosing spondylitis), 696.* (Psoriasis)
714.1	Rheumatoid arthritis	714.0-714.2	
714.2	Felty's syndrome	714.1	

Other groups have used different groupings, or no groupings, of ICD codes when performing PheWAS. CCS groupings have also been used successfully in PheWAS (Warner et al., 2013a). Neuraz et al. (2013) used ICD-10 codes from Hôpital Européen Georges-Pompidou mapped to both the native ICD-10 hierarchy (analogous to three-digit ICD-9-CM codes) and via an ICD-10 → ICD-9-CM mapping to the PheWAS code groupings mentioned above. They found that the PheWAS code groupings provided better phenotype specificity than the native ICD-10 hierarchy. In addition to aggregated ICD codes, other groups have used fully specified ICD-9-CM codes successfully in PheWAS (Hebbring et al., 2013). A potential upside to using raw ICD-9-CM codes is that it eliminates the possibility of false negatives when finding associations with rare phenotypes. A potential downside of this method is that it increases the number of statistical comparisons (increasing the type 1 error at a given *p*-value threshold) and requires a proportionally larger cohort to achieve adequate statistical power.

Another important aspect to using billing codes for diagnoses is the number of codes used to instantiate a disease. Requiring multiple ICD codes can improve the positive predictive value of the phenotype, without losing too many cases (because, for instance, an ICD code might be used once or twice as a "rule-out" and thus would have been a false positive). Most EHR-based PheWAS require at least two ICD-9-CM codes to be considered a case for a disease (Denny et al., 2013).

3.2 Software available for performing PheWAS

The original PheWAS paper in 2010 made available a PERL program for performing PheWAS and the code translation table at http://phewascatalog.org. However, this PERL code only performed simple Chi-square analysis and does not support the most recent hierarchical structure of the PheWAS codes. More recently, a software package was developed for the statistical language R. This R package (RPheWAS) provides options for performing PheWAS on different PheWAS code groupings and a variety of statistical methods, and is also available at this Web site. The R package supports continuous or categorical independent variables (eg, for PheWAS of laboratory values and other nongenetic input) and can also be used to graph the results (Carroll et al., 2014). Vignettes and an example are provided for converting ICD-9-CM, demographic, and genetic data into a PheWAS. PheWAS-View is another package that can be used to graphically display PheWAS results and includes a number of display options; it is a stand-alone Ruby program designed to support genetic PheWAS derived from either EHRs or non-EHR data (Pendergrass et al., 2012). PhenoGram can be used to graphically display phenotypes along chromosomes ideograms (Wolfe et al., 2013). Additionally, standard genetic analysis tools such as PLINK and PLATO also support the testing of multiple phenotypes against genotypes if the phenotypes have been aggregated previously (Purcell et al., 2007; Grady et al., 2010).

3.3 An overview of the current landscape of PheWAS studies

In a 2013 study, we systematically applied the PheWAS approach to each of 3144 SNPs that were previously implicated by GWAS as being important mediators of human disease traits (Denny et al., 2013). These SNPs were selected from the NHGRI catalog, with the requirement that they pass quality control and be represented on the Illumina Human660W-Quadv1_A GWAS chip. The study population consisted of 13,835 individuals of European ancestry who underwent genotyping at one of five original eMERGE sites and phenotypes were from ICD-9-CM codes mapped to one of the 1689 PheWAS groupings. The goal of the study was twofold: first we sought to replicate 751 known prior associations using PheWAS methods. Second, we sought to discover new findings. As shown in Fig. 4, the method replicated 210/751 known associations, including 66% of those for which the study was adequately powered, and identified 63 novel associations using a false discovery rate of 10%. The strongest of these were replicated in another population.

PheWAS has proven to be a valuable tool to elucidate biology of new GWAS discoveries. Linked to a GWAS on cardiac conduction, some SNP variants associated with slower cardiac conduction were found by PheWAS to associate with atrial fibrillation, while others do not (Ritchie et al., 2013). eMERGE investigators used PheWAS to analyze SNPs associated with platelet count and size and noted these variants had pleiotropic associations with myocardial infarction, autoimmune diseases, and hematologic disorders (Shameer et al., 2014). Other PheWAS results have confirmed findings in GWAS (Denny et al., 2011). Recently, PheWAS was used to investigate functional variants, identifying a nonsense variant in ARMS2 associated with age-related macular degeneration (Ye et al., 2015).

PheWAS approaches have also been successful in data collected from observational cohorts. Pendergrass et al. (2013) studied more than 70,000 individuals across the Population Architecture using Genomics and Epidemiology (PAGE) network using 4706 phenotypes. They noted 33 novel phenotypes at $p < 0.01$ in two or more PAGE sites.

Several investigators have deployed PheWAS for nongenetic investigations. Boland et al. (2013a) used PheWAS methods to investigation associations with periodontitis, noting associations with hypertension, hyperlipidemia, and benign prostatic hypertrophy. Neuraz et al. (2013) used PheWAS on thiopurine methyltransferase activity in patients with inflammatory bowel disease to suggest those with higher activity may not be adequately treated with thiopurines.

In 2014 the first systemic review of PheWAS was published (Hebbring, 2014). Since that time, several additional studies have been published, and an overview of published studies is presented in Table 3.

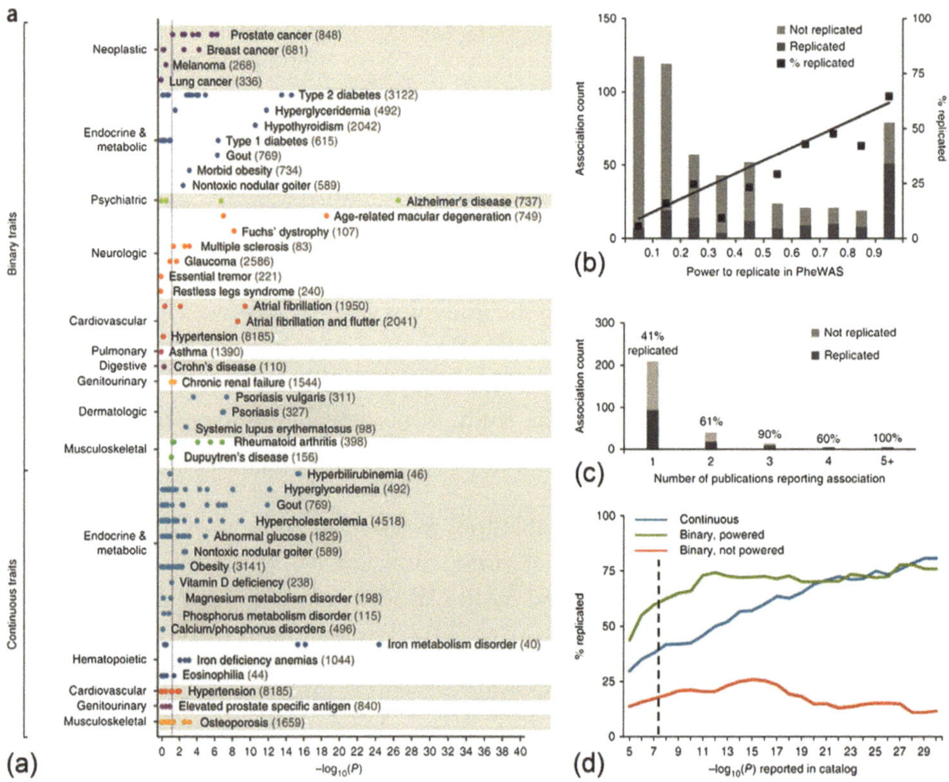

Figure 4 (a) Each point represents the $-\log10(P)$ of a single SNP-phenotype association tested with PheWAS. This study is restricted to SNP-phenotype associations that achieved genome-wide significance ($P \leq 5 \times 10^{-8}$) in at least one prior GWAS study that included individuals of European ancestry. Numbers in parentheses beside each phenotype represent the sample size within the PheWAS data set. The vertical blue line represents $P=0.05$. Binary traits refer to all adequately powered, binary traits in the NHGRI catalog with exact matches to a PheWAS phenotype. For example, 5/5 catalog SNPs associated with rheumatoid arthritis were replicated at $P<0.05$ in PheWAS, and 9/15 SNPs associated with T2DM were replicated. Continuous traits are those numerically defined traits in the NHGRI catalog that are related to PheWAS diseases (eg, "iron deficiency anemia" was the PheWAS trait paired with the "serum iron level" catalog trait). (b) Replication rates of SNP-phenotype associations at different bins of statistical power. Association count refers to the number of SNP-phenotype associations replicated or not replicated at each bin of statistical power (eg, all tested associations with power <0.1, power 0.1–0.2). The black line represents a linear regression weighted using the number of associations in each bin ($y=0.64\times$, $r^2=0.96$). (c) Replication rate of NHGRI catalog associations by number of unique publications citing the original SNP-phenotype association. Association count refers to the number of SNP-phenotype associations (among either adequately powered binary or continuous traits) with the corresponding number of publications. (d) Replication rate of NHGRI catalog associations by discovery P-value. The dashed line indicates $P=5 \times 10^{-8}$. *(Denny et al. (2013), by permission of the Nature Publishing Group).*

Table 3 A list of PheWAS studies published to date, with description of the study population(s), the number of independent variables studied, the number of phenotypes evaluated, and the significant phenotypes reported. Phenotypes labeled "ICD-9-CM" are ICD-9-CM-based but may have been grouped

Study	Population	Independent variables	Number of phenotypes	Number of patients	Significant phenotypes
Denny et al. (2010)	BioVU (European-Americans)	5 SNPs	776 (ICD-9-CM)	6005	23 (4 replicated, 19 novel)
Denny et al. (2011)	eMERGE (European ancestry)	1 SNP (near *FOXE1*)	866 (ICD-9-CM)	13,617	hypothyroidism, other thyroid diseases
Pathak et al. (2012)	Mayo Clinic Biobank	4 SNPs	285 (ICD-9-CM)	6307	diabetes, disorders of lipid metabolism
Warner and Alterovitz (2012)	MIMIC II	1: peak WBC count	5675 (ICD-9-CM)	36,095 (*)	26 (eg, unspecified septicemia)
Boland et al. (2013a)	New Yorkers (largely Hispanic)	1: presence of periodontitis	993 (ICD-9-CM)	2475	9 (eg, diabetes mellitus types 1 and 2)
Denny et al. (2013)	eMERGE (European ancestry)	3144 SNPs from NHGRI GWAS catalog	1358 (ICD-9-CM)	21,241	263 (210 replicated $p < 0.05$, 63 novel FDR < 0.1)
Hebbring et al. (2013)	Marshfield Clinic patients	1 SNP (tagging HLA-DRB1*1501)	4841 (ICD-9-CM)	4235	MS, alcohol-induced cirrhosis, erythematous conditions, benign neoplasms of respiratory organs
Liao et al. (2013)	RA cases; non-RA controls	1: presence of autoantibody	512 (RA cases); 698 (RA controls) (ICD-9-CM)	1290 (RA cases); 1236 (RA controls)	hypothyroidism, Sjögren/sicca, chronic nonalcoholic liver disease
Neuraz et al. (2013)	Patients treated by thiopurine drugs	1: TPMT activity	445 (ICD10)	442	diabetes mellitus, nutritional anemia

Continued

Table 3 A list of PheWAS studies published to date, with description of the study population(s), the number of independent variables studied, the number of phenotypes evaluated, and the significant phenotypes reported. Phenotypes labeled "ICD-9-CM" are ICD-9-CM-based but may have been grouped—Cont'd

Study	Population	Independent variables	Number of phenotypes	Number of patients	Significant phenotypes
Pendergrass et al. (2013)	PAGE network (using NHANES individuals)	83 SNPs	105 (Cohort)	70,061	111 (26 replicated, 33 novel)
Ritchie et al. (2013)	eMERGE (European ancestry)	23 SNPs	778 (ICD-9-CM)	13,859	SCN5A: cardiac arrhythmias; SCN10A: cardiac arrhythmias, atrial fibrillation
Warner et al. (2013b)	MIMIC II (adults)	1: length of hospitalization	5675 (ICD-9-CM)	24,580	191 (eg, hospital-acquired complications)
Warner et al. (2013a)	MIMIC II & SHRINE	1: presence of myeloma	407 (MIMIC II); 24 (SHRINE) (ICD-9-CM)	85 (MIMIC II); 3307 (SHRINE)	24 (eg, pathologic fracture)
Cronin et al. (2014)	eMERGE + BioVU	54 SNPs (all in FTO gene)	1645(ICD-9-CM)	24,198	obesity, T2D, fibrocystic breast disease
Hall et al. (2014)	Genetic NHANES	80 SNPs	1008 (Cohort)	14,042	69 (21 novel associations)
Mitchell et al. (2014)	BioVU (African Americans)	130 mtSNPs	8 (EMR derived)	11,519	T2D, total cholesterol level
Namjou et al. (2014)	Pediatric patients of European ancestry	2476 SNPs	539 (ICD-9-CM)	4268	Multiple
Shameer et al. (2014)	eMERGE	81 SNPs (associated with platelet parameters)	1368 (ICD-9-CM)	13,582	myocardial infarction, autoimmune, hematologic disorders
Ye et al. (2015)	Marshfield Clinic patients	105 stop-gain and stop-loss SNPs	4841 (ICD-9-CM)	14,875	ARMS2: age-related macular degeneration

Note that the threshold of significance is defined slightly differently across the studies; see the individual papers for details.

4. OTHER APPLICATIONS OF PheWAS

4.1 Continuous feature PheWAS

Many variables of phenotypic relevance may be ordinal, categorical, or continuous. Although continuous features such as many laboratory test measures can be compared across populations using a statistical test such as logistic regression, this has the effect of collapsing a dynamic range into a single *p*-value and odds ratio. This may still be useful for comparing populations when a lab test is expected to be monotonic or otherwise smooth in its distribution. For example, while serum sodium is a continuous laboratory measure, it may only matter that the value is high, or low, or within normal limits. Other laboratory values may not follow such a distribution. To investigate the hypothesis that certain ranges of laboratory tests may be associated with certain phenotypes, we developed a two-dimensional approach to PheWAS, called phenome mapping.

In this approach, a continuous feature is compartmentalized into a number of bins. These bins can be of any size and can be divided based on the range of the continuous feature or on a percentile split based on the underlying data. The advantage of the latter approach is twofold: (1) nonparametric distributions are naturally split at sensible cut points and (2) each bin will have an equal number of subjects. The advantage of the former approach is that outlier populations can be examined in finer detail. However, in both cases the optimal number of bins must be selected to ensure that adequate power exists to detect meaningful differences between populations.

If adequate power is unlikely to exist for any realistic number of bins, another option that we have employed is bounding; eg, consecutively redefining a subpopulation based upon a cutoff value of some sort. For example, we defined subpopulations of patients based on their peak white blood cell (WBC) count, with cases being those patients with a value above a certain threshold (eg, 50 k/μl) and controls being all other patients (Warner and Alterovitz, 2012). As with binning, bounding can be based on the range of the laboratory value or on percentiles seen in the observed population.

An additional complication arises when a patient has multiple measures of the laboratory measure under consideration. Patterns of laboratory tests over time can be very important to the definition of phenotype; for example, consider that the difference between acute kidney injury and chronic kidney disease is defined in large part by the tempo of the rise in serum creatinine, and the pattern of rise and fall of uric acid concentrations may differentiate gout from leukemia (Lasko et al., 2013). To simplify the phenome mapping analysis, we typically calculate a single measure in the case of multiple measurements over time; eg, the median observed lab value, or the maximum subtracted from the minimum observed lab value. Although this type of transformation admittedly limits the analysis, it is still possible to gain insights.

Visualization in this approach also becomes more difficult, as there is now an additional dimension of data to contend with. To address this, we essentially turn the

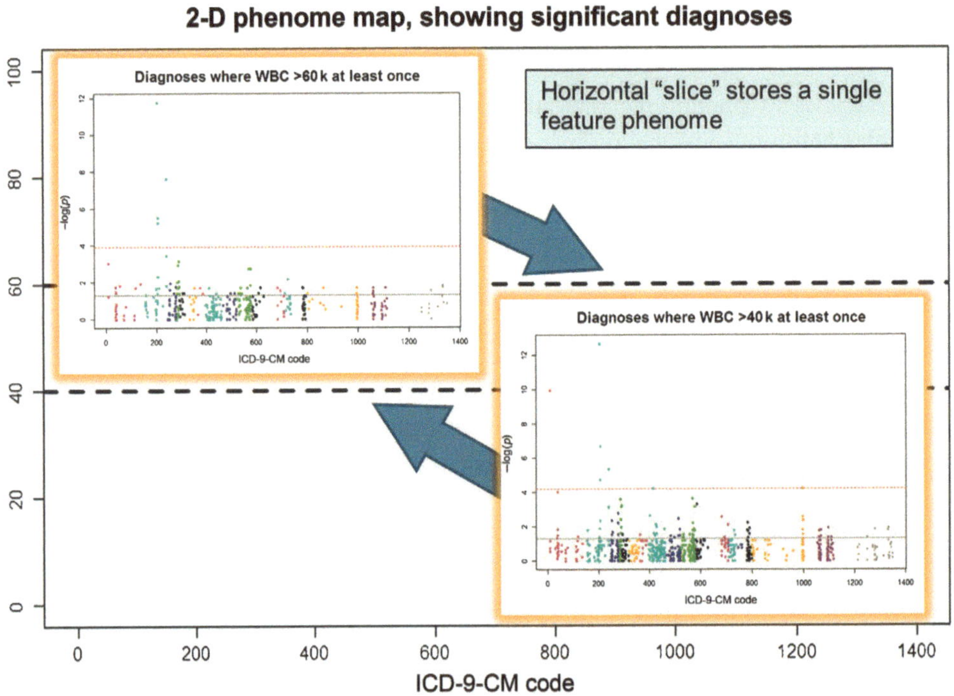

Figure 5 Building a phenome map. In this plot, the horizontal access is the same as that shown in a conventional Manhattan plot, in this case being the range of ICD-9-CM codes (with V-codes and E-codes numerically transformed and placed on the far right). The vertical axis is a bounding parameter, in this case a lower bound. Each horizontal layer of data on the map thus recapitulates a Manhattan plot analysis. In this case we are interested in the peak WBC count, so for example the horizontal line at a WBC lower bound of 40 k/μl represents the PheWAS where cases are patients who have at least one WBC measure exceeding the lower bound, and controls are all other patients.

Manhattan plot "on its side" as illustrated in Fig. 5; we are now essentially not just looking at a skyline from a distance, but at a cityscape, from above. In order to present a form that is visually comprehensible, two further modifications are used: (1) *p*-values not meeting a predetermined threshold (eg, the Bonferroni correction) are suppressed visually, essentially creating a fog layer that enshrouds the lower buildings in the cityscape and (2) points are sized proportionate to the inverse of the *p*-value, such that smaller *p*-values lead to "larger" prominences in the cityscape. Fig. 6 shows a complete WBC phenome map, using MIMIC II as the data source (Saeed et al., 2011).

4.2 Networked PheWAS

It would be convenient if Occam's razor applied to all patients; that is, any given patient would only have one "pure" phenotype. Of course, this is not the case for at least the

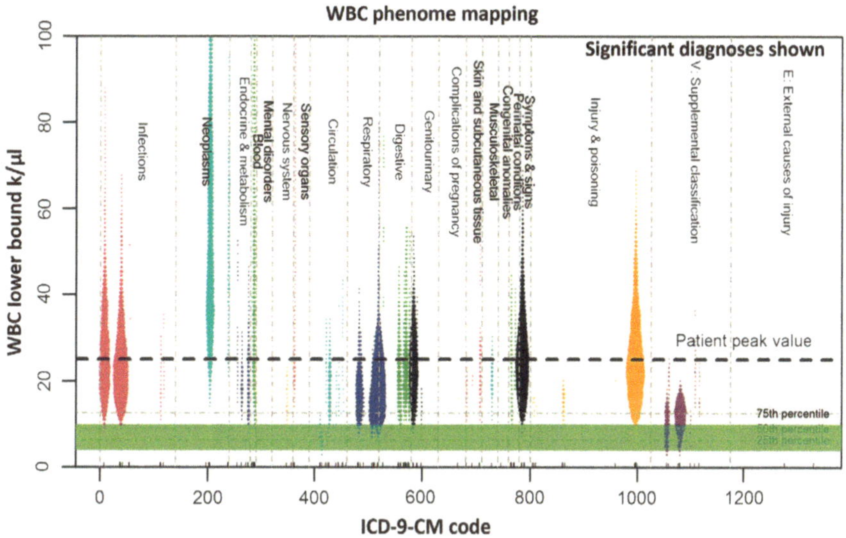

Figure 6 Phenome map of peak WBC count observed over the course of a hospitalization for critical illness, in the MIMIC II cohort. The green band toward the bottom of the graph represents the "normal range" for WBC count. The 25th, 50th, and 75th percentile peak values for the populations are also shown, suggesting that the "normal range" does not apply to this critically ill cohort. A hypothetical patient's peak WBC count is shown as the horizontal dashed line. Several diagnosis codes appear to be significantly associated with peak WBC count over differing ranges. For example, the ICD-9-CM code 038.9: Unspecified septicemia is associated with the range of 10–45 k/µl, whereas code 204.10: Chronic lymphocytic leukemia is associated with the range 15–100 k/µl.

following reasons: (1) a phenotype may induce another phenotype by the nature of the disease process; (2) the treatment for a phenotype may induce new phenotypes (treatment-related complications); and (3) various phenotypes may cluster together (syndromes). These three scenarios are illustrated in Fig. 7.

This linkage of distinct phenotypes is often also readily apparent in pairwise PheWAS analyses, especially with the extra dimension introduced in phenome mapping. For example, the *p*-values of 038.9: Unspecified septicemia in Fig. 6 appear to correlate very closely to the orange area toward the right of the map. In fact, this orange area represents 995.92: Severe sepsis. While this correlation is not surprising, given that the terms are nearly synonymous, it should be noted that these codes are not aggregated in the AHRQ CCS. What this suggests is that a network analytic approach may yield further insights into phenotype relationships.

There is published precedence for the potential utility of this approach (Rzhetsky et al., 2007). Hidalgo et al. (2009) analyzed >32 million claims from >13 million individuals enrolled in Medicare to develop a phenotype disease network. Barabasi et al. developed a networked human "diseasome" based on a bipartite graph where two

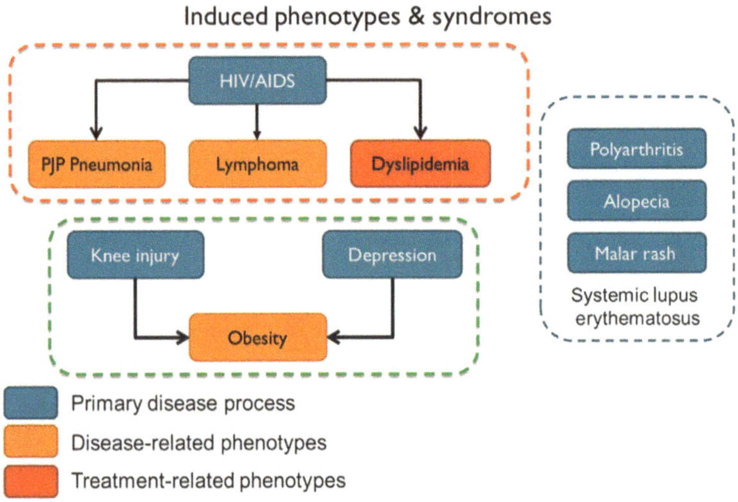

Figure 7 Three examples of the interrelatedness of phenotypes. In the top left, a disease process (HIV/AIDS) mediates the development of other disease processes, such as opportunistic infections and HIV-associated malignancies. The treatment for HIV also can induce a phenotype (eg, HAART-mediated dyslipidemia and lipodystrophy). At the bottom left, two unrelated disease processes can mediate a third process; in this case depression and a knee injury collaborate to decrease physical activity, leading to weight gain and obesity. On the right, three apparently unrelated phenotypes can be clustered into the syndrome of SLE.

diseases were considered connected if they shared a mutual genetic etiology (Goh et al., 2007; Barabasi et al., 2011). Xu et al. (2014) applied a semisupervised iterative pattern learning approach to >21 million MEDLINE records to construct a disease relationship network. We have applied a networked version of PheWAS to EHR data, showing that when secondary connections are considered, a potentially explanatory phenotype cluster emerges that was not readily apparent (Warner et al., 2015). An example of a phenotype network is shown in Fig. 8.

4.3 Future phenomic analysis beyond the EHR

To date, PheWAS approaches have used either EHR data or cohort data. A future is imagined with both denser EHR phenotypes as well as the integration of other streams of data with EHR data. In fact, there are a panoply of data sources that could be used to develop phenotyping measures, ultimately leading to deeper and perhaps more meaningful PheWAS analyses. These include but are not limited to personal health records, ambulatory monitoring devices (eg, Fitbit® and Apple Watch), geospatial data, environmental exposures, and social media (Fig. 9) (Weber et al., 2014). It is widely accepted that to achieve a true "human phenome project" requires the incorporation of a vast array of data sources, including much more information about environmental exposures than is

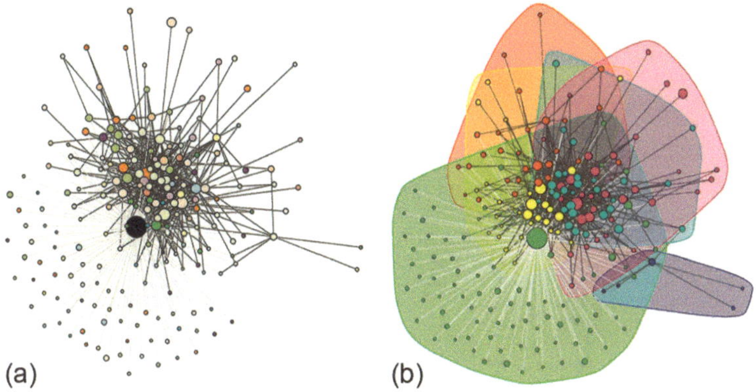

Figure 8 Networked phenotypes. In panel (a), the primary phenotype is the large black node; all primary connections are shown in light gray. Secondary connections are shown in darker gray; node size is proportionate to the prevalence of the recorded phenotype, and node color is by ICD-9-CM chapter. In this example, approximately half of the nodes are singly connected to the primary node, while the others appear to be more connected to each other than to the primary phenotype. In panel (b), a community-finding algorithm is applied and it becomes apparent that what may have visually appeared to be a single cluster can in fact be broken down into multiple clusters. This algorithm suggests that the nodes labeled green should be considered as those most likely to be correlated directly with the primary phenotype. Minor differences in layout between the panels are due to the underlying force-based layout algorithm.

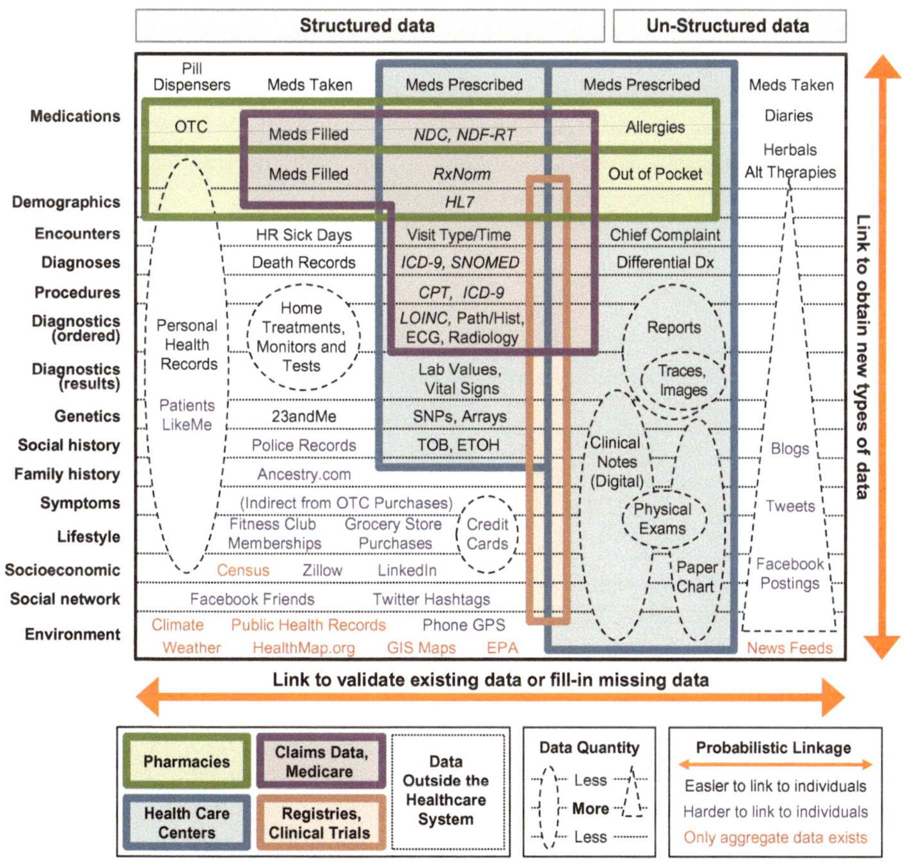

Figure 9 Information sources available for future phenomic studies. *(Image adapted from Weber et al. (2014), and provided courtesy of Dr. Weber).*

currently contained within EHRs (Houle et al., 2010). The breadth and quality of phenome analyses will also be aided by additional biologic knowledge that may or may not reside in the EHR environment: eg, the protein-protein "interactome" of an individual and their disease processes (Feng et al., 2015); the "methylome," which can quantify biological age (Hannum et al., 2013); the characteristics of an individual's microbiome, which is beginning to be appreciated as a cause and protector of human disease (Human Microbiome Project, 2012); and so forth.

5. CONCLUSION

We are fortunate to live in a time when the knowledge of the human medical condition is expanding so quickly. Along with ready access to comprehensive genotyping information at relatively low cost, our understanding of the molecular mechanisms through which disease occurs is building apace. At the same time, advances in the structured and unstructured data captured from the clinical "front lines" have made large-scale phenotyping increasingly feasible. PheWAS represents a methodological attempt to incorporate information "from bench to bedside." While the limitations in the resolution of phenotyping and our understanding of the underlying biological processes make PheWAS primarily a hypothesis-generating tool, it is nevertheless an important tool for the translational bioinformatician. With the advent of open source statistical packages and visualization tools, use of PheWAS may become commonplace for many clinical and genomic applications, and an era of "Big Data" in biomedicine will provide increasingly large populations with dense phenomes for analysis.

REFERENCES

American Psychiatric Association, 2013. The Diagnostic and Statistical Manual of Mental Disorders: DSM 5, bookpointUS.

Aramaki, E., Miura, Y., Tonoike, M., Ohkuma, T., Masuichi, H., Waki, K., Ohe, K., 2010. Extraction of adverse drug effects from clinical records. Stud. Health Technol. Inform. 160, 739–743.

Barabasi, A.L., Gulbahce, N., Loscalzo, J., 2011. Network medicine: a network-based approach to human disease. Nat. Rev. Genet. 12, 56–68.

Blumenthal, D., 2010. Launching HITECH. N. Engl. J. Med. 362, 382–385.

Boland, M.R., Hripcsak, G., Albers, D.J., Wei, Y., Wilcox, A.B., Wei, J., Li, J., Lin, S., Breene, M., Myers, R., Zimmerman, J., Papapanou, P.N., Weng, C., 2013a. Discovering medical conditions associated with periodontitis using linked electronic health records. J. Clin. Periodontol. 40, 474–482.

Boland, M.R., Hripcsak, G., Shen, Y., Chung, W.K., Weng, C., 2013b. Defining a comprehensive verotype using electronic health records for personalized medicine. J. Am. Med. Inform. Assoc. 20, e232–e238.

Carroll, R.J., Thompson, W.K., Eyler, A.E., Mandelin, A.M., Cai, T., Zink, R.M., Pacheco, J.A., Boomershine, C.S., Lasko, T.A., Xu, H., Karlson, E.W., Perez, R.G., Gainer, V.S., Murphy, S.N., Ruderman, E.M., Pope, R.M., Plenge, R.M., Kho, A.N., Liao, K.P., Denny, J.C., 2012. Portability of an algorithm to identify rheumatoid arthritis in electronic health records. J. Am. Med. Inform. Assoc. 19, e162–e169.

Carroll, R.J., Bastarache, L., Denny, J.C., 2014. R PheWAS: data analysis and plotting tools for phenome-wide association studies in the R environment. Bioinformatics 30, 2375–2376.

Cimino, J.J., 1998. Desiderata for controlled medical vocabularies in the twenty-first century. Methods Inf. Med. 37, 394–403.

Cowen, M.E., Dusseau, D.J., Toth, B.G., Guisinger, C., Zodet, M.W., Shyr, Y., 1998. Casemix adjustment of managed care claims data using the clinical classification for health policy research method. Med. Care 36, 1108–1113.

Cronin, R.M., Field, J.R., Bradford, Y., Shaffer, C.M., Carroll, R.J., Mosley, J.D., Bastarache, L., Edwards, T.L., Hebbring, S.J., Lin, S., Hindorff, L.A., Crane, P.K., Pendergrass, S.A., Ritchie, M.D., Crawford, D.C., Pathak, J., Bielinski, S.J., Carrell, D.S., Crosslin, D.R., Ledbetter, D.H., Carey, D.J., Tromp, G., Williams, M.S., Larson, E.B., Jarvik, G.P., Peissig, P.L., Brilliant, M.H., McCarty, C.A., Chute, C.G., Kullo, I.J., Bottinger, E., Chisholm, R., Smith, M.E., Roden, D.M., Denny, J.C., 2014. Phenome-wide association studies demonstrating pleiotropy of genetic variants within FTO with and without adjustment for body mass index. Front. Genet. 5, 250.

Danciu, I., Cowan, J.D., Basford, M., Wang, X., Saip, A., Osgood, S., Shirey-Rice, J., Kirby, J., Harris, P.A., 2014. Secondary use of clinical data: the Vanderbilt approach. J. Biomed. Inform. 52, 28–35.

Denny, J.C., Ritchie, M.D., Basford, M.A., Pulley, J.M., Bastarache, L., Brown-Gentry, K., Wang, D., Masys, D.R., Roden, D.M., Crawford, D.C., 2010. PheWAS: demonstrating the feasibility of a phenome-wide scan to discover gene-disease associations. Bioinformatics 26, 1205–1210.

Denny, J.C., Crawford, D.C., Ritchie, M.D., Bielinski, S.J., Basford, M.A., Bradford, Y., Chai, H.S., Bastarache, L., Zuvich, R., Peissig, P., Carrell, D., Ramirez, A.H., Pathak, J., Wilke, R.A., Rasmussen, L., Wang, X., Pacheco, J.A., Kho, A.N., Hayes, M.G., Weston, N., Matsumoto, M., Kopp, P.A., Newton, K.M., Jarvik, G.P., Li, R., Manolio, T.A., Kullo, I.J., Chute, C.G., Chisholm, R.L., Larson, E.B., McCarty, C.A., Masys, D.R., Roden, D.M., De Andrade, M., 2011. Variants near FOXE1 are associated with hypothyroidism and other thyroid conditions: using electronic medical records for genome- and phenome-wide studies. Am. J. Hum. Genet. 89, 529–542.

Denny, J.C., Bastarache, L., Ritchie, M.D., Carroll, R.J., Zink, R., Mosley, J.D., Field, J.R., Pulley, J.M., Ramirez, A.H., Bowton, E., Basford, M.A., Carrell, D.S., Peissig, P.L., Kho, A.N., Pacheco, J.A., Rasmussen, L.V., Crosslin, D.R., Crane, P.K., Pathak, J., Bielinski, S.J., Pendergrass, S.A., Xu, H., Hindorff, L.A., Li, R., Manolio, T.A., Chute, C.G., Chisholm, R.L., Larson, E.B., Jarvik, G.P., Brilliant, M.H., McCarty, C.A., Kullo, I.J., Haines, J.L., Crawford, D.C., Masys, D.R., Roden, D.M., 2013. Systematic comparison of phenome-wide association study of electronic medical record data and genome-wide association study data. Nat. Biotechnol. 31, 1102–1110.

Feng, S., Zhou, L., Huang, C., Xie, K., Nice, E.C., 2015. Interactomics: toward protein function and regulation. Expert. Rev. Proteomics 12, 37–60.

Fung, K.W., Richesson, R.L., Bodenreider, O., 2014. Coverage of rare disease names in standard terminologies and implications for patients, providers, and research. AMIA Annu. Symp. Proc., 2014, 564–572.

Goh, K.I., Cusick, M.E., Valle, D., Childs, B., Vidal, M., Barabasi, A.L., 2007. The human disease network. Proc. Natl. Acad. Sci. U.S.A. 104, 8685–8690.

Gottesman, O., Kuivaniemi, H., Tromp, G., Faucett, W.A., Li, R., Manolio, T.A., Sanderson, S.C., Kannry, J., Zinberg, R., Basford, M.A., Brilliant, M., Carey, D.J., Chisholm, R.L., Chute, C.G., Connolly, J.J., Crosslin, D., Denny, J.C., Gallego, C.J., Haines, J.L., Hakonarson, H., Harley, J., Jarvik, G.P., Kohane, I., Kullo, I.J., Larson, E.B., McCarty, C., Ritchie, M.D., Roden, D.M., Smith, M.E., Bottinger, E.P., Williams, M.S., eMERGE Network, 2013. The Electronic Medical Records and Genomics (eMERGE) Network: past, present, and future. Genet. Med. 15, 761–771.

Grady, B.J., Torstenson, E., Dudek, S.M., Giles, J., Sexton, D., Ritchie, M.D., 2010. Finding unique filter sets in PLATO: a precursor to efficient interaction analysis in GWAS data. Pac. Symp. Biocomput., 315–326.

Graunt, J., 1662. Natural and Political Observations Made upon the Bills of Mortality. The Johns Hopkins Press, Baltimore, Maryland.

Hall, M.A., Verma, A., Brown-Gentry, K.D., Goodloe, R., Boston, J., Wilson, S., McClellan, B., Sutcliffe, C., Dilks, H.H., Gillani, N.B., Jin, H., Mayo, P., Allen, M., Schnetz-Boutaud, N., Crawford, D.C., Ritchie, M.D., Pendergrass, S.A., 2014. Detection of pleiotropy through a phenome-wide association study (PheWAS) of epidemiologic data as part of the environmental architecture for genes linked to environment (EAGLE) study. PLoS Genet. 10, e1004678.

Hannum, G., Guinney, J., Zhao, L., Zhang, L., Hughes, G., Sadda, S., Klotzle, B., Bibikova, M., Fan, J.B., Gao, Y., Deconde, R., Chen, M., Rajapakse, I., Friend, S., Ideker, T., Zhang, K., 2013. Genome-wide methylation profiles reveal quantitative views of human aging rates. Mol. Cell 49, 359–367.

Hebbring, S.J., 2014. The challenges, advantages and future of phenome-wide association studies. Immunology 141, 157–165.

Hebbring, S.J., Schrodi, S.J., Ye, Z., Zhou, Z., Page, D., Brilliant, M.H., 2013. A PheWAS approach in studying HLA-DRB1*1501. Genes Immun. 14, 187–191.

Hidalgo, C.A., Blumm, N., Barabasi, A.L., Christakis, N.A., 2009. A dynamic network approach for the study of human phenotypes. PLoS Comput. Biol. 5, e1000353.

Hobbes, T., 1651. Leviathan, or the Matter, Forme and Power of a Commonwealth Ecclesiasticall and Civil. Yale University Press, New Haven, Connecticut.

Houle, D., Govindaraju, D.R., Omholt, S., 2010. Phenomics: the next challenge. Nat. Rev. Genet. 11, 855–866.

Human Microbiome Project, C., 2012. A framework for human microbiome research. Nature 486, 215–221.

Humphreys, B.L., Lindberg, D.A., Schoolman, H.M., Barnett, G.O., 1998. The unified medical language system: an informatics research collaboration. J. Am. Med. Inform. Assoc. 5, 1–11.

Ingenerf, J., Linder, R., 2009. Assessing applicability of ontological principles to different types of biomedical vocabularies. Methods Inf. Med. 48, 459–467.

Jablensky, A., 1988. Methodological issues in psychiatric classification. Br. J. Psychiatry Suppl. 152, 15–20.

Kho, A.N., Hayes, M.G., Rasmussen-Torvik, L., Pacheco, J.A., Thompson, W.K., Armstrong, L.L., Denny, J.C., Peissig, P.L., Miller, A.W., Wei, W.Q., Bielinski, S.J., Chute, C.G., Leibson, C.L., Jarvik, G.P., Crosslin, D.R., Carlson, C.S., Newton, K.M., Wolf, W.A., Chisholm, R.L., Lowe, W.L., 2012. Use of diverse electronic medical record systems to identify genetic risk for type 2 diabetes within a genome-wide association study. J. Am. Med. Inform. Assoc. 19, 212–218.

Kibbe, W.A., Arze, C., Felix, V., Mitraka, E., Bolton, E., Fu, G., Mungall, C.J., Binder, J.X., Malone, J., Vasant, D., Parkinson, H., Schriml, L.M., 2015. Disease Ontology 2015 update: an expanded and updated database of human diseases for linking biomedical knowledge through disease data. Nucleic Acids Res. 43, D1071–D1078.

Kohane, I.S., 2011. Using electronic health records to drive discovery in disease genomics. Nat. Rev. Genet. 12, 417–428.

Kohane, I.S., Churchill, S.E., Murphy, S.N., 2012. A translational engine at the national scale: informatics for integrating biology and the bedside. J. Am. Med. Inform. Assoc. 19, 181–185.

Kohler, S., Doelken, S.C., Mungall, C.J., Bauer, S., Firth, H.V., Bailleul-Forestier, I., Black, G.C., Brown, D.L., Brudno, M., Campbell, J., Fitzpatrick, D.R., Eppig, J.T., Jackson, A.P., Freson, K., Girdea, M., Helbig, I., Hurst, J.A., Jahn, J., Jackson, L.G., Kelly, A.M., Ledbetter, D.H., Mansour, S., Martin, C.L., Moss, C., Mumford, A., Ouwehand, W.H., Park, S.M., Riggs, E.R., Scott, R.H., Sisodiya, S., Van Vooren, S., Wapner, R.J., Wilkie, A.O., Wright, C.F., Vulto-Van Silfhout, A.T., De Leeuw, N., De Vries, B.B., Washingthon, N.L., Smith, C.L., Westerfield, M., Schofield, P., Ruef, B.J., Gkoutos, G.V., Haendel, M., Smedley, D., Lewis, S.E., Robinson, P.N., 2014. The Human Phenotype Ontology project: linking molecular biology and disease through phenotype data. Nucleic Acids Res. 42, D966–D974.

Lanktree, M.B., Hassell, R.G., Lahiry, P., Hegele, R.A., 2010. Phenomics: expanding the role of clinical evaluation in genomic studies. J. Investig. Med. 58, 700–706.

Lasko, T.A., Denny, J.C., Levy, M.A., 2013. Computational phenotype discovery using unsupervised feature learning over noisy, sparse, and irregular clinical data. PLoS One 8, e66341.

Liao, K.P., Cai, T., Gainer, V., Goryachev, S., Zeng-Treitler, Q., Raychaudhuri, S., Szolovits, P., Churchill, S., Murphy, S., Kohane, I., Karlson, E.W., Plenge, R.M., 2010. Electronic medical records for discovery research in rheumatoid arthritis. Arthritis Care Res. (Hoboken) 62, 1120–1127.

Liao, K.P., Kurreeman, F., Li, G., Duclos, G., Murphy, S., Guzman, R., Cai, T., Gupta, N., Gainer, V., Schur, P., Cui, J., Denny, J.C., Szolovits, P., Churchill, S., Kohane, I., Karlson, E.W., Plenge, R.M.,

2013. Associations of autoantibodies, autoimmune risk alleles, and clinical diagnoses from the electronic medical records in rheumatoid arthritis cases and non-rheumatoid arthritis controls. Arthritis Rheum. 65, 571–581.

Lin, C., Karlson, E.W., Dligach, D., Ramirez, M.P., Miller, T.A., Mo, H., Braggs, N.S., Cagan, A., Gainer, V., Denny, J.C., Savova, G.K., 2014. Automatic identification of methotrexate-induced liver toxicity in patients with rheumatoid arthritis from the electronic medical record. J. Am. Med. Inform. Assoc. 22, e151–e161.

McCarty, C.A., Chisholm, R.L., Chute, C.G., Kullo, I.J., Jarvik, G.P., Larson, E.B., Li, R., Masys, D.R., Ritchie, M.D., Roden, D.M., Struewing, J.P., Wolf, W.A., eMERGE Team, 2011. The eMERGE Network: a consortium of biorepositories linked to electronic medical records data for conducting genomic studies. BMC Med. Genomics 4, 13.

Meyer-Lindenberg, A., 2010. Intermediate or brainless phenotypes for psychiatric research? Psychol. Med. 40, 1057–1062.

Meystre, S.M., Savova, G.K., Kipper-Schuler, K.C., Hurdle, J.F., 2008. Extracting information from textual documents in the electronic health record: a review of recent research. Yearb. Med. Inform., 128–144.

Mitchell, S.L., Hall, J.B., Goodloe, R.J., Boston, J., Farber-Eger, E., Pendergrass, S.A., Bush, W.S., Crawford, D.C., 2014. Investigating the relationship between mitochondrial genetic variation and cardiovascular-related traits to develop a framework for mitochondrial phenome-wide association studies. BioData Min. 7, 6.

Moriyama, I.M., Loy, R.M., Robb-Smith, A.H.T., Rosenberg, H.M., Hoyert, D.L., 2011. History of the statistical classification of diseases and causes of death. US Department of Health and Human Services, Centers for Disease Control and Prevention, National Center for Health Statistics.

Muggah, E., Graves, E., Bennett, C., Manuel, D.G., 2013. Ascertainment of chronic diseases using population health data: a comparison of health administrative data and patient self-report. BMC Public Health 13, 16.

Murff, H.J., Fitzhenry, F., Matheny, M.E., Gentry, N., Kotter, K.L., Crimin, K., Dittus, R.S., Rosen, A.K., Elkin, P.L., Brown, S.H., Speroff, T., 2011. Automated identification of postoperative complications within an electronic medical record using natural language processing. JAMA 306, 848–855.

Murphy, S.N., Weber, G., Mendis, M., Gainer, V., Chueh, H.C., Churchill, S., Kohane, I., 2010. Serving the enterprise and beyond with informatics for integrating biology and the bedside (i2b2). J. Am. Med. Inform. Assoc. 17, 124–130.

Nadkarni, P.M., Ohno-Machado, L., Chapman, W.W., 2011. Natural language processing: an introduction. J. Am. Med. Inform. Assoc. 18, 544–551.

Namjou, B., Marsolo, K., Caroll, R.J., Denny, J.C., Ritchie, M.D., Verma, S.S., Lingren, T., Porollo, A., Cobb, B.L., Perry, C., Kottyan, L.C., Rothenberg, M.E., Thompson, S.D., Holm, I.A., Kohane, I.S., Harley, J.B., 2014. Phenome-wide association study (PheWAS) in EMR-linked pediatric cohorts, genetically links PLCL1 to speech language development and IL5-IL13 to Eosinophilic Esophagitis. Front. Genet. 5, 401.

Neuraz, A., Chouchana, L., Malamut, G., Le Beller, C., Roche, D., Beaune, P., Degoulet, P., Burgun, A., Loriot, M.A., Avillach, P., 2013. Phenome-wide association studies on a quantitative trait: application to TPMT enzyme activity and thiopurine therapy in pharmacogenomics. PLoS Comput. Biol. 9, e1003405.

Orueta, J.F., Nuno-Solinis, R., Mateos, M., Vergara, I., Grandes, G., Esnaola, S., 2012. Monitoring the prevalence of chronic conditions: which data should we use? BMC Health Serv. Res. 12, 365.

Pathak, J., Kiefer, R.C., Bielinski, S.J., Chute, C.G., 2012. Applying semantic web technologies for phenome-wide scan using an electronic health record linked Biobank. J. Biomed. Semantics 3, 10.

Pathak, J., Kho, A.N., Denny, J.C., 2013. Electronic health records-driven phenotyping: challenges, recent advances, and perspectives. J. Am. Med. Inform. Assoc. 20, e206–e211.

Peissig, P.L., Rasmussen, L.V., Berg, R.L., Linneman, J.G., McCarty, C.A., Waudby, C., Chen, L., Denny, J.C., Wilke, R.A., Pathak, J., Carrell, D., Kho, A.N., Starren, J.B., 2012. Importance of multi-modal approaches to effectively identify cataract cases from electronic health records. J. Am. Med. Inform. Assoc. 19, 225–234.

Pendergrass, S.A., Dudek, S.M., Crawford, D.C., Ritchie, M.D., 2012. Visually integrating and exploring high throughput phenome-wide association study (PheWAS) results using PheWAS-View. BioData Min. 5, 5.

Pendergrass, S.A., Brown-Gentry, K., Dudek, S., Frase, A., Torstenson, E.S., Goodloe, R., Ambite, J.L., Avery, C.L., Buyske, S., Buzkova, P., Deelman, E., Fesinmeyer, M.D., Haiman, C.A., Heiss, G., Hindorff, L.A., Hsu, C.N., Jackson, R.D., Kooperberg, C., Le Marchand, L., Lin, Y., Matise, T.C., Monroe, K.R., Moreland, L., Park, S.L., Reiner, A., Wallace, R., Wilkens, L.R., Crawford, D.C., Ritchie, M.D., 2013. Phenome-wide association study (PheWAS) for detection of pleiotropy within the population architecture using genomics and epidemiology (PAGE) network. PLoS Genet. 9, e1003087.

Perlis, R.H., Iosifescu, D.V., Castro, V.M., Murphy, S.N., Gainer, V.S., Minnier, J., Cai, T., Goryachev, S., Zeng, Q., Gallagher, P.J., Fava, M., Weilburg, J.B., Churchill, S.E., Kohane, I.S., Smoller, J.W., 2012. Using electronic medical records to enable large-scale studies in psychiatry: treatment resistant depression as a model. Psychol. Med. 42, 41–50.

Purcell, S., Neale, B., Todd-Brown, K., Thomas, L., Ferreira, M.A., Bender, D., Maller, J., Sklar, P., De Bakker, P.I., Daly, M.J., Sham, P.C., 2007. PLINK: a tool set for whole-genome association and population-based linkage analyses. Am. J. Hum. Genet. 81, 559–575.

Ritchie, M.D., Denny, J.C., Zuvich, R.L., Crawford, D.C., Schildcrout, J.S., Bastarache, L., Ramirez, A.H., Mosley, J.D., Pulley, J.M., Basford, M.A., Bradford, Y., Rasmussen, L.V., Pathak, J., Chute, C.G., Kullo, I.J., McCarty, C.A., Chisholm, R.L., Kho, A.N., Carlson, C.S., Larson, E.B., Jarvik, G.P., Sotoodehnia, N., Cohorts For, H., Aging Research In Genomic Epidemiology, Q.R.S.G., Manolio, T.A., Li, R., Masys, D.R., Haines, D.L., Roden, D.M., 2013. Genome- and phenome-wide analyses of cardiac conduction identifies markers of arrhythmia risk. Circulation 127, 1377–1385.

Roden, D.M., Pulley, J.M., Basford, M.A., Bernard, G.R., Clayton, E.W., Balser, J.R., Masys, D.R., 2008. Development of a large-scale de-identified DNA biobank to enable personalized medicine. Clin. Pharmacol. Ther. 84, 362–369.

Rosenbloom, S.T., Kiepek, W., Belletti, J., Adams, P., Shuxteau, K., Johnson, K.B., Elkin, P.L., Shultz, E.K., 2004. Generating complex clinical documents using structured entry and reporting. Stud. Health Technol. Inform. 107, 683–687.

Rosenbloom, S.T., Denny, J.C., Xu, H., Lorenzi, N., Stead, W.W., Johnson, K.B., 2011. Data from clinical notes: a perspective on the tension between structure and flexible documentation. J. Am. Med. Inform. Assoc. 18, 181–186.

Rosenbloom, S.T., Miller, R.A., Adams, P., Madani, S., Khan, N., Shultz, E.K., 2013. Implementing an interface terminology for structured clinical documentation. J. Am. Med. Inform. Assoc. 20, e178–e182.

Rzhetsky, A., Wajngurt, D., Park, N., Zheng, T., 2007. Probing genetic overlap among complex human phenotypes. Proc. Natl. Acad. Sci. U.S.A. 104, 11694–11699.

Saeed, M., Villarroel, M., Reisner, A.T., Clifford, G., Lehman, L.W., Moody, G., Heldt, T., Kyaw, T.H., Moody, B., Mark, R.G., 2011. Multiparameter Intelligent Monitoring in Intensive Care II: a public-access intensive care unit database. Crit. Care Med. 39, 952–960.

Schildcrout, J.S., Basford, M.A., Pulley, J.M., Masys, D.R., Roden, D.M., Wang, D., Chute, C.G., Kullo, I.J., Carrell, D., Peissig, P., Kho, A., Denny, J.C., 2010. An analytical approach to characterize morbidity profile dissimilarity between distinct cohorts using electronic medical records. J. Biomed. Inform. 43, 914–923.

Schulz, S., Suntisrivaraporn, B., Baader, F., Boeker, M., 2009. SNOMED reaching its adolescence: ontologists' and logicians' health check. Int. J. Med. Inform. 78 (Suppl. 1), S86–S94.

Shameer, K., Denny, J.C., Ding, K., Jouni, H., Crosslin, D.R., De Andrade, M., Chute, C.G., Peissig, P., Pacheco, J.A., Li, R., Bastarache, L., Kho, A.N., Ritchie, M.D., Masys, D.R., Chisholm, R.L., Larson, E.B., McCarty, C.A., Roden, D.M., Jarvik, G.P., Kullo, I.J., 2014. A genome- and phenome-wide association study to identify genetic variants influencing platelet count and volume and their pleiotropic effects. Hum. Genet. 133, 95–109.

Shivade, C., Raghavan, P., Fosler-Lussier, E., Embi, P.J., Elhadad, N., Johnson, S.B., Lai, A.M., 2014. A review of approaches to identifying patient phenotype cohorts using electronic health records. J. Am. Med. Inform. Assoc. 21, 221–230.

Srigley, J.R., Mcgowan, T., Maclean, A., Raby, M., Ross, J., Kramer, S., Sawka, C., 2009. Standardized synoptic cancer pathology reporting: a population-based approach. J. Surg. Oncol. 99, 517–524.

Sun, W., Rumshisky, A., Uzuner, O., 2013. Temporal reasoning over clinical text: the state of the art. J. Am. Med. Inform. Assoc. 20, 814–819.

Tapuria, A., Kalra, D., Kobayashi, S., 2013. Contribution of clinical archetypes, and the challenges, towards achieving semantic interoperability for EHRs. Healthc. Inform. Res. 19, 286–292.

Turing, A.M., 1950. Computing machinery and intelligence. Mind 49, 433–460.

Warner, J.L., Alterovitz, G., 2012. Phenome-based analysis as a means for discovering context-dependent clinical reference ranges. AMIA Annu. Symp. Proc. 2012, 1441–1449.

Warner, J.L., Alterovitz, G., Bodio, K., Joyce, R.M., 2013a. External phenome analysis enables a rational federated query strategy to detect changing rates of treatment-related complications associated with multiple myeloma. J. Am. Med. Inform. Assoc. 20, 696–699.

Warner, J.L., Zollanvari, A., Ding, Q., Zhang, P., Snyder, G.M., Alterovitz, G., 2013b. Temporal phenome analysis of a large electronic health record cohort enables identification of hospital-acquired complications. J. Am. Med. Inform. Assoc. 20, e281–e287.

Warner, J.L., Denny, J.C., Kreda, D.A., Alterovitz, G., 2015. Seeing the forest through the trees: uncovering phenomic complexity through interactive network visualization. J. Am. Med. Inform. Assoc. 22, 324–329.

Weber, G.M., Mandl, K.D., Kohane, I.S., 2014. Finding the missing link for big biomedical data. JAMA 311, 2479–2480.

Wellcome Trust Case Control Consortium, 2007. Genome-wide association study of 14,000 cases of seven common diseases and 3,000 shared controls. Nature 447, 661–678.

Wolfe, D., Dudek, S., Ritchie, M.D., Pendergrass, S.A., 2013. Visualizing genomic information across chromosomes with PhenoGram. BioData Min. 6, 18.

Wrenn, J.O., Stein, D.M., Bakken, S., Stetson, P.D., 2010. Quantifying clinical narrative redundancy in an electronic health record. J. Am. Med. Inform. Assoc. 17, 49–53.

Wright, A., Pang, J., Feblowitz, J.C., Maloney, F.L., Wilcox, A.R., Ramelson, H.Z., Schneider, L.I., Bates, D.W., 2011. A method and knowledge base for automated inference of patient problems from structured data in an electronic medical record. J. Am. Med. Inform. Assoc. 18, 859–867.

Xu, H., Stenner, S.P., Doan, S., Johnson, K.B., Waitman, L.R., Denny, J.C., 2010. MedEx: a medication information extraction system for clinical narratives. J. Am. Med. Inform. Assoc. 17, 19–24.

Xu, R., Li, L., Wang, Q., 2014. dRiskKB: a large-scale disease-disease risk relationship knowledge base constructed from biomedical text. BMC Bioinformatics 15, 105.

Ye, Z., Mayer, J., Ivacic, L., Zhou, Z., He, M., Schrodi, S.J., Page, D., Brilliant, M.H., Hebbring, S.J., 2015. Phenome-wide association studies (PheWASs) for functional variants. Eur. J. Hum. Genet. 23, 523–529.

CHAPTER 4

TCR Repertoire Analysis

Y.N. Lee
Division of Immunology, Children's Hospital, Harvard Medical School, Boston, MA, United States

Contents

1. INTRODUCTION

T cell receptor (TCR) is expressed on the surface of T cells as a heterodimer of either TCR alpha and beta chains or TCR gamma and delta chains, and it is critical for the recognition of a peptide bound to the major histocompatibility complex. The capability of TCR to bind a vast array of antigens both foreign and self is due to the fact that the antigen recognition site (or variable region) is generated by a unique process of somatic recombination. The variable regions in TCR alpha and gamma chains are encoded by recombination of various V gene segments to J gene segments. Whereas in the TCR beta and delta chains various D gene segments join to J gene segments and then V gene segments join to DJ. In addition to the recombination among various V(D)J gene segments, which allows for a diverse combination, the combinatorial pairing of the two subunits increases the diversity to a mathematical prediction of $\sim 10^{15}$ different TCR$\alpha\beta$ molecules

Translational Immunology
http://dx.doi.org/10.1016/B978-0-12-801577-3.00005-8

(Turner et al., 2006). However, with thymic positive and negative selection we remain with an estimate of $\sim 2 \times 10^7$ TCR$\alpha\beta$ molecules.

Furthermore, the recombination of the various chains is developmentaly dependant, where V(D)J genes of TCR gamma, delta, and beta start rearranging at the double negative stage of T cell development followed by a recombination TCR alpha chain (Sleckman et al., 1998). T cells that express the TCR gamma and delta chains give rise to $\gamma\delta$T cells, which appear first in the fetal thymic development (Turner et al., 2006) and in the double negative stage of T cell development. On the other hand, the $\alpha\beta$T cells express the TCR alpha and beta chains, which are expressed in the double positive and single positive stages in the T cell development. Therefore, the expression of TCR repertoire is a timely and spatially regulated process to allow expression of either a TCR alpha and beta or TCR gamma and delta, with many regulating factors, from transcription factors to modifiers of accessibility of the various TCR loci (Krangel et al., 2004; Wang et al., 2008; Bonnet et al., 2009; Spicuglia et al., 2010; Chaumeil and Skok, 2013).

The TCR repertoires are not solely generated by the combinatorial joining of various V, D, and J genes and pairing of two different TCR chains as described above. One must not forget the junctional diversity that is generated in the CDR3 region during the VDJ recombination process (Turner et al., 2006; Thai and Kearney, 2005; Helmink and Sleckman, 2012). Briefly, the recombination activating genes 1 and 2 (*RAG1* and *RAG2*) are specifically recruited and bind to the recombination signaling sequences (RSS) that are flanking the V, D, and J gene segments. *RAG1* and *RAG2* generate double-strand breaks at the end of the V, D, and J gene segments (Fig. 1A). These double-strand breaks activate the NHEJ pathway for DNA repair. One of the factors that is recruited is Artemis (genome browser) and it is important in the initiation of the DNA repair as it opens the hairpin at the ends of the double-strand breaks (Fig. 1A). Artemis can open the hairpin either by opening symmetrically at the end with no overhangs, or asymmetrically with overhangs that generate palindromic nucleotides, known as P-nucleotides. Additionally, Artemis can generate two nicks, which then leads to deletions contributing to the overall trimming at the 3'V, 5'D, 3'D, and 5'J gene ends, which may occur during the joining process by other nuclease. Before the ends are ligated, nontemplate nucleotides (N nucleotides) can be added by the terminal deoxynucleotidyl transferase, TdT (Fig. 1A). Therefore, junctional diversity is generated by P and N nucleotide additions and deletions of nucleotides at the joining of the V, D, and J gene segments (Fig. 1B). These components should be taken into consideration when analyzing the TCR repertoire, especially when there is a direct affect on the NHEJ pathway.

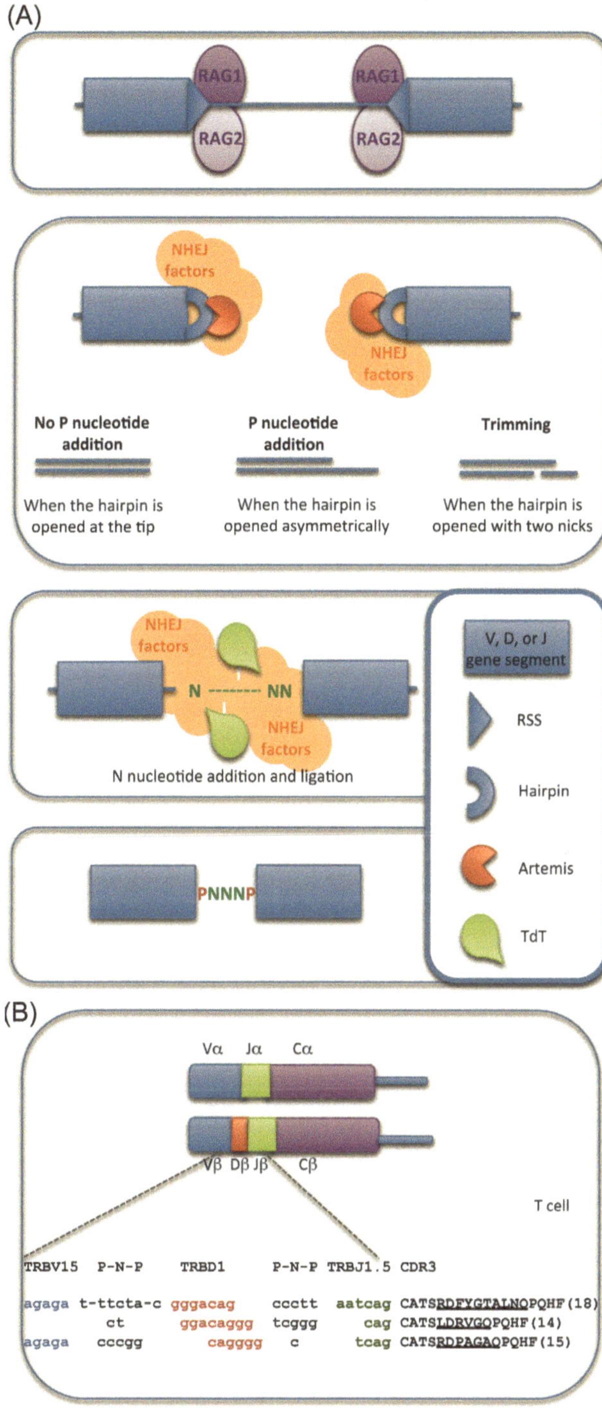

Figure 1 VDJ recombination. (A) Schematic diagram representing the processes in VDJ recombination where Artemis and TdT play a key role in generating junctional diversity. (B) Demonstration of junctional diversity generated by P and N nucleotide additions and trimming at the TRBV, TRBD, and TRBJ genes on three VDJ joining product from a TCR repertoire of healthy infant donor. The components of TRBV gene, P and N nucleotides, TRBD and TRBJ genes are shown in nucleotides, and the corresponding amino acids for the CDR3 region are represented with the amino acid length of the CDR3 in parenthesis. The nucleotides shown correspond to the underlined amino acids.

2. STUDYING THE TCR REPERTOIRE

Until recently the TCR repertoire was studied by sampling a relatively small portion of the predicted estimates by cloning and Sanger sequencing expression libraries. Determining the TCR repertoire by FACS using antibodies against various TRBV families allowed for a more rapid and quantitative measure; however, information on the actual sequence was not possible to obtain from the same experiment. These studies were critical in understanding the mechanisms shaping the immune repertoire from fetal development to immunodeficiencies and immune reconstitution after bone marrow transplant (Zemlin et al., 2002; Sarzotti et al., 2003). However, recent technical advancement and the emergence of next generation sequencing (NGS) not only allowed a robust and accurate study on TCR repertoire due to the capture of up to millions of rearrangement from a single sample, but also allowed one to obtain TRBV family and gene usage, detailed information on the sequence such as P and N nucleotide additions and CDR3 amino acid and nucleotide sequences and lengths in a quantitative manner (Meier et al., 2013; Krell et al., 2013; Yu et al., 2014; O'Connell et al., 2014; Becattini et al., 2015; Rechavi et al., 2015; van Heijst et al., 2013). A nice example is the study of fetal immune repertoire where in the past materials from a fetal spleen or liver sample were used to generate hundreds of rearrangements in the IGH and TRB loci (Schroeder et al., 2001; George and Schroeder, 1992). However, a recent study shows that from fetal blood as early as 12 weeks gestational age thousands of both IGH and TRB sequences were obtained from a single sample (Rechavi et al., 2015). As mentioned by Rechavi et al., it is important to note that NGS data confirmed results reported using direct cloning and Sanger sequencing methods. However, from the NGS data, one can learn comprehensively about the diversity of the repertoire; CDR3 length and composition: public/shared clones; and TRBV, TRBD, and TRBJ gene usages. In addition, the combination study of both IGH and TRB repertoires from the same sample allowed one to see the delayed development of the TRB repertoire compared to the IGH repertoire [Fig. 4 in Rechavi et al. (2015)].

Due to the large number of factors that control the generation of the TCR repertoire, it changes with age, infections, cancer, genetic disorders, and treatments such as bone marrow transplant and cancer treatments (Meier et al., 2013; Krell et al., 2013; Yu et al., 2014; O'Connell et al., 2014; Becattini et al., 2015; Rechavi et al., 2015; Gil et al., 2015; Bajor et al., 2014; van Heijst et al., 2013). For studies involving infections and cancer the analyses are focussed on the clonal expansion of T cells, whereas in the studies involving genetic disorders such as primary immunodeficiency the focus is more on the generation of a diverse repertoire, preferential V-D-J gene usages, P and N nucleotide additions, and CDR3 lengths. Furthermore, the TCR repertoire is different among the different subpopulations of T cells, especially among the naïve and memory (O'Connell et al., 2014).

Although there are numerous studies reporting the TCR repertoire of the β chain, thus the TRB repertoire, there are very limited reports on the TCR repertoire of the α chains, thus the TRA repertoire, and even less reports on the TCR repertoires of γ and δ chains (TRG and TRD repertoires). The limited reports on the TRG and TRD repertoires may be due to the low number of circulating γδT cells in addition to the ubiquity of their role in the immune system. However, the γδT subset is nevertheless a very intriguing subset (Chien et al., 2014). The information incorporated in the TCR repertoire may be valuable in understanding the mechanisms behind various diseases, development, maturation, and function of T cells.

3. DIVERSITY INDICES

As a general description, diversity takes into account the total number of entities in a data set, the number of unique types to which the entities belong, and the abundance of an entity in each of the types, where a diversity index is a quantitative measurement of such diversity. Thus diversity increases when the number of unique types and evenness increases. Evenness describes how the abundances of the entities are distributed among the different types; thus, maximum diversity may be reached when the entities are equally abundant, with abundance 2 and above. If the abundance is 1 and it is even then the repertoire may be not sampled enough and there may still be new types to be sampled. Once there are types with abundances two and above, most of the types are sampled and perhaps only the very rare types are still to be discovered.

Diversity indices are often used in ecology and quantitatively measure how many different species are in an ecosystem and how they are distributed among the various species. These diversity indices were recently adapted by molecular immunologists and became very useful once immune repertoires of TCR and B cell receptor (BCR) were determined using NGS sequencing technologies that generate up to millions of sequences from one sample. Each sequence is treated as an entity, and the list of the abundance of each sequence can be grouped by types or species that all originate from a single sample (individual), analogous to an ecosystem in ecology. With such a large number of data it is very difficult to compare the repertoire as a whole between different samples and even with the diversity indices it is not enough to use any one but a combination of different diversity indices to characterize the immune repertoire. Presented here are few examples of such diversity indices that are commonly used and are essential in understanding the different aspects of the immune repertoires. Furthermore, these indices allow us to easily compare different samples, individuals, and between data generated by different experiments and technical platforms.

Various diversity indices are divided by order, where the higher the order the more weight is put on abundance (Fig. 2A). Therefore in a diversity of order one, such as richness, the number of species in a data set or number of unique sequences in a TCR

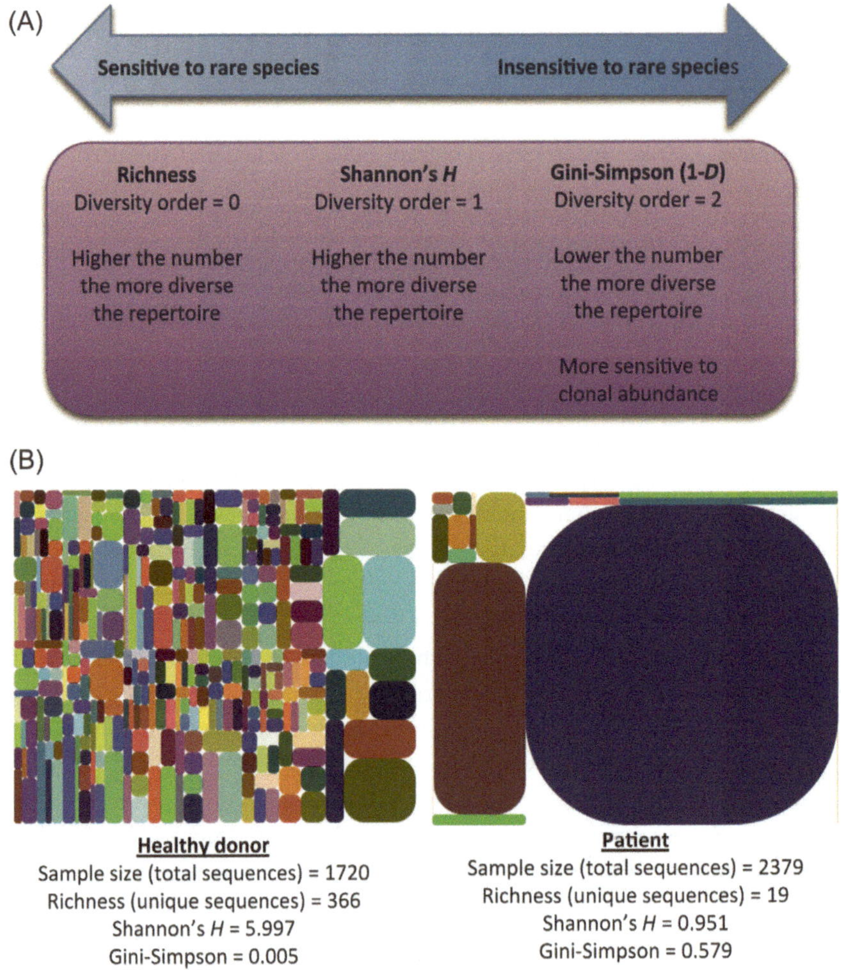

Figure 2 Diversity of TCR repertoire. (A) Diversity indices and degree of weights on rare sequences. (B) Tree maps of TRB repertoires from a healthy infant donor and a patient.

repertoire, abundance is not taken into account when determining this diversity index. On the other hand, Shannon's *H* and Gini-Simpson indices are diversity indices of order one and two, respectively, as they take into account the distribution of the various abundances (see below). It is important to know how much weight is put on the abundance so that the information that we get from these indices can be further differentiated. If we are looking at TCR repertoire that has many clonal expansions compared to a few but large clonal expansion then diversity index of order one may not depict these differences; therefore, a higher order of diversity index should also be considered.

For diversity indices we only need the abundance information of the TCR repertoire, so a list of the numbers for each of the unique VDJ recombination is sufficient. The calculations of the various diversity indices can be calculated from the formulas or using programs available online such as PAST (http://folk.uio.no/ohammer/past/) (Hammer et al., 2001).

3.1 Richness and sample size, diversity indices of order zero for the TCR repertoire

Sample size is the sum of these abundances, so corresponding to the number of total sequences and richness of the repertoire is the sum of unique VDJ recombination thus corresponding to the number of unique sequences. These indices are simple; however, they do not take into account the different unique sequences and the abundance of each of the unique sequences. Therefore, higher order of diversity indices should be considered as well.

3.2 Shannon's *H*, diversity index of order one for the TCR repertoire

Shannon's *H* entropy index, also known as Shannon's diversity index, the Shannon–Wiener index, the Shannon–Weaver index, and the Shannon entropy, was originally developed to measure the uncertainty in strings of text in information sciences. Therefore, the more equal the proportional abundances of various letters in a string of text the more difficult to correctly predict which letter will be the next one in the string, and the higher the level of uncertainty and Shannon's *H*. The proportional abundances in a string of text reaches equal distribution as the length of the string of text grows, thus leading to higher diversity. Simply, if we take two strings of text where the lengths are equal but the proportional abundances are different so that the first string of text has five letters that are more abundant, this may not affect the overall representation of the letters in the string but if there was a rare letter then that letter may be lost to account for the more abundant letter. As there are five letters that are more abundant than other letters, one can predict with a lower level of uncertainly that the next letter in the string of text would be one of the five. This demonstrates that Shannon's *H* is more sensitive to the rare species and more informative as the sample size grows. In addition, it is important to note that this entropy has no relation to the more commonly known entropy of thermodynamics.

Shannon's *H* is very popular in ecology, to study the diversity of an ecosystem in relation to the proportional abundances of various species to which individual entities belong, where the higher the Shannon's *H* the more equal are the abundances of the different types and species and thus the bigger the overall sampled and actual diversity. Therefore, it is more difficult to predict (higher the uncertainty) which species the next sampled individual entity will belong to and so the uncertainty level is increased as Shannon's *H* increases. Furthermore, as one type becomes very abundant, the Shannon's *H* decreases as it becomes easier to predict which type the next sampled individual entity will belong to; most probably, it will belong to the most abundant type.

Shannon's *H* determined for a TCR repertoire measures the diversity of the sampled repertoire taking into account the clonal size distribution in the overall repertoire. The higher the index, the more diverse the repertoire; however, a lower index is not only affected by the unique number of sequences but also by clonal expansion. For example, there are three repertoires with an equal number of sequences; the first repertoire data set has 10 unique sequences with abundance of 1 for each; the second repertoire data set has nine unique sequences with abundance of 1 except for one unique sequences, which has abundance of 2; and the third repertoire data set has five unique sequences with abundance of 2 for each. The Shannon's *H* for these repertoires equals 2.303, 2.164, and 1.582, respectively, reflecting the reduced diversity due to the reduced richness; in other words, unique sequences of 10, 9, and 5. Although the richness of the third repertoire is half of the first repertoire, the Shannon's *H* is not reduced by half because there is a weight on the distribution of abundance or proportional abundances. Therefore, Shannon's *H* is affected by the way the abundances are distributed. If we look at a fourth repertoire with the same unique and total sequences as the third repertoire but the distribution of the abundance is different so that there is a large clonal expansion, then the Shannon's *H* is adversely affected (Table 1).

By looking at the Shannon's *H* of two other repertoires that have the same unique sequences, equal proportional abundances but higher total sequences (repertoires 5 and 6 in Table 1), we can understand that it is similar to Shannon's *H* of repertoire 1. In

Table 1 Example data sets and their diversity indices

	Data set abundances	Richness unique sequences	Sample size total sequences	Shannon's *H*	Gini–Simpson (Simpson's *D*)
Repertoire 1	1, 1, 1, 1, 1, 1, 1, 1, 1, 1	10	10	2.303 (10/10)	0 (1)
Repertoire 2	1, 1, 1, 1, 1, 1, 1, 1,2	9	10	2.164 (9/10)	0.022 (0.978)
Repertoire 3	2, 2, 2, 2, 2	5	10	1.582 (0/10)	0.111 (0.889)
Repertoire 4	1, 1, 1, 1, 6	5	10	1.228 (4/5)	0.333 (0.667)
Repertoire 5	2, 2, 2, 2, 2, 2, 2, 2, 2, 2	10	20	2.303 (0/10)	0.053 (0.947)
Repertoire 6	10,10,10,10,10, 10,10,10,10,10	10	100	2.303 (0/10)	0.091 (0.909)
Repertoire 7	19,15,10,10,10, 10,10,10,5,1	10	100	2.177 (1/10)	0.112 (0.888)
Repertoire 8	91, 1, 1, 1, 1, 1, 1, 1, 1, 1	10	100	0.500 (9/10)	0.827 (0.173)

addition, if we compare it to a repertoire with the same unique and total sequences but the distribution of the abundances are different, it results in different Shannon's *H*, reducing with the presence of more common and rare species (repertoires 6 and 7, Table 1). Thus, Shannon's *H* is mostly affected by the unique sequences and distribution of the abundances. This is especially important in determining the diversity of TCR repertoire determined by NGS, as depending on the platforms used such as 454 versus illumina where illumine generates significantly more total sequence reads per sample, input RNA or gDNA used, the total number of sequences can range from thousands to millions, not necessarily each sequence being a unique sequence. However, Shannon's *H* determines the diversity in the sampled repertoire taking into account the unique sequences and distribution of clonal size, regardless of the total sequences.

Hence, it is important to determine whether the sampled sequences of a TCR repertoire are enough. One option is to sequence until one does not see an abundance of 1, which means that we have captured almost entirely the TCR repertoire. However, this is not always possible, especially when there are numerous samples in a study where the number of sequences obtained from each individual or sample is reduced due to pooling together multiple samples in a single NGS sequencing reaction. Another option is to characterize the repertoire as a whole, including several diversity indices and taking into account how deep the sampling of the TCR repertoire was. One of the easiest options was to not count the abundances of one in the data set. This will give an idea regarding the sampling of the repertoire. Thus, we can see that data sets 3, 5, and 6 in Table 1 are most likely sampled enough and any additional sampling may just increase the abundance of already existing types and will not increase the types. However, for the other repertoires in the table, especially repertoire 1, it is hard to predict whether the next sample will be a new type or one that already has been sampled.

3.3 Gini–Simpson index, diversity index of order two for the TCR repertoire

The Gini–Simpson index originates from the Simpson's *D* index, which determines the probability that two entities taken randomly from the data set are from different types. Therefore, the Gini–Simpson index, which is 1-D, calculates the probability that two entities are from same type. The Gini–Simpson index for the TCR repertoire represents the probability that two sequences of a data set are from the same unique sequence, due to higher abundances of certain sequences. As can be seen in repertoires 6, 7, and 8 in Table 1, these repertoires all have similar total and unique sequences but the distribution of the proportional abundances of the sequences are different and the Gini–Simpson index increases as there are clones that are highly abundant. Therefore, the higher the Gini–Simpson index, the more uneven the distribution of the abundances of the sequences in a TCR repertoire and thus the higher the diversity of the overall repertoire.

Furthermore, the Gini–Simpson index changes very quickly when there are dominant clones such as in repertoire 8; thus, the Gini–Simpson index is less sensitive to rare clones and sequences (Fig. 2A).

3.4 Top 10 and 100 frequencies

For the TCR repertoire it is important to graph the frequencies of the most abundant clones, showing the distribution and size of the top clones (O'Connell et al., 2014; Rechavi et al., 2015). This type of analysis either shows that the distribution does not vary among the top clones and they are of equal and low frequency, as seen for healthy donors, or emphasizes the clones with higher abundances, depicting clonal expansion due to an infection or disease. Depending on the study and data, it may be enough to present the top 10, when there are only a few expanded clones.

3.5 Tree map

Often, graphical presentations are most intuitive and readily understood. The graphical presentation of the TCR sequencing data in the form of a tree map, where each CDR3 is represented by a different colored dot and the size of the dot corresponding to the abundance of the CDR3 (Fig. 2B) (Lee et al., 2014; Rechavi et al., 2015), can be instantly informative and appealing. Therefore, representing graphically the CDR3 repertoire of TCR by a tree map and then quantifying the overall repertoire using diversity indices to compare between samples most comprehensively describes the diversity of a repertoire, both qualitatively and quantitatively.

4. ANALYSIS OF GENE USAGES IN TCR REPERTOIRE

As there are many genes involved in generating the TCR, the information on gene usages may be overwhelming. Based on the international ImMunoGeneTics information system® (IMGT), for TRB repertoire there are 48 TRBV, 2 TRBD, and 11 TRBJ known functional genes; for TRA and TRD repertoire (because the genes for TRA and TRD are present in the same locus) there are 48 TRADV, 3 TRDD, 4 TRDJ, and 50 TRAJ known functional genes. The TRG repertoire is generated with six TRGV and five TRGJ genes, from the repertoire of the least number of gene segments.

4.1 Unique versus total gene usages

The analysis of the gene usages need to be defined whether it is using the unique sequence data set or the total sequence data set. If the sequences are organized in a table with each sequence with the corresponding V, J, and/or D genes and abundances, then gene usages on the unique sequence data set is counting each sequence once and gene usages on the total sequence data set is counting each sequence by the number of abundances. The differences in the gene usages according to unique versus total sequences can be shown most effectively using the donut diagrams as seen in Fig. 3A. In healthy controls, the distribution of the unique sequence is similar to total sequence (Fig. 3A) (O'Connell et al., 2014). However, when there are dominant clones, then the donut diagram of the total sequences will be shifted from the donut diagram of the unique sequences (Fig. 3B). These differences can be statistically tested by correlation tests, comparing the frequencies of the unique sequences to the frequencies of the total sequences. As the gene usages of the unique and total sequences are similar, the correlation index will be high (Fig. 3C). However, when gene usages of the unique and total are different, the correlation index will be low (Fig. 3D).

In addition to comparing the distribution of the frequencies of unique and total sequences, we can determine whether there are genes that are preferentially used. It is

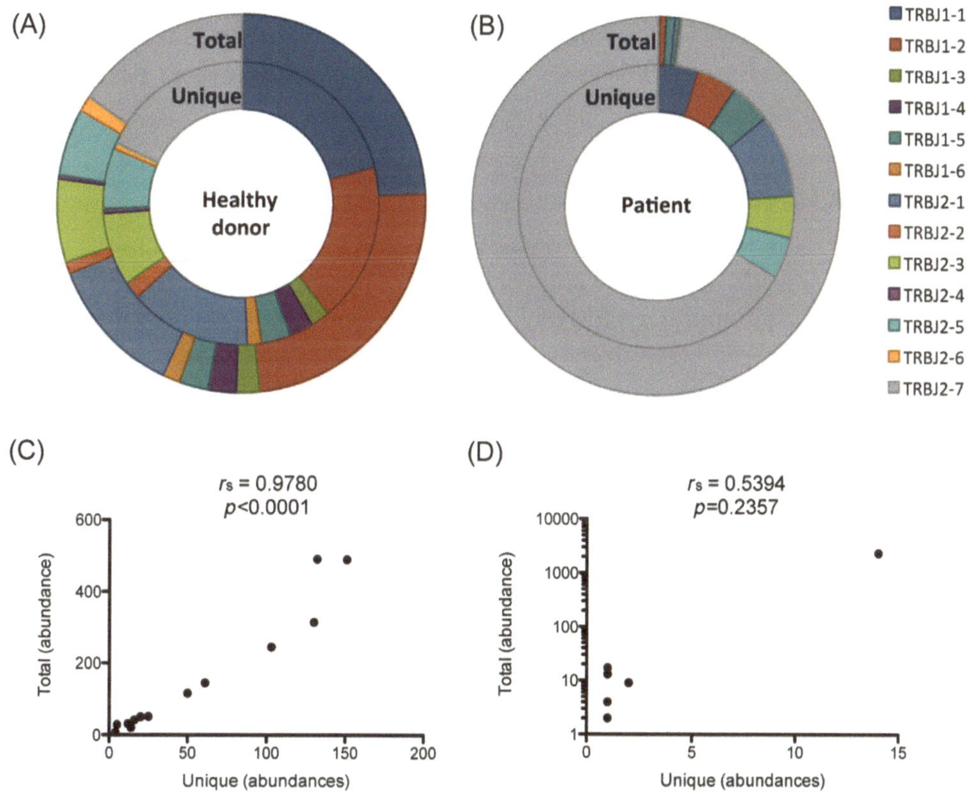

Figure 3 Gene usage analysis. Donut diagrams of unique (*inner circle*) versus total (*outer circle*) TRBJ gene usages from a healthy donor (A) and from a patient (B). The genes TRBJ1-3, 1-4, 1-6, 2-2, 2-4, and 2-6 are not present in the patient's TRB repertoire. Spearman's correlation of unique versus total in the healthy donor (C) and in the patient (D). The data sets used for healthy donor and patient shown in this figure are the same data set used for Fig. 2B.

important to note that unique sequences may reflect the genetic effect and the total sequences reflect the environmental effect. Thus, if the preferential usages are both in the unique and total sequences, then the effect is on the genetic level. If the preferential usages are only in total sequences, then this effect is due to the environment. However, if the preferential usages are only in the unique sequences, then there may be a negative selection to the specific genetic effect. Miles et al. (2011) have comprehensively summarized gene usage biases that have been observed with certain pathogens or disease, and such lists should be updated as new findings emerge.

4.2 D-proximal V and J genes usages

Because the D genes rearrange to J genes first and then the V genes rearrange to the DJ, and the rearrangement proceeds with the genes that are most proximal to each other, it is important to organize the gene usages according to their position in the genomic loci. These types of analyses are most important when studying the repertoire with regards to factors affecting either the accessibility of the genomic loci (Guo et al., 2002) (preferential TRAV proximal TRAJ usages in mice) or T cell ontogeny and development (Rechavi et al., 2015).

5. CHARACTERISTICS OF CDR3

The CDR3 region is not only composed of V, D, and J genes, but additionally determined by junctional diversity, generating the highest diversity for this region. The function of CDR3 is to bind to a vast array of ligands. Therefore, it is very important to characterize CDR3 to best understand the functions of the whole repertoire. For instance, we can determine whether a repertoire is abundant for a specific CDR3 that are known to bind to certain antigens or in the presence of a viral infection. Furthermore, even if there is no increase in abundance of a TCR molecule with a specific CDR3, other characteristics such as CDR3 length and composition, amino acid hydrophobicity, and composition can be studied. These analyses can be done using the HighV-QUEST of IMGT (Li et al., 2013) for determining the gene usage, CDR3 amino acid and nucleotide, CDR3 length and IgAT (Rogosch et al., 2012), which automatically performs additional analysis using the output files of HighV-QUEST. These additional analyses focus on the characterization of the CDR3 region such as amino acid composition and hydrophobicity, Shannon's *H* for the amino acid used in each of the position of the CDR3, CDR3 length distribution, and deconstruction maps. These are freely available to nonprofit academic communities.

5.1 CDR3 length distribution

In fetal blood, distributions of CDR3 lengths of the TRB repertoire are relatively shorter than in infants (Rechavi et al., 2015), and they gradually get longer as the fetus matures.

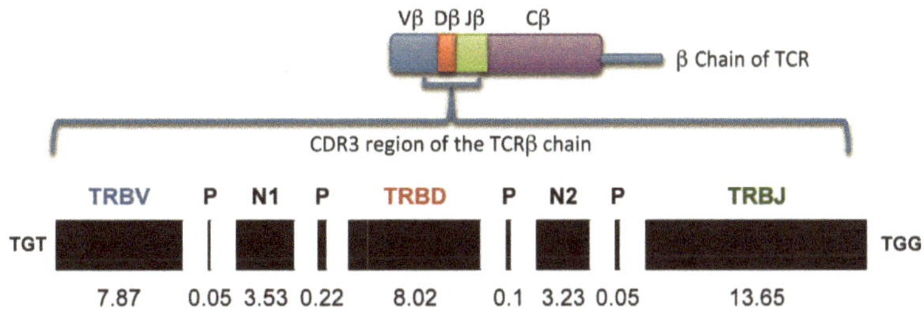

Figure 4 Deconstruction map representing the CDR3 region of healthy donors. The numbers represent the average length of each segment in nucleotides.

Abnormal distribution of CDR3 lengths may represent underlying immune abnormalities from block in development and maturation to skewed gene usages due to infections and diseases.

5.2 Deconstruction map to understand P and N nucleotide addition

Deconstruction map provides a detailed description of the junctional diversity, from the contribution in length of the various V, D, and J genes to the P and N nucleotide additions (Fig. 4) (Rogosch et al., 2012). These analyses may shed light on the possible mechanisms behind observed abnormalities in the CDR3 length distributions.

5.3 Amino acid usage and distribution and hydrophobicity

Differential gene usage and abnormal distribution of CDR3 lengths may change the amino acid composition and hydrophobicity, thus altering the ability to interact with various ligands. Analyses of amino acid composition and hydrophobicity may provide explanations for an underlying immune deregulation. As NGS technology allows us to obtain a large number of sequences, subtle differences that may have been missed may now be significant. The power of such analyses lies in the number of the sequences. Therefore, it is important to study the composition of the CDR3 region, especially on TCR repertoire data generated using the NGS technologies.

5.4 Clonal sharing/public clones

Determining which clones are shared among various patient groups is probably the most valuable information toward development of a targeted therapy. In addition, collection of data listing which shared clones are commonly found in various conditions will possibly aid in understanding of yet unknown mechanisms of diseases and processes (Krell et al., 2013; Rechavi et al., 2015).

6. CONCLUDING REMARKS

In this chapter about TCR repertoire analysis, few basic analyses were discussed. Depending on the specificity of the study and emerging new questions, other types of analyses certainly will be needed. However, the analyses that were mentioned here should be carried out almost systematically by all research involving TCR repertoires determined by NGS, so that new studies can be effortlessly compared to previous studies. Furthermore, although TCR repertoire was discussed here, similar analyses can be and should be done for BCR repertoires.

The combination of in-depth knowledge of the immune system and TCR repertoire analyses will lead to insightful findings and will further our knowledge about the complexity in generating the immune repertoires.

REFERENCES

Bajor, D.L., Xu, X., Torigian, D.A., Mick, R., Garcia, L.R., Richman, L.P., Desmarais, C., Nathanson, K.L., Schuchter, L.M., Kalos, M., Vonderheide, R.H., 2014. Immune activation and a 9-year ongoing complete remission following CD40 antibody therapy and metastasectomy in a patient with metastatic melanoma. Cancer Immunol. Res. 2, 1051–1058.

Becattini, S., Latorre, D., Mele, F., Foglierini, M., De Gregorio, C., Cassotta, A., Fernandez, B., Kelderman, S., Schumacher, T.N., Corti, D., Lanzavecchia, A., Sallusto, F., 2015. T cell immunity. Functional heterogeneity of human memory CD4(+) T cell clones primed by pathogens or vaccines. Science 347, 400–406.

Bonnet, M., Ferrier, P., Spicuglia, S., 2009. Molecular genetics at the T-cell receptor beta locus: insights into the regulation of V(D)J recombination. Adv. Exp. Med. Biol. 650, 116–132.

Chaumeil, J., Skok, J.A., 2013. A new take on v(d)j recombination: transcription driven nuclear and chromatin reorganization in rag-mediated cleavage. Front. Immunol. 4, 423.

Chien, Y.H., Meyer, C., Bonneville, M., 2014. Gammadelta T cells: first line of defense and beyond. Annu. Rev. Immunol. 32, 121–155.

George Jr., J.F., Schroeder Jr., H.W., 1992. Developmental regulation of D beta reading frame and junctional diversity in T cell receptor-beta transcripts from human thymus. J. Immunol. 148, 1230–1239.

Gil, A., Yassai, M.B., Naumov, Y.N., Selin, L.K., 2015. Narrowing of human influenza A virus specific T cell receptor alpha and beta repertoire with increasing age. J. Virol. 89 (8), 4102–4116.

Guo, J., Hawwari, A., Li, H., Sun, Z., Mahanta, S.K., Littman, D.R., Krangel, M.S., He, Y.W., 2002. Regulation of the TCRalpha repertoire by the survival window of CD4(+)CD8(+) thymocytes. Nat. Immunol. 3, 469–476.

Hammer, Ø., Harper, D.A.T., Ryan, 2001. PAST: paleontological statistics software package for education and data analysis. Palaeontol. Electron. 4.

Helmink, B.A., Sleckman, B.P., 2012. The response to and repair of RAG-mediated DNA double-strand breaks. Annu. Rev. Immunol. 30, 175–202.

Krangel, M.S., Carabana, J., Abbarategui, I., Schlimgen, R., Hawwari, A., 2004. Enforcing order within a complex locus: current perspectives on the control of V(D)J recombination at the murine T-cell receptor alpha/delta locus. Immunol. Rev. 200, 224–232.

Krell, P.F., Reuther, S., Fischer, U., Keller, T., Weber, S., Gombert, M., Schuster, F.R., Asang, C., Stepensky, P., Strahm, B., Meisel, R., Stoye, J., Borkhardt, A., 2013. Next-generation-sequencing-spectratyping reveals public T-cell receptor repertoires in pediatric very severe aplastic anemia and identifies a beta chain CDR3 sequence associated with hepatitis-induced pathogenesis. Haematologica 98, 1388–1396.

Lee, Y.N., Frugoni, F., Dobbs, K., Walter, J.E., Giliani, S., Gennery, A.R., Al-Herz, W., Haddad, E., Ledeist, F., Bleesing, J.H., Henderson, L.A., Pai, S.Y., Nelson, R.P., El-Ghoneimy, D.H., El-Feky, R.A., Reda, S.M., Hossny, E., Soler-Palacin, P., Fuleihan, R.L., Patel, N.C., Massaad, M.J., Geha, R.S., Puck, J.M., Palma, P., Cancrini, C., Chen, K., Vihinen, M., Alt, F.W., Notarangelo, L.D., 2014. A systematic analysis of recombination activity and genotype-phenotype

correlation in human recombination-activating gene 1 deficiency. J. Allergy Clin. Immunol. 133, 1099–1108.
Li, S., Lefranc, M.P., Miles, J.J., Alamyar, E., Giudicelli, V., Duroux, P., Freeman, J.D., Corbin, V.D., Scheerlinck, J.P., Frohman, M.A., Cameron, P.U., Plebanski, M., Loveland, B., Burrows, S.R., Papenfuss, A.T., Gowans, E.J., 2013. IMGT/HighV QUEST paradigm for T cell receptor IMGT clonotype diversity and next generation repertoire immunoprofiling. Nat. Commun. 4, 2333.
Meier, J., Roberts, C., Avent, K., Hazlett, A., Berrie, J., Payne, K., Hamm, D., Desmarais, C., Sanders, C., Hogan, K.T., Archer, K.J., Manjili, M.H., Toor, A.A., 2013. Fractal organization of the human T cell repertoire in health and after stem cell transplantation. Biol. Blood Marrow Transplant. 19, 366–377.
Miles, J.J., Douek, D.C., Price, D.A., 2011. Bias in the alphabeta T-cell repertoire: implications for disease pathogenesis and vaccination. Immunol. Cell Biol. 89, 375–387.
O'Connell, A.E., Volpi, S., Dobbs, K., Fiorini, C., Tsitsikov, E., De Boer, H., Barlan, I.B., Despotovic, J.M., Espinosa-Rosales, F.J., Hanson, I.C., Kanariou, M.G., Martinez-Beckerat, R., Mayorga-Sirera, A., Mejia-Carvajal, C., Radwan, N., Weiss, A.R., Pai, S.Y., Lee, Y.N., Notarangelo, L.D., 2014. Next generation sequencing reveals skewing of the T and B cell receptor repertoires in patients with Wiskott-Aldrich syndrome. Front. Immunol. 5, 340.
Rechavi, E., Lev, A., Lee, Y.N., Simon, A.J., Yinon, Y., Lipitz, S., Amariglio, N., Weisz, B., Notarangelo, L.D., Somech, R., 2015. Timely and spatially regulated maturation of B and T cell repertoire during human fetal development. Sci. Transl. Med. 7 (276), 276ra25.
Rogosch, T., Kerzel, S., Hoi, K.H., Zhang, Z., Maier, R.F., Ippolito, G.C., Zemlin, M., 2012. Immunoglobulin analysis tool: a novel tool for the analysis of human and mouse heavy and light chain transcripts. Front. Immunol. 3, 176.
Sarzotti, M., Patel, D.D., Li, X., Ozaki, D.A., Cao, S., Langdon, S., Parrott, R.E., Coyne, K., Buckley, R.H., 2003. T cell repertoire development in humans with SCID after nonablative allogeneic marrow transplantation. J. Immunol. 170, 2711–2718.
Schroeder Jr., H.W., Zhang, L., Philips 3rd, J.B., 2001. Slow, programmed maturation of the immunoglobulin HCDR3 repertoire during the third trimester of fetal life. Blood 98, 2745–2751.
Sleckman, B.P., Bassing, C.H., Bardon, C.G., Okada, A., Khor, B., Bories, J.C., Monroe, R., Alt, F.W., 1998. Accessibility control of variable region gene assembly during T-cell development. Immunol. Rev. 165, 121–130.
Spicuglia, S., Pekowska, A., Zacarias-Cabeza, J., Ferrier, P., 2010. Epigenetic control of Tcrb gene rearrangement. Semin. Immunol. 22, 330–336.
Thai, T.H., Kearney, J.F., 2005. Isoforms of terminal deoxynucleotidyltransferase: developmental aspects and function. Adv. Immunol. 86, 113–136.
Turner, S.J., Doherty, P.C., McCluskey, J., Rossjohn, J., 2006. Structural determinants of T-cell receptor bias in immunity. Nat. Rev. Immunol. 6, 883–894.
Van Heijst, J.W., Ceberio, I., Lipuma, L.B., Samilo, D.W., Wasilewski, G.D., Gonzales, A.M., Nieves, J.L., Van Den Brink, M.R., Perales, M.A., Pamer, E.G., 2013. Quantitative assessment of T cell repertoire recovery after hematopoietic stem cell transplantation. Nat. Med. 19, 372–377.
Wang, X., Xiao, G., Zhang, Y., Wen, X., Gao, X., Okada, S., Liu, X., 2008. Regulation of Tcrb recombination ordering by c-Fos-dependent RAG deposition. Nat. Immunol. 9, 794–801.
Yu, X., Almeida, J.R., Darko, S., Van Der Burg, M., Deravin, S.S., Malech, H., Gennery, A., Chinn, I., Markert, M.L., Douek, D.C., Milner, J.D., 2014. Human syndromes of immunodeficiency and dysregulation are characterized by distinct defects in T-cell receptor repertoire development. J. Allergy Clin. Immunol. 133, 1109–1115.
Zemlin, M., Schelonka, R.L., Bauer, K., Schroeder Jr., H.W., 2002. Regulation and chance in the ontogeny of B and T cell antigen receptor repertoires. Immunol. Res. 26, 265–278.

SECTION B

Emerging Pharmacological Targets

CHAPTER 5

Th17 Cells

Jianfei Yang
GlaxoSmithKline, Cambridge, MA, United States

Contents

1. INTRODUCTION

Naïve $CD4^+$ T helper (Th) cells are activated and differentiated to different subsets upon antigen stimulation via MHC class II on antigen presenting cells (APCs) and cytokine costimulation. In 1986, Mosmann and Coffman discovered that $CD4^+$ T cells are divided into two subsets, Th1 and Th2 cells, based on their production of cytokines (Mosmann et al., 1986; Mosmann and Coffman, 1989). $CD4^+$ Th cells are differentiated to Th1 cells in the presence of interleukin-12 (IL-12). Th1 cells produce interferon-γ (IFNγ) and are dependent on STAT4 and the master transcription factor T-bet (Tbx21). Th2 cells are differentiated upon activation of STAT6 and the master transcription factor GATA3

Translational Immunology
http://dx.doi.org/10.1016/B978-0-12-801577-3.00006-X

upon stimulation by IL-4. Th2 are marked by the expression of IL-4, IL-5, and IL13. Th1 cells play a critical role in host immunity to intracellular pathogens and viruses while Th2 cells are important for humoral immune responses. Overactivation or deregulation of Th1 or Th2 cells was thought to be the key cause of autoimmune and allergic inflammatory diseases (Mosmann and Coffman, 1989; Murphy and Reiner, 2002).

The Th1 cytokine IL-12 is composed of two subunits: IL-12 p35 and IL-12 p40. The critical role of IL-12 in Th cell development was discovered by Murphy and colleagues, showing that IL-12 induces the differentiation of Th1 cells (Hsieh et al., 1993). Indeed, IL-12 p40-deficient mice are defective in IFNγ production and type 1 cytokine responses (Magram et al., 1996). Genetically resistant mice lacking IL-12 are susceptible to infection with *Leishmania major* and mount a polarized Th2 cell response (Mattner et al., 1996). Experimental autoimmune encephalomyelitis (EAE), an animal model of multiple sclerosis (MS), was believed to be a Th1-mediated neuroinflammation. MS-like prolonged and relapsing EAE in dark agouti rats is associated with a prolonged expression of proinflammatory cytokines including IL-12 (Issazadeh et al., 1996). Increased IL-12 production in progressive MS has been reported (Balashov et al., 1997). Mice treated with recombinant IL-12 *in vivo* after the transfer of antigen-stimulated lymph node cells developed a more severe and prolonged course of disease compared with vehicle-treated control animals. In contrast, treatment of mice with an antibody to murine IL-12 after cell transfer completely prevented paralysis, with only 40% of the mice developing mild disease (Leonard et al., 1995). In addition, DBA/1 mice deficient in IL-12 p40 showed reduced incidence and severity of collagen-induced arthritis (CIA), an animal model of rheumatoid arthritis (RA) (McIntyre et al., 1996). In an inflammatory bowel disease (IBD) model, administration of monoclonal anti-IL-12 p40 antibodies to the TNBS-treated mice both early (at day 5) and late (at day 20) after induction of colitis led to a striking improvement in both the clinical and histopathological aspects of the disease and frequently abrogated the established colitis completely (Neurath et al., 1995). These observations indicate that the Th1 cytokine IL-12 and Th1 cells play a critical role in the pathogenesis of several autoimmune diseases.

However, Oppmann et al. discovered that IL-12 p40 is also a component of IL-23, in combination with its p19 subunit (Oppmann et al., 2000). Therefore, the effect of IL-12 p40-deficiency or anti-IL-12 p40 antibodies could be due to the loss of function of IL-23. In order to address this question, Cua and colleagues tested mice deficient in each of the three subunits (IL-12 $p35^{-/-}$, IL-12/IL-23 $p40^{-/-}$, and IL-23 $p19^{-/-}$) in a CIA model. IL-12/IL-23 p40-deficient or IL-23 p19-deficient mice protected from induction of CIA while IL-12 $p35^{-/-}$ mice showed similar disease induction to wild-type mice (Murphy et al., 2003). Thus, IL-23 but not IL-12 plays a critical role in the pathogenesis of the autoimmune diseases such as CIA. Importantly, Cua and colleagues later demonstrated that IL-23 induces IL-17 (formerly known as IL-17A) expression by $CD4^+$ T cells from lymph node cells immunized with MOG antigen. These cells were later named Th17 cells. The investigators discovered that IL-23-induced Th17 cells (Th_{IL-17} or Th17 cells) transferred EAE disease much more efficiently than IL-12-induced Th1 cells (Langrish et al., 2005). Since then, Th17 cells have been demonstrated to be critical in protective immunity as well as autoimmune inflammatory diseases.

2. Th17 CELL DIFFERENTIATION

As discussed above, IL-23 induces the generation of Th17 cells *ex vivo*. *In vitro*, the groups of Weaver and Dong demonstrated IL-23 induces the differentiation of Th17 cells from lymph node or spleen cells in the absence of IFNγ and IL-4 (Harrington et al., 2005; Park et al., 2005), demonstrating the IFNγ and IL-4 are negative regulators of Th17 cells. In addition to IL-17, Th17 cells also express IL-17F, IL-21, IL-22, and CCL20. The role of IL-23 in the differentiation of Th17 cells is complicated as IL-23 alone cannot induce the differentiation of Th17 cells from naïve $CD4^+$ T cells (Bettelli et al., 2006). Instead, Bettelli et al. and Veldhoen et al. simultaneously discovered that IL-6 and TGFβ1 are critical factors for the differentiation of Th17 cells from naïve $CD4^+$ cells (Bettelli et al., 2006; Veldhoen et al., 2006). Although TGFβ1 is believed to be a differentiation factor for the generation of inducible T regulatory cells, it is also required for the generation of Th17 cells. Significantly enhanced Th17 cells were observed from TGFβ1-transgenic mice immunized with MOG_{33-35} peptide (Bettelli et al., 2006). In TGFβ1-deficient mice, the development of Th17 cells were significantly impaired (Mangan et al., 2006). Another cytokine, IL-21, has also been shown to induce the differentiation of Th17 cells in the presence of TGFβ1. Th17 cells themselves produce IL-21, which then plays an autocrine role in Th17 cell development (Bauquet et al., 2009; Nurieva et al., 2007). In addition to cytokines, high concentrations of sodium have been reported to promote the generation of Th17 cells (Wu et al., 2013).

In humans, IL-6 and TGFβ1 failed to induce Th17 cell differentiation *in vitro*. Instead, IL-1β/IL-6 or IL-1β/IL-23 can induce the differentiation of naïve $CD4^+$ T cells into Th17 cells, indicating TGFβ1 is not required in human Th17 cell development. However, culture conditions contain serum in the medium, in which TGFβ1 may exist. Indeed, in serum-free medium, TGFβ1 is required for the differentiation of human Th17 cells. Th17 cells can be induced by costimulation with TGFβ1/IL1β/IL-6. Addition of IL-23 could further differentiate Th17 cells and maintain the phenotype of Th17 cells. In addition, TGFβ1 and IL-21 were also found to induce the generation of human Th17 cells (Korn et al., 2007; Yang et al., 2008b). For more details, the readers are referred to the review by Kuchroo and colleagues (Korn et al., 2009).

While IL-1β, IL-6, IL-23, and TGFβ1 are important for the differentiation of Th17 cells, several different cytokines inhibit the development of Th17 cells. Murine naïve $CD4^+$ T cells when cultured in the presence of APC can differentiate into Th17 cells by IL-23 stimulation and neutralization of IFNγ and/or IL-4 (Harrington et al., 2005;

Park et al., 2005). IL-10 has been demonstrated to negatively regulate cytokine expression and inflammation. A significantly high level of IL-17 was produced by splenic cells or macrophages from mice deficient in IL-10 or IL-10R (Gu et al., 2008). In addition, IL-27 can also act directly on effector T cells to suppress the development of IL-17-producing Th cells mediated by IL-6 and TGFβ1. IL-27Rα-deficient mice generated more IL-17-producing Th cells (Batten et al., 2006; Stumhofer et al., 2006). IL-27 inhibits Th17 cell differentiation by downmodulating RORγt expression (Diveu et al., 2009). Interestingly, EBI3-deficent cells produced significantly higher level of IL-17 (Yang et al., 2008a). Negative regulation of IL-17 by EBI3 could be due to the role of IL-27 because IL-27 is composed with EBI3 and p28. EBI3 also associates with IL-12 p35 to form IL-35. In line with this, IL-35 inhibited the differentiation of Th17 cells *in vitro*. *In vivo*, IL-35 effectively attenuated established CIA in mice, with concomitant suppression of IL-17 production (Niedbala et al., 2007). Taken together, IL-1β, IL-6, IL-23, and TGFβ1 promote the differentiation of Th17 cells while IL-10, IL-27, IL-35, IL-4, and IFNγ negatively regulate IL-17 production and Th17 cell development. Fig. 1 illustrates the complex pathway leading to differentiation of Th17 cells.

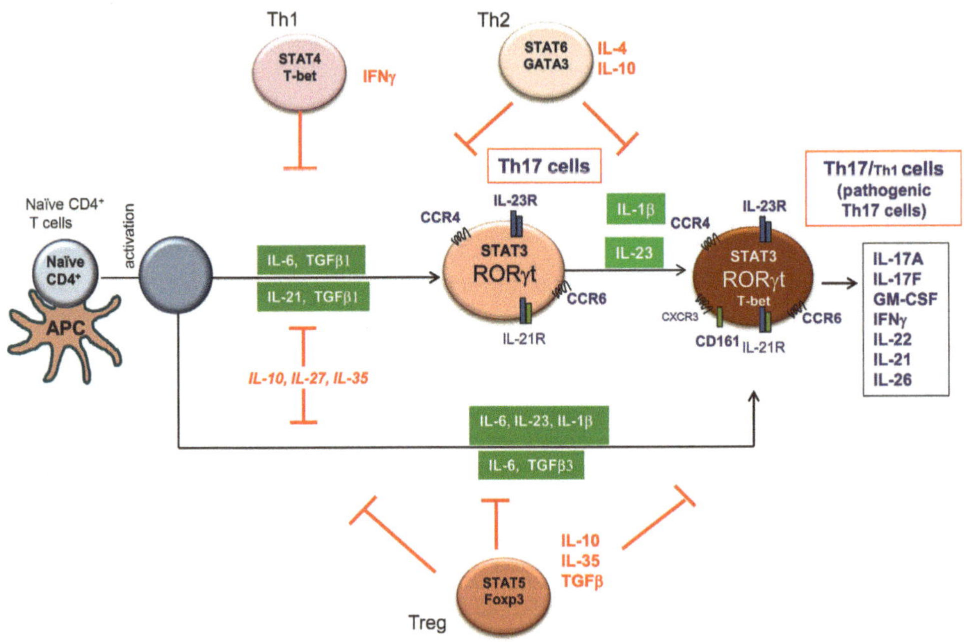

Figure 1 Regulation of Th17 cells. TCR signaling plus the costimulation of several cytokines, such as IL-6, TGFβ, IL-1β, IL-23, and IL-21, induce RORγt expression and Th17 cell differentiation. IL-23 signaling is critical for the generation of pathogenic Th17 cells. Th1, Th2, and regulatory T cells (Tregs) cytokines can inhibit the differentiation of Th17 cells.

After the discovery of IL-17-producing $CD4^+$ Th17 cells, various immune cells have been found to express IL-17, including $CD8^+$ Tc17 cell, γδ T cells, innate lymphoid cells (ILCs), natural killer T (NKT) cells, B cells, macrophages, and neutrophils. This chapter will focus on Th17 cells as they are believed to be the major IL-17-producing cells responsible for numerous autoimmune and inflammatory diseases.

3. TRANSCRIPTIONAL REGULATION OF Th17 CELLS

Transcription factors drive the lineage differentiation of Th cells. For example, STAT3 and T-bet drive Th1 differentiation while STAT6 and GATA3 are required for the development of Th2 cells. For Th17 cells, Littman, Cua and colleagues first discovered that orphan nuclear receptor RORγt is a key regulator of Th17 cell differentiation. RORγt is differentially expressed in Th17 cells and it is both necessary and sufficient for IL-17 expression as well as Th17 cell differentiation in mouse and human $CD4^+$ T cells (Ivanov et al., 2006; Manel et al., 2008). T cells lacking RORγt ($Rorc^{-/-}$) fail to induce EAE (Ivanov et al., 2006). RORα is also expressed in Th17 cells and was shown to be important for Th17 cell differentiation (Yang et al., 2008c), although it is unclear whether RORα and RORγt have redundant or unique activities in regulating gene expression in Th17 cells. RORγt binds and activates the *Il-17* and *Il-17f* promoter (Yang et al., 2014). The signaling of IL-6 receptor (IL-6R), IL-23R, or IL-21R after cytokine engagement induces phosphorylation and subsequent dimerization of STAT3. The activated STAT3 then moves to the nucleus and activates the RORγt promoter along with other transcription factors. STAT3 deficiency in T cells decreases the expression of RORγt and abrogates the induction of Th17 cells while a hyperactive form of STAT3 promotes Th17 cell development (Harris et al., 2007; Yang et al., 2007). Accordingly, mice with conditional deficiency of STAT3 in $CD4^+$ T cells are resistant to Th17-mediated EAE and autoimmune pneumonitis (Harris et al., 2007).

The AP-1 transcription factor BATF has been demonstrated to be required for the differentiation of Th17 cells (Schraml et al., 2009). $Batf^{-/-}$ mice have normal Th1 and Th2 differentiation, but show a defect in Th17 differentiation, and are resistant to EAE. $Batf^{-/-}$ T cells fail to induce known factors required for Th17 differentiation, such as RORγt. Overexpression of RORγt did not fully restore IL17 production in $Batf^{-/-}$ T cells likely because BATF also binds conserved intergenic elements in the *Il17a-Il17f* locus (Schraml et al., 2009). Interferon regulatory factor 4 (IRF4) is also critical for the generation of Th17 cells. *Irf4*-deficient mice did not develop EAE, and Th cells from such mice failed to differentiate into Th17 cells. $Irf4^{-/-}$ T helper cells had less expression of RORγt and more expression of Foxp3 (Brustle et al., 2007). The ligand-dependent transcription factor aryl hydrocarbon receptor (AHR) has also been shown to be important for the Th17 cell differentiation. AHR is expressed in both human and mouse Th17 cells. Activation of AHR boosts Th17 cell differentiation. However, $CD4^+$ T cells from AHR-deficient mice can develop

Th17 cell responses (Quintana et al., 2008; Veldhoen et al., 2008). Transcription factor Runx1 influences Th17 differentiation by inducing RORγt expression and by binding to and acting together with RORγt during *Il17* transcription (Zhang et al., 2008).

In addition, IKKα and IκBζ are also required for the differentiation of Th17 cell (Li et al., 2011; Okamoto et al., 2010). TGFβ1 promotes Foxp3 expression, a master transcription factor for the differentiation of Treg cells (see chapter 8, Regulatory T Cells). Treg cells can antagonize the function of Th17, Th1, and Th2 cells. RORγt and Foxp3 are coexpressed in $CD4^+$ T cells exposed to TGFβ1 upon TCR stimulation (Zhou et al., 2008). TGFβ1-induced Foxp3 physically antagonizes RORγt function, while IL-6, IL-21, or IL-23 relive Foxp3-medicated inhibition of RORγt (Zhou et al., 2008). Foxp3 could also bind to RORα and antagonizes its function (Du et al., 2008). In addition, Foxp3 suppresses Runx1-induced *Il17* activation (Zhang et al., 2008). Another transcription factor IRF8 also inhibits RORγt function through binding to RORγt. Indeed, IRF-8-deficiency enhances Th17 cell differentiation (Ouyang et al., 2011).

4. PATHOGENIC Th17 CELLS

Th17 cells are responsible for a variety of autoimmune inflammatory diseases. The discovery of Th17 cells by Cua and colleagues showed that adoptive transfer of MOG-specific Th17 cells induces the development of EAE much more significantly than Th1 cells (Langrish et al., 2005). However, not all Th17 cells function similarly. Although IL-6/TGFβ1-treated lymph node cells from mice immunized with $PLP_{139-151}$ produce high level of IL-17, these cells fail to induce EAE. IL-23 plus IL-6/TGFβ1-treated IL-17-producing cells also fail to induce disease, indicating a non-pathogenic role for TGFβ1 (McGeachy et al., 2007). Rather, it is the IL-23-induced Th17 cells that play a critical role in the pathogenesis of EAE. This phenomenon was further confirmed by O'Shea and colleagues (Ghoreschi et al., 2010). These investigators found IL-23-induced $ROR\gamma t^+T\text{-}bet^+$ Th17 cells during CNS inflammation are more pathogenic than IL-6/TGFβ1-induced $ROR\gamma t^+T\text{-}bet^-$ Th17 cells. As it turns out, TGFβ1 inhibits the expression of IL-23-induced upregulation of *Il23r*. IL-23-induced pathogenic Th17 cells express a high level of *Ccl9, Cxcr3, Il2, Il33, Il18r1, Tbx21,* and *Hlx1*. In addition, the following genes were downregulated in pathogenic Th17 cells: *Ccl20, Cxcr6, Il9, Il10, Irf8, Ahr,* and *Maf* (Ghoreschi et al., 2010). Finally, Kuchroo and colleagues further discovered that Th17 cells induced by IL-6 and TGFβ3 but not TGFβ1 could transfer the disease in the EAE model (Lee et al., 2012). These pathogenic Th17 cells show unique gene signatures such as upregulation of *Cxcl3, Il22, Il3, Ccl4,* and *Gzmb* (Lee et al., 2012).

In humans, multidrug resistance type 1 $(MDR1)^+$ Th17 cells have been indicated to be pathogenic Th17 cells (Ramesh et al., 2014). These cells express both Th17 (IL-17, IL-17F, IL-22) and Th1 (IFN-γ) cytokines. $MDR1^+$ Th17 cells are enriched and activated in the gut of Crohn's disease (CD) patients. Furthermore, $MDR1^+$ Th17 cells are refractory to several glucocorticoids, indicating a possible mechanism of steroid resistance in CD patients (Ramesh et al., 2014).

5. Th17 IN PROTECTIVE IMMUNITY AGAINST INFECTIONS

The Th17 cytokines IL-17 and IL-23 are believed to be important for the protective immunity against infections caused by bacteria, parasites, or fungi. IL-23 and IL-17 are critical in the establishment of protective pulmonary $CD4^+$ T cell responses after vaccination and during *Mycobacterium tuberculosis* challenge (Khader et al., 2007). Overexpression of IL-17 in the pulmonary compartment using an adenovirus encoding murine IL-17 resulted in the local induction of TNFα, IL-1β, MIP2, and G-CSF, augmented polymorphonuclear leukocyte recruitment and enhanced bacterial clearance and survival after challenge with *Klebsiella pneumonia* (Ye et al., 2001). Lung IL-17 and IL-17F production in IL-23p19$^{-/-}$ mice was dramatically reduced, and the mice showed substantial mortality from a sub-lethal dose of *K. pneumonia*. A study using *Il17a*- and/or *Il17f*-deficient mice demonstrated that both IL-17F and IL-17 are involved in host defense against mucoepithelial infection by *Staphylococcus aureus* and *Citrobacter rodentium* (Ishigame et al., 2009). In an experimental model of cutaneous *S. aureus* infection, IL-17, which is produced by epidermal γδ T cells, is critical for the clearance of the infection (Cho et al., 2010). Administration of IL-17 restored bacterial control in IL-23p19$^{-/-}$ mice (Happel et al., 2005).

In vitro, stimulation of alveolar macrophages with *Pneumocystis carinii* induced IL-23, and *Il23p19* mRNA was expressed in lungs of mice infected with *P. carinii*. IL-23p19$^{-/-}$ mice displayed transient but impaired clearance of infection of *P. carinii* in the lung. Administration of either anti-IL-23p19 or anti-IL-17 neutralizing antibody to wild-type mice infected with *P. carinii* also caused increases in fungal burdens (Rudner et al., 2007).

IL-17R-deficient mice have been utilized to demonstrate the importance of IL-17 and IL-17F in the host defense to systemic fungal *Candida albicans* infection (Huang et al., 2004). IL-23p19$^{-/-}$ and IL-17RA$^{-/-}$ mice experienced severe oropharyngeal candidiasis, whereas IL-12p35$^{-/-}$ mice showed low fungal burdens and no overt disease (Conti et al., 2009). Natural Th17 and γδ T cells, but not ILCs, are key mucosal sentinels that control oral pathogens such as *C. albicans* (Conti et al., 2014).

6. Th17 CELLS IN AUTOIMMUNE AND INFLAMMATORY DISEASES

6.1 Multiple sclerosis

MS is a chronic inflammatory autoimmune disease of the central nervous system that leads to brain inflammation and myelin destruction. Previously, MS was believed to be predominantly driven by Th1 cells. For example, IFNβ therapy has been suggested to benefit MS patients by skewing Th1 response to Th2 response. However, studies found no evidence of a Th1- or Th2-mRNA-promoting effect of IFNβ therapy in clinic (Krakauer et al., 2008). Instead, accumulating evidence supports Th17 cells and Th17 cytokines as being critical for the pathogenesis of MS. *Il17a* mRNA expressing mononuclear cells in blood and cerebrospinal fluid were augmented in MS patients compared to control individuals (Matusevicius et al., 1999). IL-23 mRNA expression in blood mononuclear cells and serum IL-23 production were both elevated in MS patients (Alexander et al., 2010; Krakauer et al., 2008). Interestingly, Th17 promoting proinflammatory cytokine IL-1β was elevated in both cerebrospinal fluid and sera in MS patients compared to controls (Dujmovic et al., 2009). Cerebrospinal fluid IL-1β correlates with cortical pathology load in MS at clinical onset (Seppi et al., 2014). Detection of IL-1β in the cerebrospinal fluid at the time of remission appears to be a potential negative prognostic factor in relapsing-remitting MS patients (Rossi et al., 2014).

EAE has been widely used as an animal model of MS. Pathogenic Th17 cells and IL-23 are critical for the pathogensis of EAE as discussed above (Langrish et al., 2005; McGeachy et al., 2007; Ghoreschi et al., 2010; Lee et al., 2012). In addition, the Th17-promoting cytokines IL-1β and IL-6 play an important role in EAE. In the Lewis rat EAE model, 10 days after immunization, IL-1β immunoreactivity was found in brains of animals that at this time showed mild clinical signs. On day 13, animals had developed full-blown EAE. At this stage the number of lesions with IL-1β-positive cells had increased (Bauer et al., 1993). MS has been mainly attributed to white matter as well as gray matter in the brain. IL-1β is also expressed in affected gray matter and white matter regions in the brain and spinal cord of chronic-relapsing EAE (Prins et al., 2013). IL-1β receptor antagonist suppresses EAE in rats by influencing the activation and proliferation of encephalitogenic cells including T cells (Badovinac et al., 1998). IL-6 is also critical for the induction of EAE. IL-6 blockade by treatment with an anti-IL-6 receptor monoclonal antibody (mAb) inhibited the development of EAE and inhibited the induction of MOG peptide-specific CD4-positive, CD8-positive, and Th17 T cells, in inguinal lymph nodes (Serada et al., 2008).

6.2 Systemic lupus erythematosus

Systemic lupus erythematosus (SLE) is a prototypical systemic autoimmune disease in which several vital organs and tissues such as the CNS, heart, small-blood vessels, and the kidney are indiscriminately affected (Tsokos, 2011). Genetic, environmental, immune-regulatory, hormonal, and epigenetic factors are thought to collectively contribute to the generation of autoantibodies, immune complexes, autoreactive or inflammatory T cells, and inflammatory cytokines, which may initiate and amplify inflammation and damage to various organs (Tsokos, 2011). Numerous studies have suggested a potential link between IL-17/Th17 cells and SLE. Wong et al. showed that plasma IL-17, IL-23, IL-12, and CXCL10 concentrations and the number of Th17 cells in the blood were significantly elevated in SLE patients than in control subjects. The elevated IL-17, IL-12, and CXCL10 concentrations correlated positively and significantly with the SLE Disease Activity Index (SLEDAI) (Wong et al., 2008). Another report showed that serum IL-17 levels in SLE patients were higher than those of controls. Correlation analysis indicated that plasma IL-17 levels were positively correlated with SLEDAI (Chen et al., 2010).

Patients with SLE also displayed an increased frequency of IL-17$^+$CD4$^+$T cells compared with healthy subjects. Further, SLE patients had an increased frequency of CCR6$^+$CCR4$^+$CD4$^+$ T cells that are known to be memory Th17 cells. The frequency of IL-17$^+$CD4$^+$T cells and CCR6$^+$CCR4$^+$CD4$^+$ T cells correlated with disease activity (Shah et al., 2010). The higher levels of Th17-promoting cytokine IL-6 were also observed in SLE patients compared with healthy subjects (Linker-Israeli et al., 1991; Shah et al., 2010). In addition to CD4$^+$ Th17 cells, IL-17-producing CD3$^+$CD4$^-$CD8$^-$ T cells (double negative T cells) were thought to be involved in the pathogenesis of SLE (Crispin et al., 2008). Double negative T cells from patients with SLE produced significant amounts of IL-17 and IFNγ. Furthermore, IL-17 and double negative T cells were found in kidney biopsies of patients with lupus nephritis. However, no direct evidence had been shown that the IL-17 was produced by double negative T cells in the kidneys (Crispin et al., 2008).

The pathophysiological findings on IL-17/Th17 cells in SLE have been discovered from several mouse models. IL-23R-deficient lupus-prone C57BL/6-*lpr/lpr* mice display decreased numbers of IL-17-producing cells in the lymph nodes. These mice produced fewer anti-DNA Abs and had less immune complexes and C3 deposition in renal glomeruli. In addition, clinical and pathology measures of lupus nephritis were abrogated (Kyttaris et al., 2010). Increased production of IL-17 family cytokines and their signaling via the adaptor protein CIKS (TRAF3 interacting protein 2) critically contributed to lethal pathology in an FcγR2β-deficient mouse model of lupus. Mice lacking IL-17 and especially those lacking CIKS showed greatly improved survival and were largely protected from development of glomerulonephritis (Pisitkun et al., 2012). These findings suggest the IL-17-CIKS axis might serve as promising therapeutic targets for the treatment of SLE, especially in cases with kidney involvement (Pisitkun et al., 2012).

6.3 Inflammatory bowel disease

IBD is a chronic inflammatory disorder that is comprised of both CD and ulcerative colitis (UC). CD is characterized by focal and transmural inflammation that can occur anywhere along the length of the gastrointestinal system, which may include B2 stricturing (gut luminal narrowing), B3 penetrating (bowel perforation, fistula, inflammatory mass/abscess), and with possible perianal disease. UC is characterized by colonic mucosal inflammation along the entire colon and involving the rectum (Wallace et al., 2014). The cause of IBD is complicated. An abnormal immune response in the gut may be responsible for the disease in genetically susceptible individuals. Both innate and adaptive immune responses are involved in the pathogenesis of IBD (Geremia et al., 2011).

IL-17 production by organ culture biopsies was higher in IBD inflamed mucosa than IBD uninflamed mucosa and controls. Anti-CD3/CD28-stimulated IBD lamina propria mononuclear cells produced higher IL-17 amounts compared to controls. The percentages of Th17 and Th1/Th17 cells were increased in patients with IBD (Rovedatti et al., 2009). IL-17 expression by immunohistochemistry was not detected in gut tissue samples from normal colonic mucosa, infectious colitis, or ischaemic colitis. In the inflamed mucosa of active UC and CD patients, IL-17 expression was clearly detectable in $CD3^+$ T cells or $CD68^+$ monocytes/macrophages. The average number of IL-17^+ cells was significantly increased in active UC and CD patients compared with inactive patients. IL-17 was not detected in the sera from normal individuals, infectious colitis, or ischemic colitis patients but IL-17 levels were significantly elevated in IBD patients (Fujino et al., 2003). *Il17a* mRNA was significantly elevated in the active but not the inactive mucosa region of CD and UC (Sugihara et al., 2010). One report showed that CD patients had statistically significantly higher levels of IL-17-, IL-21-, and IL-22-producing $CD45RO^+CD4^+$ T cells in both active and quiescent disease compared with health controls (Dige et al., 2013).

In a model of acute trinitrobenzenesulfonic acid (TNBS)-induced colitis, Zhang et al. discovered that IL-17 was produced in colon tissue at 24 and 48 hours after TNBS treatment, and IL-17R knockout mice were significantly protected against TNBS-induced weight loss, IL-6 production, colonic inflammation, and local macrophage inflammatory protein-2 (MIP-2) induction (Zhang et al., 2006). Naïve $CD4^+$ T cells from IL-10–/– mice induce colitis after adoptive transfer of the T cells into RAG–/– mice. This colitis is significantly reduced after treatment with neutralizing antibody to IL-17 (Yen et al., 2006). However, Flavell and colleagues reported that IL-17-deficient $CD45RB^{hi}$ T cells induce an aggressive wasting disease in *Rag1*$^{-/-}$ recipient mice, indicating protective role of IL-17 in T cell-mediated intestinal inflammation (O'Connor et al., 2009). This protective role could be due to the suppressive function of IL-17 in the development of Th1 cells, which is critical in the T cell-mediated intestinal inflammation (O'Connor et al., 2009). In the mouse dextran sulfate sodium-induced colitis model, anti-IL-17 neutralizing mAb markedly enhanced the severity of colitis. The mucosal infiltration of CD4-positive helper T cells and CD11b-positive granulocytes-monocytes was increased in the anti-IL-17 mAb-treated mice. Treatment with the anti-IL-17 mAb increased the mucosal expression of mRNAs of TNFα, IFNγ, IL-6, RANTES, and IP-10 (Ogawa et al., 2004). In the *Helicobacter bilis*-infected *Mdr1a*$^{-/-}$ mouse model of colitis, IL-23 inhibition provided strong efficacy while IL-17 or IL-17RA inhibition exacerbated disease. IL-17RA inhibition increased expression of many genes including IFNγ and TNFα. This study further supports that Th17 cells shift to Th1 cells in colitis after blockade of IL-17 signaling (Maxwell et al., 2013).

Another study found adoptive transfer of IL-17-, IL-17F-, or IL-22-deficient T lymphocytes into RAG1-deficient mice all failed to protect mice from developing colitis. In contrast, transfer of $ROR\gamma^{-/-}$ T cells failed to increase mucosal IL-17 cytokine levels and did not induce colitis. Treatment with recombinant IL-17 was able to restore colitis after transfer of $ROR\gamma^{-/-}$ T cells, indicating a crucial role for Th17 cells in pathogenesis. Treatment of $RAG1^{-/-}$ mice that received $IL\text{-}17F^{-/-}$, but not wild-type, T cells with a neutralizing anti-IL-17 antibody significantly suppressed disease, indicating redundant biological effects of IL-17 and IL-17F (Leppkes et al., 2009). Finally, a clinical trial using anti-IL-17 mAb secukinumab for the treatment of active CD showed that blockade of IL-17 was ineffective and higher rates of adverse events were noted compared with placebo (Hueber et al., 2012). Thus, the role of IL-17 in the pathogenesis of colitis/IBD is very complicated. Further evaluation is needed.

The critical role of IL-23-IL-23R signaling in IBD is supported by several studies. Genome-wide association studies (GWAS) found significant association between IBD and the *IL23R* gene in independent cohorts of patients (Duerr et al., 2006). IL-23 is not only essential for the generation of protective Th17 cells, it is also important for the pathogenic role of ILCs in human IBD patients. Although the gene expression of *Il17a* and *Il17f* was increased among intestinal $CD3^-$ cells in IBD, IL-17 and IL-17F expression is restricted to CD56-ILCs, On the other hand, IL-23 induces IL-22 and IL-26 expression in the $CD56^+$ ILC compartment (Geremia et al., 2011). Significant *Il17a* mRNA upregulation in lamina propria (LP) $CD4^+$ cells was found in UC, while IFNγ was increased in CD. IL23R and RORC were upregulated in LP $CD4^+$ cells isolated from both UC and CD. However, IL-17 production was significantly increased by IL-23 stimulation in LP $CD4^+$ cells from UC but not CD. Upregulated *Il23p19* mRNA expression was correlated with IL-17 in UC and IFNγ in CD (Kobayashi et al., 2008). Thus, IL-23 may play important roles in controlling the differential Th1/Th17 balance in both UC and CD, although Th17 cells may exist in both diseases (Kobayashi et al., 2008).

In the TNBS-induced colitis model, neutralizing antibodies against IL-12 p40 abrogated established experimental colitis in mice (Neurath et al., 1995). It was believed that this phenomenon was due to antagonism of IL-12. However, IL-12 p40 also forms IL-23 with IL-23 p19. Indeed, in a T cell-mediated colitis model in $RAG^{-/-}$ mice, IL-23 is essential for the pathogenesis of colitis and promotes inflammation via IL-17 and IL-6 (Yen et al., 2006). $IL\text{-}10^{-/-}$ or IL-12 $p35^{-/-}$/$IL\text{-}10^{-/-}$, but not IL-23 $p19^{-/-}$/$IL\text{-}10^{-/-}$, mice develop spontaneous colitis, while recombinant IL-23 accelerates T cell transfer colitis through promoting memory-activated T cell production of IL-6 and IL-17. Blockade of IL-6 or IL-17 by neutralizing mAbs also ameliorates colitis (Yen et al., 2006). In the clinic, treatment with a mAb against IL-12 p40 induced clinical responses and remission in patients with active CD. This treatment is associated with decreases in Th1-mediated inflammatory cytokines at the site of disease (Mannon et al., 2004).

In sum, although the role of IL-23- and IL-17-producing T cells in the pathogenesis of IBD is clear, the Th17 cytokine IL-17 could play a protective in IBD. It is possible another Th17 effector cytokine, IL-26, could contribute to the pathogenesis of IBD. Indeed, IL-26 induces phosphorylation of STAT1/3, ERK-1/2, SAPK/JNK-1/2, and Akt in intestinal epithelial cells. It also increases gene expression of proinflammatory cytokines IL-8 and TNFα by intestinal epithelial cells. Importantly, IL-26 expression is upregulated in active CD and UC (Dambacher et al., 2009).

6.4 Psoriasis and psoriatic arthritis

Psoriasis is a chronic inflammatory skin disorder affecting approximately 2% of the population (Nestle et al., 2009). The exact pathophysiology of psoriasis has not been fully elucidated. Genetic susceptibility, environmental factors, and immune dysregulation have been shown to contribute to the disease onset. T cells, dendritic cells, macrophages, and keratinocytes are critically involved in the pathogenesis of psoriasis (Nestle et al., 2009). Initially, psoriasis was believed to be caused by dysregulation of Th1 cells. Indeed, a Phase I study first demonstrated the efficacy of human IL-12 p40 antibody in the treatment of plaque psoriasis (Kauffman et al., 2004). Further clinical trials demonstrated that human IL-12p40 antibodies Stelara® (ustekinumab) and briakinumab (ABT-874) are efficacious in the treatment of psoriasis. Importantly, ustekinumab has received US FDA approval for treatment of psoriasis (Leonardi et al., 2008; Papp et al., 2008).

Although the above studies clearly demonstrate the critical role of IL-12 in the pathogenesis of psoriasis subsequent studies also revealed an important role for IL-23/Th17 cells. Psoriatic lesions contain near-normal expression of IL-12p35, whereas IL-12p40 expression is increased. Interestingly, IL-23p19 expression is significantly increased in psoriatic lesions, suggesting that IL-23(p19/p40) but not IL-12 (p35/p40) is the critical cause of psoriasis (Fitch et al., 2007). Furthermore, a large-scale genetic association study identified *Il12p40* and *Il23r* as psoriasis-risk genes (Cargill et al., 2007). In this regard, cells with *Il23r* SNP Arg381Gln produce less IL-17 upon stimulation (Oosting et al., 2011). Indeed, *Il23r* Arg381Gln mutation leads to the protection from psoriatic arthritis (Rahman et al., 2009).

In the dermis of psoriasis lesions, there were significantly higher numbers of Th17 cells than in control lesions (Lowes et al., 2008). The expression of Th17-associated genes including *Keratin 16, Il17a, Ifng,* and *Il22* was increased in psoriatic skin, but reduced to normal level after 8 weeks of treatment with cyclosporine (Lowes et al., 2008). IL-17-producing γδ T cells are also implicated in the pathogenesis of psoriasis. In psoriasis patients, γδ T cells were greatly increased in affected skin and produced large amounts of IL-17 (Cai et al., 2011). IL-23 predominantly stimulates dermal γδ T cells to produce IL-17, which leads to disease progression. Dermal γδ T cells constitutively express

IL-23R and RORγt. IL-17 production from dermal γδ T cells is independent of αβ T cells. The epidermal hyperplasia and inflammation induced by IL-23 were significantly decreased in T cell receptor δ-deficient and IL-17R-deficient mice but occurred normally in *Tcrα*$^{-/-}$ mice (Cai et al., 2011). In addition to IL-17, IL-22 mediates IL-23-induced dermal inflammation and acanthosis (Zheng et al., 2007). Further, overrepresentation of IL-17- and IL-22-producing $CD8^+$ T cells in psoriatic lesional skin suggests the involvement of $CD8^+$ T cells in the pathogenesis of psoriasis (Res et al., 2010).

An emerging picture of how IL-17-producing cells contribute to psoriasis can now be appreciated. Briefly, innate immune cells produce key cytokines (TNF-α, IFN-α, IFN-γ, IL-1β, and IL-6) that activate myeloid dendritic cells. Activated dendritic cells present antigens and secrete mediators including IL-23, leading to the differentiation of Th17 cells and Tc17 cells or the expansion of IL-17-producing γδ T cells. IL-17-producing cells, in turn, secrete mediators (eg, IL-17, IL-17F, and IL-22) that activate keratinocytes and induce the production of antimicrobial peptides (eg, LL-37 cathelicidin and β-defensins), proinflammatory cytokines (TNF-α, IL-1β, and IL-6), chemokines (CXCL8, CXCL11, and CCL20), and S100 proteins. These soluble mediators feed back into the proinflammatory disease cycle and shape the inflammatory infiltrate (Nestle et al., 2009).

The role of IL-17 in the pathogenesis of psoriasis has been demonstrated by several clinical trial studies. A 12-week study for anti-IL17A mAb ixekizumab showed improvement of clinical symptoms in chronic plaque psoriasis (Leonardi et al., 2012). Both the anti-IL-17 antibody secukinumab (AIN457) and anti-IL-17RA antibody brodalumab (AMG827) have significantly improved moderate-to-severe psoriasis (Papp et al., 2012, 2013).

A 76-week result from a randomized, double-blind, placebo-controlled trial has demonstrated that human anti-IL-12/23 p40 antibody ustekinumab has clinical efficacy in psoriasis patients (Leonardi et al., 2008). Another 52-week clinical trial for ustekinumab demonstrates similar efficacy in psoriasis (Papp et al., 2008). Ustekinumab, under the commercial name of Stelara®, has received US FDA approval for treatment of psoriasis. The drug now may be prescribed for psoriatic arthritis in adults, used alone or in combination with methotrexate, based on findings from two Phase III studies (McInnes et al., 2013). Briakinumab, another anti-IL-12/23 p40 antibody, despite demonstrating superb efficacy in psoriasis, has been withdrawn from application with the FDA due to safety concerns including increased incidence of major cardiac events (Traczewski and Rudnicka, 2012).

However, anti-IL-12/23 p40 antibodies block the function of both IL-23 and IL-12. Thus, antibodies targeting the IL-23 p19 subunit have the advantage of neutralizing IL-23 in a more specific manner. Merck Sharp & Dohme Corp. developed anti-IL-23 p19 antibody SCH 900222 (MK3222) that has been tested in plaque psoriasis. A Phase II study to determine the optimal dose of SCH 900222 for the treatment of moderate-to-severe chronic plaque psoriasis has been completed, although the data have not yet been published [ClinicalTrials.gov Identifier: NCT01225731]. Nonetheless, a Phase III study with SCH 900222 has been initiated [ClinicalTrials.gov Identifier: NCT01225731]. Another anti-IL-23p19 antibody from Eli Lilly, LY3074828, is now in a Phase I, randomized, placebo-controlled study in subjects with psoriasis [ClinicalTrials.gov Identifier: NCT01947933]. Boehringer Ingelheim has initiated a Phase II study for their anti-IL-23 p19 antibody (BI 655066) in moderate-to-severe CD [ClinicalTrials.gov Identifier: NCT02031276].

6.5 Rheumatoid arthritis

RA is a chronic inflammatory disease of the joints, in which infiltration of the joint synovium membrane leads to bone and cartilage destruction. IL-17 potently induces osteoclastogenesis. It first acts on osteoblasts, which stimulates both COX-2-dependent prostaglandin E2 (PGE2) synthesis and osteoclast differentiation factor gene expression, which in turn induces differentiation of osteoclast progenitors into mature osteoclasts (Kotake et al., 1999). IL-17 titers in synovial fluids were significantly higher in RA patients than osteoarthritis (OA) patients; anti-IL-17 antibody significantly inhibited osteoclast formation induced by culture media of RA synovial tissues (Kotake et al., 1999). Functional IL-17 was spontaneously produced by RA but not OA or normal synovial tissue pieces cultured *ex vivo*. By immunostaining, IL-17-producing cells were found in the T cell-rich area of RA but not OA synovium. Addition of exogenous IL-17 to RA synovium resulted in an increase in IL-6 production, whereas that of a blocking anti-IL-17 antibody reduced production of IL-6 (Chabaud et al., 1999). Another study showed that both IL-17 and the Th17 chemokine CCL20 were elevated in synovial fluid from RA but not OA patients (Hirota et al., 2007).

The SKG mouse model spontaneously develops T cell-mediated autoimmune arthritis, which clinically and immunologically resembles human RA. The numbers of $CCR6^+$Th17 cells were significantly higher in lymph nodes of arthritic SKG mice than control mice. Higher levels of IL-17 and CCL20 were observed in the joints of arthritic mice. The CCL20 production by synoviocytes was augmented *in vitro* by IL-1β, IL-17, or TNFα, and was suppressed by IFNγ or IL-4. IL-1 receptor antagonist-deficient (IL-$1Ra^{-/-}$) mice spontaneously develop an inflammatory and destructive arthritis due to unopposed excess IL-1 signaling. IL-17 expression is greatly enhanced in IL-$1Ra^{-/-}$ mice, suggesting that IL-17 activity is involved in the pathogenesis of arthritis in these mice. Indeed, the spontaneous development of arthritis did not occur in mice deficient in both IL-1Ra and IL-17 (Nakae et al., 2003b). In CIA model, IL-17 is responsible for the priming of collagen-specific T cells and collagen-specific IgG2a production. Further, CIA was markedly suppressed in IL-$17^{-/-}$ mice (Nakae et al., 2003a). On the other hand, the development of proteoglycan-induced arthritis (PGIA) seems to be dependent on IFNγ but not IL-17 (Doodes et al., 2008). Further study shows that both IFNγ and

IL-17 contribute to arthritis, as T-bet$^{-/-}$ mice lacking IL-17 (T-bet/IL-17$^{-/-}$) were resistant, whereas wild-type, T-bet$^{-/-}$, and IL-17$^{-/-}$ mice were susceptible to PGIA (Doodes et al., 2010).

Several different biologics intended to inhibit IL-17 activity have progressed into RA clinical trials, but results have been inconsistent.

6.6 Ankylosing spondylitis

Ankylosing spondylitis (AS) is a chronic immune-mediated inflammatory disease characterized by spinal inflammation, progressive spinal ankylosis due to new bone formation, peripheral arthritis and enthesitis, extraarticular manifestations, familial clustering, and a strong genetic association with human leucocyte antigen-B27 (Baeten et al., 2013). GWAS showed the association of IL-23R variants with AS. The primary SNP of interest in a previous study of IBD (Arg381Gln; rs11209026) was found to be protective against AS. The strongest association, however, was with SNP rs11465804 (Rahman et al., 2008). CD4^{+} T cells and CD8^{+} T cells from Arg381Gln IL23R carriers showed decreased IL-23-dependent IL-17 and IL-22 production relative to WT IL23R individuals (Sarin et al., 2011). The frequencies of IL-17$\pm$ and IL-22$\pm$ CD4^{+} T cells were increased in PBMCs from patients with AS (Shen et al., 2009). A randomized, double-blind, placebo-controlled trial showed that anti-IL-17 mAb secukinumab rapidly reduced clinical or biological signs of active AS and was well tolerated (Baeten et al., 2013).

6.7 Chronic obstructive pulmonary disease

Chronic obstructive pulmonary disease (COPD) is defined by airflow obstruction and is associated with an exaggerated inflammatory response to noxious stimuli, such as cigarette smoke. Inflammation and recruitment of immune cells drives the underlying pathophysiology (Holloway and Donnelly, 2013). COPD is the fourth leading cause of death in the world and current therapeutic strategies have shown little success at addressing inflammation and disease progression. Macrophages, neutrophils, and lymphocytes are increased in the airways of COPD patients and may be critically involved in the pathogenesis and disease progress (Holloway and Donnelly, 2013). The role of Th17 cells in COPD has been recently suggested. In peripheral blood, an increase of Th17 cells was observed in patients with COPD compared with current smokers without COPD and healthy subjects (Vargas-Rojas et al., 2011). Increased Th17 cells predicted the presence and severity of airflow limitation (Vargas-Rojas et al., 2011). In bronchial biopsies, the number of IL-23^{+} and IL-22^{+} cells was increased in the bronchial epithelium of stable COPD compared with control groups. In addition, the number of IL-17^{+} and IL-22^{+} immunoreactive cells was increased in the bronchial submucosa of stable COPD compared with control nonsmokers (Di et al., 2009). Intranasal stimulation of mice with IL-17 increased the concentration of biologically active MMP-9 as well as its precursor molecule in bronchoalveolar lavage (BAL) fluid (Prause et al., 2004). We have also discovered that MMP-9 expression is dependent on RORγt *in vivo* (Skepner et al., 2015). MMP-9 is significantly increased in BAL fluid from COPD patients and may be destructive to the airway in COPD (Demedts et al., 2005). The pathogenic role of IL-17 and IL-17-producing cells in COPD need to be further elucidated.

6.8 Asthma

Asthma is a chronic inflammatory disease of the airways characterized by bronchial hyperreactivity, mucus overproduction, airway wall remodeling, and airway narrowing caused by dysregulation of innate and adaptive immune cells acting together with epithelial cells. The majority of the patient's symptoms can be controlled by the combination of an inflammation-inhibiting corticosteroid and a β2-adrenergic agonist, which opens the constricting bronchial smooth muscle. However, there are about 5–10% of patients (about 15–30 million patients in a total of 300 million patients worldwide) who are resistant to steroid treatment and require hospitalization.

Asthma was believed to be caused by deregulation of Th2 cells. Recently, Woodruff discovered that asthma can be divided into at least two distinct molecular phenotypes defined by the degree of Th2 inflammation: Th2-high and Th2-low asthma subgroups. The lung function improvements expected with inhaled corticosteroids were restricted to Th2-high asthma, while Th2-low asthma responds poorly to corticosteroid treatment (Woodruff et al., 2009). The Th2-low asthma patients usually display predominant bronchial neutrophilic inflammation. Neutrophilic inflammation is largely responsible for sudden onset fatal asthma in the absence of eosinophils. IL-17 has been reported to be involved in the neutrophilic inflammation and airway remodeling processes, a characteristic of severe and steroid-resistant asthma (Al-Ramli et al., 2009; Bullens et al., 2006). Intratracheal instillation of recombinant IL-17 selectively recruited neutrophils into the airways. This recruitment of neutrophils into the airways was inhibited by an anti-IL-17 antibody (Laan et al., 1999). Using Th17-deficient mice with genetic disruption of gp130 in T cells, it was discovered that Th17 cells induce airway remodeling independent of the Th2 response (Zhao et al., 2013). IL-17 induces the expression of several cytokines and chemokines by bronchial epithelia cells, such as IL-6, CXCL1–3, 5, and 6. This activation of epithelial cells is critical for airway inflammation. Allergic sensitization through the airway primes modest Th2 responses but strong Th17 responses, which promote airway neutrophilia and acute airway hyperresponsiveness (AHR) (Wilson et al., 2009).

Transfer of Th2 cells to mice challenged with ovalbumin (OVA) protein resulted in lymphocyte and eosinophil emigration into the lung that was markedly reduced by dexamethasone treatment, whereas Th17 transfer resulted in increased CXC chemokine secretion and neutrophil influx that was not attenuated by dexamethasone. Both Th2 and Th17 cells are able to induce AHR, whereas Th17 cell-mediated airway inflammation and AHR are steroid resistant (McKinley et al., 2008). In an OVA-sensitized/

challenged AHR model, Th2 transcription factor GATA-3-overexpressing mice exhibited steroid-sensitive eosinophilic inflammation with goblet cell hyperplasia and mucus hyperproduction under Th2-biased conditions, whereas Th17 transcription factor RORγt-overexpressing mice developed steroid-insensitive neutrophilic inflammation under Th17-biased conditions. This AHR accompanied by neutrophilic airway inflammation in RORγt-overexpressing mice was effectively suppressed by anti-IL-17 Ab, CXCR2 antagonist, or anti-IL-6R Ab administration (Ano et al., 2013).

Many clinical studies indicate that IL-17 in the asthmatic airway is related to the severity of asthma (Chesne et al., 2014). IL-17, IL-17F, Th17 cells, and IL-17-producing ILC3 cells in the sputum, BAL, lung biopsies, and peripheral blood have been positively correlated with asthma severity in adults and children (Chesne et al., 2014). Bronchial inflammation and airway resistance increased in healthy subjects after exposure to diesel exhaust particles (DEPs). In patients with mild-to-moderate asthma, just 2 hour exposure to streets with high diesel traffic reduced airway function compared with that seen in patients who walked for 2 hours in an area not exposed to traffic (McCreanor et al., 2007). In mice, exposure to DEPs alone did not induce asthma. DEP and house dust mite coexposure markedly enhanced AHR compared with house dust mite exposure alone and generated a mixed Th2 and Th17 response. IL-17 neutralization prevented DEP-induced exacerbation of ARH (Brandt et al., 2013). Additionally, high DEP-exposed children with allergic asthma had nearly 6 times higher serum IL-17 levels compared with low DEP-exposed children (Brandt et al., 2013).

7. Th17 CELLS IN OTHER DISEASES

The pathogenic role of Th17 cytokines and IL-17-producing cells such as Th17 cells is not limited to the diseases discussed above. They may play critical pathogenic roles in diseases such as allergic contact dermatitis (Peiser, 2013), vasculitis and atherosclerosis, and autoimmune myositis (Miossec and Kolls, 2012). There is an emerging role of Th17 cells in organ transplantation (Sullivan et al., 2014). Finally, IL-17 and Th17 have potential antitumorigenic and protumorigenic roles depending on the type and organ of the cancer. Several pieces of evidence demonstrate that Th17 cytokines and IL-17-producing cells have a protumorigenic role in colon cancer (Grivennikov et al., 2012; Zou and Restifo, 2010).

8. TARGETING Th17 CELLS AND TH17 CYTOKINES FOR AUTOIMMUNE INFLAMMATORY DISEASES AND CANCER

There are a variety of targets and methods to block pathogenic Th17 cell differentiation. These include anti-IL-23/12 p40 Ab, anti-IL-23p19 Ab, anti-IL-23R Ab, IL-23R signaling inhibitors, anti-IL-1β Ab, anti-IL-6 Ab, and STAT3 inhibitor. Antibodies against Th17 effector cytokines are also promising agents, including anti-IL-17 Ab, anti-IL17/IL-17F Ab, anti-IL-21 Ab, anti-IL-22 Ab, and anti-IL-26 Ab. Anti-IL-17R Ab and IL-17R signaling inhibitors could block the IL-17 and IL-17F signaling. Alternatively, recombinant IL-10, IL-27, or IL-35 could inhibit both Th17 cell differentiation and effector cytokine production. Chemotaxis inhibitors targeting CCR6 or CCR4 could block the pathogenic Th17 migration to the inflammatory tissues. Depleting pathogenic Th17 cells using anti-CCR6 and/or anti-CD161 could also be a good approach. Fig. 2 summarizes the possible targets and avenues for therapeutic intervention.

8.1 Anti-IL-23 antibodies

IL-23 is a key cytokine for the generation of pathogenic Th17 cells. As discussed above, human anti-IL-12/23 p40 antibody ustekinumab has clinical efficacy in psoriasis patients (Leonardi et al., 2008; Papp et al., 2008). Stelara® (ustekinumab) has received FDA approval for the treatment of psoriasis and psoriatic arthritis in adults (McInnes et al., 2013). Several anti-IL-23 p19 antibodies are in clinical development for the treatment of psoriasis, arthritis, or CD [ClinicalTrials.gov Identifier: NCT01225731, NCT01947933, NCT02031276].

8.2 IL-6 signaling blockade

IL-6 is a Th17-promoting cytokine and plays a critical role in the pathogenesis of RA. Inhibition of IL-6 signaling by the humanized anti-IL-6 receptor antibody, tocilizumab, significantly improved the signs and symptoms of RA in the initial Phase II trials (Choy

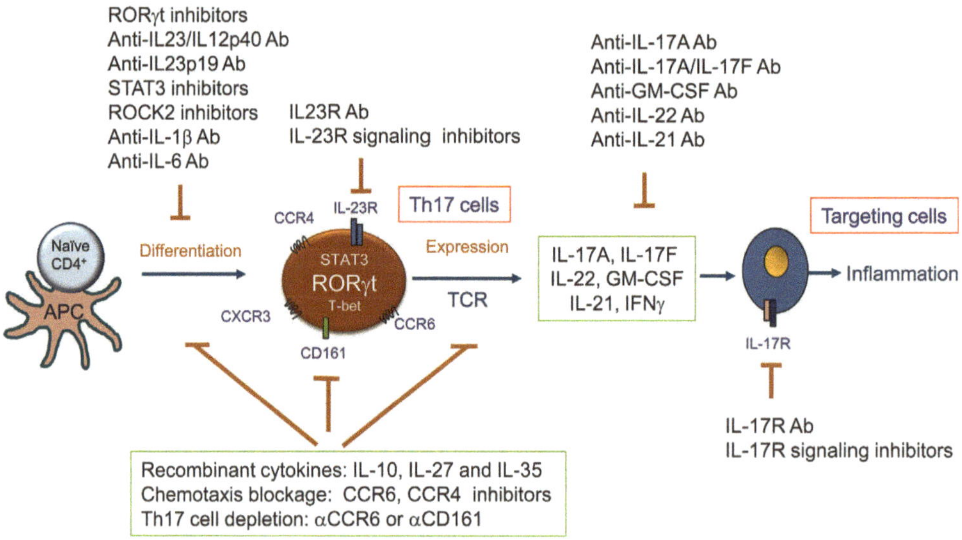

Figure 2 Targeting Th17 cells and Th17 cytokine pathways.

et al., 2002; Nishimoto et al., 2004). Seven Phase III clinical trials verified the outstanding efficacy of tocilizumab in the suppression of disease activity and progression of joint destruction associated with RA. Actemra® (tocilizumab) is currently approved for the treatment of RA in more than 130 countries (Tanaka et al., 2014).

Sirukumab is a human anti-IL-6 mAb. A Phase II study showed that neutralizing IL-6 function by sirukumab improves signs and symptoms of RA patients (Smolen et al., 2014).

8.3 RORγt inverse agonists

ROR is a member of the nuclear receptor superfamily containing an N-terminal A/B domain, a DNA-binding domain (DBD), a hinge region (D), a ligand-binding domain (LBD), and a variable C-terminal region. In most nuclear receptors, ligand binding to the LBD induces a conformation change, recruitment of transcriptional coactivators, and activation of transcriptional activity. There are three members of the ROR family: RORα (or RORA), RORβ (or RORB), and RORγ (or RORC) (Jetten, 2009). Two different forms of RORγ are present in mammalian cells: RORγ (or RORC) and RORγt (or RORC2), with only a variable N-terminus differing between the two isoforms (Jetten, 2009).

RORγt has been found to be the master transcription factor for IL-17-producing cells such as Th17 cells, Tc17 cells, ILC3, IL-17-producing γδ T cells, and IL-17-producing NKT cells. The RORγ/RORγt LBD is an ideal domain to target via small molecules. Small molecules targeting RORs come in at least two flavors: inverse agonists, which block ROR-dependent transcriptional activity, and agonists, which enhance the transactivation of RORs (Solt and Burris, 2012). We and several other groups discovered that RORγt inverse agonists blocks Th17 cell differentiation, IL-17 production, EAE induction, adjuvant-induced arthritis, and skin inflammation (Cascao et al., 2012; Huh et al., 2011; Skepner et al., 2014; Solt et al., 2011; Xiao et al., 2014; Xu et al., 2011; Yang et al., 2013; Yang et al., 2014). However, development of clinical quality RORγt inverse agonists may be a challenging task. Many current small molecules targeting RORγt are inverse agonists that bind the LBD, a domain present in both RORγ and RORγt. RORγ, unlike RORγt, is broadly expressed across many human tissues (liver, kidney, skeletal muscle, heart, brain, and adipose), opening the possibility that RORγt inverse agonists could impact nonimmune tissues.

8.4 Anti-IL-17 or IL-17R antibodies

Secukinumab (AIN457), ixekizumab (LY2439821), SCH-900117, and RG4934 have been developed as neutralizing mAbs against IL-17. As IL-17 and IL-17F can form IL-17/IL-17F heterodimers, RG7624 was developed to interact with both IL-17 and IL-17F. Targeting IL-17 receptor is another way to block the IL-17/IL-17R interaction.

Brodalumab (AMG827) binds to IL-17RA, a subunit of functional IL-17R together with IL-17RC, and inhibits IL-17 binding to the functional receptor complex.

In psoriasis, a Phase II study with a single injection of secukinumab reduced the number of IL-17-positive cells in skin biopsy samples with significant efficacy of the psoriatic skin lesions (Hueber et al., 2010). Multiple injection of ixekizumab showed significant effects as early as 1 week and were sustained through 20 weeks (Leonardi et al., 2012). Targeting IL-17RA with brodalumab also showed significant improvement in plaque psoriasis at 12 weeks (Papp et al., 2012). Phase III studies have been completed for secukinumab [ClinicalTrials.gov Identifier: NCT01406938], ixekizumab [ClinicalTrials.gov Identifier: NCT01597245], and brodalumab [ClinicalTrials.gov Identifier: NCT00975637] although the results have not yet been released. A Phase II trial with secukinumab rapidly reduced clinical and biological signs of moderate-to-severe ankylosing spondylitis (AS), and demonstrated significant improvement in ASAS20 at 6 weeks (Baeten et al., 2013).

In a clinical study with RA patients, secukinumab injection significantly reduced inflammation in the joints, and showed improvement in ACR20, DAS28, and CRP scores (Hueber et al., 2010). A Phase I study with ixekizumab added to oral DMARDs improved signs, symptoms, and DAS28 scores of RA, with no significant adverse safety signals (Genovese et al., 2010). However, an exploratory efficacy analysis in Phase IB with brodalumab based on ACR20 and DAS28 criteria did not reveal significant clinical responses with moderate-to-severe RA patients (Martin et al., 2013). Further, a Phase II study revealed RA patients with inadequate response to methotrexate did not achieve significant ACR20 response to secukinumab after 16 weeks (Genovese et al., 2013). Thus, the role of the IL-17-IL17R pathway in RA needs to be further evaluated. Choosing the right subpopulation of RA patients for further clinical trials could be the key for the success of these mAbs.

Clinical trials of brodalumab and secukinumab in CD failed to improve disease symptoms, and even increased disease activity in some patients, indicating that the IL-17/IL-17R pathway may not be pathogenic in IBD (Hueber et al., 2012; Symons et al., 2012).

Finally, Rho-associated kinase 2 (ROCK2) inhibitors have been developed to inhibit IL-17 and IL-21 secretion. ROCK2 is activated in mouse T cells under Th17 skewing conditions. It phosphorylates Th17 transcription factor IRF4 (Biswas et al., 2010), which is important for the development of Th17 cells (Brustle et al., 2007). ROCK2 haploinsufficiency impairs Th17 differentiation. The expression of IL-17, IL-21, and RORγt were significantly lower in *Rock2*$^{+/-}$ T cells than *Rock2*$^{+/+}$ T cells (Biswas et al., 2010). ROCK inhibitor Fasudil decreases IL-17 and IL-21 production *in vivo* and ameliorates arthritis development in *Def6*$^{trap/trap}$ DO11.10 mice (Biswas et al., 2010). In humans, oral administration of selective ROCK2 inhibitor KD025 downregulates the secretion of IL-17 and IL-21 but not IFNγ in human PBMCs (Zanin-Zhorov et al., 2014). KD025 downregulates proinflammatory responses with concurrent effects on

STAT3 and STAT5 phosphorylation and a shift in Th17/Treg balance in human T cells (Zanin-Zhorov et al., 2014).

9. CONCLUDING REMARKS

Th17 cells and IL-17-producing cells are key effectors of autoimmune inflammatory diseases. Neutralizing antibodies against IL-23, IL-6/IL-6R, IL-17, IL-17F, and IL-17R have been developed to target the lineage of Th17 cells or effector cytokines, and their therapeutic potential are being realized in the clinic. Small-molecules agents such as inverse agonists of RORγt and ROCK2 inhibitors are promising alternative approaches to modulate Th17 cells, which could find broader therapeutic applications.

REFERENCES

Alexander, J.S., Harris, M.K., Wells, S.R., Mills, G., Chalamidas, K., Ganta, V.C., McGee, J., Jennings, M.H., Gonzalez-Toledo, E., Minagar, A., 2010. Alterations in serum MMP-8, MMP-9, IL-12p40 and IL-23 in multiple sclerosis patients treated with interferon-beta1b. Mult. Scler. 16 (7), 801–809, available from: PM:20621951.

Al-Ramli, W., Prefontaine, D., Chouiali, F., Martin, J.G., Olivenstein, R., Lemiere, C., Hamid, Q., 2009. T(H)17-associated cytokines (IL-17A and IL-17F) in severe asthma. J. Allergy Clin. Immunol. 123 (5), 1185–1187, available from: PM:19361847.

Ano, S., Morishima, Y., Ishii, Y., Yoh, K., Yageta, Y., Ohtsuka, S., Matsuyama, M., Kawaguchi, M., Takahashi, S., Hizawa, N., 2013. Transcription factors GATA-3 and RORgammat are important for determining the phenotype of allergic airway inflammation in a murine model of asthma. J. Immunol. 190 (3), 1056–1065, available from: PM:23293351.

Badovinac, V., Mostarica-Stojkovic, M., Dinarello, C.A., Stosic-Grujicic, S., 1998. Interleukin-1 receptor antagonist suppresses experimental autoimmune encephalomyelitis (EAE) in rats by influencing the activation and proliferation of encephalitogenic cells. J. Neuroimmunol. 85 (1), 87–95, available from: PM:9627001.

Baeten, D., Baraliakos, X., Braun, J., Sieper, J., Emery, P., van der Heijde, D., McInnes, I., van Laar, J.M., Landewe, R., Wordsworth, P., Wollenhaupt, J., Kellner, H., Paramarta, J., Wei, J., Brachat, A., Bek, S., Laurent, D., Li, Y., Wang, Y.A., Bertolino, A.P., Gsteiger, S., Wright, A.M., Hueber, W., 2013. Anti-interleukin-17A monoclonal antibody secukinumab in treatment of ankylosing spondylitis: a randomised, double-blind, placebo-controlled trial. Lancet 382 (9906), 1705–1713, available from: PM:24035250.

Balashov, K.E., Smith, D.R., Khoury, S.J., Hafler, D.A., Weiner, H.L., 1997. Increased interleukin 12 production in progressive multiple sclerosis: induction by activated CD4+ T cells via CD40 ligand. Proc. Natl. Acad. Sci. U. S. A. 94 (2), 599–603, available from: PM:9012830.

Batten, M., Li, J., Yi, S., Kljavin, N.M., Danilenko, D.M., Lucas, S., Lee, J., de Sauvage, F.J., Ghilardi, N., 2006. Interleukin 27 limits autoimmune encephalomyelitis by suppressing the development of interleukin 17-producing T cells. Nat. Immunol. 7 (9), 929–936, available from: PM:16906167.

Bauer, J., Berkenbosch, F., Van Dam, A.M., Dijkstra, C.D., 1993. Demonstration of interleukin-1 beta in Lewis rat brain during experimental allergic encephalomyelitis by immunocytochemistry at the light and ultrastructural level. J. Neuroimmunol. 48 (1), 13–21, available from: PM:8227304.

Bauquet, A.T., Jin, H., Paterson, A.M., Mitsdoerffer, M., Ho, I.C., Sharpe, A.H., Kuchroo, V.K., 2009. The costimulatory molecule ICOS regulates the expression of c-Maf and IL-21 in the development of follicular T helper cells and TH-17 cells. Nat. Immunol. 10 (2), 167–175, available from: PM:19098919.

Bettelli, E., Carrier, Y., Gao, W., Korn, T., Strom, T.B., Oukka, M., Weiner, H.L., Kuchroo, V.K., 2006. Reciprocal developmental pathways for the generation of pathogenic effector TH17 and regulatory T cells. Nature 441 (7090), 235–238, available from: PM:16648838.

Biswas, P.S., Gupta, S., Chang, E., Song, L., Stirzaker, R.A., Liao, J.K., Bhagat, G., Pernis, A.B., 2010. Phosphorylation of IRF4 by ROCK2 regulates IL-17 and IL-21 production and the development of autoimmunity in mice. J. Clin. Invest. 120 (9), 3280–3295, available from: PM:20697158.

Brandt, E.B., Kovacic, M.B., Lee, G.B., Gibson, A.M., Acciani, T.H., Le Cras, T.D., Ryan, P.H., Budelsky, A.L., Khurana Hershey, G.K., 2013. Diesel exhaust particle induction of IL-17A contributes to severe asthma. J. Allergy Clin. Immunol. 132 (5), 1194–1204, available from: PM:24060272.

Brustle, A., Heink, S., Huber, M., Rosenplanter, C., Stadelmann, C., Yu, P., Arpaia, E., Mak, T.W., Kamradt, T., Lohoff, M., 2007. The development of inflammatory T(H)-17 cells requires interferon-regulatory factor 4. Nat. Immunol. 8 (9), 958–966, available from: PM:17676043.

Bullens, D.M., Truyen, E., Coteur, L., Dilissen, E., Hellings, P.W., Dupont, L.J., Ceuppens, J.L., 2006. IL-17 mRNA in sputum of asthmatic patients: linking T cell driven inflammation and granulocytic influx? Respir. Res. 7, 135, available from: PM:17083726.

Cai, Y., Shen, X., Ding, C., Qi, C., Li, K., Li, X., Jala, V.R., Zhang, H.G., Wang, T., Zheng, J., Yan, J., 2011. Pivotal role of dermal IL-17-producing gammadelta T cells in skin inflammation. Immunity 35 (4), 596–610, available from: PM:21982596.

Cargill, M., Schrodi, S.J., Chang, M., Garcia, V.E., Brandon, R., Callis, K.P., Matsunami, N., Ardlie, K.G., Civello, D., Catanese, J.J., Leong, D.U., Panko, J.M., McAllister, L.B., Hansen, C.B., Papenfuss, J., Prescott, S.M., White, T.J., Leppert, M.F., Krueger, G.G., Begovich, A.B., 2007. A large-scale genetic association study confirms IL12B and leads to the identification of IL23R as psoriasis-risk genes. Am. J. Hum. Genet. 80 (2), 273–290, available from: PM:17236132.

Cascao, R., Vidal, B., Raquel, H., Neves-Costa, A., Figueiredo, N., Gupta, V., Fonseca, J.E., Moita, L.F., 2012. Effective treatment of rat adjuvant-induced arthritis by celastrol. Autoimmun. Rev. 11 (12), 856–862, available from: PM:22415021.

Chabaud, M., Durand, J.M., Buchs, N., Fossiez, F., Page, G., Frappart, L., Miossec, P., 1999. Human interleukin-17: a T cell-derived proinflammatory cytokine produced by the rheumatoid synovium. Arthritis Rheum. 42 (5), 963–970, available from: PM:10323452.

Chen, X.Q., Yu, Y.C., Deng, H.H., Sun, J.Z., Dai, Z., Wu, Y.W., Yang, M., 2010. Plasma IL-17A is increased in new-onset SLE patients and associated with disease activity. J. Clin. Immunol. 30 (2), 221–225, available from: PM:20107878.

Chesne, J., Braza, F., Mahay, G., Brouard, S., Aronica, M., Magnan, A., 2014. IL-17 in severe asthma. Where do we stand? Am. J. Respir. Crit. Care Med. 190 (10), 1094–1101, available from: PM:25162311.

Cho, J.S., Pietras, E.M., Garcia, N.C., Ramos, R.I., Farzam, D.M., Monroe, H.R., Magorien, J.E., Blauvelt, A., Kolls, J.K., Cheung, A.L., Cheng, G., Modlin, R.L., Miller, L.S., 2010. IL-17 is essential for host defense against cutaneous staphylococcus aureus infection in mice. J. Clin. Invest. 120 (5), 1762–1773, available from: PM:20364087.

Choy, E.H., Isenberg, D.A., Garrood, T., Farrow, S., Ioannou, Y., Bird, H., Cheung, N., Williams, B., Hazleman, B., Price, R., Yoshizaki, K., Nishimoto, N., Kishimoto, T., Panayi, G.S., 2002. Therapeutic benefit of blocking interleukin-6 activity with an anti-interleukin-6 receptor monoclonal antibody in rheumatoid arthritis: a randomized, double-blind, placebo-controlled, dose-escalation trial. Arthritis Rheum. 46 (12), 3143–3150, available from: PM:12483717.

Conti, H.R., Shen, F., Nayyar, N., Stocum, E., Sun, J.N., Lindemann, M.J., Ho, A.W., Hai, J.H., Yu, J.J., Jung, J.W., Filler, S.G., Masso-Welch, P., Edgerton, M., Gaffen, S.L., 2009. Th17 cells and IL-17 receptor signaling are essential for mucosal host defense against oral candidiasis. J. Exp. Med. 206 (2), 299–311, available from: PM:19204111.

Conti, H.R., Peterson, A.C., Brane, L., Huppler, A.R., Hernandez-Santos, N., Whibley, N., Garg, A.V., Simpson-Abelson, M.R., Gibson, G.A., Mamo, A.J., Osborne, L.C., Bishu, S., Ghilardi, N., Siebenlist, U., Watkins, S.C., Artis, D., McGeachy, M.J., Gaffen, S.L., 2014. Oral-resident natural Th17 cells and gammadelta T cells control opportunistic Candida albicans infections. J. Exp. Med. 211 (10), 2075–2084, available from: PM:25200028.

Crispin, J.C., Oukka, M., Bayliss, G., Cohen, R.A., Van Beek, C.A., Stillman, I.E., Kyttaris, V.C., Juang, Y.T., Tsokos, G.C., 2008. Expanded double negative T cells in patients with systemic lupus erythematosus produce IL-17 and infiltrate the kidneys. J. Immunol. 181 (12), 8761–8766, available from: PM:19050297.

Dambacher, J., Beigel, F., Zitzmann, K., De Toni, E.N., Goke, B., Diepolder, H.M., Auernhammer, C.J., Brand, S., 2009. The role of the novel Th17 cytokine IL-26 in intestinal inflammation. Gut 58 (9), 1207–1217, available from: PM:18483078.

Demedts, I.K., Brusselle, G.G., Bracke, K.R., Vermaelen, K.Y., Pauwels, R.A., 2005. Matrix metalloproteinases in asthma and COPD. Curr. Opin. Pharmacol. 5 (3), 257–263, available from: PM:15907912.

Di, S.A., Caramori, G., Gnemmi, I., Contoli, M., Vicari, C., Capelli, A., Magno, F., D'Anna, S.E., Zanini, A., Brun, P., Casolari, P., Chung, K.F., Barnes, P.J., Papi, A., Adcock, I., Balbi, B., 2009. T helper type 17-related cytokine expression is increased in the bronchial mucosa of stable chronic obstructive pulmonary disease patients. Clin. Exp. Immunol. 157 (2), 316–324, available from: PM:19604272.

Dige, A., Stoy, S., Rasmussen, T.K., Kelsen, J., Hvas, C.L., Sandahl, T.D., Dahlerup, J.F., Deleuran, B., Agnholt, J., 2013. Increased levels of circulating Th17 cells in quiescent versus active Crohn's disease. J. Crohns Colitis 7 (3), 248–255, available from: PM:22784949.

Diveu, C., McGeachy, M.J., Boniface, K., Stumhofer, J.S., Sathe, M., Joyce-Shaikh, B., Chen, Y., Tato, C.M., McClanahan, T.K., de Waal, M.R., Hunter, C.A., Cua, D.J., Kastelein, R.A., 2009. IL-27 blocks RORc expression to inhibit lineage commitment of Th17 cells. J. Immunol. 182 (9), 5748–5756, available from: PM:19380822.

Doodes, P.D., Cao, Y., Hamel, K.M., Wang, Y., Farkas, B., Iwakura, Y., Finnegan, A., 2008. Development of proteoglycan-induced arthritis is independent of IL-17. J. Immunol. 181 (1), 329–337, available from: PM:18566398.

Doodes, P.D., Cao, Y., Hamel, K.M., Wang, Y., Rodeghero, R.L., Mikecz, K., Glant, T.T., Iwakura, Y., Finnegan, A., 2010. IFN-gamma regulates the requirement for IL-17 in proteoglycan-induced arthritis. J. Immunol. 184 (3), 1552–1559, available from: PM:20028652.

Du, J., Huang, C., Zhou, B., Ziegler, S.F., 2008. Isoform-specific inhibition of ROR alpha-mediated transcriptional activation by human FOXP3. J. Immunol. 180 (7), 4785–4792, available from: PM:18354202.

Duerr, R.H., Taylor, K.D., Brant, S.R., Rioux, J.D., Silverberg, M.S., Daly, M.J., Steinhart, A.H., Abraham, C., Regueiro, M., Griffiths, A., Dassopoulos, T., Bitton, A., Yang, H., Targan, S., Datta, L.W., Kistner, E.O., Schumm, L.P., Lee, A.T., Gregersen, P.K., Barmada, M.M., Rotter, J.I., Nicolae, D.L., Cho, J.H., 2006. A genome-wide association study identifies IL23R as an inflammatory bowel disease gene. Science 314 (5804), 1461–1463, available from: PM:17068223.

Dujmovic, I., Mangano, K., Pekmezovic, T., Quattrocchi, C., Mesaros, S., Stojsavljevic, N., Nicoletti, F., Drulovic, J., 2009. The analysis of IL-1 beta and its naturally occurring inhibitors in multiple sclerosis: the elevation of IL-1 receptor antagonist and IL-1 receptor type II after steroid therapy. J. Neuroimmunol. 207 (1-2), 101–106, available from: PM:19162335.

Fitch, E., Harper, E., Skorcheva, I., Kurtz, S.E., Blauvelt, A., 2007. Pathophysiology of psoriasis: recent advances on IL-23 and Th17 cytokines. Curr. Rheumatol. Rep. 9 (6), 461–467, available from: PM:18177599.

Fujino, S., Andoh, A., Bamba, S., Ogawa, A., Hata, K., Araki, Y., Bamba, T., Fujiyama, Y., 2003. Increased expression of interleukin 17 in inflammatory bowel disease. Gut 52 (1), 65–70, available from: PM:12477762.

Genovese, M.C., Van den Bosch, F., Roberson, S.A., Bojin, S., Biagini, I.M., Ryan, P., Sloan-Lancaster, J., 2010. LY2439821, a humanized anti-interleukin-17 monoclonal antibody, in the treatment of patients with rheumatoid arthritis: a phase I randomized, double-blind, placebo-controlled, proof-of-concept study. Arthritis Rheum. 62 (4), 929–939, available from: PM:20131262.

Genovese, M.C., Durez, P., Richards, H.B., Supronik, J., Dokoupilova, E., Mazurov, V., Aelion, J.A., Lee, S.H., Codding, C.E., Kellner, H., Ikawa, T., Hugot, S., Mpofu, S., 2013. Efficacy and safety of secukinumab in patients with rheumatoid arthritis: a phase II, dose-finding, double-blind, randomised, placebo controlled study. Ann. Rheum. Dis. 72 (6), 863–869, available from: PM:22730366.

Geremia, A., Arancibia-Carcamo, C.V., Fleming, M.P., Rust, N., Singh, B., Mortensen, N.J., Travis, S.P., Powrie, F., 2011. IL-23-responsive innate lymphoid cells are increased in inflammatory bowel disease. J. Exp. Med. 208 (6), 1127–1133, available from: PM:21576383.

Ghoreschi, K., Laurence, A., Yang, X.P., Tato, C.M., McGeachy, M.J., Konkel, J.E., Ramos, H.L., Wei, L., Davidson, T.S., Bouladoux, N., Grainger, J.R., Chen, Q., Kanno, Y., Watford, W.T., Sun, H.W., Eberl, G., Shevach, E.M., Belkaid, Y., Cua, D.J., Chen, W., O'Shea, J.J., 2010. Generation of pathogenic T(H)17 cells in the absence of TGF-beta signalling. Nature 467 (7318), 967–971, available from: PM:20962846.

Grivennikov, S.I., Wang, K., Mucida, D., Stewart, C.A., Schnabl, B., Jauch, D., Taniguchi, K., Yu, G.Y., Osterreicher, C.H., Hung, K.E., Datz, C., Feng, Y., Fearon, E.R., Oukka, M., Tessarollo, L., Coppola, V., Yarovinsky, F., Cheroutre, H., Eckmann, L., Trinchieri, G., Karin, M., 2012. Adenoma-linked barrier defects and microbial products drive IL-23/IL-17-mediated tumour growth. Nature 491 (7423), 254–258, available from: PM:23034650.

Gu, Y., Yang, J., Ouyang, X., Liu, W., Li, H., Yang, J., Bromberg, J., Chen, S.H., Mayer, L., Unkeless, J.C., Xiong, H., 2008. Interleukin 10 suppresses Th17 cytokines secreted by macrophages and T cells. Eur. J. Immunol. 38 (7), 1807–1813, available from: PM:18506885.

Happel, K.I., Dubin, P.J., Zheng, M., Ghilardi, N., Lockhart, C., Quinton, L.J., Odden, A.R., Shellito, J.E., Bagby, G.J., Nelson, S., Kolls, J.K., 2005. Divergent roles of IL-23 and IL-12 in host defense against Klebsiella pneumoniae. J. Exp. Med. 202 (6), 761–769, available from: PM:16157683.

Harrington, L.E., Hatton, R.D., Mangan, P.R., Turner, H., Murphy, T.L., Murphy, K.M., Weaver, C.T., 2005. Interleukin 17-producing CD4+ effector T cells develop via a lineage distinct from the T helper type 1 and 2 lineages. Nat. Immunol. 6 (11), 1123–1132, available from: PM:16200070.

Harris, T.J., Grosso, J.F., Yen, H.R., Xin, H., Kortylewski, M., Albesiano, E., Hipkiss, E.L., Getnet, D., Goldberg, M.V., Maris, C.H., Housseau, F., Yu, H., Pardoll, D.M., Drake, C.G., 2007. Cutting edge: an in vivo requirement for STAT3 signaling in TH17 development and TH17-dependent autoimmunity. J. Immunol. 179 (7), 4313–4317, available from: PM:17878325.

Hirota, K., Yoshitomi, H., Hashimoto, M., Maeda, S., Teradaira, S., Sugimoto, N., Yamaguchi, T., Nomura, T., Ito, H., Nakamura, T., Sakaguchi, N., Sakaguchi, S., 2007. Preferential recruitment of CCR6-expressing Th17 cells to inflamed joints via CCL20 in rheumatoid arthritis and its animal model. J. Exp. Med. 204 (12), 2803–2812, available from: PM:18025126.

Holloway, R.A., Donnelly, L.E., 2013. Immunopathogenesis of chronic obstructive pulmonary disease. Curr. Opin. Pulm. Med. 19 (2), 95–102, available from: PM:23325031.

Hsieh, C.S., Macatonia, S.E., Tripp, C.S., Wolf, S.F., O'Garra, A., Murphy, K.M., 1993. Development of TH1 CD4+ T cells through IL-12 produced by Listeria-induced macrophages. Science 260 (5107), 547–549, [see comments].

Huang, W., Na, L., Fidel, P.L., Schwarzenberger, P., 2004. Requirement of interleukin-17A for systemic anti-Candida albicans host defense in mice. J. Infect. Dis. 190 (3), 624–631, available from: PM:15243941.

Hueber, W., Patel, D.D., Dryja, T., Wright, A.M., Koroleva, I., Bruin, G., Antoni, C., Draelos, Z., Gold, M.H., Durez, P., Tak, P.P., Gomez-Reino, J.J., Foster, C.S., Kim, R.Y., Samson, C.M., Falk, N.S., Chu, D.S., Callanan, D., Nguyen, Q.D., Rose, K., Haider, A., Di, P.F., 2010. Effects of AIN457, a fully human antibody to interleukin-17A, on psoriasis, rheumatoid arthritis, and uveitis. Sci.Transl.Med. 2 (52), 52ra72, available from: PM:20926833.

Hueber, W., Sands, B.E., Lewitzky, S., Vandemeulebroecke, M., Reinisch, W., Higgins, P.D., Wehkamp, J., Feagan, B.G., Yao, M.D., Karczewski, M., Karczewski, J., Pezous, N., Bek, S., Bruin, G., Mellgard, B., Berger, C., Londei, M., Bertolino, A.P., Tougas, G., Travis, S.P., 2012. Secukinumab, a human anti-IL-17A monoclonal antibody, for moderate to severe Crohn's disease: unexpected results of a randomised, double-blind placebo-controlled trial. Gut 61 (12), 1693–1700, available from: PM:22595313.

Huh, J.R., Leung, M.W., Huang, P., Ryan, D.A., Krout, M.R., Malapaka, R.R., Chow, J., Manel, N., Ciofani, M., Kim, S.V., Cuesta, A., Santori, F.R., Lafaille, J.J., Xu, H.E., Gin, D.Y., Rastinejad, F., Littman, D.R., 2011. Digoxin and its derivatives suppress TH17 cell differentiation by antagonizing RORgammat activity. Nature 472 (7344), 486–490, available from: PM:21441909.

Ishigame, H., Kakuta, S., Nagai, T., Kadoki, M., Nambu, A., Komiyama, Y., Fujikado, N., Tanahashi, Y., Akitsu, A., Kotaki, H., Sudo, K., Nakae, S., Sasakawa, C., Iwakura, Y., 2009. Differential roles of interleukin-17A and -17F in host defense against mucoepithelial bacterial infection and allergic responses. Immunity 30 (1), 108–119, available from: PM:19144317.

Issazadeh, S., Lorentzen, J.C., Mustafa, M.I., Hojeberg, B., Mussener, A., Olsson, T., 1996. Cytokines in relapsing experimental autoimmune encephalomyelitis in DA rats: persistent mRNA expression of proinflammatory cytokines and absent expression of interleukin-10 and transforming growth factor-beta. J. Neuroimmunol. 69 (1-2), 103–115, available from: PM:8823381.

Ivanov, I.I., McKenzie, B.S., Zhou, L., Tadokoro, C.E., Lepelley, A., Lafaille, J.J., Cua, D.J., Littman, D.R., 2006. The orphan nuclear receptor RORgammat directs the differentiation program of proinflammatory IL-17+ T helper cells. Cell 126 (6), 1121–1133, available from: PM:16990136.

Jetten, A.M., 2009. Retinoid-related orphan receptors (RORs): critical roles in development, immunity, circadian rhythm, and cellular metabolism. Nucl. Recept. Signal. 7, e003, available from: PM:19381306.

Kauffman, C.L., Aria, N., Toichi, E., McCormick, T.S., Cooper, K.D., Gottlieb, A.B., Everitt, D.E., Frederick, B., Zhu, Y., Graham, M.A., Pendley, C.E., Mascelli, M.A., 2004. A phase I study evaluating the safety, pharmacokinetics, and clinical response of a human IL-12 p40 antibody in subjects with plaque psoriasis. J. Invest. Dermatol. 123 (6), 1037–1044, available from: PM:15610511.

Khader, S.A., Bell, G.K., Pearl, J.E., Fountain, J.J., Rangel-Moreno, J., Cilley, G.E., Shen, F., Eaton, S.M., Gaffen, S.L., Swain, S.L., Locksley, R.M., Haynes, L., Randall, T.D., Cooper, A.M., 2007. IL-23 and IL-17 in the establishment of protective pulmonary CD4+ T cell responses after vaccination and during Mycobacterium tuberculosis challenge. Nat. Immunol. 8 (4), 369–377, available from: PM:17351619.

Kobayashi, T., Okamoto, S., Hisamatsu, T., Kamada, N., Chinen, H., Saito, R., Kitazume, M.T., Nakazawa, A., Sugita, A., Koganei, K., Isobe, K., Hibi, T., 2008. IL23 differentially regulates the Th1/Th17 balance in ulcerative colitis and Crohn's disease. Gut 57 (12), 1682–1689, available from: PM:18653729.

Korn, T., Bettelli, E., Gao, W., Awasthi, A., Jager, A., Strom, T.B., Oukka, M., Kuchroo, V.K., 2007. IL-21 initiates an alternative pathway to induce proinflammatory T(H)17 cells. Nature 448 (7152), 484–487, available from: PM:17581588.

Korn, T., Bettelli, E., Oukka, M., Kuchroo, V.K., 2009. IL-17 and Th17 cells. Annu. Rev. Immunol. 27, 485–517, available from: PM:19132915.

Kotake, S., Udagawa, N., Takahashi, N., Matsuzaki, K., Itoh, K., Ishiyama, S., Saito, S., Inoue, K., Kamatani, N., Gillespie, M.T., Martin, T.J., Suda, T., 1999. IL-17 in synovial fluids from patients with rheumatoid arthritis is a potent stimulator of osteoclastogenesis. J. Clin. Invest. 103 (9), 1345–1352, available from: PM:10225978.

Krakauer, M., Sorensen, P., Khademi, M., Olsson, T., Sellebjerg, F., 2008. Increased IL-10 mRNA and IL-23 mRNA expression in multiple sclerosis: interferon-beta treatment increases IL-10 mRNA expression while reducing IL-23 mRNA expression. Mult. Scler. 14 (5), 622–630, available from: PM:18424480.

Kyttaris, V.C., Zhang, Z., Kuchroo, V.K., Oukka, M., Tsokos, G.C., 2010. Cutting edge: IL-23 receptor deficiency prevents the development of lupus nephritis in C57BL/6-lpr/lpr mice. J. Immunol. 184 (9), 4605–4609, available from: PM:20308633.

Laan, M., Cui, Z.H., Hoshino, H., Lotvall, J., Sjostrand, M., Gruenert, D.C., Skoogh, B.E., Linden, A., 1999. Neutrophil recruitment by human IL-17 via C-X-C chemokine release in the airways. J. Immunol. 162 (4), 2347–2352, available from: PM:9973514.

Langrish, C.L., Chen, Y., Blumenschein, W.M., Mattson, J., Basham, B., Sedgwick, J.D., McClanahan, T., Kastelein, R.A., Cua, D.J., 2005. IL-23 drives a pathogenic T cell population that induces autoimmune inflammation. J. Exp. Med. 201 (2), 233–240, available from: PM:15657292.

Lee, Y., Awasthi, A., Yosef, N., Quintana, F.J., Xiao, S., Peters, A., Wu, C., Kleinewietfeld, M., Kunder, S., Hafler, D.A., Sobel, R.A., Regev, A., Kuchroo, V.K., 2012. Induction and molecular signature of pathogenic T(H)17 cells. Nat. Immunol. 13 (10), 991–999, available from: PM:22961052.

Leonard, J.P., Waldburger, K.E., Goldman, S.J., 1995. Prevention of experimental autoimmune encephalomyelitis by antibodies against interleukin 12. J. Exp. Med. 181 (1), 381–386, available from: PM:7528773.

Leonardi, C.L., Kimball, A.B., Papp, K.A., Yeilding, N., Guzzo, C., Wang, Y., Li, S., Dooley, L.T., Gordon, K.B., 2008. Efficacy and safety of ustekinumab, a human interleukin-12/23 monoclonal antibody, in patients with psoriasis: 76-week results from a randomised, double-blind, placebo-controlled trial (PHOENIX 1). Lancet 371 (9625), 1665–1674, available from: PM:18486739.

Leonardi, C., Matheson, R., Zachariae, C., Cameron, G., Li, L., Edson-Heredia, E., Braun, D., Banerjee, S., 2012. Anti-interleukin-17 monoclonal antibody ixekizumab in chronic plaque psoriasis. N. Engl. J. Med. 366 (13), 1190–1199, available from: PM:22455413.

Leppkes, M., Becker, C., Ivanov, I.I., Hirth, S., Wirtz, S., Neufert, C., Pouly, S., Murphy, A.J., Valenzuela, D.M., Yancopoulos, G.D., Becher, B., Littman, D.R., Neurath, M.F., 2009. ROR-gamma-expressing Th17 cells induce murine chronic intestinal inflammation via redundant effects of IL-17A and IL-17F. Gastroenterology 136 (1), 257–267, available from: PM:18992745.

Li, L., Ruan, Q., Hilliard, B., Devirgiliis, J., Karin, M., Chen, Y.H., 2011. Transcriptional regulation of the Th17 immune response by IKK(alpha). J. Exp. Med. 208 (4), 787–796, available from: PM:21402739.

Linker-Israeli, M., Deans, R.J., Wallace, D.J., Prehn, J., Ozeri-Chen, T., Klinenberg, J.R., 1991. Elevated levels of endogenous IL-6 in systemic lupus erythematosus. A putative role in pathogenesis. J. Immunol. 147 (1), 117–123, available from: PM:2051017.

Lowes, M.A., Kikuchi, T., Fuentes-Duculan, J., Cardinale, I., Zaba, L.C., Haider, A.S., Bowman, E.P., Krueger, J.G., 2008. Psoriasis vulgaris lesions contain discrete populations of Th1 and Th17 T cells. J. Invest. Dermatol. 128 (5), 1207–1211, available from: PM:18200064.

Magram, J., Connaughton, S.E., Warrier, R.R., Carvajal, D.M., Wu, C.Y., Ferrante, J., Stewart, C., Sarmiento, U., Faherty, D.A., Gately, M.K., 1996. IL-12-deficient mice are defective in IFN gamma production and type 1 cytokine responses. Immunity 4 (5), 471–481, available from: PM:8630732.

Manel, N., Unutmaz, D., Littman, D.R., 2008. The differentiation of human T(H)-17 cells requires transforming growth factor-beta and induction of the nuclear receptor RORgammat. Nat. Immunol. 9 (6), 641–649, available from: PM:18454151.

Mangan, P.R., Harrington, L.E., O'Quinn, D.B., Helms, W.S., Bullard, D.C., Elson, C.O., Hatton, R.D., Wahl, S.M., Schoeb, T.R., Weaver, C.T., 2006. Transforming growth factor-beta induces development of the T(H)17 lineage. Nature 441 (7090), 231–234, available from: PM:16648837.

Mannon, P.J., Fuss, I.J., Mayer, L., Elson, C.O., Sandborn, W.J., Present, D., Dolin, B., Goodman, N., Groden, C., Hornung, R.L., Quezado, M., Yang, Z., Neurath, M.F., Salfeld, J., Veldman, G.M., Schwertschlag, U., Strober, W., 2004. Anti-interleukin-12 antibody for active Crohn's disease. N. Engl. J. Med. 351 (20), 2069–2079, available from: PM:15537905.

Martin, D.A., Churchill, M., Flores-Suarez, L., Cardiel, M.H., Wallace, D., Martin, R., Phillips, K., Kaine, J.L., Dong, H., Salinger, D., Stevens, E., Russell, C.B., Chung, J.B., 2013. A phase Ib multiple ascending dose study evaluating safety, pharmacokinetics, and early clinical response of brodalumab, a human anti-IL-17R antibody, in methotrexate-resistant rheumatoid arthritis. Arthritis Res.Ther. 15 (5), R164, available from: PM:24286136.

Mattner, F., Magram, J., Ferrante, J., Launois, P., Di, P.K., Behin, R., Gately, M.K., Louis, J.A., Alber, G., 1996. Genetically resistant mice lacking interleukin-12 are susceptible to infection with Leishmania major and mount a polarized Th2 cell response. Eur. J. Immunol. 26 (7), 1553–1559, available from: PM:8766560.

Matusevicius, D., Kivisakk, P., He, B., Kostulas, N., Ozenci, V., Fredrikson, S., Link, H., 1999. Interleukin-17 mRNA expression in blood and CSF mononuclear cells is augmented in multiple sclerosis. Mult. Scler. 5 (2), 101–104, available from: PM:10335518.

Maxwell, J., Zhang, Y., Rottman, J., Budelsky, A., 2013. Modeling the distinct roles for IL-23 and IL-17 in inflammatory bowel disease using Mdr1a-/- Mice. In: The 16th International Congress of, Mucosal Immunology, p. OR.57.

McCreanor, J., Cullinan, P., Nieuwenhuijsen, M.J., Stewart-Evans, J., Malliarou, E., Jarup, L., Harrington, R., Svartengren, M., Han, I.K., Ohman-Strickland, P., Chung, K.F., Zhang, J., 2007. Respiratory effects of exposure to diesel traffic in persons with asthma. N. Engl. J. Med. 357 (23), 2348–2358, available from: PM:18057337.

McGeachy, M.J., Bak-Jensen, K.S., Chen, Y., Tato, C.M., Blumenschein, W., McClanahan, T., Cua, D.J., 2007. TGF-beta and IL-6 drive the production of IL-17 and IL-10 by T cells and restrain T(H)-17 cell-mediated pathology. Nat. Immunol. 8 (12), 1390–1397, available from: PM:17994024.

McInnes, I.B., Kavanaugh, A., Gottlieb, A.B., Puig, L., Rahman, P., Ritchlin, C., Brodmerkel, C., Li, S., Wang, Y., Mendelsohn, A.M., Doyle, M.K., 2013. Efficacy and safety of ustekinumab in patients with active psoriatic arthritis: 1 year results of the phase 3, multicentre, double-blind, placebo-controlled PSUMMIT 1 trial. Lancet 382 (9894), 780–789, available from: PM:23769296.

McIntyre, K.W., Shuster, D.J., Gillooly, K.M., Warrier, R.R., Connaughton, S.E., Hall, L.B., Arp, L.H., Gately, M.K., Magram, J., 1996. Reduced incidence and severity of collagen-induced arthritis in interleukin-12-deficient mice. Eur. J. Immunol. 26 (12), 2933–2938, available from: PM:8977288.

McKinley, L., Alcorn, J.F., Peterson, A., Dupont, R.B., Kapadia, S., Logar, A., Henry, A., Irvin, C.G., Piganelli, J.D., Ray, A., Kolls, J.K., 2008. TH17 cells mediate steroid-resistant airway inflammation and airway hyperresponsiveness in mice. J. Immunol. 181 (6), 4089–4097, available from: PM:18768865.

Miossec, P., Kolls, J.K., 2012. Targeting IL-17 and TH17 cells in chronic inflammation. Nat. Rev. Drug Discov. 11 (10), 763–776, available from: PM:23023676.

Mosmann, T.R., Coffman, R.L., 1989. TH1 and TH2 cells: different patterns of lymphokine secretion lead to different functional properties. Annu. Rev. Immunol. 7, 145–173, available from: PM:2523712.

Mosmann, T.R., Cherwinski, H., Bond, M.W., Giedlin, M.A., Coffman, R.L., 1986. Two types of murine helper T cell clone. I. Definition according to profiles of lymphokine activities and secreted proteins. J. Immunol. 136 (7), 2348–2357.

Murphy, K.M., Reiner, S.L., 2002. The lineage decisions of helper T cells [Review] [122 refs]. Nat. Rev. Immunol. 2 (12), 933–944.

Murphy, C.A., Langrish, C.L., Chen, Y., Blumenschein, W., McClanahan, T., Kastelein, R.A., Sedgwick, J.D., Cua, D.J., 2003. Divergent pro- and antiinflammatory roles for IL-23 and IL-12 in joint autoimmune inflammation. J. Exp. Med. 198 (12), 1951–1957, available from: PM:14662908.

Nakae, S., Nambu, A., Sudo, K., Iwakura, Y., 2003a. Suppression of immune induction of collagen-induced arthritis in IL-17-deficient mice. J. Immunol. 171 (11), 6173–6177, available from: PM:14634133.

Nakae, S., Saijo, S., Horai, R., Sudo, K., Mori, S., Iwakura, Y., 2003b. IL-17 production from activated T cells is required for the spontaneous development of destructive arthritis in mice deficient in IL-1 receptor antagonist. Proc. Natl. Acad. Sci. U. S. A. 100 (10), 5986–5990, available from: PM:12721360.

Nestle, F.O., Kaplan, D.H., Barker, J., 2009. Psoriasis. N. Engl. J. Med. 361 (5), 496–509, available from: PM:19641206.

Neurath, M.F., Fuss, I., Kelsall, B.L., Stuber, E., Strober, W., 1995. Antibodies to interleukin 12 abrogate established experimental colitis in mice. J. Exp. Med. 182 (5), 1281–1290, available from: PM:7595199.

Niedbala, W., Wei, X.Q., Cai, B., Hueber, A.J., Leung, B.P., McInnes, I.B., Liew, F.Y., 2007. IL-35 is a novel cytokine with therapeutic effects against collagen-induced arthritis through the expansion of regulatory T cells and suppression of Th17 cells. Eur. J. Immunol. 37 (11), 3021–3029, available from: PM:17874423.

Nishimoto, N., Yoshizaki, K., Miyasaka, N., Yamamoto, K., Kawai, S., Takeuchi, T., Hashimoto, J., Azuma, J., Kishimoto, T., 2004. Treatment of rheumatoid arthritis with humanized anti-interleukin-6 receptor antibody: a multicenter, double-blind, placebo-controlled trial. Arthritis Rheum. 50 (6), 1761–1769, available from: PM:15188351.

Nurieva, R., Yang, X.O., Martinez, G., Zhang, Y., Panopoulos, A.D., Ma, L., Schluns, K., Tian, Q., Watowich, S.S., Jetten, A.M., Dong, C., 2007. Essential autocrine regulation by IL-21 in the generation of inflammatory T cells. Nature 448 (7152), 480–483, available from: PM:17581589.

O'Connor Jr., W., Kamanaka, M., Booth, C.J., Town, T., Nakae, S., Iwakura, Y., Kolls, J.K., Flavell, R.A., 2009. A protective function for interleukin 17A in T cell-mediated intestinal inflammation. Nat. Immunol. 10 (6), 603–609, available from: PM:19448631.

Ogawa, A., Andoh, A., Araki, Y., Bamba, T., Fujiyama, Y., 2004. Neutralization of interleukin-17 aggravates dextran sulfate sodium-induced colitis in mice. Clin. Immunol. 110 (1), 55–62, available from: PM:14962796.

Okamoto, K., Iwai, Y., Oh-Hora, M., Yamamoto, M., Morio, T., Aoki, K., Ohya, K., Jetten, A.M., Akira, S., Muta, T., Takayanagi, H., 2010. IkappaBzeta regulates T(H)17 development by cooperating with ROR nuclear receptors. Nature 464 (7293), 1381–1385, available from: PM:20383124.

Oosting, M., Ter, H.H., van de Veerdonk, F.L., Sturm, P., Kullberg, B.J., van der Meer, J.W., Netea, M.G., Joosten, L.A., 2011. Role of interleukin-23 (IL-23) receptor signaling for IL-17 responses in human Lyme disease. Infect. Immun. 79 (11), 4681–4687, available from: PM:21896776.

Oppmann, B., Lesley, R., Blom, B., Timans, J.C., Xu, Y., Hunte, B., Vega, F., Yu, N., Wang, J., Singh, K., Zonin, F., Vaisberg, E., Churakova, T., Liu, M.R., Gorman, D., Wagner, J., Zurawski, S., Liu, Y.J., Abrams, J.S., Moore, K.W., Rennick, D., de Waal-Malefyt, R., Hannum, C., Bazan, J.F., Kastelein, R.A., 2000. Novel p19 protein engages IL-12p40 to form a cytokine, IL-23, with biological activities similar as well as distinct from IL-12. Immunity 13 (5), 715–725.

Ouyang, X., Zhang, R., Yang, J., Li, Q., Qin, L., Zhu, C., Liu, J., Ning, H., Shin, M.S., Gupta, M., Qi, C.F., He, J.C., Lira, S.A., Morse III, H.C., Ozato, K., Mayer, L., Xiong, H., 2011. Transcription factor IRF8 directs a silencing programme for TH17 cell differentiation. Nat. Commun. 2, 314, available from: PM:21587231.

Papp, K.A., Langley, R.G., Lebwohl, M., Krueger, G.G., Szapary, P., Yeilding, N., Guzzo, C., Hsu, M.C., Wang, Y., Li, S., Dooley, L.T., Reich, K., 2008. Efficacy and safety of ustekinumab, a human interleukin-12/23 monoclonal antibody, in patients with psoriasis: 52-week results from a randomised, double-blind, placebo-controlled trial (PHOENIX 2). Lancet 371 (9625), 1675–1684, available from: PM:18486740.

Papp, K.A., Leonardi, C., Menter, A., Ortonne, J.P., Krueger, J.G., Kricorian, G., Aras, G., Li, J., Russell, C.B., Thompson, E.H., Baumgartner, S., 2012. Brodalumab, an anti-interleukin-17-receptor antibody for psoriasis. N. Engl. J. Med. 366 (13), 1181–1189, available from: PM:22455412.

Papp, K.A., Langley, R.G., Sigurgeirsson, B., Abe, M., Baker, D.R., Konno, P., Haemmerle, S., Thurston, H.J., Papavassilis, C., Richards, H.B., 2013. Efficacy and safety of secukinumab in the treatment of moderate-to-severe plaque psoriasis: a randomized, double-blind, placebo-controlled phase II dose-ranging study. Br. J. Dermatol. 168 (2), 412–421, available from: PM:23106107.

Park, H., Li, Z., Yang, X.O., Chang, S.H., Nurieva, R., Wang, Y.H., Wang, Y., Hood, L., Zhu, Z., Tian, Q., Dong, C., 2005. A distinct lineage of CD4 T cells regulates tissue inflammation by producing interleukin 17. Nat. Immunol. 6 (11), 1133–1141, available from: PM:16200068.

Peiser, M., 2013. Role of Th17 cells in skin inflammation of allergic contact dermatitis. Clin. Dev. Immunol. 2013, 261037, available from: PM:24023564.

Pisitkun, P., Ha, H.L., Wang, H., Claudio, E., Tivy, C.C., Zhou, H., Mayadas, T.N., Illei, G.G., Siebenlist, U., 2012. Interleukin-17 cytokines are critical in development of fatal lupus glomerulonephritis. Immunity 37 (6), 1104–1115, available from: PM:23123062.

Prause, O., Bozinovski, S., Anderson, G.P., Linden, A., 2004. Increased matrix metalloproteinase-9 concentration and activity after stimulation with interleukin-17 in mouse airways. Thorax 59 (4), 313–317, available from: PM:15047951.

Prins, M., Eriksson, C., Wierinckx, A., Bol, J.G., Binnekade, R., Tilders, F.J., Van Dam, A.M., 2013. Interleukin-1beta and interleukin-1 receptor antagonist appear in grey matter additionally to white matter lesions during experimental multiple sclerosis. PLoS One 8 (12), e83835, available from: PM:24376764.

Quintana, F.J., Basso, A.S., Iglesias, A.H., Korn, T., Farez, M.F., Bettelli, E., Caccamo, M., Oukka, M., Weiner, H.L., 2008. Control of T(reg) and T(H)17 cell differentiation by the aryl hydrocarbon receptor. Nature 453 (7191), 65–71, available from: PM:18362915.

Rahman, P., Inman, R.D., Gladman, D.D., Reeve, J.P., Peddle, L., Maksymowych, W.P., 2008. Association of interleukin-23 receptor variants with ankylosing spondylitis. Arthritis Rheum. 58 (4), 1020–1025, available from: PM:18383363.

Rahman, P., Inman, R.D., Maksymowych, W.P., Reeve, J.P., Peddle, L., Gladman, D.D., 2009. Association of interleukin 23 receptor variants with psoriatic arthritis. J. Rheumatol. 36 (1), 137–140, available from: PM:19040306.

Ramesh, R., Kozhaya, L., McKevitt, K., Djuretic, I.M., Carlson, T.J., Quintero, M.A., McCauley, J.L., Abreu, M.T., Unutmaz, D., Sundrud, M.S., 2014. Pro-inflammatory human Th17 cells selectively express P-glycoprotein and are refractory to glucocorticoids. J. Exp. Med. 211 (1), 89–104, available from: PM:24395888.

Res, P.C., Piskin, G., de Boer, O.J., van der Loos, C.M., Teeling, P., Bos, J.D., Teunissen, M.B., 2010. Overrepresentation of IL-17A and IL-22 producing CD8 T cells in lesional skin suggests their involvement in the pathogenesis of psoriasis. PLoS One 5 (11), e14108, available from: PM:21124836.

Rossi, S., Studer, V., Motta, C., Germani, G., Macchiarulo, G., Buttari, F., Mancino, R., Castelli, M., De, C.V., Weiss, S., Martino, G., Furlan, R., Centonze, D., 2014. Cerebrospinal fluid detection of interleukin-1beta in phase of remission predicts disease progression in multiple sclerosis. J. Neuroinflammation 11, 32, available from: PM:24548694.

Rovedatti, L., Kudo, T., Biancheri, P., Sarra, M., Knowles, C.H., Rampton, D.S., Corazza, G.R., Monteleone, G., Di, S.A., MacDonald, T.T., 2009. Differential regulation of interleukin 17 and interferon gamma production in inflammatory bowel disease. Gut 58 (12), 1629–1636, available from: PM:19740775.

Rudner, X.L., Happel, K.I., Young, E.A., Shellito, J.E., 2007. Interleukin-23 (IL-23)-IL-17 cytokine axis in murine Pneumocystis carinii infection. Infect. Immun. 75 (6), 3055–3061, available from: PM:17403873.

Sarin, R., Wu, X., Abraham, C., 2011. Inflammatory disease protective R381Q IL23 receptor polymorphism results in decreased primary CD4+ and CD8+ human T-cell functional responses. Proc. Natl. Acad. Sci. U. S. A. 108 (23), 9560–9565, available from: PM:21606346.

Schraml, B.U., Hildner, K., Ise, W., Lee, W.L., Smith, W.A., Solomon, B., Sahota, G., Sim, J., Mukasa, R., Cemerski, S., Hatton, R.D., Stormo, G.D., Weaver, C.T., Russell, J.H., Murphy, T.L., Murphy, K.M., 2009. The AP-1 transcription factor Batf controls T(H)17 differentiation. Nature 460 (7253), 405–409, available from: PM:19578362.

Seppi, D., Puthenparampil, M., Federle, L., Ruggero, S., Toffanin, E., Rinaldi, F., Perini, P., Gallo, P., 2014. Cerebrospinal fluid IL-1beta correlates with cortical pathology load in multiple sclerosis at clinical onset. J. Neuroimmunol. 270 (1-2), 56–60, available from: PM:24657029.

Serada, S., Fujimoto, M., Mihara, M., Koike, N., Ohsugi, Y., Nomura, S., Yoshida, H., Nishikawa, T., Terabe, F., Ohkawara, T., Takahashi, T., Ripley, B., Kimura, A., Kishimoto, T., Naka, T., 2008. IL-6 blockade inhibits the induction of myelin antigen-specific Th17 cells and Th1 cells in experimental autoimmune encephalomyelitis. Proc. Natl. Acad. Sci. U. S. A. 105 (26), 9041–9046, available from: PM:18577591.

Shah, K., Lee, W.W., Lee, S.H., Kim, S.H., Kang, S.W., Craft, J., Kang, I., 2010. Dysregulated balance of Th17 and Th1 cells in systemic lupus erythematosus. Arthritis Res. Ther. 12 (2), R53, available from: PM:20334681.

Shen, H., Goodall, J.C., Hill Gaston, J.S., 2009. Frequency and phenotype of peripheral blood Th17 cells in ankylosing spondylitis and rheumatoid arthritis. Arthritis Rheum. 60 (6), 1647–1656, available from: PM:19479869.

Skepner, J., Ramesh, R., Trocha, M., Schmidt, D., Baloglu, E., Lobera, M., Carlson, T., Hill, J., Orband-Miller, L.A., Barnes, A., Boudjelal, M., Sundrud, M., Ghosh, S., Yang, J., 2014. Pharmacologic inhibition of RORgammat regulates Th17 signature gene expression and suppresses cutaneous inflammation *in vivo*. J. Immunol, 192 (6), 2564–2575, available from: PM:24516202.

Skepner, J., Trocha, M., Ramesh, R., Qu, X.A., Schmidt, D., Baloglu, E., Lobera, M., Davis, S., Nolan, M.A., Carlson, T.J., Hill, J., Ghosh, S., Sundrud, M.S., Yang, J., 2015. In vivo regulation of gene expression and Th17 differentiation by RORgammat inverse agonists. Immunology 145 (3), 347–356, (Epub ahead of print) available from: PM:25604624.

Smolen, J.S., Weinblatt, M.E., Sheng, S., Zhuang, Y., Hsu, B., 2014. Sirukumab, a human anti-interleukin-6 monoclonal antibody: a randomised, 2-part (proof-of-concept and dose-finding), phase II study in patients with active rheumatoid arthritis despite methotrexate therapy. Ann. Rheum. Dis. 73 (9), 1616–1625, available from: PM:24699939.

Solt, L.A., Burris, T.P., 2012. Action of RORs and their ligands in (patho)physiology. Trends Endocrinol. Metab. 23 (12), 619–627, available from: PM:22789990.

Solt, L.A., Kumar, N., Nuhant, P., Wang, Y., Lauer, J.L., Liu, J., Istrate, M.A., Kamenecka, T.M., Roush, W.R., Vidovic, D., Schurer, S.C., Xu, J., Wagoner, G., Drew, P.D., Griffin, P.R., Burris, T.P., 2011. Suppression of TH17 differentiation and autoimmunity by a synthetic ROR ligand. Nature 472 (7344), 491–494, available from: PM:21499262.

Stumhofer, J.S., Laurence, A., Wilson, E.H., Huang, E., Tato, C.M., Johnson, L.M., Villarino, A.V., Huang, Q., Yoshimura, A., Sehy, D., Saris, C.J., O'Shea, J.J., Hennighausen, L., Ernst, M., Hunter, C.A., 2006. Interleukin 27 negatively regulates the development of interleukin 17-producing T helper cells during chronic inflammation of the central nervous system. Nat. Immunol. 7 (9), 937–945, available from: PM:16906166.

Sugihara, T., Kobori, A., Imaeda, H., Tsujikawa, T., Amagase, K., Takeuchi, K., Fujiyama, Y., Andoh, A., 2010. The increased mucosal mRNA expressions of complement C3 and interleukin-17 in inflammatory bowel disease. Clin. Exp. Immunol. 160 (3), 386–393, available from: PM:20089077.

Sullivan, J.A., Adams, A.B., Burlingham, W.J., 2014. The emerging role of TH17 cells in organ transplantation. Transplantation 97 (5), 483–489, available from: PM:24212502.

Symons, A., Budelsky, A.L., Towne, J.E., 2012. Are Th17 cells in the gut pathogenic or protective? Mucosal Immunol. 5 (1), 4–6, available from: PM:22071661.

Tanaka, T., Hishitani, Y., Ogata, A., 2014. Monoclonal antibodies in rheumatoid arthritis: comparative effectiveness of tocilizumab with tumor necrosis factor inhibitors. Biologics 8, 141–153, available from: PM:24741293.

Traczewski, P., Rudnicka, L., 2012. Briakinumab for the treatment of plaque psoriasis. BioDrugs 26 (1), 9–20, available from: PM:22077474.

Tsokos, G.C., 2011. Systemic lupus erythematosus. N. Engl. J. Med. 365 (22), 2110–2121, available from: PM:22129255.

Vargas-Rojas, M.I., Ramirez-Venegas, A., Limon-Camacho, L., Ochoa, L., Hernandez-Zenteno, R., Sansores, R.H., 2011. Increase of Th17 cells in peripheral blood of patients with chronic obstructive pulmonary disease. Respir. Med. 105 (11), 1648–1654, available from: PM:21763119.

Veldhoen, M., Hocking, R.J., Atkins, C.J., Locksley, R.M., Stockinger, B., 2006. TGFbeta in the context of an inflammatory cytokine milieu supports de novo differentiation of IL-17-producing T cells. Immunity 24 (2), 179–189, available from: PM:16473830.

Veldhoen, M., Hirota, K., Westendorf, A.M., Buer, J., Dumoutier, L., Renauld, J.C., Stockinger, B., 2008. The aryl hydrocarbon receptor links TH17-cell-mediated autoimmunity to environmental toxins. Nature 453 (7191), 106–109, available from: PM:18362914.

Wallace, K.L., Zheng, L.B., Kanazawa, Y., Shih, D.Q., 2014. Immunopathology of inflammatory bowel disease. World J. Gastroenterol. 20 (1), 6–21, available from: PM:24415853.

Wilson, R.H., Whitehead, G.S., Nakano, H., Free, M.E., Kolls, J.K., Cook, D.N., 2009. Allergic sensitization through the airway primes Th17-dependent neutrophilia and airway hyperresponsiveness. Am. J. Respir. Crit. Care Med. 180 (8), 720–730, available from: PM:19661246.

Wong, C.K., Lit, L.C., Tam, L.S., Li, E.K., Wong, P.T., Lam, C.W., 2008. Hyper production of IL-23 and IL-17 in patients with systemic lupus erythematosus: implications for Th17-mediated inflammation in auto-immunity. Clin. Immunol. 127 (3), 385–393, available from: PM:18373953.

Woodruff, P.G., Modrek, B., Choy, D.F., Jia, G., Abbas, A.R., Ellwanger, A., Koth, L.L., Arron, J.R., Fahy, J.V., 2009. T-helper type 2-driven inflammation defines major subphenotypes of asthma. Am. J. Respir. Crit. Care Med. 180 (5), 388–395, available from: PM:19483109.

Wu, C., Yosef, N., Thalhamer, T., Zhu, C., Xiao, S., Kishi, Y., Regev, A., Kuchroo, V.K., 2013. Induction of pathogenic TH17 cells by inducible salt-sensing kinase SGK1. Nature 496 (7446), 513–517, available from: PM:23467085.

Xiao, S., Yosef, N., Yang, J., 2014. Chemical Inhibition of the RORgammat-dependent transcriptional network in T helper 17 cells. Immunity 40 (4), 477–489.

Xu, T., Wang, X., Zhong, B., Nurieva, R.I., Ding, S., Dong, C., 2011. Ursolic acid suppresses interleukin-17 (IL-17) production by selectively antagonizing the function of RORgamma t protein. J. Biol. Chem. 286 (26), 22707–22710, available from: PM:21566134.

Yang, X.O., Panopoulos, A.D., Nurieva, R., Chang, S.H., Wang, D., Watowich, S.S., Dong, C., 2007. STAT3 regulates cytokine-mediated generation of inflammatory helper T cells. J. Biol. Chem. 282 (13), 9358–9363, available from: PM:17277312.

Yang, J., Yang, M., Htut, T.M., Ouyang, X., Hanidu, A., Li, X., Sellati, R., Jiang, H., Zhang, S., Li, H., Zhao, J., Ting, A.T., Mayer, L., Unkeless, J.C., Labadia, M.E., Hodge, M., Li, J., Xiong, H., 2008a. Epstein-Barr virus-induced gene 3 negatively regulates IL-17, IL-22 and RORgamma t. Eur. J. Immunol. 38 (5), 1204–1214, available from: PM:18412165.

Yang, L., Anderson, D.E., Baecher-Allan, C., Hastings, W.D., Bettelli, E., Oukka, M., Kuchroo, V.K., Hafler, D.A., 2008b. IL-21 and TGF-beta are required for differentiation of human T(H)17 cells. Nature 454 (7202), 350–352, available from: PM:18469800.

Yang, X.O., Pappu, B.P., Nurieva, R., Akimzhanov, A., Kang, H.S., Chung, Y., Ma, L., Shah, B., Panopoulos, A.D., Schluns, K.S., Watowich, S.S., Tian, Q., Jetten, A.M., Dong, C., 2008c. T helper 17 lineage differentiation is programmed by orphan nuclear receptors ROR alpha and ROR gamma. Immunity 28 (1), 29–39, available from: PM:18164222.

Yang, J., Skepner, J., Mark, T., Ghosh, S., 2013. Small molecule inhibitors targeting the Th17 cell transcription factor RORgammat for the treatment of autoimmune diseases. J. Clin. Cell Immunol. 4 (3), e111.

Yang, J., Sundrud, M.S., Skepner, J., Yamagata, T., 2014. Targeting Th17 cells in autoimmune diseases. Trends Pharmacol. Sci. 35 (10), 493–500, available from: PM:25131183.

Ye, P., Garvey, P.B., Zhang, P., Nelson, S., Bagby, G., Summer, W.R., Schwarzenberger, P., Shellito, J.E., Kolls, J.K., 2001. Interleukin-17 and lung host defense against Klebsiella pneumoniae infection. Am. J. Respir. Cell Mol. Biol. 25 (3), 335–340, available from: PM:11588011.

Yen, D., Cheung, J., Scheerens, H., Poulet, F., McClanahan, T., McKenzie, B., Kleinschek, M.A., Owyang, A., Mattson, J., Blumenschein, W., Murphy, E., Sathe, M., Cua, D.J., Kastelein, R.A., Rennick, D., 2006. IL-23 is essential for T cell-mediated colitis and promotes inflammation via IL-17 and IL-6. J. Clin. Invest. 116 (5), 1310–1316, available from: PM:16670770.

Zanin-Zhorov, A., Weiss, J.M., Nyuydzefe, M.S., Chen, W., Scher, J.U., Mo, R., Depoil, D., Rao, N., Liu, B., Wei, J., Lucas, S., Koslow, M., Roche, M., Schueller, O., Weiss, S., Poyurovsky, M.V., Tonra, J., Hippen, K.L., Dustin, M.L., Blazar, B.R., Liu, C.J., Waksal, S.D., 2014. Selective oral ROCK2 inhibitor down-regulates IL-21 and IL-17 secretion in human T cells via STAT3-dependent mechanism. Proc. Natl. Acad. Sci. U. S. A. 111 (47), 16814–16819, available from: PM:25385601.

Zhang, Z., Zheng, M., Bindas, J., Schwarzenberger, P., Kolls, J.K., 2006. Critical role of IL-17 receptor signaling in acute TNBS-induced colitis. Inflamm. Bowel Dis. 12 (5), 382–388, available from: PM:16670527.

Zhang, F., Meng, G., Strober, W., 2008. Interactions among the transcription factors Runx1, RORgammat and Foxp3 regulate the differentiation of interleukin 17-producing T cells. Nat. Immunol. 9 (11), 1297–1306, available from: PM:18849990.

Zhao, J., Lloyd, C.M., Noble, A., 2013. Th17 responses in chronic allergic airway inflammation abrogate regulatory T-cell-mediated tolerance and contribute to airway remodeling. Mucosal Immunol. 6 (2), 335–346, available from: PM:22892938.

Zheng, Y., Danilenko, D.M., Valdez, P., Kasman, I., Eastham-Anderson, J., Wu, J., Ouyang, W., 2007. Interleukin-22, a T(H)17 cytokine, mediates IL-23-induced dermal inflammation and acanthosis. Nature 445 (7128), 648–651, available from: PM:17187052.

Zhou, L., Lopes, J.E., Chong, M.M., Ivanov, I.I., Min, R., Victora, G.D., Shen, Y., Du, J., Rubtsov, Y.P., Rudensky, A.Y., Ziegler, S.F., Littman, D.R., 2008. TGF-beta-induced Foxp3 inhibits T(H)17 cell differentiation by antagonizing RORgammat function. Nature 453 (7192), 236–240, available from: PM:18368049.

Zou, W., Restifo, N.P., 2010. T(H)17 cells in tumour immunity and immunotherapy. Nat. Rev. Immunol. 10 (4), 248–256, available from: PM:20336152.

CHAPTER 6

Th9 Cells as Targets for Immunotherapy

O. Awe[1,2], M.H. Kaplan[1,2]
[1]Herman B Wells Center for Pediatric Research, Indianapolis, IN, United States
[2]Indiana University School of Medicine, Indianapolis, IN, United States

Contents

1. INTRODUCTION TO T HELPER CELLS

T helper (Th) cells are one component of the finely tuned immune system. Th cells have diverse functions within the immune system including providing help to B cells allowing for the production of high-affinity antibodies and upon differentiation into specific effector subsets, Th cells are crucial for the elimination of infectious agents and foreign proteins. The differentiation of Th cells is largely dependent upon the cytokines present within the microenvironment during an active immune response. Cytokines such as interleukin (IL)-12 and IL-4 polarize T cells to become Th1 and Th2 cells, respectively (Mosmann et al., 1986). Furthermore, transforming growth factor (TGF)-β signaling alone or in combination with IL-6 promotes the differentiation of T regulatory or Th17 cells, respectively. The most recently discovered Th subset is the Th9 subset, which primarily secretes IL-9 and differentiates in response to TGF-β and IL-4 (Dardalhon et al., 2008; Veldhoen et al., 2008; Schmitt et al., 1994). Th9 cells are an important part of the immune response against parasites and have antitumor properties;

Translational Immunology
http://dx.doi.org/10.1016/B978-0-12-801577-3.00007-1

however, Th9 cells have also been implicated in promoting asthma and autoimmunity (Nicolaides et al., 1997; Jager et al., 2009; Shimbara et al., 2000). Although the contribution of IL-9 in various disease pathologies requires further investigation, preclinical data suggest that IL-9 may be a promising immunotherapy target for the treatment of certain diseases.

The goal of this chapter is to describe the proinflammatory environments that regulate the development of the Th9 cell subset and to summarize the disease scenarios where Th9 cells and IL-9 are known to have effects. As part of this summary, we will highlight how current and in trial patient therapies might be used to modulate Th9 cell inflammatory activity and ultimately disease phenotypes in patients.

1.1 Th9 cell differentiation and activity

IL-9 was first described as a T cell growth factor but has since been shown to target a variety of cell types including mast cells, astrocytes, keratinocytes, and lung epithelial cells (Kearley et al., 2011; Jager et al., 2009; Temann et al., 2007; Ma et al., 2014; Goswami and Kaplan, 2011). The cytokines IL-4 and TGF-β induce a network of transcription factors within naïve $CD4^+$ T cells necessary for IL-9 production in both mice and humans (Kaplan, 2013). In addition to the requirement of TGF-β and IL-4, other costimulatory molecules and cytokines have been shown to augment or inhibit IL-9 production by Th9 cells (Fig. 1). Both murine and human Th9 cells increase IL-9 production in response to IL-1β, nitric oxide, and thymic stromal lymphopoietin (TSLP; Anuradha et al., 2013; Niedbala et al., 2014; Yao et al., 2013) and downregulate IL-9 production in response to interferon (IFN)-γ and IL-27 (Murugaiyan et al., 2012; Ye et al., 2012; Wong et al., 2010). Cultured human Th9 cells also increase IL-9 production when exposed to IL-6, IL-10, IFN-α, IFN-β, and IL-21 (Wong et al., 2010); however, the relative importance of these cytokines in regulating Th9 cellular activity during the onset and progression of different disease states is still in question.

Th9 cells act in a proinflammatory or an anti-inflammatory manner depending on the experimental disease model being tested. The inflammatory nature of Th9 cells is often directly related to the ability of IL-9 to act on various cell types within the lung, skin, brain, and other nonimmune privileged organs. IL-9 can also enhance the effector function of other Th cell subsets. For example, the binding of IL-9 in combination with TGF-β and IL-6 to human $CD4^+$ T cells leads to higher levels of $CD4^+IL\text{-}17A^+$ cells compared to cultures without IL-9 (Singh et al., 2013). A similar observation was made in mice but IL-6 was not required (Elyaman et al., 2009). Conversely, IL-9 has been associated with promoting the activity of T regulatory cells, which are a subset of Th cells that through the expression of anti-inflammatory cytokines IL-10 and TGF-β dampen the immune response (Smith et al., 2011; Elyaman et al., 2009). The impact of IL-9 on human T regulatory cells has not been closely examined and will require further study

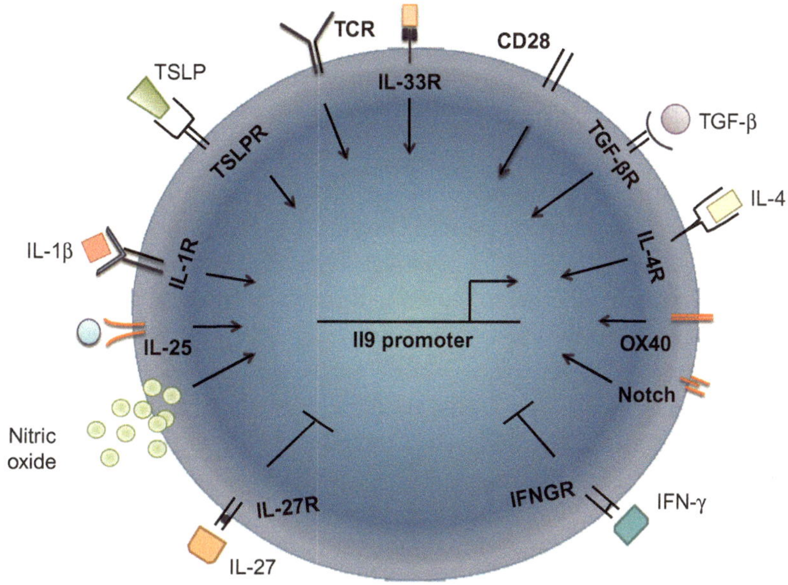

Figure 1 Factors regulating human and mouse Th9 differentiation. Th9 cells are a distinct subset of T helper (Th) cells that require a combination of factors for proper differentiation. Signaling through the IL-4 and TGF-β receptors induces intracellular signaling that induces the transcriptional network that establishes the Th9 phenotype in mouse and humans. Signaling through other cytokines and costimulatory molecules such as IL-1β, IL-25, IL-33, TSLP, OX40, notch, and nitric oxide can enhance various aspects of the Th9 phenotype, most notably IL-9 expression (Anuradha et al., 2013; Angkasekwinai et al., 2010; Blom et al., 2011; Uyttenhove et al., 2010; Yao et al., 2013; Xiao et al., 2012; Elyaman et al., 2012; Niedbala et al., 2014; Gerlach et al., 2014). Cytokines such as IFN-γ and IL-27 have been shown to negatively regulate the development of Th9 cells. Factors that have not yet been shown to promote human Th9 cell development are indicated in red.

to determine if observations made using murine cells can be expanded to humans. The proclivity of Th9 cells to lead to enhanced or reduced inflammation may depend on the dominant cell type within the immediate environment.

1.2 Alternative sources of IL-9

Although Th9 cells produce high levels of IL-9, other Th subsets can produce lesser amounts of IL-9. Th2 cells were initially believed to be the predominant producers of IL-9. Some of the first observations that connected IL-9 to Th2 cells were during helminthic parasite infections and allergic inflammation, pathologies that are dependent on Th2-associated cytokines. In more recent studies where IL-9 is attributed to Th9 cells, IL-9 production can be detected in the absence of other Th2-associated cytokines, including IL-4, IL-5, and IL-13 (Chang et al., 2010). Similarly, in cultures using human peripheral blood mononuclear cells (PBMCs) treated with IL-4 and TGF-β, IL-9-single positive cells that lack IL-4 production predominate over IL-9^+ cells that coexpress Th2-

associated cytokines (Wong et al., 2010). Th17 cells have also been found to secrete IL-9 (Stephens et al., 2011). Human naïve $CD4^+$ T cells stimulated under Th17-polarizing conditions (ie, TGF-β, IL-6, IL-1β, IL-23^+IL-21), produced a similar frequency of IL-9 single positive cells compared to naïve cells stimulated under standard Th9-inducing cytokines (ie, IL-4 and TGF-β; Beriou et al., 2010). Cells that coexpressed IL-9 and IL-17A were not observed after the first round of culture but were observed after multiple rounds of culture. Similar observations were made using murine naïve cells cultured *in vitro* under Th17 conditions; however, IL-$17A^+$IL-9^+ cells were present after the first round of culture. There are conflicting reports as to whether or not T regulatory cells produce IL-9. One report states that IL-9 mRNA could not be detected in T regulatory cells and Foxp3 repressed IL-9 production (Veldhoen et al., 2008; Goswami et al., 2012) while others report detecting IL-9 at the mRNA and protein levels in cells that are either T regulatory cells or cells that phenotypically match T regulatory cells (Liu et al., 2006; Lu et al., 2006; Nowak et al., 2009). In addition to $CD4^+$ T helper cells, other cell types such as innate lymphoid cells (ILCs), mast cells, eosinophils, basophils, and neurons have been shown to produce IL-9 (Wilhelm et al., 2011; Hultner et al., 2000; Gounni et al., 2004; Blom et al., 2011; Fontaine et al., 2008).

The importance of Th9 cells during various inflammatory processes in the human body is still not well defined. In the following paragraphs, we review disease pathologies in humans where IL-9 correlated with disease severity and in analogous experimental mouse models where IL-9 was found to be a prominent factor linked to the observed pathology. In some situations, the production of IL-9 precedes the subsequent cytokine cascade that further advances the pathology observed. This may suggest that IL-9 may be a practical target for the treatment of the diseases discussed in this chapter and possibly in diseases that have yet to be examined.

2. ALLERGY AND ATOPIC DISEASE

The prevalence of allergic and atopic disease is steadily increasing (Kay, 2001). There is considerable evidence that diseases such as asthma, allergic rhinitis, and atopic dermatitis are partially mediated by Th2-associated cytokines and increased levels of IgE specific to antigens that are commonly inhaled. IL-9 was initially one of the cytokines associated with the Th2 response because it was linked to diseases traditionally attributed to Th2 cells. However, recent studies using Th9 cell transfer models in mice and corroborating *in vitro* studies using human primary cells and cell lines have suggested that the observations made involving IL-9 could possibly be due to the newly discovered Th9 lineage. Although, it is difficult to isolate the exact cell type that may be producing IL-9 *in vivo*, IL-9-producing T cells are often detected in the absence of other cytokines suggesting that in diseases mediated in part by $CD4^+$ T cells, such as asthma and atopic dermatitis, Th9 cells may be the source of IL-9. Ahead we review the preclinical mouse studies and human data that support the notion that IL-9 is a crucial cytokine in the initiation and progression of various atopic diseases.

2.1 IL-9 and inflammation of the lung

The study of IL-9 as a potential target for the treatment of asthma was triggered by genetic association studies, which linked asthma to genes located on chromosome 5q31-33 in humans (Postma et al., 1995; Marsh et al., 1994). Genes located in this region were found to be divided among chromosomes 11, 13, and 18 in mice (DeBry and Seldin, 1996). IL-9 is located in 5q31.1 and on mouse chromosome 13 (Nicolaides et al., 1997). Different strains of mice have varying levels of bronchial hyperresponsiveness (BHR) that have been associated with genes located on mouse chromosome 13. Using mice that are known to demonstrate a range of BHR from hyporesponsiveness to hyperresponsiveness, it was determined that protein and mRNA levels of IL-9 in the lungs of these mice correlated with the level of BHR (Levitt et al., 1999). A similar correlation was not found for other genes surrounding the IL-9 locus. Correlative studies in humans have also linked IL-9 to asthma and atopic disease. Immunohistochemistry of endobronchial specimens from patients with asthma, chronic bronchitis, sarcoidosis, atopic nonasthmatic disease, and healthy controls showed patients with asthma had significantly higher levels of IL-9 mRNA and protein within their specimens compared to patients with chronic bronchitis, sarcoidosis, atopic nonasthmatic disease, and healthy controls (Shimbara et al., 2000). Many of the cells that stained positive for IL-9 also stained positive for CD3 suggesting that $CD4^+$ Th cells are a major source of IL-9 in asthmatic patients. The level of IL-9 detected in the lungs of asthmatic patients also correlated to the decline in lung function. Similar to IL-9 protein, the amount of IL-9 receptor (IL-9R) protein was increased in asthmatic specimens (Shimbara et al., 2000). These studies also showed that individuals with atopic disease expressed significantly higher levels of IL-9 mRNA and protein compared to nonatopic patients (Shimbara et al., 2000). Analogous to the increased levels of IL-9 in atopic individuals found in this study, another study looking at IL-9 production by PBMCs from atopic infants and nonatopic infants stimulated with specific antigens and nonspecifically with PMA (phorbol 12-myristate 13-acetate) and Ionomycin found that PBMCs from atopic infants produced higher levels of IL-9 protein but not other cytokines associated with the Th1, Th2, and Th17 lineages (Yao et al., 2011). In the same study, naïve $CD4^+$ cells from atopic and nonatopic infants cultured under Th9-skewing conditions, expressed more IL-9 at the mRNA and protein levels after restimulation with α-CD3. These studies have demonstrated that $CD4^+$ cells in individuals with asthmatic and atopic disease produce IL-9 at a level that is significantly greater than individuals with other lung-associated diseases and healthy controls. To further understand how IL-9 impacts the pathology of asthma and atopic dermatitis, the target cells of IL-9 must also be studied.

2.2 Targets of IL-9 during lung inflammation

IL-9 has been found to have an impact on a variety of cells including epithelial and structural cells of the lungs as well as cells of the hematopoietic system. One principal IL-9 target is mast cells, one of the principal cell types involved in the pathology of asthma and atopic disease. Through the production of proteins, proteases, and monocyte chemotactic proteins (MCP1-5), mast cells increase tissue remodeling, mucus production, and overall can lead to the worsening of an inflammatory response. The impact of IL-9 on mast cells was initially studied using mouse bone marrow-derived mast cells (BMMC; Hultner et al., 1990). IL-9 was found to enhance proliferation of BMMC and their production of IL-6 *in vitro*. In murine models where IL-9 is constitutively expressed within the lungs, mast cells were found in both the epithelium and subepithelium of the upper respiratory tracts and the epithelium of the lower respiratory tract, features not found in the lungs of nontransgenic control mice (Temann et al., 1998). IL-9 has also been shown to impact the activity of mast cells in the context of allergic inflammation of the lung. A study that looked at acute and chronic allergic inflammation of the lung found that allergen challenge induced an increase in the mast cell protease mMCP-1 in the serum, which could be abrogated with anti-IL-9 antibody treatment (Kearley et al., 2011). The decrease in mMCP-1 was not accompanied by a reduction in the number of mast cells, suggesting that in the context of lung inflammation IL-9 can enhance mast cell protease production. IL-9 has also been shown to impact human mast cell progenitors. In conjunction with stem cell factor (SCF), IL-9 has been shown to increase the expansion of uncultured $CD34^+$ mast cells from cord blood compared to SCF alone (Matsuzawa et al., 2003). The effect of IL-9 appeared to be limited to increasing cell numbers because the amount of histamine and chemical mediators within the mast cell culture medium was not impacted by the presence of IL-9. Interestingly, when $CD34^+$ cells were taken from the peripheral blood of asthmatics and healthy donors, cells from asthmatics expanded more when cultured with SCF alone when compared to healthy donors, and this difference was augmented when IL-9 was added. These results suggest mast cells from asthma patients may be altered in some way that makes them hyperresponsive to growth stimuli, allowing for greater expansion during an allergic response.

Other potential targets of IL-9 during atopic disease include eosinophils and $CD4^+$ Th cell subsets. IL-9 enhances the survival and differentiation of eosinophils by increasing the expression of the IL-5Rα (Levitt et al., 1999). During allergic pulmonary inflammation, IL-9 leads to the production of IL-5, an eosinophil activator. In some studies, the production of IL-9 has been found to precede the production of Th2-associated cytokines such as IL-4, IL-5, and IL-13. In fact, blocking IL-9 has been shown to limit the expression of such cytokines and others, thereby attenuating the development of allergic inflammation of the lung (Temann et al., 2002). However, treating asthma patients with an IL-9 blocking antibody was not as efficacious as seen in mice (Oh et al., 2013).

2.3 Efficacy of an IL-9 blocking antibody in asthma

In a study where patients with moderate to severe asthma were given either placebo or the anti-IL-9 monoclonal antibody, MEDI-528, patients who received the placebo experienced the same level of improvement that patients who received the monoclonal antibody experienced (Oh et al., 2013). There was no improvement in lung function in patients that received MEDI-528 compared to patients that received placebo. Despite the lack of improvement reported in this study, earlier clinical trials looking at the effect of MEDI-528 on asthma control in patients with mild asthma reported a trend toward fewer asthma exacerbations in patients that received MEDI-528 (Parker et al., 2011). A similar result was also seen when the effect of MEDI-528 on exercise-induced bronchoconstriction was tested. Patients who received MEDI-528 showed improved lung function after receiving the monoclonal antibody. The subjects in both of these studies belonged to different subgroups of individuals with asthma or some form of uncontrolled bronchoconstriction and two of the three studies showed that MEDI-528 treatment could be beneficial. The disparity in efficacy of MEDI-528 could be due to a difference in the contribution of IL-9 in the pathogenesis of these subgroups of asthma. Further study will be required to pinpoint individuals who would benefit from MEDI-528 and other IL-9 targeted therapies that may be developed in the future.

It is quite clear that IL-9 participates in the pathogenesis of allergic disease. However, the mechanistic requirement for IL-9 during the pathogenesis of such diseases is still unclear. IL-9 targets several cell types that are the primary mediators of disease progression and exacerbation in asthma and atopic disease. Mast cells and eosinophils are both targets of IL-9 and both cell types contribute to the pathogenesis of allergic disease by releasing inflammation-promoting molecules at the site of inflammation. IL-9 also appears to have the ability to regulate the production of inflammation-promoting cytokines produced by Th2 cells. One question that remains to be answered is whether IL-9 expression changes during the development and progression of allergic diseases such as asthma. In animal models of allergic inflammation of the lung and other inflammatory processes the expression of IL-9 seems to be transient (Tan et al., 2010). The possible transient nature of IL-9 expression may be the cause of the ineffectiveness of anti-IL-9 monoclonal antibody treatment in patients with moderate-to-severe asthma, an outcome that contrasted to the beneficial effect of MEDI-528 in patients with mild asthma. In patients with mild asthma the importance of IL-9 in the maintenance of this disease stage may be greater than the importance of IL-9 in maintaining disease in individuals with moderate-to-severe asthma. Determining if IL-9 is a cytokine important for setting the foundation of the inflammatory process in diseases such as asthma will be an interesting finding and may provide a prophylactic target for preventing the cascade of inflammatory events that lead to the development of allergic disease.

3. Th9 CELLS AND GUT IMMUNITY AND INFLAMMATION

3.1 Th9 cells and helminthic parasite immunity

Helminthic parasite infections affect billions of people and animals worldwide and are a great cause of morbidity and mortality, especially in developing countries

(Macdonald et al., 2002). The burden of helminthic parasite infections is likely to be persistent due to the absence of effective vaccines. It is thought that helminthic parasite infections are able to advance from acute to chronic infections without being lethal to the host because of the host's ability to initiate a type 2 immune response mediated by cytokines such as IL-4, IL-9, IL-10, and IL-13. The mechanism by which a type 2 immune response is triggered by helminthic parasite infections is not completely understood but the importance of IL-4 and IL-10 in limiting injury to the host has been demonstrated in experimental mouse models of infection (Brunet et al., 1997; Fallon et al., 2000; Hoffmann et al., 1999).

In helminthic parasite infections, the ability of IL-9 to promote worm expulsion is highlighted in IL-9 transgenic mice (IL-9-Tg mice) infected with either *Trichuris muris* (Faulkner et al., 1998) or *Trichinella spiralis* (Faulkner et al., 1997). Upon infection with *T. spiralis*, IL-9-Tg mice were able to clear all worms by day 8 postinfection compared to minimal clearance observed in control mice. Similar but less striking results were observed in IL-9-Tg mice infected with *T. muris*. In these studies, IL-9-Tg mice had eliminated the parasite within 34 days while *T. muris* worms persisted in the control animals. Mast cells, an important cell type in helminthic parasite resistance and a known target of IL-9, were suggested to play a prominent role in facilitating worm expulsion during both infections. Increases in mast cell numbers were accompanied by increases in serum levels of mast cell protease-1 (MMCP-1). Another possible explanation for the accelerated clearance of *T. muris* in IL-9-Tg mice is the induction of intestinal muscle hypercontractility by IL-9 (Khan et al., 2003). Treatment of wild-type (WT) mice with recombinant IL-9 has been shown to induce contraction of the smooth muscle of the small intestine in mice possibly by increasing the expression of IL-4 and IL-13. To demonstrate the importance of IL-9 in promoting intestinal muscle hypercontractility, mice were infected with either *T. spiralis* or *T. muris* and treated with antibodies against IL-9. Interestingly, neutralization of IL-9 only limited the expulsion of *T. muris* and not *T. spiralis*. In addition to the attenuation of *T. muris* expulsion, these mice also showed less intestinal muscle hypercontractility. The selective necessity of IL-9 for clearing different helminthic parasite infections suggests that although many infections induce a type 2 immune response, there are distinct mechanistic requirements for the expulsion of specific helminthic parasites. Furthermore, there is limited data demonstrating the contribution of IL-9 during human infection. A study looking at the prevalence and expansion of $IL\text{-}9^{+}IL\text{-}10^{+}IL\text{-}4^{-}$ cells, identified as human Th9 cells, in patients with filarial disease found that stimulation with parasite-antigen caused greater expansion of Th9 cells compared to $IL\text{-}9^{+}IL\text{-}4^{+}$ Th2 cells (Anuradha et al., 2013). Th9 cells from patients with active filarial disease expanded to a greater extent then Th9 cells from patients who were infected but asymptomatic, suggesting that in contrast to the protective role associated with IL-9 in the context of *T. muris* or *T. spiralis* infection, Th9 cells may be pathogenic in nature in human filarial disease.

One common theme in IL-9 biology is that the expression of IL-9 in many instances precedes the expression of other type 2 cytokines. During infection with *Nippostrongylus brasiliensis*, IL-9 levels peak 2–4 days after initial infections in the lungs, mediastinal lymph nodes, and mesenteric lymph nodes (Licona-Limon et al., 2013). However, IL-4, IL-5, and IL-13 levels continue to increase and peak 7 days after initial infection. Infection with *T. muris* and *T. spiralis* is associated with a similar sequential pattern of cytokine expression (Faulkner et al., 1997, 1998; Angkasekwinai et al., 2013). Although, there is significant evidence indicating that IL-9 can play a protective or possibly a pathogenic role in parasitic immunity, there is also evidence suggesting that IL-9 may be expendable during certain infections (Townsend et al., 2000). Mice deficient in the expression of IL-9 showed a comparable disease course and higher Th2-associated cytokine levels when compared to WT mice during infection with *N. brasiliensis*. IL-9-deficient mice had a trend of less mast cell infiltration and goblet cell hyperplasia compared to WT mice, supporting the belief that IL-9 plays an important part in promoting such phenotypes. Thus, effective expulsion of *N. brasiliensis* in the absence of IL-9 may suggest that although IL-9 plays an active role during helminth immunity, there are other mechanisms in place that can compensate when IL-9 is not available.

3.2 Th9 cells and colitis

In addition to enhancing immunity in the context of helminthic parasite infections, Th9 cells have also been found to be pathogenic in human and experimental colitis (Nalleweg et al., 2015; Gerlach et al., 2014). One of the first papers to describe Th9 cells demonstrated a pathogenic role for Th9 cells in colitis using a transfer model (Dardalhon et al., 2008). When IL-9^+IL-10^+ cells were transferred into naïve mice with Foxp3^-CD45RB^{hi} effector cells, the mice lost the most weight and histologically showed signs of more severe colitis compared to WT mice that received effector cells alone, suggesting that the IL-9^+ cells worsened disease. More recently, a study looking at patients with ulcerative colitis (UC) reported increased levels of IL-9 mRNA and protein in inflamed UC lesions compared to mucosal tissue from healthy control patients and noninflamed mucosal tissue from UC patients (Gerlach et al., 2014). The amount of IL-9 mRNA also correlated with disease activity. The expression of the transcription factor PU.1, which is vital for Th9 development, was also increased in patients with UC. The association between IL-9, PU.1, and colitis severity was confirmed using mouse models of colitis. Similar results were found in patients with Crohn's disease, but the association with IL-9 was not statistically significant.

4. Th9 CELLS AND CNS DISEASE

The opposing functions of T regulatory cells and the proinflammatory Th1, Th2, and Th17 subsets regulate the balance between tolerance and inflammation. Th9 cells likely impact this balance as well. When the balance between tolerance and inflammation is tipped to favor proinflammatory effector cells, autoimmune diseases can arise. Experimental autoimmune encephalomyelitis (EAE), a mouse model of the human disease multiple sclerosis characterized by demyelination within the central nervous system (CNS), has been used to demonstrate the impact of the Th subsets on the initiation and progression of autoimmune conditions. Currently, there are conflicting views on the contribution of Th9 cells during EAE because it is thought that IL-9 can promote either a proinflammatory or anti-inflammatory state depending on the microenvironment of expression. Adoptive transfer experiments demonstrated that naïve T cells from mice expressing a myelin oligodendrocyte glycoprotein-specific-TCR (T cell receptor) skewed under Th9 conditions can induce EAE (Jager et al., 2009).

The pathogenic capability of Th9 cells contrasts the reported ability of IL-9 to augment the activity of T regulatory cells (Elyaman et al., 2009). In one study, mice deficient in the expression of the IL-9R showed earlier onset of EAE and increased disease severity compared to WT mice. When *Il9r*$^{-/-}$ or *Il9r*$^{+/+}$ $CD4^+CD25^+$ regulatory T (Treg) cells were adoptively transferred into WT mice after induction of EAE, IL-9R-deficient Tregs had a reduced capacity to suppress T cell proliferation suggesting that the absence of IL-9 signaling during EAE diminishes Treg activity and exacerbates CNS disease (Elyaman et al., 2009). The protective role of IL-9 in this study differs from the pathogenic role of IL-9 presented in other studies. One study links IL-9 production in the CNS to the production of CCL20 (CC chemokine ligand 20) by astrocytes expressing the IL-9R and suggests that the CCL20 produced can lead to the migration of Th17 cells (Zhou et al., 2011). In other studies that utilized IL-9 blocking antibodies, *Il9*$^{-/-}$ mice, and *Il9r*$^{-/-}$ mice observed delayed onset of disease and decreased disease severity (Nowak et al., 2009; Li et al., 2011; Elyaman et al., 2012). The proposed mechanisms employed by IL-9 in promoting EAE pathology in these different models include activation of STAT1 and STAT3 pathways, increasing mast cell numbers in the CNS, and enabling activation of antigen-specific T cells. The diverging observations concerning the significance of IL-9 in the pathology of EAE will require further investigation. However, a study conducted by Elyaman et al. (2012) provides a possible explanation for the conflicting results. Signaling by Jagged2-stimulated notch receptors can induce the production of IL-9. Pretreating WT mice with Jagged2 before the induction of EAE led to less severe disease and simultaneous treatment with Jagged2 and induction of EAE led to greater disease severity. The authors suggest that the disparity in outcomes is due to changes in the Treg/Th17 ratio brought on by differing cell targets for IL-9. When mice are pretreated with Jagged2, the Treg/Th17 ratio increased suggesting that in this relatively noninflammatory microenvironment where Tregs may predominate, IL-9 is able to promote Treg activity and dampen subsequent CNS inflammation. However, the presence of IL-9 as the immune response is being initiated leads to even greater inflammation, possibly by expanding proinflammatory cells such as Th17 cells. Currently, Th17 and Th1 cells are the primary Th subsets found to be associated with the human disease multiple sclerosis. However, increasing amounts of evidence in mouse models suggest that further study into the possible contribution of Th9 cells during multiple sclerosis would be revealing.

5. Th9 CELLS AND TUMOR IMMUNITY

Cancer immunotherapy is advancing at a rapid pace. The potential use of T cells for targeting tumors is actively being pursued (Restifo et al., 2012). The presence of $CD4^+$ and $CD8^+$ cells within the tumor microenvironment in certain cancers is used as an indicator of positive prognosis (Hadrup et al., 2013). Interestingly, metastatic tissue from patients with advanced melanoma contained fewer IL-9-producing T cells than skin tissue and blood from healthy controls (Purwar et al., 2012). Although, $CD8^+$ are thought to be the more beneficial of the two cell types because of their ability to directly kill caner cells, $CD4^+$ T cells are becoming increasingly viewed as an important cancer fighting cell type. $CD4^+$ T cells are important for the activation of $CD8^+$ cells, they help recruit other immune cell types to the tumor microenvironment, and in some cases, $CD4^+$ cells can directly kill tumor cells (Knutson and Disis, 2005; Lu et al., 2012). Th9 cells appear to be a cell type that possesses each of these attributes, making Th9 cells an excellent candidate for cancer immunotherapy.

The potential of Th9 cells or IL-9 to promote antitumor phenotypes has been explored by a number of groups and preclinical results suggest that Th9 cells may be efficacious in the treatment of certain cancers (Purwar et al., 2012; Lu et al., 2012; Vegran et al., 2014). Th9 cells can induce tumor tissues to produce CCL20, which leads to the recruitment of $CD8\alpha^+$ and $CD11b^+$ dendritic cells that travel to tumor-draining lymph nodes and prime $CD8^+$ cytotoxic lymphocytes to kill tumor cells (Lu et al., 2012). Th9 cells can also produce IL-3 supporting the survival of dendritic cells that can further promote antitumor immune responses (Park et al., 2014).

Adoptive transfer of differing OT-II Th subsets (cells recognizing an epitope in ovalbumin (OVA)) into WT or $Rag^{-/-}$ mice challenged with the metastatic melanoma cell line B16F10 that overexpress OVA demonstrated that OT-II-Th9 cells were able to suppress tumor growth better than mice that received no cells, Th1, Th2, and Th17 cells (Purwar et al., 2012). That result suggested that Th9 cells have superior antitumor capabilities compared to other effector subsets and the antitumor activity of Th9 cells does not require endogenous T cells, including $CD8^+$ cells, which are thought to be crucial tumor fighting immune cells. Multiple studies have demonstrated that neutralization of IL-9 after mice are challenged with tumor cell lines abrogates the ability of Th9 cells to limit tumor growth compared to mice receiving antibody controls (Purwar et al., 2012; Lu et al., 2012; Vegran et al., 2014). Importantly, this was seen when mice received OT-II-Th9 cells after being challenged with the melanoma cell line overexpressing OVA. Th9 cells are able to limit tumor growth through the production of IL-9 and not another cytokine or molecule. However, a recent study looking at the antitumor capabilities of Th9 cells challenges the idea that Th9 cells developing in situ during a tumor immune response have a phenotype similar to Th9 cells cultured *in vitro* (Vegran et al., 2014). Th9 cells sorted from cells taken directly from tumor-draining lymph nodes have a molecular signature similar to Th9 cells that have been cultured in the presence of IL-1β, which require interferon regulatory factor 1 (IRF1) for their antitumor phenotype. In addition to being dependent on IRF1 expression, these cells also express high levels of IL-9 and IL-21. Neutralizing IL-9 did not inhibit the ability of OT-II-Th9 cells skewed in the presence of IL-1β to kill tumor cells. However, blockade of IL-21 in the same experiments abrogated tumor killing. These findings suggest that the tumor microenvironment can impact the phenotype of Th9 cells but does not eliminate their ability to be tumoricidal.

However, there are some concerns that should be addressed before Th9 cells reach the cancer therapeutic stage. The ability of Th9 cells to be proinflammatory and anti-inflammatory in distinct settings will be a concern. There is some evidence that IL-9 can promote tumor survival, again by acting on Tregs (Smith et al., 2011). This dichotomy in IL-9 activity may be a concern when proposing IL-9 as a potential target for disease treatment as it might have differing effects at progressing stages of disease. Despite the findings that IL-9 can negatively impact tumor killing, the preponderance of literature demonstrates the ability of Th9 cells to promote tumor killing.

The cell types targeted by IL-9 that promote the Th9 anticancer phenotype are still unclear. The requirement for mast cells and $CD8^+$ cells have been reported, suggesting that there may be several parallel pathways (Fig. 2; Purwar et al., 2012; Vegran et al., 2014). These findings may be due to the pleiotropic nature of IL-9 and support that IL-9 induces multiple aspects of the immune system eliciting a substantial antitumor immune response. Whether human Th9 cells possess the same anticancer abilities observed in murine Th9 cells remains to be determined.

6. POTENTIAL DRUGS FOR LIMITING Th9 DEVELOPMENT

Th9 differentiation can be enhanced by a variety of factors, many of which are drug targets for the treatment of different inflammatory diseases (Table 1). In disease states where Th9 cells are thought to promote inflammation limiting Th9 development would be advantageous. The cytokines present in an inflammatory microenvironment play a pivotal role in directing the differentiation of activated T cells toward a specific phenotype. Thus, treatment modalities that block cytokines such as IL-4, TGF-β, IL-33, TSLP, and IL-1β, which promote Th9 development, may work to constrain activated T cells from adopting the proinflammatory Th9 phenotype. In addition to cytokines, costimulatory molecules, transcription factors, and signaling molecules are also important factors in Th9 differentiation; therefore, therapies that target such factors may also be valuable.

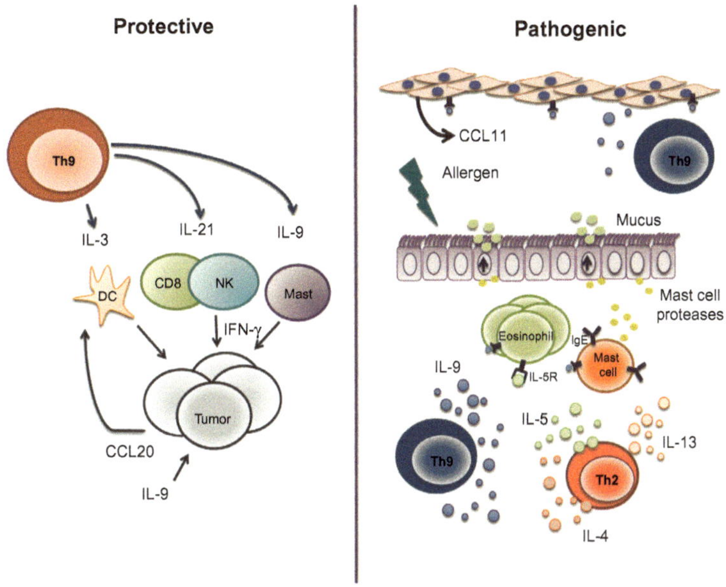

Figure 2 Th9 cells can be protective or pathogenic. In tumor immunity (*left*), through the production of cytokines, Th9 cells can limit tumor growth. IL-3, produced by Th9 cells, targets dendritic cells and promotes their survival allowing for a more potent antitumor immune response. IL-21, another Th9 cytokine, can also promote tumor immunity by binding the IL-21R on the surface of $CD8^+$ and NK cells leading to increased production of IFN-γ and enhanced tumor immunity. The hallmark cytokine of Th9 cells, IL-9, can also mediate protection against tumor growth. The mechanism of action required for IL-9 antitumor activity is unclear but may involve IL-9 targeting mast cells or IL-9 promoting CCL20 expression by tumor cells allowing for dendritic cell recruitment. The pathogenic function of Th9 cells is exemplified by allergic inflammation of the lung (*right*). Mast cells are one of the major targets of IL-9 during allergic inflammation of the lung. Through the production of proteases and cytokines, mast cells can increase mucus secretion by lung epithelial cells. Additionally, eosinophils and airway smooth muscle cells are targets of IL-9. IL-9 signaling in eosinophils leads to increased survival and maturation of via upregulation of the IL-5R. IL-9R signaling in airway smooth muscle cells increases CCL11 expression in humans (Gounni et al., 2004; Yamasaki et al., 2010), increasing the recruitment of inflammatory cells to the lung. The production of IL-9 is also thought to contribute to the production of Th2 cytokines during allergic inflammation of the lung, allowing for continued progression of the inflammatory response.

OX40 is a costimulatory molecule expressed on the surface of activated T cells and through interactions with its ligand partner, OX40L, located on the surface of antigen-presenting cells, promotes T cell survival, expansion, and cytokine production (Croft et al., 2009). OX40 has been shown to augment the expression of a variety of proinflammatory cytokines including IL-9 expression by Th9 cells (Xiao et al., 2012). OX40L antagonists have shown efficacy in limiting lung inflammation in mice (Salek-Ardakani et al., 2003); however, results of clinical trials of OX40L antagonist in patients

Table 1 Potential for pharmaceutical intervention of Th9 development and function

Drug target	Mechanism of action	Current usage and development stage	References
IL-1 (Anakinra)	IL-1R antagonist, blocks IL-1 signaling	Currently used for rheumatoid arthritis treatment	Zitvogel et al. (2012)
IL-4 (Pascolizumab)	IL-4 antagonist, inhibits binding to IL-4R	Completed phase II clinical trials	Akdis (2012); Hart et al. (2002)
IL-4Rα (Pitrakinra and Altrakincept)	Mutated form of IL-4 that blocks the IL-4Rα chain inhibiting IL-4 and IL-13 binding (Pitrakinra); soluble form of the IL-4R that inactivates IL-4 (Altrakincept)	Phase II of clinical trials have been completed (Pitrakinra); phase III of clinical trials have been completed (Altrkincept)	Pelaia et al. (2012)
IL-33	IL-33 inhibitor (mice only)	Preclinical stage	Liu et al. (2009)
JAK1/JAK3 (Tofacitinib)	Kinase inhibitor	Currently used for rheumatoid arthritis treatment	Kyttaris (2012)
IL-9 (MEDI-528)	IL-9 inhibitor	Phase II of clinical trials	Oh et al. (2013); Parker et al. (2011)
α-TSLP	TSLP inhibitor	Phase II of development, previous study results are very promising	Gauvreau et al. (2014b)
OX40L antagonist	Blocks OX40–OX40L interactions	Completed phase II clinical trials	Gauvreau et al. (2014a)
STAT6 (Teriflunomide)	STAT6 inhibitor (Anuradha et al., 2013)	Currently being used to treat multiple sclerosis	Olsan et al. (2011)
TGF-β (many types)	Block TGF-β and TGF-β receptors	Variable stages of development	Akhurst and Hata (2012)

with atopic asthma have not been as promising (Gauvreau et al., 2014a). Despite poor efficacy in atopic asthma treatment, OX40L antagonist may be more effective in treating other inflammatory conditions such as multiple sclerosis as blocking the OX40–OX40L interaction has been effective in EAE mouse models (Nohara et al., 2001; Weinberg et al., 1999). Another potential target is STAT6, a downstream transcription factor of IL-4R signaling in Th9 cells. In mice, STAT6 signaling has been shown to be required for Th9 differentiation (Goswami et al., 2012). Teriflunomide, a metabolite of the drug flunomide, has been shown to inhibit STAT6 although nonspecifically. There are currently no drugs that specifically inhibit STAT6 but such inhibitors may be in development. For STAT6 activation to occur, phosphorylation by kinases in the Janus kinase family must occur. Therefore, inhibition of Jak kinases may potentially be effective in limiting Th9 development. In addition to regulating Th9 development, inhibition of Jak kinases may also impact the function of Th9 cells because of their ability to mediate the downstream signaling of cytokines such as IL-9 and IL-21, which are produced by Th9 cells. Jak kinase inhibitors such as Tofacitinib are currently used in diseases such as rheumatoid arthritis.

7. CONCLUSION

The recent discovery of Th9 cells identifies a primary source of the cytokine IL-9. Whether Th9 cells are a distinct Th lineage on their own was initially questioned, but studies both in humans and in mice provide support for Th9 cells being a unique subset of cells that produce IL-9 without coexpression of other cytokines (Goswami and Kaplan, 2011; Kaplan, 2013). Many of the studies looking at the involvement of Th9 cells during various pathologies have been preclinical, utilizing mouse models of atopic disease, autoimmune disease, and tumor immunity to elucidate the contribution of Th9 cells during disease pathology. However, there is growing evidence of Th9 cells contributing to human disease. As the primary cytokine secreted by Th9 cells, IL-9 has become a target for drug development. An IL-9-blocking antibody has been shown to have some efficacy in patients with asthma but no effect in patients with severe asthma. More clinical trials will be required to fully determine the efficacy of this drug and the subset of patients that can receive the greatest benefit. Also, whether this antibody will be efficacious in other disease contexts is yet to be determined. The use of therapeutics to modulate IL-9 activity will require a thorough understanding of the contribution of IL-9 during a disease process due to the ability of IL-9 to be proinflammatory and anti-inflammatory depending on the inflammatory microenvironment (Fig. 2). Particularly, in the context of tumor immunity and multiple sclerosis treatment, IL-9 therapeutics will require rigorous preclinical testing and cautious clinical application. If the development of Th9 cells can be therapeutically modulated, altering Th9/IL-9 activity could be used to treat inflammatory disease and enhance protective immunity.

REFERENCES

Akdis, C.A., 2012. Therapies for allergic inflammation: refining strategies to induce tolerance. Nat. Med. 18, 736–749.

Akhurst, R.J., Hata, A., 2012. Targeting the TGFbeta signaling pathway in disease. Nat. Rev. Drug Discov. 11, 790–811.

Angkasekwinai, P., Chang, S.H., Thapa, M., Watarai, H., Dong, C., 2010. Regulation of IL-9 expression by IL-25 signaling. Nat. Immunol. 11, 250–256.

Angkasekwinai, P., Srimanote, P., Wang, Y.H., Pootong, A., Sakolvaree, Y., Pattanapanyasat, K., Chaicumpa, W., Chaiyaroj, S., Dong, C., 2013. Interleukin-25 (IL-25) promotes efficient protective immunity against Trichinella spiralis infection by enhancing the antigen-specific IL-9 response. Infect. Immun. 81, 3731–3741.

Anuradha, R., George, P.J., Hanna, L.E., Chandrasekaran, V., Kumaran, P., Nutman, T.B., Babu, S., 2013. IL-4-, TGF-beta-, and IL-1-dependent expansion of parasite antigen-specific Th9 cells is associated with clinical pathology in human lymphatic filariasis. J. Immunol. 191, 2466–2473.

Beriou, G., Bradshaw, E.M., Lozano, E., Costantino, C.M., Hastings, W.D., Orban, T., Elyaman, W., Khoury, S.J., Kuchroo, V.K., Baecher-Allan, C., Hafler, D.A., 2010. TGF-beta induces IL-9 production from human Th17 cells. J. Immunol. 185, 46–54.

Blom, L., Poulsen, B.C., Jensen, B.M., Hansen, A., Poulsen, L.K., 2011. IL-33 induces IL-9 production in human CD4+ T cells and basophils. PLoS One 6, e21695.

Brunet, L.R., Finkelman, F.D., Cheever, A.W., Kopf, M.A., Pearce, E.J., 1997. IL-4 protects against TNF-alpha-mediated cachexia and death during acute schistosomiasis. J. Immunol. 159, 777–785.

Chang, H.-C., Sehra, S., Goswami, R., Yao, W., Yu, Q., Stritesky, G.L., Jabeen, R., Mckinley, C., Ahyi, A.-N., Han, L., Nguyen, E.T., Robertson, M.J., Perumal, N.B., Tepper, R.S., Nutt, S.L., Kaplan, M.H., 2010. The transcription factor PU.1 is required for the development of IL-9-producing T cells and allergic inflammation. Nat. Immunol. 11, 527–534.

Croft, M., So, T., Duan, W., Soroosh, P., 2009. The significance of OX40 and OX40L to T-cell biology and immune disease. Immunol. Rev. 229 (1), 173–191.

Dardalhon, V., Awasthi, A., Kwon, H., Galileos, G., Gao, W., Sobel, R.A., Mitsdoerffer, M., Strom, T.B., Elyaman, W., Ho, I.C., Khoury, S., Oukka, M., Kuchroo, V.K., 2008. IL-4 inhibits TGF-[beta]-induced Foxp3+ T cells, and together with TGF-[beta], generates IL-9+ IL-10+ Foxp3- effector T cells. Nat. Immunol. 9, 1347–1355.

Debry, R.W., Seldin, M.F., 1996. Human/mouse homology relationships. Genomics 33, 337–351.

Elyaman, W., Bradshaw, E.M., Uyttenhove, C., Dardalhon, V., Awasthi, A., Imitola, J., Bettelli, E., Oukka, M., Van Snick, J., Renauld, J.C., Kuchroo, V.K., Khoury, S.J., 2009. IL-9 induces differentiation of TH17 cells and enhances function of FoxP3+ natural regulatory T cells. Proc. Natl. Acad. Sci. USA 106, 12885–12890.

Elyaman, W., Bassil, R., Bradshaw, E.M., Orent, W., Lahoud, Y., Zhu, B., Radtke, F., Yagita, H., Khoury, S.J., 2012. Notch receptors and Smad3 signaling cooperate in the induction of interleukin-9-producing T cells. Immunity 36, 623–634.

Fallon, P.G., Richardson, E.J., Mckenzie, G.J., Mckenzie, A.N., 2000. Schistosome infection of transgenic mice defines distinct and contrasting pathogenic roles for IL-4 and IL-13: IL-13 is a profibrotic agent. J. Immunol. 164, 2585–2591.

Faulkner, H., Humphreys, N., Renauld, J.C., Van Snick, J., Grencis, R., 1997. Interleukin-9 is involved in host protective immunity to intestinal nematode infection. Eur. J. Immunol. 27, 2536–2540.

Faulkner, H., Renauld, J.C., Van Snick, J., Grencis, R.K., 1998. Interleukin-9 enhances resistance to the intestinal nematode Trichuris muris. Infect. Immun. 66, 3832–3840.

Fontaine, R.H., Cases, O., Lelièvre, V., Mesplès, B., Renauld, J.C., Loron, G., Degos, V., Dournaud, P., Baud, O., Gressens, P., 2008. IL-9/IL-9 receptor signaling selectively protects cortical neurons against developmental apoptosis. Cell Death Differ. 15, 1542–1552.

Gauvreau, G.M., Boulet, L.P., Cockcroft, D.W., Fitzgerald, J.M., Mayers, I., Carlsten, C., Laviolette, M., Killian, K.J., Davis, B.E., Larché, M., Kipling, C., Dua, B., Mosesova, S., Putnam, W., Zheng, Y.,

Scheerens, H., Mcclintock, D., Matthews, J.G., O'byrne, P.M., 2014a. OX40L blockade and allergen-induced airway responses in subjects with mild asthma. Clin. Exp. Allergy 44, 29–37.
Gauvreau, G.M., O'Byrne, P.M., Boulet, L.P., Wang, Y., Cockcroft, D., Bigler, J., Fitzgerald, J.M., Boedigheimer, M., Davis, B.E., Dias, C., Gorski, K.S., Smith, L., Bautista, E., Comeau, M.R., Leigh, R., Parnes, J.R., 2014b. Effects of an anti-TSLP antibody on allergen-induced asthmatic responses. N. Engl. J. Med. 370, 2102–2110.
Gerlach, K., Hwang, Y., Nikolaev, A., Atreya, R., Dornhoff, H., Steiner, S., Lehr, H.A., Wirtz, S., Vieth, M., Waisman, A., Rosenbauer, F., Mckenzie, A.N., Weigmann, B., Neurath, M.F., 2014. TH9 cells that express the transcription factor PU.1 drive T cell-mediated colitis via IL-9 receptor signaling in intestinal epithelial cells. Nat. Immunol. 15, 676–686.
Goswami, R., Kaplan, M.H., 2011. A brief history of IL-9. J. Immunol. 186, 3283–3288.
Goswami, R., Jabeen, R., Yagi, R., Pham, D., Zhu, J., Goenka, S., Kaplan, M.H., 2012. STAT6-dependent regulation of Th9 development. J. Immunol. 188, 968–975.
Gounni, A.S., Hamid, Q., Rahman, S.M., Hoeck, J., Yang, J., Shan, L., 2004. IL-9-mediated induction of eotaxin1/CCL11 in human airway smooth muscle cells. J. Immunol. 173 (4), 2771–2779.
Gounni, A.S., Nutku, E., Koussih, L., Aris, F., Louahed, J., Levitt, R.C., Nicolaides, N.C., Hamid, Q., 2000. IL-9 expression by human eosinophils: regulation by IL-1beta and TNF-alpha. J. Allergy Clin. Immunol. 106, 460–466.
Hadrup, S., Donia, M., Thor Straten, P., 2013. Effector CD4 and CD8 T cells and their role in the tumor microenvironment. Cancer Microenviron. 6, 123–133.
Hart, T.K., Blackburn, M.N., Brigham-Burke, M., Dede, K., Al-Mahdi, N., Zia-Amirhosseini, P., Cook, R.M., 2002. Preclinical efficacy and safety of pascolizumab (SB 240683): a humanized anti-interleukin-4 antibody with therapeutic potential in asthma. Clin. Exp. Immunol. 130, 93–100.
Hoffmann, K.F., James, S.L., Cheever, A.W., Wynn, T.A., 1999. Studies with double cytokine-deficient mice reveal that highly polarized Th1- and Th2-type cytokine and antibody responses contribute equally to vaccine-induced immunity to Schistosoma mansoni. J. Immunol. 163, 927–938.
Hultner, L., Druez, C., Moeller, J., Uyttenhove, C., Schmitt, E., Rude, E., Dormer, P., Van Snick, J., 1990. Mast cell growth-enhancing activity (MEA) is structurally related and functionally identical to the novel mouse T cell growth factor P40/TCGFIII (interleukin 9). Eur. J. Immunol. 20, 1413–1416.
Hultner, L., Kolsch, S., Stassen, M., Kaspers, U., Kremer, J.P., Mailhammer, R., Moeller, J., Broszeit, H., Schmitt, E., 2000. In activated mast cells, IL-1 up-regulates the production of several Th2-related cytokines including IL-9. J. Immunol. 164, 5556–5563.
Jager, A., Dardalhon, V., Sobel, R.A., Bettelli, E., Kuchroo, V.K., 2009. Th1, Th17, and Th9 effector cells induce experimental autoimmune encephalomyelitis with different pathological phenotypes. J. Immunol. 183, 7169–7177.
Kaplan, M.H., 2013. Th9 cells: differentiation and disease. Immunol. Rev. 252, 104–115.
Kay, A.B., 2001. Allergy and allergic diseases. First of two parts. N. Engl. J. Med. 344, 30–37.
Kearley, J., Erjefalt, J.S., Andersson, C., Benjamin, E., Jones, C.P., Robichaud, A., Pegorier, S., Brewah, Y., Burwell, T.J., Bjermer, L., Kiener, P.A., Kolbeck, R., Lloyd, C.M., Coyle, A.J., Humbles, A.A., 2011. IL-9 governs allergen-induced mast cell numbers in the lung and chronic remodeling of the airways. Am. J. Respir. Crit. Care Med. 183, 865–875.
Khan, W.I., Richard, M., Akiho, H., Blennerhasset, P.A., Humphreys, N.E., Grencis, R.K., Van Snick, J., Collins, S.M., 2003. Modulation of intestinal muscle contraction by interleukin-9 (IL-9) or IL-9 neutralization: correlation with worm expulsion in murine nematode infections. Infect. Immun. 71, 2430–2438.
Knutson, K.L., Disis, M.L., 2005. Tumor antigen-specific T helper cells in cancer immunity and immunotherapy. Cancer Immunol. Immunother. 54, 721–728.
Kyttaris, V.C., 2012. Kinase inhibitors: a new class of antirheumatic drugs. Drug Des. Devel. Ther. 6, 245–250.
Levitt, R.C., Mclane, M.P., Macdonald, D., Ferrante, V., Weiss, C., Zhou, T., Holroyd, K.J., Nicolaides, N.C., 1999. IL-9 pathway in asthma: new therapeutic targets for allergic inflammatory disorders. J. Allergy Clin. Immunol. 103, S485–S491.

Li, H., Nourbakhsh, B., Cullimore, M., Zhang, G.X., Rostami, A., 2011. IL-9 is important for T-cell activation and differentiation in autoimmune inflammation of the central nervous system. Eur. J. Immunol. 41, 2197–2206.

Licona-Limon, P., Henao-Mejia, J., Temann, A.U., Gagliani, N., Licona-Limon, I., Ishigame, H., Hao, L., Herbert, D.R., Flavell, R.A., 2013. Th9 cells drive host immunity against gastrointestinal worm infection. Immunity 39, 744–757.

Liu, Y., Teige, I., Birnir, B., Issazadeh-Navikas, S., 2006. Neuron-mediated generation of regulatory T cells from encephalitogenic T cells suppresses EAE. Nat. Med. 12, 518–525.

Liu, X., Li, M., Wu, Y., Zhou, Y., Zeng, L., Huang, T., 2009. Anti-IL-33 antibody treatment inhibits airway inflammation in a murine model of allergic asthma. Biochem. Biophys. Res. Commun. 386, 181–185.

Lu, L.F., Lind, E.F., Gondek, D.C., Bennett, K.A., Gleeson, M.W., Pino-Lagos, K., Scott, Z.A., Coyle, A.J., Reed, J.L., Van Snick, J., Strom, T.B., Zheng, X.X., Noelle, R.J., 2006. Mast cells are essential intermediaries in regulatory T-cell tolerance. Nature 442, 997–1002.

Lu, Y., Hong, S., Li, H., Park, J., Hong, B., Wang, L., Zheng, Y., Liu, Z., Xu, J., He, J., Yang, J., Qian, J., Yi, Q., 2012. Th9 cells promote antitumor immune responses in vivo. J. Clin. Invest. 122, 4160–4171.

Ma, L., Xue, H.B., Guan, X.H., Shu, C.M., Zhang, J.H., Yu, J., 2014. Possible pathogenic role of T helper type 9 cells and interleukin (IL)-9 in atopic dermatitis. Clin. Exp. Immunol. 175, 25–31.

Macdonald, A.S., Araujo, M.I., Pearce, E.J., 2002. Immunology of parasitic helminth infections. Infect. Immun. 70, 427–433.

Marsh, D.G., Neely, J.D., Breazeale, D.R., Ghosh, B., Freidhoff, L.R., Ehrlich-Kautzky, E., Schou, C., Krishnaswamy, G., Beaty, T.H., 1994. Linkage analysis of IL4 and other chromosome 5q31.1 markers and total serum immunoglobulin E concentrations. Science 264, 1152–1156.

Matsuzawa, S., Sakashita, K., Kinoshita, T., Ito, S., Yamashita, T., Koike, K., 2003. IL-9 enhances the growth of human mast cell progenitors under stimulation with stem cell factor. J. Immunol. 170, 3461–3467.

Mosmann, T.R., Cherwinski, H., Bond, M.W., Giedlin, M.A., Coffman, R.L., 1986. Two types of murine helper T cell clone. I. Definition according to profiles of lymphokine activities and secreted proteins. J. Immunol. 136, 2348–2357.

Murugaiyan, G., Beynon, V., Pires Da Cunha, A., Joller, N., Weiner, H.L., 2012. IFN-gamma limits Th9-mediated autoimmune inflammation through dendritic cell modulation of IL-27. J. Immunol. 189, 5277–5283.

Nalleweg, N., Chiriac, M.T., Podstawa, E., Lehmann, C., Rau, T.T., Atreya, R., Krauss, E., Hundorfean, G., Fichtner-Feigl, S., Hartmann, A., Becker, C., Mudter, J., 2015. IL-9 and its receptor are predominantly involved in the pathogenesis of UC. Gut 64 (5), 743–755.

Nicolaides, N.C., Holroyd, K.J., Ewart, S.L., Eleff, S.M., Kiser, M.B., Dragwa, C.R., Sullivan, C.D., Grasso, L., Zhang, L.Y., Messler, C.J., Zhou, T., Kleeberger, S.R., Buetow, K.H., Levitt, R.C., 1997. Interleukin 9: a candidate gene for asthma. Proc. Natl. Acad. Sci. USA 94, 13175–13180.

Niedbala, W., Besnard, A.G., Nascimento, D.C., Donate, P.B., Sonego, F., Yip, E., Guabiraba, R., Chang, H.D., Fukada, S.Y., Salmond, R.J., Schmitt, E., Bopp, T., Ryffel, B., Liew, F.Y., 2014. Nitric oxide enhances Th9 cell differentiation and airway inflammation. Nat. Commun. 5, 4575.

Nohara, C., Akiba, H., Nakajima, A., Inoue, A., Koh, C.S., Ohshima, H., Yagita, H., Mizuno, Y., Okumura, K., 2001. Amelioration of experimental autoimmune encephalomyelitis with anti-OX40 ligand monoclonal antibody: a critical role for OX40 ligand in migration, but not development, of pathogenic T cells. J. Immunol. 166, 2108–2115.

Nowak, E.C., Weaver, C.T., Turner, H., Begum-Haque, S., Becher, B., Schreiner, B., Coyle, A.J., Kasper, L.H., Noelle, R.J., 2009. IL-9 as a mediator of Th17-driven inflammatory disease. J. Exp. Med. 206, 1653–1660.

Oh, C.K., Leigh, R., Mclaurin, K.K., Kim, K., Hultquist, M., Molfino, N.A., 2013. A randomized, controlled trial to evaluate the effect of an anti-interleukin-9 monoclonal antibody in adults with uncontrolled asthma. Respir. Res. 14, 93.

Olsan, E.E., Mukherjee, S., Wulkersdorfer, B., Shillingford, J.M., Giovannone, A.J., Todorov, G., Song, X., Pei, Y., Weimbs, T., 2011. Signal transducer and activator of transcription-6 (STAT6) inhibition suppresses renal cyst growth in polycystic kidney disease. Proc. Natl. Acad. Sci. USA 108, 18067–18072.

Park, J., Li, H., Zhang, M., Lu, Y., Hong, B., Zheng, Y., He, J., Yang, J., Qian, J., Yi, Q., 2014. Murine Th9 cells promote the survival of myeloid dendritic cells in cancer immunotherapy. Cancer Immunol. Immunother. 63, 835–845.

Parker, J.M., Oh, C.K., Laforce, C., Miller, S.D., Pearlman, D.S., Le, C., Robbie, G.J., White, W.I., White, B., Molfino, N.A., Group M.-C. T., 2011. Safety profile and clinical activity of multiple subcutaneous doses of MEDI-528, a humanized anti-interleukin-9 monoclonal antibody, in two randomized phase 2a studies in subjects with asthma. BMC Pulm. Med. 11, 14.

Pelaia, G., Vatrella, A., Maselli, R., 2012. The potential of biologics for the treatment of asthma. Nat. Rev. Drug Discov. 11, 958–972.

Postma, D.S., Bleecker, E.R., Amelung, P.J., Holroyd, K.J., Xu, J., Panhuysen, C.I., Meyers, D.A., Levitt, R.C., 1995. Genetic susceptibility to asthma–bronchial hyperresponsiveness coinherited with a major gene for atopy. N. Engl. J. Med. 333, 894–900.

Purwar, R., Schlapbach, C., Xiao, S., Kang, H.S., Elyaman, W., Jiang, X., Jetten, A.M., Khoury, S.J., Fuhlbrigge, R.C., Kuchroo, V.K., Clark, R.A., Kupper, T.S., 2012. Robust tumor immunity to melanoma mediated by interleukin-9-producing T cells. Nat. Med. 18, 1248–1253.

Restifo, N.P., Dudley, M.E., Rosenberg, S.A., 2012. Adoptive immunotherapy for cancer: harnessing the T cell response. Nat. Rev. Immunol. 12, 269–281.

Salek-Ardakani, S., Song, J., Halteman, B.S., Jember, A.G., Akiba, H., Yagita, H., Croft, M., 2003. OX40 (CD134) controls memory T helper 2 cells that drive lung inflammation. J. Exp. Med. 198, 315–324.

Schmitt, E., Germann, T., Goedert, S., Hoehn, P., Huels, C., Koelsch, S., Kühn, R., Müller, W., Palm, N., Rüde, E., 1994. IL-9 production of naive CD4+ T cells depends on IL-2, is synergistically enhanced by a combination of TGF-beta and IL-4, and is inhibited by IFN-gamma. J. Immunol. 153, 3989–3996.

Shimbara, A., Christodoulopoulos, P., Soussi-Gounni, A., Olivenstein, R., Nakamura, Y., Levitt, R.C., Nicolaides, N.C., Holroyd, K.J., Tsicopoulos, A., Lafitte, J.-J., Wallaert, B., Hamid, Q.A., 2000. IL-9 and its receptor in allergic and nonallergic lung disease: increased expression in asthma. J. Allergy Clin. Immunol. 105, 108–115.

Singh, T.P., Schön, M.P., Wallbrecht, K., Gruber-Wackernagel, A., Wang, X.J., Wolf, P., 2013. Involvement of IL-9 in Th17-associated inflammation and angiogenesis of psoriasis. PLoS One 8 (1), e51752. http://dx.doi.org/10.1371/journal.pone.0051752.

Smith, S.E., Hoelzinger, D.B., Dominguez, A.L., Van Snick, J., Lustgarten, J., 2011. Signals through 4-1BB inhibit T regulatory cells by blocking IL-9 production enhancing antitumor responses. Cancer Immunol. Immunother. 60, 1775–1787.

Stephens, G.L., Swerdlow, B., Benjamin, E., Coyle, A.J., Humbles, A., Kolbeck, R., Fung, M., 2011. IL-9 is a Th17-derived cytokine that limits pathogenic activity in organ-specific autoimmune disease. Eur. J. Immunol. 41, 952–962.

Tan, C., Aziz, M.K., Lovaas, J.D., Vistica, B.P., Shi, G., Wawrousek, E.F., Gery, I., 2010. Antigen-specific Th9 cells exhibit uniqueness in their kinetics of cytokine production and short retention at the inflammatory site. J. Immunol. 185, 6795–6801.

Temann, U.A., Geba, G.P., Rankin, J.A., Flavell, R.A., 1998. Expression of interleukin 9 in the lungs of transgenic mice causes airway inflammation, mast cell hyperplasia, and bronchial hyperresponsiveness. J. Exp. Med. 188, 1307–1320.

Temann, U.A., Ray, P., Flavell, R.A., 2002. Pulmonary overexpression of IL-9 induces Th2 cytokine expression, leading to immune pathology. J. Clin. Invest. 109, 29–39.

Temann, U.-A., Laouar, Y., Eynon, E.E., Homer, R., Flavell, R.A., 2007. IL9 leads to airway inflammation by inducing IL13 expression in airway epithelial cells. Int. Immunol. 19, 1–10.

Townsend, J.M., Fallon, G.P., Matthews, J.D., Smith, P., Jolin, E.H., Mckenzie, N.A., 2000. IL-9-deficient mice establish fundamental roles for IL-9 in pulmonary mastocytosis and goblet cell hyperplasia but not T cell development. Immunity 13, 573–583.

Uyttenhove, C., Brombacher, F., Van Snick, J., 2010. TGF-beta interactions with IL-1 family members trigger IL-4-independent IL-9 production by mouse CD4(+) T cells. Eur. J. Immunol. 40, 2230–2235.

Vegran, F., Berger, H., Boidot, R., Mignot, G., Bruchard, M., Dosset, M., Chalmin, F., Rebe, C., Derangere, V., Ryffel, B., Kato, M., Prevost-Blondel, A., Ghiringhelli, F., Apetoh, L., 2014. The transcription factor IRF1 dictates the IL-21-dependent anticancer functions of TH9 cells. Nat. Immunol. 15, 758–766.

Veldhoen, M., Uyttenhove, C., Van Snick, J., Helmby, H., Westendorf, A., Buer, J., Martin, B., Wilhelm, C., Stockinger, B., 2008. Transforming growth factor-[beta] 'reprograms' the differentiation of T helper 2 cells and promotes an interleukin 9-producing subset. Nat. Immunol. 9, 1341–1346.
Weinberg, A.D., Wegmann, K.W., Funatake, C., Whitham, R.H., 1999. Blocking OX-40/OX-40 ligand interaction in vitro and in vivo leads to decreased T cell function and amelioration of experimental allergic encephalomyelitis. J. Immunol. 162, 1818–1826.
Wilhelm, C., Hirota, K., Stieglitz, B., Van Snick, J., Tolaini, M., Lahl, K., Sparwasser, T., Helmby, H., Stockinger, B., 2011. An IL-9 fate reporter demonstrates the induction of an innate IL-9 response in lung inflammation. Nat. Immunol. 12, 1071–1077.
Wong, M.T., Ye, J.J., Alonso, M.N., Landrigan, A., Cheung, R.K., Engleman, E., Utz, P.J., 2010. Regulation of human Th9 differentiation by type I interferons and IL-21. Immunol. Cell Biol. 88, 624–631.
Xiao, X., Balasubramanian, S., Liu, W., Chu, X., Wang, H., Taparowsky, E.J., Fu, Y.X., Choi, Y., Walsh, M.C., Li, X.C., 2012. OX40 signaling favors the induction of T(H)9 cells and airway inflammation. Nat. Immunol. 13, 981–990.
Yamasaki, A., Saleh, A., Koussih, L., Muro, S., Halayko, A.J., Gounni, A.S., 2010. IL-9 induces CCL11 expression via STAT3 signaling in human airway smooth muscle cells. PLoS One 5, e9178.
Yao, W., Tepper, R.S., Kaplan, M.H., 2011. Predisposition to the development of IL-9-secreting T cells in atopic infants. J. Allergy Clin. Immunol. 128 (1357-1360), e5.
Yao, W., Zhang, Y., Jabeen, R., Nguyen, E.T., Wilkes, D.S., Tepper, R.S., Kaplan, M.H., Zhou, B., 2013. Interleukin-9 is required for allergic airway inflammation mediated by the cytokine TSLP. Immunity 38, 360–372.
Ye, Z.-J., Yuan, M.-L., Zhou, Q., Du, R.-H., Yang, W.-B., Xiong, X.-Z., Zhang, J.-C., Wu, C., Qin, S.-M., Shi, H.-Z., 2012. Differentiation and recruitment of Th9 cells stimulated by pleural mesothelial cells in human Mycobacterium tuberculosis infection. PLoS One 7, e31710.
Zhou, Y., Sonobe, Y., Akahori, T., Jin, S., Kawanokuchi, J., Noda, M., Iwakura, Y., Mizuno, T., Suzumura, A., 2011. IL-9 promotes Th17 cell migration into the central nervous system via CC chemokine ligand-20 produced by astrocytes. J. Immunol. 186, 4415–4421.
Zitvogel, L., Kepp, O., Galluzzi, L., Kroemer, G., 2012. Inflammasomes in carcinogenesis and anticancer immune responses. Nat. Immunol. 13, 343–351.

CHAPTER 7

T Follicular Helper Cells as a Therapeutic Target for Autoimmune Diseases

H. Ueno
Baylor Institute for Immunology Research, Dallas, TX, United States

Contents

1. INTRODUCTION

T follicular helper (Tfh) cells constitute one of the expanding families of $CD4^+$ T cell subsets. Tfh cells are specialized to provide help to B cells and to induce durable antibody response (Crotty, 2011; Tangye et al., 2013). Tfh cells are essential for the formation of germinal centers (GCs) (Linterman et al., 2010; Zotos et al., 2010; Victora et al., 2010), where high-affinity B cells are selected and differentiate into long-lived memory B cells and plasma cells (Tarlinton, 2008; MacLennan, 1994).

Translational Immunology
http://dx.doi.org/10.1016/B978-0-12-801577-3.00008-3

While the presence of $CD4^+$ T cells in GCs was discovered more than three decades ago, their biological properties remained largely unknown until the early 2000s, when ~50% of $CD4^+$ T cells isolated from human tonsils were found to express the chemokine receptor CXCR5 (Breitfeld et al., 2000; Schaerli et al., 2000; Kim et al., 2001). Furthermore, tonsillar $CXCR5^+$ $CD4^+$ T cells were shown to display a superior capacity to induce B cells to produce immunoglobulins *in vitro* as compared to the $CXCR5^-$ counterparts. Based on their localization and functions, $CXCR5^+$ $CD4^+$ T cells in lymphoid organs were originally designated T follicular B helper cells (Breitfeld et al., 2000; Schaerli et al., 2000; Kim et al., 2001). Yet, only a fraction of $CXCR5^+$ $CD4^+$ T cells in tonsils are localized within GCs. Early studies suggested that CD57 is a marker for $CD4^+$ T cells in GC in humans (Porwit-Ksiazek et al., 1983). However, recent studies show that CD57 is expressed by only approximately 30% of GC Tfh cells, and also expressed by a fraction (~10%) of $CD4^+$ T cells localized outside GCs (Rasheed et al., 2006; Bentebibel et al., 2011). Tfh cells in human GCs are currently defined by the high expression of CXCR5, ICOS, and PD-1 (Rasheed et al., 2006; Bentebibel et al., 2011; Ma et al., 2009). Later, the transcription repressor Bcl-6 was discovered as an essential factor for Tfh cell generation *in vivo* in mice (Nurieva et al., 2009; Johnston et al., 2009; Yu et al., 2009), and Tfh cells are established as an independent $CD4^+$ T cell subset.

Our knowledge on the biology of Tfh cells has significantly increased during the past decade (reviewed in Tangye et al., 2013; Crotty, 2011; Ueno et al., 2015). In this chapter, we will first summarize our current knowledge of the biology of Tfh cells and their association with the pathogenesis of autoimmune diseases. Then, we will discuss potential strategies to target Tfh cells and/or Tfh molecules as a therapeutic modality of autoimmune diseases.

2. BIOLOGY OF Tfh CELLS

2.1 Molecules associated with Tfh functions

Tfh cells are equipped with molecules important for provision help to B cells. CXCR5 expressed by Tfh cells guides their migration toward B cell follicles (Breitfeld et al., 2000; Schaerli et al., 2000; Kim et al., 2001; Rasheed et al., 2006). Tfh cells express high levels of inducible costimulator (ICOS), a costimulatory molecule critical in many aspects including development (Akiba et al., 2005; Bossaller et al., 2006; Choi et al., 2011), migration into follicles (Xu et al., 2013), and functions (Hutloff et al., 1999; Vogelzang et al., 2008). Tfh cells support the survival of GC B cells and their differentiation into memory cells and plasma cells through secretion of interleukin(IL)-21 (Bryant et al., 2007; Bentebibel et al., 2011) and by providing signals through CD40 (Banchereau et al., 1994). Tfh cells also highly express several inhibitory receptors including PD-1 and BTLA, which regulate the activity of Tfh cells in GCs by downregulating their survival and proliferation (Cubas et al., 2013; Kashiwakuma et al., 2010).

2.2 Three phases in the development of Tfh cells

As with other $CD4^+$ T cell subsets, Tfh cells differentiate from naïve T cells (Fig. 1). However, the differentiation and maturation process of Tfh cells is more complicated than that of other subsets, and composed of three phases: (1) initial differentiation toward the Tfh lineage; (2) migration into B cell follicles; and (3) maturation in GCs (Fig. 2).

2.2.1 *Initial differentiation toward the Tfh lineage*

The first differentiation process initiates when naïve $CD4^+$ T cells interact with dendritic cells (DCs) loaded with antigens in secondary lymphoid organs. Programming toward the Tfh cell lineage occurs as early as the first few divisions (Kitano et al., 2011; Choi et al., 2011; Baumjohann et al., 2011; Kerfoot et al., 2011). The key event in this initial process is to upregulate the chemokine receptor CXCR5 (Ansel et al., 1999; Flynn et al., 1998) (mediated at least in mice by increased expression of the transcription factors Bcl-6 (Kerfoot et al., 2011; Kitano et al., 2011) and Ascl2 (Liu et al., 2014b)), while downregulating the chemokine receptor CCR7 (Haynes et al., 2007) and the cell adhesion

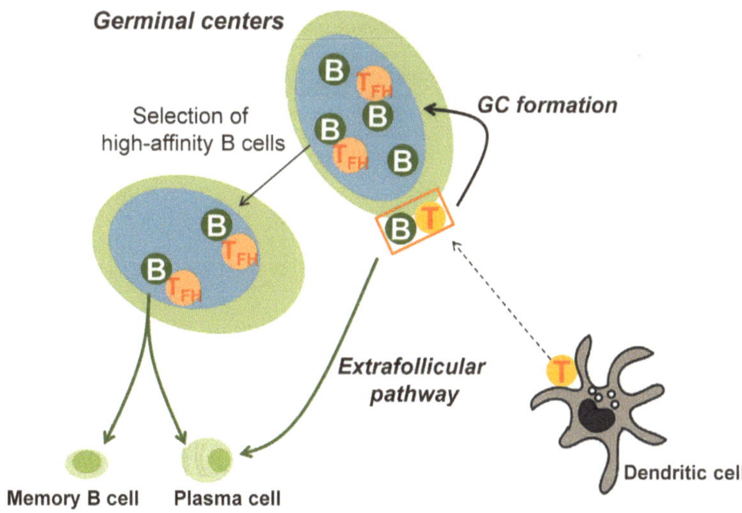

Figure 1 T-dependent antibody responses. In secondary lymphoid organs, naïve $CD4^+$ T cells interact with DCs loaded with antigens at T cell zones. A fraction of activated $CD4^+$ T cells initiate the program to differentiate into the Tfh lineage, migrate toward B cell follicles, and interact with B cells typically at the T:B border. T and B cell interaction initiates the B cell differentiation process toward two different paths: extrafollicular short-lived plasma cells and cells forming GCs. Inside the GCs, Tfh cells provide help to high-affinity B cells and support their differentiation into long-lived plasma cells or memory B cells.

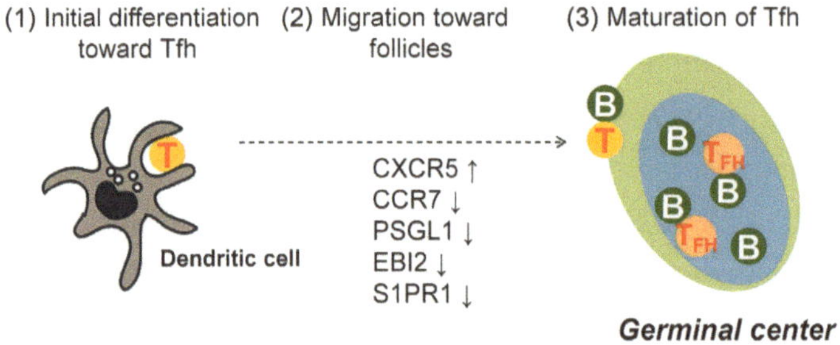

Figure 2 Three phases in Tfh cell generation. The differentiation and maturation process of Tfh cells is composed of three phases: (1) initial differentiation toward the Tfh lineage; (2) migration into B cell follicles; and (3) maturation in GCs. In phase I, multiple factors derived from DCs and microenvironment promote activated CD4$^+$ T cells to express Batf, c-Maf, Bcl-6, and Ascl2 while suppressing the expression of Blimp-1. In phase II, these CD4$^+$ T cells upregulate CXCR5 while downregulating CCR7 and PSGL1, and migrate into B cell follicles. ICOS signaling suppresses the expression of EBI2 and S1PR1, which is also required for their entry to follicles. In phase III, high expression of CXCR5 and S1PR2 is required to retain Tfh cells within GCs. Yet, GC Tfh cells can emigrate and redistribute to other follicles and neighboring GCs.

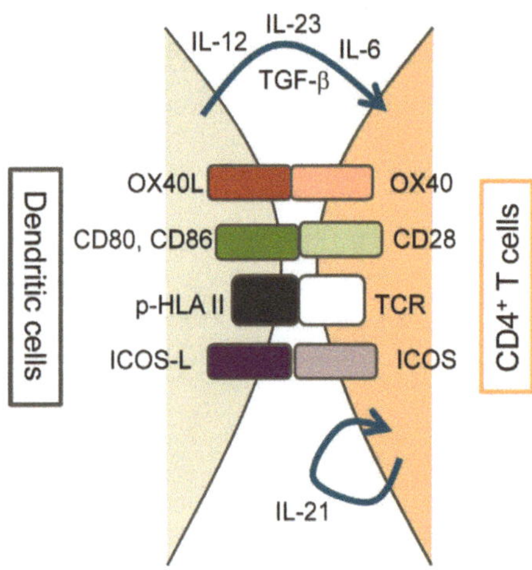

Figure 3 Signals important during phase I. Antigens are presented by DCs in the context of peptide-HLA class II complex (p-HLA II), and recognized by CD4$^+$ T cells with T cell receptor (TCR). CD28 signals delivered by CD80 and CD86 are essential for Tfh cell differentiation. Other costimulatory molecules including ICOS and OX40 provide additional signals that promote the expression of Tfh molecules. TGF-β synergizes with IL-12, IL-23, IL-21, and IL-6 to induce human CD4$^+$ T cells to express multiple Tfh molecules while inhibiting Blimp-1.

molecule PSGL-1 (Odegard et al., 2008). Such changes in the expression of surface molecules are required for their migration toward B cell follicles in the second phase.

Cytokines derived from both DCs and lymphoid microenvironment contribute to this process (Fig. 3). Importantly, recent studies suggest that the dominant cytokines associated with the development of Tfh cells differ between mice and humans. In mice, IL-6,

IL-21, and IL-27 (which activate STAT3) have dominant roles (Crotty, 2011; Sweet et al., 2012), while IL-12 (which mainly activates STAT4) can also participate in the early phase (Nakayamada et al., 2011). In contrast, in humans, IL-12 induces higher expression of IL-21, ICOS, CXCR5, and Bcl-6 on activated naïve helper T cells than IL-6, IL-21, and IL-27 (Schmitt et al., 2009, 2013, 2014b). Furthermore, in humans, the cytokine TGF-β co-operates with IL-12 and IL-23 to promote the expression of multiple Tfh molecules including CXCR5, IL-21, and Bcl-6 on activated naïve $CD4^+$ T cells (Schmitt et al., 2014b). These cytokine combinations also induce human naïve $CD4^+$ T cells to express multiple other transcription factors such as c-Maf, Batf that are essential for Tfh development, while inhibiting the expression of Blimp-1, a repressor of Bcl-6. This is in stark contrast to mouse $CD4^+$ T cells, in which TGF-β signals suppress expression of Tfh molecules including IL-21, ICOS, and Bcl-6 (Schmitt et al., 2014b; Nurieva et al., 2008, 2009; Suto et al., 2008). Of note, a recent mouse study showed that TGF-β contributes to the generation of Tfh cells also in mice *in vivo* yet *via* different mechanisms. In mice infected with influenza virus, TGF-β suppressed the expression of the high-affinity IL-2 receptor α chain (CD25) on virus-specific $CD4^+$ T cells, and inhibited IL-2-mediated activation of mammalian target of rapamycin, which inhibits the generation of Tfh cells (Marshall et al., 2014).

Several costimulatory molecules expressed by DCs are also important for Tfh cell generation. CD80 and CD86 on the surface of DCs provide essential signals *via* CD28 on T cells, and CD28-deficient mice completely lack GC formation (Ferguson et al., 1996). ICOS-L expressed by DCs interacts with ICOS expressed by activated $CD4^+$ T cells, and promotes their expression of Bcl-6 (Choi et al., 2011). OX40L-expressing DCs also promote activated $CD4^+$ T cells to express CXCR5 *via* OX40 signals (Fillatreau and Gray, 2003).

Which types of DCs promote Tfh cell generation in humans? DCs are endowed with functional plasticity, which permits them to induce different immune responses according to the microenvironment. In addition, the DC system is composed of subsets associated with the induction of different types of immunity (Ueno et al., 2007, 2010). Therefore, it is possible that distinct DC subsets play a dominant role in the generation of Tfh response according to the type of infection and/or inflammation. Nonetheless, among human skin DC subsets, $CD14^+$ dermal DCs are the most efficient at inducing human naïve $CD4^+$ T cells to become Tfh-like cells *in vitro* (Klechevsky et al., 2008). $CD4^+$ T cells primed by $CD14^+$ dermal DCs, but not by epidermal Langerhans cells (LCs), strongly induce naïve B cells to become antibody-secreting plasma cells producing IgM, as well as to switch isotypes toward IgG and IgA (Klechevsky et al., 2008). Skin DC subsets including dermal $CD14^+$ DCs migrate into the draining lymph nodes (Segura et al., 2012), and interact with T cells at the T cell zone. $CD206^+$ DCs in the lymph nodes, a proposed counterpart of migrating dermal $CD14^+$ DCs, promote naïve Th cells to produce CXCL13 (Segura et al., 2012), the chemokine abundantly expressed by Tfh cells (Kim et al., 2004; Bentebibel et al., 2011). These observations suggest the involvement of dermal CD14$^+$ DCs in the generation of Tfh cells and antibody responses in draining lymph nodes of skin. Interestingly, in mice, activated dermal DCs migrate into the outer paracortex just beneath the B cell follicles, whereas LCs migrate into the T cell rich inner paracortex (Kissenpfennig et al., 2005). Therefore, dermal DCs might also contribute to the development of humoral immunity also in mice.

2.2.2 Migration into B cell follicles

The migratory behavior of CD4$^+$ T cells following interactions with DCs is largely dependent on the balance between CXCR5 and CCR7. CXCL13, the ligand of CXCR5, is highly expressed by stromal networks including follicular DCs within follicles, and attract T and B cells expressing CXCR5. In contrast, CCL19 and CCL21, the ligand of CCR7, are highly expressed by T cell zone, and retain CCR7$^+$ lymphocytes. Thus, upregulation of CXCR5 together with downregulation of CCR7 renders CD4$^+$ T cells to migrate toward B cell follicles. Other molecules such as PSGL1, sphingosine-1-phosphate receptor 1 (S1PR1), and EBI2 also regulate the migration of activated CD4$^+$ T cells toward and into follicles (all molecules need to be downregulated).

CD4$^+$ T cells interact with antigen-primed naïve B cells typically at the border of T cell zone and follicles (Okada et al., 2005; Garside et al., 1998) (Fig. 4). Durable interactions are essential for the development of Tfh cells, as deficiency of SAP, an adaptor protein essential for durable interactions of helper T cells and B cells (Qi et al., 2008),

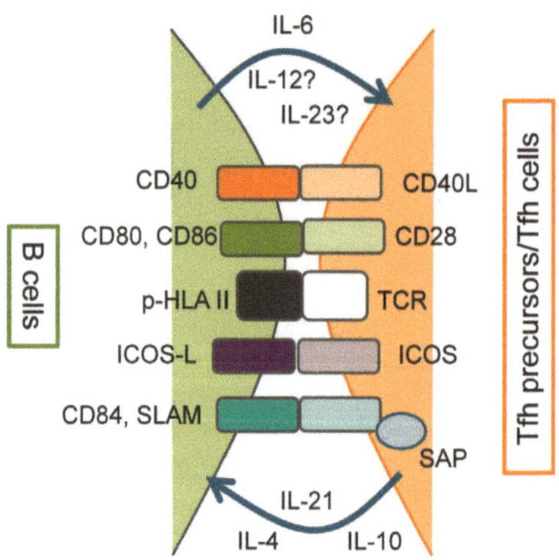

Figure 4 Signals important during Phase II. In addition to the signals *via* TCR and CD28, signals *via* ICOS are essential for CD4$^+$ T cells to migrate into and remain within the follicles. Signals mediated by SAP are required for durable interactions between T and B cells. During the interactions, B cells receive activation signals *via* CD40 and cytokine receptors such as IL-4 receptor and IL-21 receptor, and undergo proliferation and differentiation.

results in profoundly altered generation of Tfh cells and GCs (Cannons et al., 2011). The interactions with B cells induce Tfh precursors to increase and maintain Bcl-6 expression, likely mediated by B cell-derived cytokines such as IL-6 and the ICOS–ICOS ligand interaction. The ICOS ligand expressed by B cells also provides important signals for $CD4^+$ T cells to migrate into B cell follicles (Xu et al., 2013). The interactions also induce B cells to undergo a differentiation process toward two paths: extrafollicular plasma cells and cells forming GCs (MacLennan and Gray, 1986; McHeyzer-Williams et al., 1993; Jacob et al., 1991) (Fig. 1). Extrafollicular plasma cells contribute to the early generation of specific antibodies after antigen challenge (MacLennan et al., 2003). Germinal center B (GC-B) cells subsequently differentiate into either high-affinity long-lived plasma cells or memory B cells after an extensive selection step (Tarlinton, 2008; MacLennan, 1994).

2.2.3 Maturation of Tfh cells within GCs

While little was known regarding the dynamics of Tfh cells until recently, studies using intravital imaging have started revealing their unique behavior. Now we know that GC Tfh cells continuously emigrate and redistribute to other follicles and neighboring GCs (Shulman et al., 2013). This dynamics is regulated by high expression of CXCR5 and the trafficking molecule sphingosine-1-phosphate receptor 2 (S1PR2), and S1PR2 is particularly important to retain Tfh cells within GCs (Moriyama et al., 2014). A dynamic exchange of GC Tfh cells among multiple GCs and bidirectional signals between GC Tfh cells and B cells during their cognate interactions likely represent important mechanisms associated with efficient selection and expansion of high-affinity B cells during GC responses. Tfh cells in GCs interact with B cells in an antigen-specific manner, and selectively provide survival signals to B cells expressing high-affinity receptors (Victora et al., 2010). Conversely, signals derived from interacting $ICOSL^+$ B cells induce GC Tfh cells to increase intracellular Ca^{2+} and their expression of IL-4 and IL-21 (Shulman et al., 2014; Liu et al., 2014a). Importantly, both cell division and hypermutation frequency of the selected B cells are directly proportional to the amount of antigens presented to Tfh cells in GCs (Gitlin et al., 2014). These observations clearly indicate the significance of Tfh cells for the generation of high-affinity B cells in GCs.

2.3 Regulatory compartment in GCs

Mouse studies have recently identified two types of T cells that suppress Tfh/GC response: $CD8^+$ regulatory T cells (Tregs) (Kim et al., 2010) and T follicular regulatory (Tfr) cells (Linterman et al., 2011; Chung et al., 2011). $CD8^+$ Tregs were shown to inhibit Tfh response by targeting murine Qa-1 molecule expressed by the surface of Tfh cells (Kim et al., 2010). However, human cells do not express Qa-1, and therefore the significance of $CD8^+$ Tregs in the regulation of GC response in humans remains unknown. Tfr cells are derived from thymus-derived $FoxP3^+$ Tregs that migrate into GCs (Linterman et al., 2011; Chung et al., 2011). Although Bcl-6 is essential for Tfr cell development (similar to Tfh), Tfr cells lack the expression of IL-21 and CD40L, and dampen GC responses by limiting the numbers of both Tfh and B cells in GCs (Wollenberg et al., 2011; Linterman et al., 2011; Chung et al., 2011). While the role of Tfr cells in the regulation of GC response and in the selection of high-affinity B cells in GCs remains to be established, there is evidence that Tfr cells might be responsible for terminating GC response (Wollenberg et al., 2011), and repress self-reactive B cells in GCs (Linterman et al., 2011). The balance between Tfh and Tfr cells in the GC environment likely represents a key factor in the generation of high-affinity protective antibodies as well as pathogenic autoantibodies. In humans, the role and the properties of Tfr cells remain largely uncharacterized.

3. Tfh CELLS IN AUTOIMMUNE DISEASES

Generation of autoantibodies is a hallmark of autoimmune diseases. Autoantibodies target a broad range of self-antigens, including nuclear components, organ-specific antigens, and soluble factors. Autoantibodies result from a breakdown of tolerance mechanisms during B cell development (Yurasov and Nussenzweig, 2007), as well as alteration in the selection of clones within GCs (Di Zenzo et al., 2012; Vinuesa et al., 2009). Many mouse models and human studies have demonstrated that aberrant generation and/or activation of Tfh cells and extrafollicular helper T cells contributes to the pathogenesis of autoimmune diseases.

3.1 Evidence in mouse models

The first demonstration linking aberrant Tfh responses and autoimmunity came from the studies of the *sanroque* mouse model, which carries a single amino acid mutation in the RNA-binding protein Roquin1 (Vinuesa et al., 2005). Development of these diseases is accompanied by spontaneous GC formation due to excessive Tfh response and generation of high amounts of antinuclear antibodies. In *sanroque* mice, excessive expression of ICOS (Yu et al., 2007) and IFN-γ (Lee et al., 2012) by activated $CD4^+$ T cells plays a key role in Tfh cell accumulation. Genetic ablation of SAP in *sanroque* mice (which abrogates the generation of mature Tfh cells) prevents lupus pathology, whereas transfer of *sanroque* Tfh cells into wild-type mice promotes the lupus-like disease through spontaneous GC formation (Linterman et al., 2009b). These observations show that excessive Tfh response together with spontaneous GC formation is sufficient to cause autoimmunity.

Contribution of extrafollicular helper T cells in the pathogenesis of autoimmune disease is supported by findings in the MRL/lpr lupus mouse model, which is characterized by the deficiency of the proapoptotic molecule Fas (Odegard et al., 2008). Extrafollicular helper T cells that develop in the MRL/lpr mice largely share features with GC Tfh cells (Odegard et al., 2008; Lee et al., 2011).

3.2 Evidence in human studies

Increased GC response in patients with systemic lupus erythematosus (SLE) was suggested in early studies by an increased frequency of $CD27^{+}CD38^{hi}$ somatically mutated antibody-producing plasmablasts in peripheral blood (Arce et al., 2001; Jacobi et al., 2003). SLE patients are predisposed to develop a broader range of autoantibodies than healthy subjects, because SLE patients display higher frequencies of self-reactive mature naïve B cells than healthy controls (Yurasov et al., 2005, 2006). Assessing whether the increased GC response is accompanied with excessive Tfh response in human autoimmune disease has been a challenge, as the access to the lymphoid organ samples in autoimmune disease patients is extremely limited. However, recent progress in understanding the relationship between blood $CXCR5^{+}$ $CD4^{+}$ memory T cells and the Tfh lineage cells in lymphoid organs has made the monitoring of ongoing Tfh responses more feasible than before.

3.2.1 Blood memory Tfh subsets in humans

The $CD4^{+}$ T cells expressing the chemokine receptor CXCR5 were first described in human blood more than 20 years ago (Forster et al., 1994). While these cells were initially considered to be recently activated T cells (Breitfeld et al., 2000; Schaerli et al., 2001; Kim et al., 2001), recent studies indicate that blood $CXCR5^{+}$ $CD4^{+}$ T cells contain long-lived memory cells that share functional properties with Tfh cells. Accordingly, blood $CXCR5^{+}$ $CD4^{+}$ T cells are currently termed blood (or peripheral) memory Tfh cells (reviewed in Schmitt et al., 2014a). Blood memory Tfh cells do not express the Bcl-6 protein, and the molecular mechanisms by which blood memory Tfh cells maintain their Tfh characteristics remain to be established.

Another important discovery was that human blood memory Tfh cells are composed of distinct subsets with unique phenotype and functions (Schmitt et al., 2014a). These subsets can be ultimately defined by the combinations of these markers: the chemokine receptors CXCR3 and CCR6; PD-1; and ICOS. The combination of CXCR3 and CCR6 defines three major subsets: $CXCR3^{+}CCR6^{-}$ cells that share properties with Th1 cells (hereafter called blood memory Tfh1 cells), $CXCR3^{-}CCR6^{-}$ cells resembling Th2 cells (hereafter called blood memory Tfh2 cells), and $CXCR3^{-}CCR6^{+}$ cells resembling Th17 cells (hereafter called blood memory Tfh17 cells) (Morita et al., 2011). The differential expression of ICOS and PD-1 further defines developmentally and functionally distinct subpopulations within the subsets: one activated subset ($ICOS^{+}PD\text{-}1^{++}$), and two quiescent subsets ($ICOS^{-}PD\text{-}1^{+}$ and $ICOS^{-}PD\text{-}1^{-}$).

Blood memory Tfh cells can be largely subdivided into nonefficient helpers (Tfh1) and efficient helpers (Tfh2 and Tfh17). The activated $ICOS^{+}PD\text{-}1^{++}$ populations within blood memory Tfh2 and Tfh17 cells might represent the most efficient helpers. Within quiescent Tfh2 and Tfh17 subsets, the $ICOS^{-}PD\text{-}1^{+}$ population provides more prompt help to memory B cells than the $ICOS^{-}PD\text{-}1^{-}$ population (Locci et al., 2013; Boswell et al., 2014). By contrast, blood memory Tfh1 cells largely lack the capacity to help naïve or memory B cells (Locci et al., 2013; Morita et al., 2011; Boswell et al., 2014; Bentebibel et al., 2013). Blood memory Tfh1 cells appear to contribute to antibody responses, only when they become $ICOS^{+}PD\text{-}1^{++}$ activated cells. These cells produce limited amounts of IL-21, and help memory B cells, but not naïve B cells, to become antibody-producing cells (Bentebibel et al., 2013).

3.2.2 Alterations in the composition of blood memory Tfh subsets in patients with autoimmune diseases

Multiple studies demonstrated that the frequency of $ICOS^{+}$ or $PD\text{-}1^{++}$ cells among blood memory Tfh cells is increased in patients with autoantibody-mediated autoimmune diseases such as SLE (Simpson et al., 2010; He et al., 2013), Sjögren syndrome (Li et al., 2012; Simpson et al., 2010; Luo et al., 2013), rheumatoid arthritis (Wang et al., 2013; Liu et al., 2012), and autoimmune thyroid diseases (Zhu et al., 2012). Furthermore, an increase of $ICOS^{+}$ blood memory Tfh cells showed a positive correlation with serum autoantibody titers and disease activity and/or severity in these diseases (Simpson et al., 2010; He et al., 2013; Zhu et al., 2012; Wang et al., 2013; Luo et al., 2013). These studies suggest that an increase of blood memory Tfh cells with active phenotype is a common feature of autoantibody-mediated autoimmune diseases, and likely reflects aberrant Tfh responses in patients.

Accumulating evidence also indicates that patients with autoimmune disease display an alteration in the composition of blood memory Tfh1, Tfh2, and Tfh17 cells. In patients with juvenile dermatomyositis (Morita et al., 2011), adult SLE (Le Coz et al., 2013), and Sjögren syndrome (Li et al., 2012), Tfh1 cells are underrepresented among blood memory Tfh cells, whereas Tfh2 and/or Tfh17 cells are overrepresented. Such alterations were found to correlate with disease activity, serum autoantibody titers, and/or the frequency of blood plasmablasts (Morita et al., 2011; Le Coz et al., 2013; Li et al., 2012). Furthermore, while not generally considered an autoantibody-mediated autoimmune disease, patients with primary progressive multiple sclerosis (MS) also display the same alteration (low Tfh1 and high Tfh17) in the composition of blood memory Tfh subsets (Romme Christensen et al., 2013). Collectively, these observations suggest that an increase in activated Tfh2 and/or Tfh17 cell subsets and a decrease of Tfh1 cells within blood memory Tfh cells might be a common feature across multiple autoimmune diseases. Such alterations in blood memory Tfh cells might reflect an overall increase of efficient helpers that promote the generation of antibodies in lymphoid organs and/or inflammatory sites in patients with autoimmune diseases.

3.2.3 Analysis of Tfh cells in inflammatory tissues

Inflammatory sites in autoimmune diseases often develop lymphoid cell aggregation, which leads to the formation of well-structured GCs (hereafter called ectopic GCs).

Autoimmune patients with ectopic GCs often have higher disease activity and are refractory to treatment. Yet, formation of ectopic GCs does not simply reflect the extent or the duration of inflammation in the lesions, as only 20–40% of patients with chronic inflammation develop ectopic GCs (Pitzalis et al., 2014). The mechanisms that control the formation of ectopic GCs remain to be established, but might be shared with GCs in lymphoid organs. $CD4^+$ T cells found in lymphoid aggregates and ectopic GCs share properties with Tfh cells. For example, in lupus tubulointerstitial nephritis lesions, helper T cells found in lymphoid T and B cell aggregates express ICOS, PD-1, Bcl-6, and IL-21 (Liarski et al., 2014). Mouse models suggest the involvement of Th17 cells in the generation of ectopic GCs. In the experimental autoimmune encephalomyelitis model, Th17 cells induce the formation of ectopic GCs in inflammatory brain lesions *via* IL-17 and the cell surface molecule podoplanin, and then acquire features of Tfh cells in ectopic GCs (Peters et al., 2011). Given that patients with autoimmune diseases display increased activated Tfh17 cells in blood (as discussed earlier), that early developmental pathway for Tfh and Th17 cells in inflammatory environment are shared in humans (Schmitt et al., 2014b), and that in mice Th17-derived IL-17 directly promotes B cell differentiation into GC B cells, which are thought to be the source of pathogenic autoantibodies (Wu et al., 2010), it is tempting to speculate that Tfh17 cells might be involved in the formation of ectopic GCs in human autoimmune diseases.

When compared to lymphoid organs, ectopic GCs might be more enriched with autoreactive B cells (Pitzalis et al., 2014). First, organ-specific self-antigens are easily accessible by B cells in ectopic GCs, due to the abundance of damaged and/or apoptotic cells caused by the inflammatory process. Second, at variance with follicles in lymphoid tissues where the entry of autoreactive B cells is excluded due to their reduced expression of CXCR5 (Ekland et al., 2004), lymphoid aggregates in inflammatory tissues are more open in structure, and thus likely to be permissive to the entry of autoreactive B cells. Last, there is evidence that B cells in lymphoid aggregates and/or ectopic GCs indeed produce antibodies against self-antigens overexpressed at the inflammatory sites (Pitzalis et al., 2014; Kinloch et al., 2014). Therefore, ectopic GCs might represent a major site of autoantibody production in autoimmune diseases, and thus a potentially good target for therapeutics.

4. Tfh CELLS AS A THERAPEUTIC TARGET FOR AUTOIMMUNE DISEASE

4.1 Evidence from GWAS in autoimmune diseases

Autoimmune diseases result from a complex interplay between genetic and environmental factors. Genome-wide association studies (GWAS) conducted in multiple autoimmune diseases have yielded risk-associated loci (Stranger and De Jager, 2012). Furthermore, recent studies have provided a proof of principle that integration of GWAS data with other databases can identify fundamental genes, pathways, and cell types that contribute to pathogenesis, and therefore contribute to drug discovery (Okada et al., 2014).

In this regard, it is important to note that multiple risk-associated loci identified in autoimmune diseases are potentially associated with the regulation of the development and/or the function of human Tfh cells. The list includes genes associated with IL-12 and IL-23, cytokines implicated in human Tfh cell differentiation (Schmitt et al., 2009, 2013, 2014b; Ma et al., 2009), such as *IL12A*, *IL12B* (both in MS), *IL23R* (rheumatoid arthritis), *STAT3* (MS), *STAT4* (SLE, rheumatoid arthritis, Sjögren syndrome), *IRF5* (SLE, rheumatoid arthritis), and *IRF8* (SLE, rheumatoid arthritis, MS). IRF8 also contributes to TGF-β signaling, another cytokine important for the generation of human Tfh cells (Schmitt et al., 2014b) by promoting the expression of TGF-β-activating integrin αvβ8 on the surface of DCs (Yoshida et al., 2014). OX40L-coding *TNFSF4*, identified in the GWAS of SLE and Sjögren syndrome, might be also involved in the generation and/or homeostasis of Tfh cells. Overexpression of OX40L causes accumulation of T cells in B cell follicles (Brocker et al., 1999) and OX40 signals induce $CD4^+$ T cells to express CXCR5 (Flynn et al., 1998; Walker et al., 1999; Kim et al., 2003). Furthermore, GWAS identified multiple risk-associated loci encoding molecules expressed by Tfh cells including *IL21* (SLE, rheumatoid arthritis) and *CXCR5* (MS, Sjögren syndrome). In addition to Blimp-1-encoding *PRDM1* (Johnston et al., 2009), a recent study showed that *PTPN22*, a risk-associated locus identified in GWAS of SLE, rheumatoid arthritis, myasthenia gravis, and type 1 diabetes (T1D), negatively regulates the generation of Tfh and GC responses in mice (Maine et al., 2014). Although the direct link between these gene variants and aberrant Tfh responses remains to be demonstrated, these studies likely support that Tfh cells can be a good therapeutic target in autoimmune diseases. Here, two major approaches can be taken: inhibit the generation of Tfh cells, and inhibit the molecules expressed by Tfh cells (Fig. 5).

4.2 Strategies to block Tfh development

As described earlier, the initial commitment toward Tfh cells occurs when $CD4^+$ T cells encounter DCs. Therefore, cytokines and costimulatory molecules expressed by DCs can

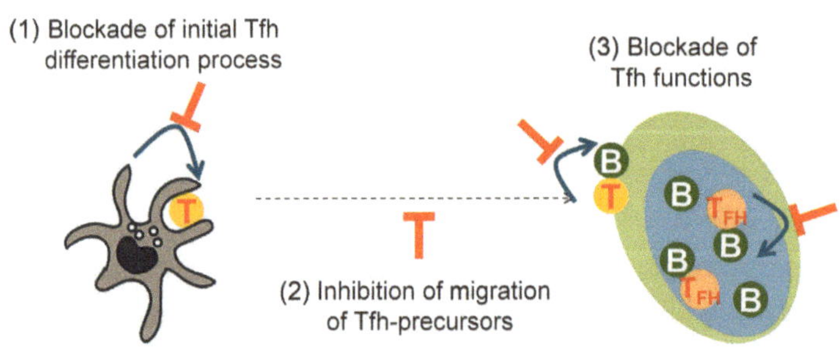

Figure 5 Strategies to inhibit Tfh responses. Two major approaches can be taken: inhibit the generation of Tfh cells, and inhibit the molecules expressed by Tfh cells. Potential target molecules are discussed in the text.

be potential therapeutic targets. The list of target cytokines includes IL-12, IL-23, and IL-6, and therefore anti-IL-12, anti-IL-23, anti-IL-12p40 (ustekinumab, which targets both IL-12 and IL-23), and anti-IL-6 (tocilizumab) might be beneficial. While STAT3 and STAT4 can be potential targets, it should be considered that both STAT3 and STAT4 contribute to human Tfh cell generation and compensate each other (Schmitt et al., 2014b). An alternative approach is to inhibit the secretion of these Tfh-promoting cytokines from antigen-presenting cells. In this context, inhibitors of IRF5 and IRF8 might be interesting candidates. Moreover, it is anticipated that blocking these molecules also inhibit the generation of pathogenic Th1 and Th17 cells.

The list of target costimulatory molecules includes CD28/CD80 and CD86, ICOS/ICOSL, and OX40/OX40L, and thus a CTLA4-Ig chimeric protein (abatacept which inhibits CD28 signals), anti-ICOS/ICOSL, and anti-OX40/OX40L might be considered. Abatacept has been approved for use in patients with rheumatoid arthritis, and a Phase II/III study of abatacept with SLE also yielded some positive outcome (Furie et al., 2014). There the treatment improved in serum anti-dsDNA titers, C3, and C4 levels, and reduced proteinuria. Two Phase I studies of an ICOSL neutralizing mAb (AMG-557) and a depleting ICOS mAb (MEDI-570) are under way with SLE patients. Anti-ICOS/ICOSL might also contribute to the inhibition of migration of Tfh precursors into follicle, given the importance of ICOS–ICOSL axis in this context (Xu et al., 2013). In the same context, as migration of Tfh precursors toward follicles is largely dependent on CXCR5, anti-CXCR5 might be beneficial to inhibit the generation of Tfh cells.

4.3 Targeting molecules expressed by Tfh cells

Many mouse models have demonstrated that inhibition of effector molecules expressed by Tfh and extrafollicular helper T cells ameliorates the generation of autoantibodies and/or the development of glomerulonephritis, thereby providing a rationale to target these molecules for therapeutics. For example, pathogenic extrafollicular helper T cells that develop in the MRL/lpr mice are dependent on IL-21 and CD40L for their functions (Odegard et al., 2008). Similarly, in the BXSB-*Yaa* mouse model, which displays a duplication of the *Tlr7* gene, aberrant Tfh responses as well as the development of glomerulonephritis is completely dependent on IL-21 signals (Bubier et al., 2009). In contrast, in *sanroque* mice IL-21 signals are not essential for pathology (Linterman et al., 2009a), but IFN-γ signaling blockade not only alleviated Tfh and GC B cell accumulation but also virtually prevented all clinical manifestations (Lee et al., 2012). This effect was more profound as compared to SAP-deficiency, which did not correct the splenomegaly nor hypergammaglobulinemia (Linterman et al., 2009b), or ICOS-deficiency, which did not eliminate autoantibody formation (Lee et al., 2012).

In humans, anti-CD40L (BG9588) was tested in Phase I/II studies with lupus nephritis about 15 years ago. The early results were encouraging and the treatment reduced serum anti-dsDNA titers, increased serum complement levels, and reduced nephritis score (Sidiropoulos and Boumpas, 2004). While the trial was prematurely terminated due to the development of thrombotic events in some patients, this observation provides evidence that interruption of T and B cell interactions can be beneficial for treatment of SLE. The potential mechanism for the thrombotic events by BG9588 is the formation of platelet aggregates due to its binding to CD40L and Fc receptor expressed by platelets. Recently, two Phase I studies of an anti-CD40L Fab fragment (CDP7657) have been completed with healthy volunteers and SLE patients [ClinicalTrials.gov: NCT01093911, NCT01764594]. No study results are posted at present. Phase I study of an IL-21 neutralizing mAb (NNC114-0005) are under way with rheumatoid arthritis.

5. CONCLUDING REMARKS

The pathogenic role of Tfh cells in autoimmunity is supported by many studies in human autoimmune diseases and mouse models. There is now little doubt that Tfh cells are an interesting therapeutic target for autoimmune diseases. Several molecules that inhibit the generation and/or the function of Tfh cells are being tested in clinical trials. Nonetheless, Tfh is still a relatively new field, and much remains to be established to develop new target molecules. What is the mechanism to cause the formation of ectopic GCs? How do Tfh cells contribute to the process? What are the precursors of Tfh cells in ectopic GCs? What is the mechanism by which the precursors mature into Tfh cells? Which transcription factors other than Bcl-6 are required for Tfh cell generations in humans? How is gene polymorphism associated with Tfh response? Answering these questions will provide significant insights into new treatments and stratification strategies for treatment options.

REFERENCES

Akiba, H., Takeda, K., Kojima, Y., Usui, Y., Harada, N., Yamazaki, T., Ma, J., Tezuka, K., Yagita, H., Okumura, K., 2005. The role of ICOS in the CXCR5+ follicular B helper T cell maintenance in vivo. J. Immunol. 175, 2340–2348.

Ansel, K.M., Mcheyzer-Williams, L.J., Ngo, V.N., Mcheyzer-Williams, M.G., Cyster, J.G., 1999. In vivo-activated CD4 T cells upregulate CXC chemokine receptor 5 and reprogram their response to lymphoid chemokines. J. Exp. Med. 190, 1123–1134.

Arce, E., Jackson, D.G., Gill, M.A., Bennett, L.B., Banchereau, J., Pascual, V., 2001. Increased frequency of pre-germinal center b cells and plasma cell precursors in the blood of children with systemic lupus erythematosus. J. Immunol. 167, 2361–2369.

Banchereau, J., Bazan, F., Blanchard, D., Briere, F., Galizzi, J.P., Van Kooten, C., Liu, Y.J., Rousset, F., Saeland, S., 1994. The CD40 antigen and its ligand. Annu. Rev. Immunol. 12, 881–922.

Baumjohann, D., Okada, T., Ansel, K.M., 2011. Cutting edge: distinct waves of BCL6 expression during T follicular helper cell development. J. Immunol. 187, 2089–2092.

Bentebibel, S.E., Schmitt, N., Banchereau, J., Ueno, H., 2011. Human tonsil B-cell lymphoma 6 (BCL6)-expressing CD4+ T-cell subset specialized for B-cell help outside germinal centers. Proc. Natl. Acad. Sci. U. S. A. 108, E488–E497.

Bentebibel, S.E., Lopez, S., Obermoser, G., Schmitt, N., Mueller, C., Harrod, C., Flano, E., Mejias, A., Albrecht, R.A., Blankenship, D., Xu, H., Pascual, V., Banchereau, J., Garcia-Sastre, A.,

Palucka, A.K., Ramilo, O., Ueno, H., 2013. Induction of ICOS + CXCR3 + CXCR5 + TH cells correlates with antibody responses to influenza vaccination. Sci. Transl. Med. 5, 176ra32.

Bossaller, L., Burger, J., Draeger, R., Grimbacher, B., Knoth, R., Plebani, A., Durandy, A., Baumann, U., Schlesier, M., Welcher, A.A., Peter, H.H., Warnatz, K., 2006. ICOS deficiency is associated with a severe reduction of CXCR5 + CD4 germinal center Th cells. J. Immunol. 177, 4927–4932.

Boswell, K.L., Paris, R., Boritz, E., Ambrozak, D., Yamamoto, T., Darko, S., Wloka, K., Wheatley, A., Narpala, S., Mcdermott, A., Roederer, M., Haubrich, R., Connors, M., Ake, J., Douek, D.C., Kim, J., Petrovas, C., Koup, R.A., 2014. Loss of circulating CD4 T cells with B cell helper function during chronic HIV infection. PLoS Pathog. 10, e1003853.

Breitfeld, D., Ohl, L., Kremmer, E., Ellwart, J., Sallusto, F., Lipp, M., Forster, R., 2000. Follicular B helper T cells express CXC chemokine receptor 5, localize to B cell follicles, and support immunoglobulin production. J. Exp. Med. 192, 1545–1552.

Brocker, T., Gulbranson-Judge, A., Flynn, S., Riedinger, M., Raykundalia, C., Lane, P., 1999. CD4 T cell traffic control: in vivo evidence that ligation of OX40 on CD4 T cells by OX40-ligand expressed on dendritic cells leads to the accumulation of CD4 T cells in B follicles. Eur. J. Immunol. 29, 1610–1616.

Bryant, V.L., Ma, C.S., Avery, D.T., Li, Y., Good, K.L., Corcoran, L.M., De Waal Malefyt, R., Tangye, S.G., 2007. Cytokine-mediated regulation of human B cell differentiation into Ig-secreting cells: predominant role of IL-21 produced by CXCR5+ T follicular helper cells. J. Immunol. 179, 8180–8190.

Bubier, J.A., Sproule, T.J., Foreman, O., Spolski, R., Shaffer, D.J., Morse 3rd., H.C., Leonard, W.J., Roopenian, D.C., 2009. A critical role for IL-21 receptor signaling in the pathogenesis of systemic lupus erythematosus in BXSB-Yaa mice. Proc. Natl. Acad. Sci. U. S. A. 106, 1518–1523.

Cannons, J.L., Tangye, S.G., Schwartzberg, P.L., 2011. SLAM family receptors and SAP adaptors in immunity. Annu. Rev. Immunol. 29, 665–705.

Choi, Y.S., Kageyama, R., Eto, D., Escobar, T.C., Johnston, R.J., Monticelli, L., Lao, C., Crotty, S., 2011. ICOS receptor instructs T follicular helper cell versus effector cell differentiation via induction of the transcriptional repressor Bcl6. Immunity 34, 932–946.

Chung, Y., Tanaka, S., Chu, F., Nurieva, R.I., Martinez, G.J., Rawal, S., Wang, Y.H., Lim, H., Reynolds, J.M., Zhou, X.H., Fan, H.M., Liu, Z.M., Neelapu, S.S., Dong, C., 2011. Follicular regulatory T cells expressing Foxp3 and Bcl-6 suppress germinal center reactions. Nat. Med. 17, 983–988.

Crotty, S., 2011. Follicular helper CD4 T cells (TFH). Annu. Rev. Immunol. 29, 621–663.

Cubas, R.A., Mudd, J.C., Savoye, A.L., Perreau, M., Van Grevenynghe, J., Metcalf, T., Connick, E., Meditz, A., Freeman, G.J., Abesada-Terk Jr., G., Jacobson, J.M., Brooks, A.D., Crotty, S., Estes, J.D., Pantaleo, G., Lederman, M.M., Haddad, E.K., 2013. Inadequate T follicular cell help impairs B cell immunity during HIV infection. Nat. Med. 19, 494–499.

Di Zenzo, G., Di Lullo, G., Corti, D., Calabresi, V., Sinistro, A., Vanzetta, F., Didona, B., Cianchini, G., Hertl, M., Eming, R., Amagai, M., Ohyama, B., Hashimoto, T., Sloostra, J., Sallusto, F., Zambruno, G., Lanzavecchia, A., 2012. Pemphigus autoantibodies generated through somatic mutations target the desmoglein-3 cis-interface. J. Clin. Invest. 122, 3781–3790.

Ekland, E.H., Forster, R., Lipp, M., Cyster, J.G., 2004. Requirements for follicular exclusion and competitive elimination of autoantigen-binding B cells. J. Immunol. 172, 4700–4708.

Ferguson, S.E., Han, S., Kelsoe, G., Thompson, C.B., 1996. CD28 is required for germinal center formation. J. Immunol. 156, 4576–4581.

Fillatreau, S., Gray, D., 2003. T cell accumulation in B cell follicles is regulated by dendritic cells and is independent of B cell activation. J. Exp. Med. 197, 195–206.

Flynn, S., Toellner, K.M., Raykundalia, C., Goodall, M., Lane, P., 1998. CD4 T cell cytokine differentiation: the B cell activation molecule, OX40 ligand, instructs CD4 T cells to express interleukin 4 and upregulates expression of the chemokine receptor, Blr-1. J. Exp. Med. 188, 297–304.

Forster, R., Emrich, T., Kremmer, E., Lipp, M., 1994. Expression of the G-protein–coupled receptor BLR1 defines mature, recirculating B cells and a subset of T-helper memory cells. Blood 84, 830–840.

Furie, R., Nicholls, K., Cheng, T.T., Houssiau, F., Burgos-Vargas, R., Chen, S.L., Hillson, J.L., Meadows-Shropshire, S., Kinaszczuk, M., Merrill, J.T., 2014. Efficacy and safety of abatacept in lupus nephritis: a twelve-month, randomized, double-blind study. Arthritis Rheumatol. 66, 379–389.

Garside, P., Ingulli, E., Merica, R.R., Johnson, J.G., Noelle, R.J., Jenkins, M.K., 1998. Visualization of specific B and T lymphocyte interactions in the lymph node. Science 281, 96–99.

Gitlin, A.D., Shulman, Z., Nussenzweig, M.C., 2014. Clonal selection in the germinal centre by regulated proliferation and hypermutation. Nature 509, 637–640.

Haynes, N.M., Allen, C.D., Lesley, R., Ansel, K.M., Killeen, N., Cyster, J.G., 2007. Role of CXCR5 and CCR7 in follicular Th cell positioning and appearance of a programmed cell death gene-1high germinal center-associated subpopulation. J. Immunol. 179, 5099–5108.

He, J., Tsai, L.M., Leong, Y.A., Hu, X., Ma, C.S., Chevalier, N., Sun, X., Vandenberg, K., Rockman, S., Ding, Y., Zhu, L., Wei, W., Wang, C., Karnowski, A., Belz, G.T., Ghali, J.R., Cook, M.C., Riminton, D.S., Veillette, A., Schwartzberg, P.L., Mackay, F., Brink, R., Tangye, S.G., Vinuesa, C.G., Mackay, C.R., Li, Z., Yu, D., 2013. Circulating precursor CCR7(lo)PD-1(hi) CXCR5(+) CD4(+) T cells indicate Tfh cell activity and promote antibody responses upon antigen reexposure. Immunity 39, 770–781.

Hutloff, A., Dittrich, A.M., Beier, K.C., Eljaschewitsch, B., Kraft, R., Anagnostopoulos, I., Kroczek, R.A., 1999. ICOS is an inducible T-cell co-stimulator structurally and functionally related to CD28. Nature 397, 263–266.

Jacob, J., Kassir, R., Kelsoe, G., 1991. In situ studies of the primary immune response to (4-hydroxy-3-nitrophenyl)acetyl. I. The architecture and dynamics of responding cell populations. J. Exp. Med. 173, 1165–1175.

Jacobi, A.M., Odendahl, M., Reiter, K., Bruns, A., Burmester, G.R., Radbruch, A., Valet, G., Lipsky, P.E., Dorner, T., 2003. Correlation between circulating CD27high plasma cells and disease activity in patients with systemic lupus erythematosus. Arthritis Rheum. 48, 1332–1342.

Johnston, R.J., Poholek, A.C., Ditoro, D., Yusuf, I., Eto, D., Barnett, B., Dent, A.L., Craft, J., Crotty, S., 2009. Bcl6 and Blimp-1 are reciprocal and antagonistic regulators of T follicular helper cell differentiation. Science 325, 1006–1010.

Kashiwakuma, D., Suto, A., Hiramatsu, Y., Ikeda, K., Takatori, H., Suzuki, K., Kagami, S., Hirose, K., Watanabe, N., Iwamoto, I., Nakajima, H., 2010. B and T lymphocyte attenuator suppresses IL-21 production from follicular Th cells and subsequent humoral immune responses. J. Immunol. 185, 2730–2736.

Kerfoot, S.M., Yaari, G., Patel, J.R., Johnson, K.L., Gonzalez, D.G., Kleinstein, S.H., Haberman, A.M., 2011. Germinal center B cell and T follicular helper cell development initiates in the interfollicular zone. Immunity 34, 947–960.

Kim, C.H., Rott, L.S., Clark-Lewis, I., Campbell, D.J., Wu, L., Butcher, E.C., 2001. Subspecialization of CXCR5 + T cells: B helper activity is focused in a germinal center-localized subset of CXCR5 + T cells. J. Exp. Med. 193, 1373–1381.

Kim, M.Y., Gaspal, F.M., Wiggett, H.E., Mcconnell, F.M., Gulbranson-Judge, A., Raykundalia, C., Walker, L.S., Goodall, M.D., Lane, P.J., 2003. CD4(+)CD3(−) accessory cells costimulate primed CD4 T cells through OX40 and CD30 at sites where T cells collaborate with B cells. Immunity 18, 643–654.

Kim, C.H., Lim, H.W., Kim, J.R., Rott, L., Hillsamer, P., Butcher, E.C., 2004. Unique gene expression program of human germinal center T helper cells. Blood 104, 1952–1960.

Kim, H.J., Verbinnen, B., Tang, X., Lu, L., Cantor, H., 2010. Inhibition of follicular T-helper cells by CD8(+) regulatory T cells is essential for self tolerance. Nature 467, 328–332.

Kinloch, A.J., Chang, A., Ko, K., Henry Dunand, C.J., Henderson, S., Maienschein-Cline, M., Kaverina, N., Rovin, B.H., Salgado Ferrer, M., Wolfgeher, D., Liarski, V., Haddon, D.J., Utz, P.J., Wilson, P.C., Clark, M.R., 2014. Vimentin is a dominant target of in situ humoral immunity in human lupus tubulointerstitial nephritis. Arthritis Rheumatol. 66, 3359–3370.

Kissenpfennig, A., Henri, S., Dubois, B., Laplace-Builhe, C., Perrin, P., Romani, N., Tripp, C.H., Douillard, P., Leserman, L., Kaiserlian, D., Saeland, S., Davoust, J., Malissen, B., 2005. Dynamics and function of Langerhans cells in vivo: dermal dendritic cells colonize lymph node areas distinct from slower migrating Langerhans cells. Immunity 22, 643–654.

Kitano, M., Moriyama, S., Ando, Y., Hikida, M., Mori, Y., Kurosaki, T., Okada, T., 2011. Bcl6 protein expression shapes pre-germinal center B cell dynamics and follicular helper T cell heterogeneity. Immunity 34, 961–972.

Klechevsky, E., Morita, R., Liu, M., Cao, Y., Coquery, S., Thompson-Snipes, L., Briere, F., Chaussabel, D., Zurawski, G., Palucka, A.K., Reiter, Y., Banchereau, J., Ueno, H., 2008. Functional specializations of human epidermal Langerhans cells and CD14+ dermal dendritic cells. Immunity 29, 497–510.

Le Coz, C., Joublin, A., Pasquali, J.L., Korganow, A.S., Dumortier, H., Monneaux, F., 2013. Circulating TFH subset distribution is strongly affected in lupus patients with an active disease. PLoS One 8, e75319.

Lee, S.K., Rigby, R.J., Zotos, D., Tsai, L.M., Kawamoto, S., Marshall, J.L., Ramiscal, R.R., Chan, T.D., Gatto, D., Brink, R., Yu, D., Fagarasan, S., Tarlinton, D.M., Cunningham, A.F., Vinuesa, C.G., 2011. B cell priming for extrafollicular antibody responses requires Bcl-6 expression by T cells. J. Exp. Med. 208, 1377–1388.

Lee, S.K., Silva, D.G., Martin, J.L., Pratama, A., Hu, X., Chang, P.P., Walters, G., Vinuesa, C.G., 2012. Interferon-gamma excess leads to pathogenic accumulation of follicular helper T cells and germinal centers. Immunity 37, 880–892.

Li, X.Y., Wu, Z.B., Ding, J., Zheng, Z.H., Li, X.Y., Chen, L.N., Zhu, P., 2012. Role of the frequency of blood CD4(+) CXCR5(+) CCR6(+) T cells in autoimmunity in patients with Sjogren's syndrome. Biochem. Biophys. Res. Commun. 422, 238–244.

Liarski, V.M., Kaverina, N., Chang, A., Brandt, D., Yanez, D., Talasnik, L., Carlesso, G., Herbst, R., Utset, T.O., Labno, C., Peng, Y., Jiang, Y., Giger, M.L., Clark, M.R., 2014. Cell distance mapping identifies functional T follicular helper cells in inflamed human renal tissue. Sci. Transl. Med. 6, 230ra46.

Linterman, M.A., Rigby, R.J., Wong, R., Silva, D., Withers, D., Anderson, G., Verma, N.K., Brink, R., Hutloff, A., Goodnow, C.C., Vinuesa, C.G., 2009a. Roquin differentiates the specialized functions of duplicated T cell costimulatory receptor genes CD28 and ICOS. Immunity 30, 228–241.

Linterman, M.A., Rigby, R.J., Wong, R.K., Yu, D., Brink, R., Cannons, J.L., Schwartzberg, P.L., Cook, M.C., Walters, G.D., Vinuesa, C.G., 2009b. Follicular helper T cells are required for systemic autoimmunity. J. Exp. Med. 206, 561–576.

Linterman, M.A., Beaton, L., Yu, D., Ramiscal, R.R., Srivastava, M., Hogan, J.J., Verma, N.K., Smyth, M.J., Rigby, R.J., Vinuesa, C.G., 2010. IL-21 acts directly on B cells to regulate Bcl-6 expression and germinal center responses. J. Exp. Med. 207, 353–363.

Linterman, M.A., Pierson, W., Lee, S.K., Kallies, A., Kawamoto, S., Rayner, T.F., Srivastava, M., Divekar, D.P., Beaton, L., Hogan, J.J., Fagarasan, S., Liston, A., Smith, K.G., Vinuesa, C.G., 2011. Foxp3+ follicular regulatory T cells control the germinal center response. Nat. Med. 17, 975–982.

Liu, R., Wu, Q., Su, D., Che, N., Chen, H., Geng, L., Chen, J., Chen, W., Li, X., Sun, L., 2012. A regulatory effect of IL-21 on T follicular helper-like cell and B cell in rheumatoid arthritis. Arthritis Res. Ther. 14, R255.

Liu, D., Xu, H., Shih, C., Wan, Z., Ma, X., Ma, W., Luo, D., Qi, H., 2014a. T-B-cell entanglement and ICOSL-driven feed-forward regulation of germinal centre reaction. Nature 517 (7533), 214–218.

Liu, X., Chen, X., Zhong, B., Wang, A., Wang, X., Chu, F., Nurieva, R.I., Yan, X., Chen, P., Van Der Flier, L.G., Nakatsukasa, H., Neelapu, S.S., Chen, W., Clevers, H., Tian, Q., Qi, H., Wei, L., Dong, C., 2014b. Transcription factor achaete-scute homologue 2 initiates follicular T-helper-cell development. Nature 507, 513–518.

Locci, M., Havenar-Daughton, C., Landais, E., Wu, J., Kroenke, M.A., Arlehamn, C.L., Su, L.F., Cubas, R., Davis, M.M., Sette, A., Haddad, E.K., International, A.V.I.P.C.P.I., Poignard, P., Crotty, S., 2013. Human circulating PD-1(+)CXCR3(−)CXCR5(+) memory Tfh cells are highly functional and correlate with broadly neutralizing HIV antibody responses. Immunity 39, 758–769.

Luo, C., Li, Y., Liu, W., Feng, H., Wang, H., Huang, X., Qiu, L., Ouyang, J., 2013. Expansion of circulating counterparts of follicular helper T cells in patients with myasthenia gravis. J. Neuroimmunol. 256 (1-2), 55–61.

Ma, C.S., Suryani, S., Avery, D.T., Chan, A., Nanan, R., Santner-Nanan, B., Deenick, E.K., Tangye, S.G., 2009. Early commitment of naive human CD4(+) T cells to the T follicular helper (T(FH)) cell lineage is induced by IL-12. Immunol. Cell Biol. 87, 590–600.

Maclennan, I.C., 1994. Germinal centers. Annu. Rev. Immunol. 12, 117–139.

Maclennan, I.C., Gray, D., 1986. Antigen-driven selection of virgin and memory B cells. Immunol. Rev. 91, 61–85.

Maclennan, I.C., Toellner, K.M., Cunningham, A.F., Serre, K., Sze, D.M., Zuniga, E., Cook, M.C., Vinuesa, C.G., 2003. Extrafollicular antibody responses. Immunol. Rev. 194, 8–18.

Maine, C.J., Marquardt, K., Cheung, J., Sherman, L.A., 2014. PTPN22 controls the germinal center by influencing the numbers and activity of T follicular helper cells. J. Immunol. 192, 1415–1424.

Marshall, H.D., Ray, J.P., Laidlaw, B.J., Zhang, N., Gawande, D., Staron, M.M., Craft, J., Kaech, S.M., 2014. The tumor growth factor beta signaling pathway is critical for the formation of CD4 T follicular helper cells and isotype-switched antibody responses in the lung mucosa. eLife 4, e04851.

Mcheyzer-Williams, M.G., Mclean, M.J., Lalor, P.A., Nossal, G.J., 1993. Antigen-driven B cell differentiation in vivo. J. Exp. Med. 178, 295–307.

Morita, R., Schmitt, N., Bentebibel, S.E., Ranganathan, R., Bourdery, L., Zurawski, G., Foucat, E., Dullaers, M., Oh, S., Sabzghabaei, N., Lavecchio, E.M., Punaro, M., Pascual, V., Banchereau, J., Ueno, H., 2011. Human blood CXCR5(+) CD4(+) T cells are counterparts of T follicular cells and contain specific subsets that differentially support antibody secretion. Immunity 34, 108–121.

Moriyama, S., Takahashi, N., Green, J.A., Hori, S., Kubo, M., Cyster, J.G., Okada, T., 2014. Sphingosine-1-phosphate receptor 2 is critical for follicular helper T cell retention in germinal centers. J. Exp. Med. 211, 1297–1305.

Nakayamada, S., Kanno, Y., Takahashi, H., Jankovic, D., Lu, K.T., Johnson, T.A., Sun, H.W., Vahedi, G., Hakim, O., Handon, R., Schwartzberg, P.L., Hager, G.L., O'shea, J.J., 2011. Early Th1 cell differentiation is marked by a Tfh cell-like transition. Immunity 35, 919–931.

Nurieva, R.I., Chung, Y., Hwang, D., Yang, X.O., Kang, H.S., Ma, L., Wang, Y.H., Watowich, S.S., Jetten, A.M., Tian, Q., Dong, C., 2008. Generation of T follicular helper cells is mediated by interleukin-21 but independent of T helper 1, 2, or 17 cell lineages. Immunity 29, 138–149.

Nurieva, R.I., Chung, Y., Martinez, G.J., Yang, X.O., Tanaka, S., Matskevitch, T.D., Wang, Y.H., Dong, C., 2009. Bcl6 mediates the development of T follicular helper cells. Science 325, 1001–1005.

Odegard, J.M., Marks, B.R., Diplacido, L.D., Poholek, A.C., Kono, D.H., Dong, C., Flavell, R.A., Craft, J., 2008. ICOS-dependent extrafollicular helper T cells elicit IgG production via IL-21 in systemic autoimmunity. J. Exp. Med. 205, 2873–2886.

Okada, T., Miller, M.J., Parker, I., Krummel, M.F., Neighbors, M., Hartley, S.B., O'garra, A., Cahalan, M.D., Cyster, J.G., 2005. Antigen-engaged B cells undergo chemotaxis toward the T zone and form motile conjugates with helper T cells. PLoS Biol. 3, e150.

Okada, Y., Wu, D., Trynka, G., Raj, T., Terao, C., Ikari, K., Kochi, Y., Ohmura, K., Suzuki, A., Yoshida, S., Graham, R.R., Manoharan, A., Ortmann, W., Bhangale, T., Denny, J.C., Carroll, R.J., Eyler, A.E., Greenberg, J.D., Kremer, J.M., Pappas, D.A., Jiang, L., Yin, J., Ye, L., Su, D.F., Yang, J., Xie, G., Keystone, E., Westra, H.J., Esko, T., Metspalu, A., Zhou, X., Gupta, N., Mirel, D., Stahl, E.A., Diogo, D., Cui, J., Liao, K., Guo, M.H., Myouzen, K., Kawaguchi, T., Coenen, M.J., Van Riel, P.L., Van De Laar, M.A., Guchelaar, H.J., Huizinga, T.W., Dieude, P., Mariette, X., Bridges Jr., S.L., Zhernakova, A., Toes, R.E., Tak, P.P., Miceli-Richard, C., Bang, S.Y., Lee, H.S., Martin, J., Gonzalez-Gay, M.A., Rodriguez-Rodriguez, L., Rantapaa-Dahlqvist, S., Arlestig, L., Choi, H.K., Kamatani, Y., Galan, P., Lathrop, M., Consortium, R., Consortium, G., Eyre, S., Bowes, J., Barton, A., De Vries, N., Moreland, L.W., Criswell, L.A., Karlson, E.W., Taniguchi, A., Yamada, R., Kubo, M., Liu, J.S., Bae, S.C., Worthington, J., Padyukov, L., Klareskog, L., Gregersen, P.K., Raychaudhuri, S., Stranger, B.E., De Jager, P.L., Franke, L., Visscher, P.M., Brown, M.A., Yamanaka, H., Mimori, T., Takahashi, A., Xu, H., Behrens, T.W., Siminovitch, K.A., Momohara, S., Matsuda, F., Yamamoto, K., Plenge, R.M., 2014. Genetics of rheumatoid arthritis contributes to biology and drug discovery. Nature 506, 376–381.

Peters, A., Pitcher, L.A., Sullivan, J.M., Mitsdoerffer, M., Acton, S.E., Franz, B., Wucherpfennig, K., Turley, S., Carroll, M.C., Sobel, R.A., Bettelli, E., Kuchroo, V.K., 2011. Th17 cells induce ectopic lymphoid follicles in central nervous system tissue inflammation. Immunity 35, 986–996.

Pitzalis, C., Jones, G.W., Bombardieri, M., Jones, S.A., 2014. Ectopic lymphoid-like structures in infection, cancer and autoimmunity. Nat. Rev. Immunol. 14, 447–462.

Porwit-Ksiazek, A., Ksiazek, T., Biberfeld, P., 1983. Leu 7+ (HNK-1+) cells. I. Selective compartmentalization of Leu 7+ cells with different immunophenotypes in lymphatic tissues and blood. Scand. J. Immunol. 18, 485–493.

Qi, H., Cannons, J.L., Klauschen, F., Schwartzberg, P.L., Germain, R.N., 2008. SAP-controlled T-B cell interactions underlie germinal centre formation. Nature 455, 764–769.

Rasheed, A.U., Rahn, H.P., Sallusto, F., Lipp, M., Muller, G., 2006. Follicular B helper T cell activity is confined to CXCR5(hi)ICOS(hi) CD4 T cells and is independent of CD57 expression. Eur. J. Immunol. 36, 1892–1903.

Romme Christensen, J., Bornsen, L., Ratzer, R., Piehl, F., Khademi, M., Olsson, T., Sorensen, P.S., Sellebjerg, F., 2013. Systemic inflammation in progressive multiple sclerosis involves follicular T-helper, Th17- and activated B-cells and correlates with progression. PLoS One 8, e57820.

Schaerli, P., Willimann, K., Lang, A.B., Lipp, M., Loetscher, P., Moser, B., 2000. CXC chemokine receptor 5 expression defines follicular homing T cells with B cell helper function. J. Exp. Med. 192, 1553–1562.

Schaerli, P., Loetscher, P., Moser, B., 2001. Cutting edge: induction of follicular homing precedes effector Th cell development. J. Immunol. 167, 6082–6086.

Schmitt, N., Morita, R., Bourdery, L., Bentebibel, S.E., Zurawski, S.M., Banchereau, J., Ueno, H., 2009. Human dendritic cells induce the differentiation of interleukin-21-producing T follicular helper-like cells through interleukin-12. Immunity 31, 158–169.

Schmitt, N., Bustamante, J., Bourdery, L., Bentebibel, S.E., Boisson-Dupuis, S., Hamlin, F., Tran, M.V., Blankenship, D., Pascual, V., Savino, D.A., Banchereau, J., Casanova, J.L., Ueno, H., 2013. IL-12 receptor beta1 deficiency alters in vivo T follicular helper cell response in humans. Blood 121, 3375–3385.

Schmitt, N., Bentebibel, S.E., Ueno, H., 2014a. Phenotype and functions of memory Tfh cells in human blood. Trends Immunol. 35, 436–442.

Schmitt, N., Liu, Y., Bentebibel, S.E., Munagala, I., Bourdery, L., Venuprasad, K., Banchereau, J., Ueno, H., 2014b. The cytokine TGF-beta co-opts signaling via STAT3-STAT4 to promote the differentiation of human TFH cells. Nat. Immunol. 15, 856–865.

Segura, E., Valladeau-Guilemond, J., Donnadieu, M.H., Sastre-Garau, X., Soumelis, V., Amigorena, S., 2012. Characterization of resident and migratory dendritic cells in human lymph nodes. J. Exp. Med. 209, 653–660.

Shulman, Z., Gitlin, A.D., Targ, S., Jankovic, M., Pasqual, G., Nussenzweig, M.C., Victora, G.D., 2013. T follicular helper cell dynamics in germinal centers. Science 341, 673–677.

Shulman, Z., Gitlin, A.D., Weinstein, J.S., Lainez, B., Esplugues, E., Flavell, R.A., Craft, J.E., Nussenzweig, M.C., 2014. Dynamic signaling by T follicular helper cells during germinal center B cell selection. Science 345, 1058–1062.

Sidiropoulos, P.I., Boumpas, D.T., 2004. Lessons learned from anti-CD40L treatment in systemic lupus erythematosus patients. Lupus 13, 391–397.

Simpson, N., Gatenby, P.A., Wilson, A., Malik, S., Fulcher, D.A., Tangye, S.G., Manku, H., Vyse, T.J., Roncador, G., Huttley, G.A., Goodnow, C.C., Vinuesa, C.G., Cook, M.C., 2010. Expansion of circulating T cells resembling follicular helper T cells is a fixed phenotype that identifies a subset of severe systemic lupus erythematosus. Arthritis Rheum. 62, 234–244.

Stranger, B.E., De Jager, P.L., 2012. Coordinating GWAS results with gene expression in a systems immunologic paradigm in autoimmunity. Curr. Opin. Immunol. 24, 544–551.

Suto, A., Kashiwakuma, D., Kagami, S., Hirose, K., Watanabe, N., Yokote, K., Saito, Y., Nakayama, T., Grusby, M.J., Iwamoto, I., Nakajima, H., 2008. Development and characterization of IL-21-producing CD4+ T cells. J. Exp. Med. 205, 1369–1379.

Sweet, R.A., Lee, S.K., Vinuesa, C.G., 2012. Developing connections amongst key cytokines and dysregulated germinal centers in autoimmunity. Curr. Opin. Immunol. 24, 658–664.

Tangye, S.G., Ma, C.S., Brink, R., Deenick, E.K., 2013. The good, the bad and the ugly—TFH cells in human health and disease. Nat. Rev. Immunol. 13, 412–426.

Tarlinton, D.M., 2008. Evolution in miniature: selection, survival and distribution of antigen reactive cells in the germinal centre. Immunol. Cell Biol. 86, 133–138.

Ueno, H., Klechevsky, E., Morita, R., Aspord, C., Cao, T., Matsui, T., Di Pucchio, T., Connolly, J., Fay, J.W., Pascual, V., Palucka, A.K., Banchereau, J., 2007. Dendritic cell subsets in health and disease. Immunol. Rev. 219, 118–142.

Ueno, H., Schmitt, N., Klechevsky, E., Pedroza-Gonzalez, A., Matsui, T., Zurawski, G., Oh, S., Fay, J., Pascual, V., Banchereau, J., Palucka, K., 2010. Harnessing human dendritic cell subsets for medicine. Immunol. Rev. 234, 199–212.

Ueno, H., Banchereau, J., Vinuesa, C.G., 2015. Pathophysiology of T follicular helper cells in humans and mice. Nat. Immunol. 16, 142–152.

Victora, G.D., Schwickert, T.A., Fooksman, D.R., Kamphorst, A.O., Meyer-Hermann, M., Dustin, M.L., Nussenzweig, M.C., 2010. Germinal center dynamics revealed by multiphoton microscopy with a photoactivatable fluorescent reporter. Cell 143, 592–605.

Vinuesa, C.G., Cook, M.C., Angelucci, C., Athanasopoulos, V., Rui, L., Hill, K.M., Yu, D., Domaschenz, H., Whittle, B., Lambe, T., Roberts, I.S., Copley, R.R., Bell, J.I., Cornall, R.J., Goodnow, C.C., 2005. A RING-type ubiquitin ligase family member required to repress follicular helper T cells and autoimmunity. Nature 435, 452–458.

Vinuesa, C.G., Sanz, I., Cook, M.C., 2009. Dysregulation of germinal centres in autoimmune disease. Nat. Rev. Immunol. 9, 845–857.

Vogelzang, A., Mcguire, H.M., Yu, D., Sprent, J., Mackay, C.R., King, C., 2008. A fundamental role for interleukin-21 in the generation of T follicular helper cells. Immunity 29, 127–137.

Walker, L.S., Gulbranson-Judge, A., Flynn, S., Brocker, T., Raykundalia, C., Goodall, M., Forster, R., Lipp, M., Lane, P., 1999. Compromised OX40 function in CD28-deficient mice is linked with failure to develop CXC chemokine receptor 5-positive CD4 cells and germinal centers. J. Exp. Med. 190, 1115–1122.

Wang, J., Shan, Y., Jiang, Z., Feng, J., Li, C., Ma, L., Jiang, Y., 2013. High frequencies of activated B cells and T follicular helper cells are correlated with disease activity in patients with new-onset rheumatoid arthritis. Clin. Exp. Immunol. 174, 212–220.

Wollenberg, I., Agua-Doce, A., Hernandez, A., Almeida, C., Oliveira, V.G., Faro, J., Graca, L., 2011. Regulation of the germinal center reaction by Foxp3+ follicular regulatory T cells. J. Immunol. 187, 4553–4560.

Wu, H.J., Ivanov, I., Darce, J., Hattori, K., Shima, T., Umesaki, Y., Littman, D.R., Benoist, C., Mathis, D., 2010. Gut-residing segmented filamentous bacteria drive autoimmune arthritis via T helper 17 cells. Immunity 32, 815–827.

Xu, H., Li, X., Liu, D., Li, J., Zhang, X., Chen, X., Hou, S., Peng, L., Xu, C., Liu, W., Zhang, L., Qi, H., 2013. Follicular T-helper cell recruitment governed by bystander B cells and ICOS-driven motility. Nature 496, 523–527.

Yoshida, Y., Yoshimi, R., Yoshii, H., Kim, D., Dey, A., Xiong, H., Munasinghe, J., Yazawa, I., O'donovan, M.J., Maximova, O.A., Sharma, S., Zhu, J., Wang, H., Morse 3rd., H.C., Ozato, K., 2014. The transcription factor IRF8 activates integrin-mediated TGF-beta signaling and promotes neuroinflammation. Immunity 40, 187–198.

Yu, D., Tan, A.H., Hu, X., Athanasopoulos, V., Simpson, N., Silva, D.G., Hutloff, A., Giles, K.M., Leedman, P.J., Lam, K.P., Goodnow, C.C., Vinuesa, C.G., 2007. Roquin represses autoimmunity by limiting inducible T-cell co-stimulator messenger RNA. Nature 450, 299–303.

Yu, D., Rao, S., Tsai, L.M., Lee, S.K., He, Y., Sutcliffe, E.L., Srivastava, M., Linterman, M., Zheng, L., Simpson, N., Ellyard, J.I., Parish, I.A., Ma, C.S., Li, Q.J., Parish, C.R., Mackay, C.R., Vinuesa, C.G., 2009. The transcriptional repressor Bcl-6 directs T follicular helper cell lineage commitment. Immunity 31, 457–468.

Yurasov, S., Nussenzweig, M.C., 2007. Regulation of autoreactive antibodies. Curr. Opin. Rheumatol. 19, 421–426.

Yurasov, S., Wardemann, H., Hammersen, J., Tsuiji, M., Meffre, E., Pascual, V., Nussenzweig, M.C., 2005. Defective B cell tolerance checkpoints in systemic lupus erythematosus. J. Exp. Med. 201, 703–711.

Yurasov, S., Tiller, T., Tsuiji, M., Velinzon, K., Pascual, V., Wardemann, H., Nussenzweig, M.C., 2006. Persistent expression of autoantibodies in SLE patients in remission. J. Exp. Med. 203, 2255–2261.

Zhu, C., Ma, J., Liu, Y., Tong, J., Tian, J., Chen, J., Tang, X., Xu, H., Lu, L., Wang, S., 2012. Increased frequency of follicular helper T cells in patients with autoimmune thyroid disease. J. Clin. Endocrinol. Metab. 97, 943–950.

Zotos, D., Coquet, J.M., Zhang, Y., Light, A., D'costa, K., Kallies, A., Corcoran, L.M., Godfrey, D.I., Toellner, K.M., Smyth, M.J., Nutt, S.L., Tarlinton, D.M., 2010. IL-21 regulates germinal center B cell differentiation and proliferation through a B cell-intrinsic mechanism. J. Exp. Med. 207, 365–378.

CHAPTER 8

Regulatory T Cells

Translational Immunology: Mechanisms and Pharmacologic Approaches

M. Monteiro[1], A. Agua-Doce[1], R.I. Azevedo[1], J.F. Lacerda[1,2], L. Graca[1]
[1]Instituto de Medicina Molecular, University of Lisbon, Lisbon, Portugal
[2]Hospital de Santa Maria, Lisbon, Portugal

Contents

Translational Immunology
http://dx.doi.org/10.1016/B978-0-12-801577-3.00009-5

1. INTRODUCTION

Permanent exposure of the organism to antigens, including self, forces the immune system to opt between mounting an effector immune response to eliminate the source of antigen, or adapting to its presence. The state of unresponsiveness to an antigen to which the system has been previously exposed is called *immune tolerance*—a property of the adaptive immune system. Tolerance is, thus, antigen specific, in contrast with therapeutic immune suppression and immunodeficiency, which affect lymphocytes of many specificities.

Healthy individuals are tolerant to their self-antigens, but tolerance can also be naturally induced to foreign, harmless antigens, such as those present in food or the environment. Breakdown of self-tolerance results in immune reactions against autologous cells and tissues, originating autoimmune diseases, and failure on the mechanisms underlying tolerance to environmental antigens can lead to allergy. Therefore, understanding how tolerance to self and nonself antigens is achieved has become a major goal of immunologists for several decades.

Several mechanisms can contribute to immune tolerance. During lymphocyte development, some B and T cells acquire receptors capable of recognizing self-antigens as a result of random B or T cell receptor rearrangements. Most of these self-reactive lymphocytes undergo clonal deletion during maturation in the bone marrow and thymus, respectively. This early self-defense mechanism is generally known as *central tolerance*. Nevertheless, self-reactive lymphocytes may escape elimination during negative selection. Several additional mechanisms ensure these mature self-reactive cells become incapable of attacking self-tissues when they reach the periphery. The manifestation of these mechanisms is called *peripheral tolerance*. For instance, when T cells encounter the specific antigen in absence of appropriate costimulatory signals, they become functionally unresponsive—a phenomenon termed *anergy*. Alternatively, self-reactive T cells may undergo apoptosis if they receive defective costimulation upon antigen exposure, or if they go through repetitive TCR stimulation, which induces the expression of death receptors and their ligands. Such *deletion* of mature T cells in consequence of antigen recognition is also called activation-induced cell death (AICD). However, the most relevant feature of peripheral tolerance is the *active regulation* (or suppression) of effector cells exerted by a specialized subset of CD4 T lymphocytes expressing the forkhead box protein 3 (Foxp3) transcription factor and called *regulatory T cells* (*Tregs*) (Josefowicz et al., 2012).

In this chapter we will review and summarize the current knowledge of Treg cells' contribution for tolerance maintenance, their mechanisms of action, their functional diversity, and their therapeutic application.

2. GENERAL FEATURES OF REGULATORY T CELLS

2.1 The discovery of regulatory T cells

For many years, scientists tried to prove the concept that a specialized subset of cells would be capable of controlling the response of other immune cells. In the 1970s, this was a hot topic, as results from many studies were consistent with the existence of a T lymphocyte population endowed with suppressor properties. At the time, although many research groups were committed to find these "suppressor cells," available techniques failed to prove their existence. In addition, discoveries made by Mosmann and Coffman in the 1980s, that CD4 T cells could differentiate toward Th1 and Th2 phenotypes that cross-regulated each other's effector functions, established the concept of immune deviation (Mosmann et al., 1986). Although immune deviation is considered today to be a function of immune regulation rather than a form of tolerance, at the time it offered a plausible explanation for many of the results that were being interpreted as immune suppression, and raised a generalized skepticism about the existence of regulatory cells.

Reliable evidence supporting the existence of Tregs was provided only in the 1990s by several independent studies. Le Douarin's group performed a series of studies using cell engraftment strategies in avian and mouse chimeras showing that thymic epithelium induces the formation of cells capable of promoting *dominant tolerance*, which can be defined as the capacity of modulating and/or suppressing the activation, proliferation, and function of cells through nondepleting, contact-dependent regulatory mechanisms [reviewed by (Le Douarin et al., 1996)]. Mason's group showed that low expression levels of CD45RC (in rats) or CD45RB (in mice) on peripheral CD4 T cells and CD4 single-positive thymocytes correlated with regulatory behavior, leading them to propose that production of Tregs would be the "third function of the thymus" [reviewed by (Seddon and Mason, 2000)]. In experimental models of transplantation tolerance, induced with CD4-blockade, it was shown tolerance was mediated by CD4 T cells that could regulate naïve T cells, namely leading to their conversion into a "regulatory" pool; a phenomenon that was termed *infectious tolerance* (Graca et al., 2000; Qin et al., 1993). However, a more specific cell-surface marker of Tregs was still lacking. It was Sakaguchi and collaborators who identified CD25, the α-chain of interleukin-2 (IL-2) receptor, as a marker that could best discriminate Tregs from other lymphocytes (Sakaguchi et al., 1995). CD25 is expressed by 5-10% of mature CD4 T lymphocytes in normal naïve mice and humans, which comprise a subpopulation of $CD45RB^{low}$ CD4 T cells. Reconstitution of athymic mice with cell suspensions depleted of $CD25^+$ CD4 T cells leads to severe multiorgan autoimmunity, which can be prevented if both $CD25^{+}$ and $CD25^{-}$ CD4 T lymphocytes are coadministered.

2.2 Phenotype of regulatory T cells

Tregs constitute approximately 10% of peripheral CD4 T lymphocytes. In addition to CD25, they express constitutively other cell-surface molecules that may be used to distinguish them from other CD4 T cells. Among others, Tregs express cytotoxic T lymphocyte antigen-4 (CTLA-4), membrane-bound transforming growth factor (TGF)-β, OX-40, glucurocorticoid-induced TNFR-related receptor (GITR), CD39, CD73, lymphocyte activation gene-3 (LAG-3), and fibrinogen-like protein-2 (FGL-2). These surface receptors are mostly involved in Treg activation, trafficking, and suppressive function.

Activated T cells can also express many of these molecules, but levels of expression are higher on Tregs than conventional T cells. This is the case, for instance, of CD25, GITR, CTLA-4, CD103, and OX40, which for being expressed at higher levels on Tregs create a competitive advantage over autoreactive T lymphocytes for accessing their respective ligands, thus providing a mechanism that favors immune suppression and tolerance over autoimmunity.

A more detailed discussion about the molecules involved in Treg-mediated immune suppression is provided in Section 4.

2.3 The Foxp3 master transcription factor

Foxp3 is the transcription factor driving the genetic program of regulatory T cell development. It is critical not only for their generation, but also for their function. Mice with a dysfunctional or deleted *foxp3* gene manifest severe multiorgan autoimmune disease associated with the absence of $CD25^{+}$ Tregs (Brunkow et al., 2001; Fontenot et al., 2003; Hori et al., 2003; Khattri et al., 2003). Several mouse models of overexpression, deletion, and report of Foxp3 gene expression were developed over the past 15 years, helping to uncover the cellular and molecular mechanisms of Treg cell development and function (Khattri et al., 2001, 2003; Fontenot et al., 2005; Miyao et al., 2012).

In humans, mutations on the *FOXP3* gene cause IPEX (immune dysregulation, polyendocrinopathy, enteropathy, X-linked syndrome), a rare condition characterized by a wide spectrum of autoimmune manifestations and associated with the absence of Treg cells (Bennett et al., 2001; Owen et al., 2003; Tommasini et al., 2002; Wildin et al., 2002). The drastic phenotype resulting from dysfunctional *FOXP3* gene expression established the importance of Treg cells for the prevention of wasting disease and death resulting from uncontrolled lymphoproliferation and attack of self-tissues. But in addition to restraining autoimmunity, the potential of Treg cells to suppress a wide range of immune responses has been progressively appreciated. They are capable of preventing collateral tissue damage triggered by immune responses against microbes or allergens, maintaining homeostasis with the commensal microbiota, facilitating maternal tolerance to allogeneic fetus during pregnancy, promoting therapeutic tolerance toward transplanted organs, and sometimes helping tumor cells or certain pathogens to escape from immune surveillance (Demengeot et al., 2006; Izcue et al., 2009; Bilate and Lafaille, 2012; Nagano et al., 2012; Nutsch and Hsieh, 2012; Aluvihare et al., 2004; Waldmann et al., 2006; Yamaguchi and Sakaguchi, 2006). Recent studies have even suggested that Treg functions go beyond regulation of immune responses and also mediate regulation of tissue homeostasis in general (Burzyn et al., 2013). Because of their critical role in several immune and nonimmune processes and because of their therapeutic potential, Treg cells have become an appealing object of research. The full understanding of mechanisms of their development and function is fundamental for the rationale of novel strategies to correct defects in Treg cells that may lead to autoimmunity, or to manipulate them in the clinic. Therapeutic modulation of specific Treg function could be used to boost their activity and ameliorate suppression of autoimmunity, or to limit Treg cell differentiation, trafficking, and/or activity to dampen their suppression effect over beneficial immune responses, such as the ones directed to tumors.

3. GENERATION OF REGULATORY T CELLS

3.1 In the thymus

Like any other T lymphocyte, Treg cells develop primarily in the thymus. Thymic commitment to the Treg lineage occurs after positive selection and development of CD4 single-positive thymocytes. These interact with epithelial and dendritic cells (DCs) in the thymic medulla that present extrathymic tissue-specific self-peptides in consequence of active expression of the gene *AIRE*. Thymocytes establishing successful interactions are selected and will establish the population of natural, thymic-derived Treg (nTreg or tTreg) cells, which have a TCR repertoire biased toward low-abundance agonist self-antigens (Weissler and Caton, 2014).

TCR stimulation is a key aspect of tTreg development. Relatively high interaction between TCRs and self-peptide/MHC is critical to provide strong signaling, but not so high as to induce apoptosis. High TCR signaling, in concert with costimulation, activates nuclear factor of activated T cells (NF-AT), activator protein-1 (AP-1), and CARMA1/Bcl10/Malt1-dependent activation of NF-κB, which directly interacts with *FOXP3* inducing its expression. Engagement of TGF-β-dependent Smad3 and IL-2-dependent signal transducer and activator of transcription 5 (STAT5) provide survival and growth signals that intensify *FOXP3* gene expression. In addition to IL-2, other γ-chain cytokines, namely IL-7 and IL-15, can contribute to the development of tTreg. However, IL-7 and IL-15 cannot fully compensate for IL-2-derived signaling, as demonstrated by reduced STAT5 phosphorylation and fewer Treg numbers in IL-2Rβ-deficient mice (Vang et al., 2008).

High levels of Foxp3 are necessary for tTreg to complete their maturation and also to induce the Treg functional program (Yuan and Malek, 2012; Morikawa and Sakaguchi, 2014). Mature tTreg cells leave the thymus and migrate to the periphery where they critically suppress self-reactive lymphocytes that have escaped negative selection in the thymus.

3.2 In the periphery

Activation of conventional CD4 T cells under specific protolerogenic conditions in the periphery induces expression of the *FOXP3* gene, resulting in the generation of peripheral Treg (pTreg cells, previously known as induced or iTreg). This process is especially important, albeit not restricted to, tolerance establishment at mucosal surfaces, where the immune system must be carefully regulated to avoid exacerbated inflammatory responses to food and airborne antigens, or to commensal microbiota. Uncontrolled immune responses to those antigens lead to severe tissue damage, which is on the basis of inflammatory bowel diseases (IBD), for instance. Those environmental antigens shape the diverse TCR repertoire of conventional CD4 T cells, selecting specificities for microflora-derived peptides. Mucosal Tregs thus contain a mixture of tTregs and pTregs, as the two populations are necessary for tolerance to be effective at those sites. Therefore, to successfully prevent autoimmunity in mice lacking a functional *foxp3* gene, the cotransfer of tTregs and conventional CD4 T cells, which can develop into pTregs, would be required (Haribhai et al., 2011).

The gut-associated lymphoid tissue (GALT) provides a particularly suitable microenvironment for the development of pTreg. First, mucosal sites are especially rich in TGF-β, produced by epithelial cells (Barnard et al., 1989, 1991). When conventional CD4 T cells receive appropriate TCR and costimulatory signals along with stimulation through the TGF-β receptors, Smad3 is phosphorylated and activates the *FOXP3* gene, prompting the differentiation of pTreg cells (Mucida et al., 2005; Tone et al., 2008; Zheng et al., 2010). Secondly, there are specialized populations of antigen-presenting cells (APCs) in the GALT that support local pTreg induction and expansion. These are CD103-expressing DCs that reside in the small intestinal *lamina propria* and mesenteric lymph nodes. $CD103^+$ DCs are able to generate bioactive TGF-β from its latent, membrane-coupled form, which has been shown to induce Foxp3 upon contact with conventional CD4 T cells. Furthermore, $CD103^+$ DCs isolated from the GALT express high amounts of retinaldehyde dehydrogenases, the necessary enzymes for the production of retinoic acid (RA) from dietary or stored vitamin A. $CD103^+$ DC-derived RA acts on CD4 T cells through RARα, promoting Foxp3 induction (Mucida et al., 2007; Coombes et al., 2007; Sun et al., 2007; Hill et al., 2008). Remarkably, release of RA by

CD103$^+$ DCs also promotes the expression of the gut homing receptors integrin α4β7 and CCR9 on Treg cells, thereby directing their homing potential to the gut (Grainger et al., 2014). In concert with CD103$^+$ DCs, a specialized population of gut-resident CX3CR1^{high} macrophages also participates in the establishment of oral tolerance. They are proficient secretors of IL-10, an antiinflammatory cytokine with reported capacity of expanding Treg cells and restraining other APCs from producing proinflammatory cytokines (Murai et al., 2009; Grainger et al., 2014).

It is relevant to note that, in addition to commensal pathogens living in the mucosa, other pathogenic organisms have developed strategies to interfere with Treg function, thereby avoiding elimination. One fine example is infection with helminth parasites, which absolutely require pTreg induction to establish chronic infection. The crucial role of Treg cells is strikingly supported by experimental evidence of parasite effective elimination upon Treg depletion in mice, and also by the observation of higher Treg cell levels in the peripheral blood of patients infected with filarial nematodes or schistosomes (Taylor et al., 2009; Nausch et al., 2011; Finlay et al., 2014). Manipulation of Treg cells is achieved through the release of excretory/secretory (ES) products by helminths, as well as specific molecules such as TGF-β homologs. These mechanisms can act directly on conventional CD4 T cells *via* TGF-β receptors, leading to Foxp3 induction and pTreg formation, or indirectly through DC modulation, promoting DC hyporesponsiveness and consequent failure on upregulation of costimulatory receptors and proinflammatory cytokines (Finlay et al., 2014).

During pregnancy, pTreg cells also play a critical role in maternal immune tolerance toward the fetus. Although inside the uterus, fetal tissues express paternal alloantigens able to induce immune responses that may lead to rejection if effective tolerance is not established. One of the mechanisms operating during pregnancy to avoid an immune attack of the fetus is an increase in Treg levels. Heightened Treg frequencies are observed in the peripheral blood at early pregnancy, being the consequence of altered Treg homing properties, which translocate Treg cells from the lymph nodes to the periphery. In addition, increased pTreg generation and accumulation in the placenta are also observed. The observation that tTreg alone fail to protect the fetus from maternal effector T cells indicated that pTreg cells are the population able to effectively contribute to tolerance establishment toward the fetus (Samstein et al., 2012; Rowe et al., 2012).

3.3 *In vitro*

Foxp3 expression can also be induced *in vitro* upon stimulation of conventional CD4 T cells in presence of TGF-β. Because they were generated *in vitro*, they were named *in vitro*-induced Treg (iTreg) cells (Chen et al., 2003). Like tTreg cells, induction of iTreg is critically dependent on TCR signal strength, TGF-β, and IL-2 (Graca et al., 2005; Davidson et al., 2007; Oliveira et al., 2011). As expected, CD28 costimulation significantly decreases the concentration of plate-bound anti-CD3 needed to achieve maximal Foxp3 expression *in vitro* (Chen et al., 2003). CD28 costimulation is important because it boosts endogenous IL-2 secretion. In conditions of low TCR signal strength, TGF-β can also be endogenously secreted by CD4 T cells at sufficient levels to induce Foxp3 expression. Experimentally, this can be achieved by stimulation of conventional CD4 T cells with reduced concentrations of plate-bound anti-CD3 or low-dose peptide-loaded DCs or, alternatively, by adding nondepleting monoclonal antibodies (MAb) that interfere with the immune synapse stability, such as anti-CD4. Of note, generation of iTreg in the absence of exogenous TGF-β is possible, but the yield of iTreg is considerably low (5- to 50-fold less than with addition of TGF-β) (Oliveira et al., 2011). Therefore, at low TCR-signal strength conditions, *in vitro* Foxp3 induction requires lower concentrations of exogenous TGF-β, and vice versa.

Due to interest of reinfusing Treg cells in patients suffering from autoimmune disorders, many studies have been trying to define the optimal conditions to generate these cells *in vitro* and to evaluate their efficacy. One of the major concerns is that iTreg cells have a TCR repertoire biased for nonself antigens. Therefore, they might have limited ability of effectively suppress autoimmune diseases that developed in consequence of a lack of Treg cells specific for self-antigens. Second, Foxp3 expression in iTreg is less stable than in tTreg, as discussed below, and several reports suggested that Foxp3 is rapidly downregulated in iTregs following their transfer *in vivo*. Third, iTreg homing potential is different from tTreg, as they lose CD62L expression during *in vitro* conversion, which might compromise their ability to enter the lymph nodes. Nonetheless, transfer of iTreg to neonatal Foxp3-deficient mice abrogates all the pathologic autoimmune manifestations in both lymphoid sites and tissues (Huter et al., 2008), and in several independent reports iTregs were shown to suppress effector function in distinct disease models including autoimmune gastritis (DiPaolo et al., 2007), experimental autoimmune encephalomyelitis (EAE) (Selvaraj and Geiger, 2008), and diabetes (Weber et al., 2006).

3.4 Regulation and stability of the *FOXP3* gene

Transcriptional regulation of *FOXP3* is controlled by factors that target the gene promoter and conserved noncoding sequence 1 (CNS1), 2 (CNS2), and 3 (CNS3) (Kim and Leonard, 2007; Tone et al., 2008; Zheng et al., 2010). CNS1 contains one enhancer whose activity is regulated by the transcription factors Smad3, NFAT, and AP-1 (Xu et al., 2010; Tone et al., 2008). A second enhancer, located in CNS2, contains highly methylated CpG sequences in Foxp3^{-} T cells, but is demethylated in Foxp3^{+} Tregs (Kim and Leonard, 2007). For this reason, CNS2 was denominated Treg cell-specific demethylated region (TSDR) (Polansky et al., 2008; Floess et al., 2007). Demethylation of the CNS2 region is mediated by the transcription factor Stat5, which critically depends upon IL-2 (Zorn et al., 2006) and TGF-β receptor signaling (Ogawa et al., 2014), thereby illustrating the importance of IL-2 and TGF-β for the development and function of Tregs. Stat5 is a key regulator of chromatin remodeling to make CNS2 region accessible for transcription, whereas AP-1 and Creb exert enhancer 2 activity (Ogawa et al., 2014).

Importantly, CNS2 was shown to be essential for heritable maintenance of Foxp3 expression in dividing Treg cells, with demethylation of TSDR correlating with the stability of Foxp3 expression (Kim and Leonard, 2007; Tone et al., 2008; Zheng et al., 2010). Notably, while tTregs and pTregs have a largely demethylated TSDR, TGF-β-induced iTregs show no or only limited TSDR demethylation (Polansky et al., 2008; Floess et al., 2007). Instable Foxp3 expression in iTregs severely limits the usefulness of iTregs adoptive transfers as a cellular therapy for immune undesired reactions (Beres et al., 2011; Rossetti et al., 2015). In fact, *ex vivo* expansion of endogenous Tregs with rapamycin has proved to be a better approach to treat autoimmune diseases than using iTregs (Rossetti et al., 2015).

Despite their stable Foxp3 expression, under lymphopenic conditions tTregs can switch from regulatory to effector phenotype (Komatsu et al., 2009) and the same can be observed in lymphoid microenvironments such as Peyer's patches (Tsuji et al., 2009).

Also, activation of conventional T cells in humans promotes a transient upregulation of Foxp3. However, such brief Foxp3 expression does not correlate with acquisition of suppressor function (Tran et al., 2007).

3.5 Discrimination of regulatory T cell populations from different origins

A marker claimed to identify tTreg cells is Helios, a member of the Ikaros transcription factor family. These transcription factor proteins bind DNA as homodimers or heterodimers, regulating gene expression through chromatin remodeling. Expression of Helios was reported to be exclusive of cells in the adult thymus (Kelley et al., 1998). Although deletion of Helios does not affect the Treg development in the thymus or their maintenance in the periphery, nor has any reported effect on Treg suppressive function, it is faithfully expressed by Foxp3$^+$ thymocytes at CD4 single-positive stage. Consequently, the first Treg cells arising in the thymus and seeding the spleen in mice during the first 12 days of life, a time frame in which only thymically derived Treg cells have an opportunity to develop, express Helios (Thornton et al., 2010; Shevach and Thornton, 2014). However, Helios expression was shown not to be restricted to tTreg, being expressed at low levels by conventional T cells under certain conditions, as antigen-specific Foxp3$^-$ CD4 T cells expressing Helios can be found at early time points after immunization. These observations strongly suggest those conventional T cells expressing Helios might sustain Helios expression when converting to Treg in the periphery or *in vitro*. Therefore, although useful to identify tTreg, the Helios-expressing population might include pTreg contaminants.

Another molecule abundantly expressed among the tTreg population is neuropilin-1 (Nrp-1) (Weiss et al., 2012; Yadav et al., 2012). This transmembrane receptor, which can be expressed by many cell types, mediates homotypic interactions between Treg and DCs expressing Nrp-1 at their surface, having a role in Treg suppressive activity and also on the activation of latent TGF-β (Sarris et al., 2008; Glinka and Prud'homme, 2008). Being a protein expressed at the cell membrane, Nrp-1 has an advantage over Helios for the isolation of viable tTreg cells. However, despite coexpression of Nrp-1 and Helios among Helios$^+$ Treg cells, a significant fraction of Helios$^-$ Treg subset (20% to 30%) expresses Nrp-1. One possible explanation is the fact that TGF-β-mediated signaling positively regulates Nrp-1 expression. Because of that, *in vitro*-generated Treg, which require TGF-β for their generation, upregulate Nrp-1. Therefore, conventional CD4 T cells activated at the periphery under inflammatory conditions in which TGF-β is present might, as well, be converted to Nrp-1$^+$ Treg cells (Thornton et al., 2010; Shevach and Thornton, 2014). This fact must be taken into account when using Nrp-1 to isolate or discriminate tTreg from other Treg populations.

4. ACTIVATION AND FUNCTIONAL DIFFERENTIATION OF REGULATORY T CELLS

4.1 Role of TCR stimulation

Anergy upon TCR engagement has been one of the hallmarks of Treg cells (Takahashi et al., 1998; Itoh et al., 1999; Kuniyasu et al., 2000). Nonetheless, studies in mice with Treg cells expressing a transgenic TCR have shown they are highly proliferative *in vivo* in response to antigen (Walker et al., 2003; Klein et al., 2003; Killebrew et al., 2011). Indeed, peptide-pulsed bone marrow-derived DCs injected under the skin have promoted Treg expansion eight- to tenfold (Yamazaki et al., 2003). In these studies, proliferating Tregs showed all the characteristics associated with a regulatory population: no production of IL-2, IFN-γ, or IL-4; no upregulation of CD40L, IL-10 production and, most notably, *in vitro* suppressive capacity (Klein et al., 2003; Walker et al., 2003).

In humans the same trend is observed, even though Treg cells *in vitro* are poor proliferators (Ng et al., 2001; Taams et al., 2001). *Ex vivo*, Treg cells defined as $CD4^+CD25^+CD127^{lo}Foxp3^+$ express the proliferation marker Ki67 fourfold higher than their $CD4^+CD25^-$ T cell counterpart (Vukmanovic-Stejic et al., 2008). In fact, Treg cells with proliferative properties, which can be found in the blood and secondary lymphoid organs, are $CD45RA^-Foxp3^{high}$ and have been called "activated Tregs" (Miyara et al., 2009; Vukmanovic-Stejic et al., 2008; Peters et al., 2013).

Despite their proliferative capacity, Treg cells have a dampened response to TCR stimulation: contrary to effector T cells, Tregs are hyporesponsive to antigenic stimuli *in vivo* and unable to flux Ca^{2+} upon TCR engagement (Gavin et al., 2002). Premature termination of TCR signaling and inhibition of phosphatidyl inositol 3-kinase (PI3K),

AKT, and mTOR induce Foxp3 expression. Conversely, persistent TCR signaling and continued PI3K/AKT/mTOR activity inhibit Foxp3 induction (Sauer et al., 2008), thus demonstrating a crucial role for the TCR/mTOR axis. In contrast to conventional T-cell proliferation and effector response, suppression by Treg does not require ZAP-70 activity (Au-Yeung et al., 2010). On the other hand, Foxp3 can regulate Glut1 through the PI3K/AKT/mTOR pathway, thereby diminishing the ability of Tregs to use glucose (Basu et al., 2015). In line with these evidences, several groups have demonstrated that Treg cells require low TCR signaling for proper differentiation and expansion (Turner et al., 2009, 2014; Long et al., 2011; Oliveira et al., 2011).

Foxp3 shapes the unique genetic program of Tregs by activating and repressing the transcription of several molecules. Hence, Foxp3 has the ability to inhibit IL-2, IL-4, and IFN-γ production through cooperation with NFAT and NF-κB (Bettelli et al., 2005; Hench and Su, 2011). It also activates the expression of genes such as GITR, CD25, and CTLA-4 through binding to the corresponding promoter region (Wu et al., 2006; Chen et al., 2006). Importantly, Treg cells are unique in that they constitutively express the high-affinity IL-2 receptor CD25.

4.2 Role of costimulatory receptors

Resting Treg cells have costimulatory receptors such as OX-40 (Xiao et al., 2012), GITR (Liao et al., 2010), 4-1BB (Schoenbrunn et al., 2012) and TNFR2 (Chen and Oppenheim, 2011). Signaling through costimulatory molecules is of paramount importance for Treg biology. The CD28/B7 signaling not only maintains Treg homeostasis (Salomon et al., 2000), but also cycling and survival (Tang et al., 2003). Inducible costimulator (ICOS), a member of the CD28 superfamily, is broadly expressed in activated and pTregs (Grinberg-Bleyer et al., 2010; Gomez de Aguero et al., 2012). Intriguingly, the expression levels of ICOS correlate with the cytokines expressed by T cells. Hence, intermediate expression of ICOS associates with production of IL-4, IL-5, and IL-13, whereas the highest ICOS expression levels correlates with secretion of IL-10 (Lohning et al., 2003), an inhibitory cytokine important for Treg-mediated suppression and further discussed in Section 4.1.

4.3 Role of cytokines

Treg cells are reliant on IL-2 for cell cycle progression and expression of antiapoptotic proteins, such as Bcl-2 (Pierson et al., 2013; Deng and Podack, 1993). In addition, some reports suggest IL-2 is also important for Treg function. In particular, IL-2 neutralization *in vivo* results in the development of autoimmune gastritis and exacerbated diabetes, whereas IL-2 administration, which increases Treg numbers, protects mice from diabetes and EAE, and induces transplantation tolerance (Setoguchi et al., 2005; Tang et al., 2008; Webster et al., 2009). The contribution of IL-2 for Treg-mediated suppression is further discussed in Section 5.1.

Despite constitutive expression of CD25, Tregs do not produce IL-2 themselves because Foxp3 associates with Runx1 and NFAT to bind to IL-2 promoter, inhibiting transcription. In consequence, Tregs depend upon IL-2 production by other cells, and especially on the balance between the rate of IL-2 production and consumption. Importantly, distinct Treg subpopulations have different requirements for IL-2, as discussed below.

4.4 Regulatory T cell subpopulations

In mice, Treg cells can be subdivided into two subsets: a quiescent $CCR7^{hi}CD44^{lo}CD62L^{hi}$ Treg population named central Treg (cT_R) and a highly proliferative $CCR7^{lo}CD44^{hi}CD62L^{lo}$ effector Treg (eT_R) population. Expression of CCR7 allows cT_R cells to localize primarily within the T cell zones of secondary lymphoid organs, gaining access to IL-2 produced by activated T cells, which is critical for their survival and function. Due to their privileged localization, cT_R cells are the Treg subset that mediates suppression of APCs and autoreactive T cell priming. Conversely, eT_R cells are the prevailing Treg cell population seeding nonlymphoid tissues, where they suppress mostly effector T cells in order to reduce inflammation. Notably, eT_R cells are highly proliferative and depend upon ICOS signaling for survival, but are independent of IL-2 (Smigiel et al., 2014).

Based on CD45RA, CD25, and Foxp3 expression levels, it is possible to identify three different Treg populations in humans. One is $CD45RA^{+}CD25^{low}Foxp3^{low}$ and exhibits a naïve-like behavior. Upon activation, $CD45RA^{+}$ Treg cells proliferate and acquire suppressive capacity, while converting from $CD45RA^{+}$ to $CD45RO^{+}$. The second Treg population is $CD45RA^{-}CD25^{hi}Foxp3^{hi}$ and is considered the subset having effective suppressive capacity. Nevertheless, contrary to the $CD45RA^{+}$ population, $CD45RA^{-}$ Treg cells are very susceptible to death. In both these populations the Foxp3 region is completely demethylated, indicating these cells have active Foxp3 gene transcription. The third Treg population can be identified as $CD45RA^{-}CD25^{low}Foxp3^{low}$. This subset is nonsuppressive, secretes cytokines, and exhibits a higher methylation status in the *FOXP3* gene promoter than the other two populations (Miyara et al., 2009).

4.5 Regulatory T cell trafficking

Efficient regulation of immune responses requires Treg and effector cell migration to be well articulated in space and time. Chemokines are pivotal orchestrators of leukocyte trafficking, defining the tissue tropism, as well as migration of cells within lymphoid organs and from these to nonlymphoid tissues. Accordingly, Treg cells selectively express a broad set of chemokine receptors, which allow them to home to different locations. Expression of those receptors is stringently regulated, as Treg recruitment to tissues results in suppression of both deleterious (eg, autoreactive) and protective (eg, antitumor) immune responses. Therefore, it is not surprising that across evolution pathogens and tumors have selected strategies to recruit Treg cells and escape immune surveillance.

Differential chemokine receptor expression enables Treg patrolling of lymphoid and nonlymphoid tissues. During inflammation, Treg migration to nonlymphoid tissues increases significantly. Engagement of chemokine receptors is defined by the tissue and the type of inflammatory response. For instance, many cytokines produced during immune responses can act directly on Tregs, shaping their functional differentiation, similar to what is observed with effector T cells [reviewed by (Campbell and Koch, 2011)]. This is the case, for instance, for IFN-γ, a cytokine produced by NK, NKT, γδT, Th1, and CD8 T cells in response to intracellular pathogen infections. Despite the active inhibition of pTreg generation by IFN-γ, signaling *via* STAT1 activation promotes T-bet expression in tTreg. T-bet was shown to be required for Treg function and homeostasis in Th1 inflammatory responses. Importantly, T-bet induces the expression of CXCR3, a chemokine receptor critical for Treg (and T effector) migration to the tissues undergoing type 1 inflammation. At the same time, IFN-γ induces the expression of CXCR3 ligands in the inflamed tissue, which are necessary for the recruitment of CXCR3-expressing cells (Koch et al., 2009; Campbell and Koch, 2011). Likewise, Treg expression of interferon regulatory factor 4 (IRF-4), a transcription factor required for the control of IL-4 production by CD4 T cells and for Th2 differentiation, is critical for the expression of CCR8, the chemokine receptor involved in the recruitment of cells during type 2 inflammation, and also for Treg-mediated suppression of IL-4 responses (Zheng et al., 2009). Genetic ablation of STAT3 selectively in Treg cells, in turn, leads to fatal intestinal inflammation triggered by excessive IL-17 production without significant differences in Th1- or Th2-associated cytokines, illustrating the selective regulation of Th17 responses by STAT3-expressing Treg cells (Chaudhry et al., 2009). As expected, STAT3 regulates the expression of CCR6, the chemokine receptor necessary for optimal cell recruitment to sites of Th17-mediated inflammation.

In addition to selective expression of chemokine receptors, T-bet, IRF-4, and STAT3 were reported to regulate the expression of Treg effector molecules, such as IL-10, ICOS, and IL-35, among others. These data suggest that Tregs use different transcriptional regulators associated with Th1, Th2, or Th17 cells to undergo phenotypic and functional specialization and acquire the molecular machinery adequate for effective suppression of specific types of inflammatory responses (Campbell and Koch, 2011). This model has important implications for the therapeutic use of Treg cells, as it implies that only specific subsets of Treg cells will be efficacious in treating Th1-, Th2-, or Th17-driven inflammatory diseases.

5. ACTIVITY OF REGULATORY T CELLS

5.1 Suppression mechanisms

Treg cells use multiple mechanisms to limit the activation of other immune players and ensure dominant tolerance. These include contact-dependent and independent mechanisms that encompass secretion of inhibitory cytokines, cytolysis of target cells, metabolic disruption, and modulation of DC maturation or function (Fig. 1).

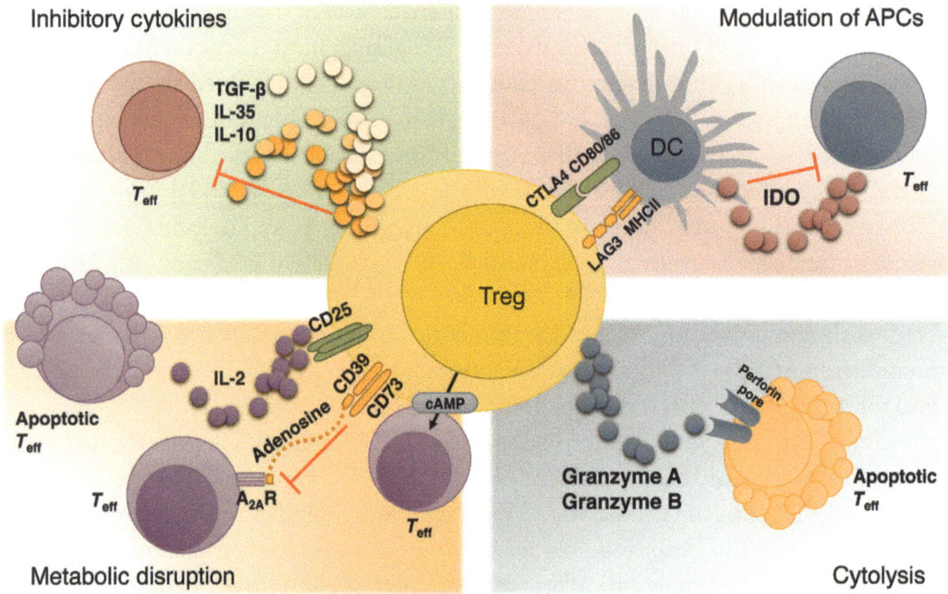

Figure 1 Mechanisms of suppression mediated by Treg cells. Treg cells have been shown capable of producing inhibitory cytokines, such as TGF-β, IL-10, and IL-35, that prevent the activity of effector T cells. In addition, Treg cells constitutively express cell surface molecules, such as CTLA-4 and LAG3, that upon engagement can decrease the ability of APCs to stimulate effector T cell responses. Furthermore, Treg cells can modulate the local availability of molecules that are critical for effector T cell responses, namely promote a decrease in IL-2 or an increase in adenosine. Finally it has been reported that Treg cells can directly trigger the lysis of target cells. Citations to primary literature are present in the main text.

Expression of surface receptors, such as CTLA-4 and LAG-3, are involved in Treg-mediated contact-dependent suppression and endow Treg cells with competitive advantage for interaction with APCs. *CTLA-4*, expressed by Tregs, competes with CD28, expressed by conventional T cells, for their common ligands CD80 and CD86 on the surface of APCs. The higher affinity of CTLA-4 for CD80/CD86 ligands deprives conventional T cells of adequate costimulation through CD28, thereby leading to defective effector T cell activation (Yokosuka et al., 2010). In addition, upon CTLA-4 interaction, expression of CD80/CD86 is downregulated from the surface of APCs, which also impacts T cell activation (Cederbom et al., 2000; Oderup et al., 2006; Wing et al., 2008). Finally, interaction with CTLA-4 activates in DCs the expression of tryptophan catabolizing enzyme indoleamine 2,3-dioxygenase (*IDO*), promoting T-cell suppression by local depletion of tryptophan and induction of apoptosis *via* tryptophan catabolites (Grohmann et al., 2002; Fallarino et al., 2003). In turn, expression of *LAG-3*, a protein that binds MHC class II with high affinity, enhances the interaction between Treg and

DCs and inhibits DC maturation, decreasing their immunostimulatory capacity (Workman et al., 2004; Huang et al., 2004; Liang et al., 2008). Hence, not only CTLA-4 and LAG-3 hamper the access of conventional T lymphocytes to APCs, but also exert on the latter immune modulator effects that prevent them from effectively activating and sustaining immune responses.

Studies with human cells suggest that Tregs may also be able to modulate the function of monocytes and macrophages (Taams et al., 2005; Tiemessen et al., 2007). Although the exact mechanism by which this is achieved is still unclear, this modulation may be mediated through cell-surface molecules such as CTLA-4 and/or cytokines such IL-10 or TGF-β.

The extent to which *suppressive cytokines*, such as TGF-β, IL-10, or IL-35, contribute to Treg-mediated suppression is still controversial. At the origin of the debate are *in vitro* studies using neutralizing antibodies or Treg cells unable to produce or respond to TGF-β or IL-10, indicating these cytokines might be dispensable for Treg function (Takahashi et al., 1998; Thornton and Shevach, 1998; Dieckmann et al., 2001; Jonuleit et al., 2001). Nevertheless, *in vivo* studies show that TGF-β and/or IL-10 might be required for Treg control of immune responses in allergy and asthma (Hawrylowicz and O'Garra, 2005; Annacker et al., 2003; Joetham et al., 2007; Rubtsov et al., 2008), infection (Stoop et al., 2007; Kursar et al., 2007), tolerance to transplants (Molitor-Dart et al., 2007), autoimmune responses (Asseman et al., 1999; Mann et al., 2007; Fahlen et al., 2005; Li et al., 2007b), cancer (Bergmann et al., 2007; Loser et al., 2007; Strauss et al., 2007; Hilchey et al., 2007; Li et al., 2007a) and fetal–maternal tolerance (Schumacher et al., 2007).

TGF-β has pleiotropic functions and can be expressed by many cell types. However, GARP, which binds to the latent form of TGF-β, is specifically expressed on Tregs (Tran et al., 2009). Surface-bound TGF-β is therefore present at high concentrations on Treg cells and is involved in the induction of IDO expression by DCs and in mediating infectious tolerance (Pallotta et al., 2011; Edwards et al., 2013). Indeed, in the absence of GARP, Treg cells show decreased ability of promoting Foxp3 expression *in vitro*. Accordingly, it is likely that, upon interaction with the same DC *in vivo*, Treg cells release activated TGF-β resulting in the conversion of nearby Foxp3^{-} conventional T cells to pTreg. In addition, TGF-β supports Treg cell maintenance, as strong TCR signaling can result in the loss of the regulatory phenotype, and TGF-β decreases T cell sensitivity to TCR stimulation (Sledzinska et al., 2013). Notably, deficient TGF-β signaling in T cells causes fatal lymphoproliferative diseases similar to Foxp3-deficient *scurfy* mice (Shull et al., 1992; Marie et al., 2005; Li et al., 2006; Liu et al., 2008).

IL-10 production by Treg cells was reported to be critical for their function at mucosal surfaces, namely for protection from colitis in mouse models of IBD (Asseman et al., 1999; Rubtsov et al., 2008). Because naïve and effector T lymphocytes express IL-10 receptor, Treg-derived IL-10 can suppress directly the differentiation and proliferation of effector T cells, and also induce the polarization of naïve T cells into IL-10-secreting cells (Huber et al., 2011; Groux et al., 1997). Tregs themselves respond to IL-10 by enhancing IL-10 production in a STAT3-dependent manner (Chaudhry et al., 2011). Suppression of DC function is another pivotal role of IL-10 produced by Tregs. Besides interfering with effective antigen presentation to conventional T cells, IL-10 induces DCs to secrete IL-27 that, in turn, promotes IL-10 production by conventional T cells, thus establishing a tolerogenic positive feedback loop (Steinbrink et al., 1997; Awasthi et al., 2007; Chattopadhyay and Shevach, 2013). Importantly, IL-10 production by Tregs seems to be dependent on ICOS signaling, as $ICOS^{-/-}$ Tregs fail to express this cytokine. Accordingly, ICOS-deficient patients show a severe reduction in IL-10 production (Kornete et al., 2012; Warnatz et al., 2006).

The immunosuppressive cytokine *IL-35* has been described as being preferentially expressed by Treg cells and required for their maximal suppressive activity (Collison et al., 2007). IL-35 halts the proliferation of conventional T cells and induces them to produce IL-35 and become "Tr35 cells" (Collison et al., 2010). However, the suppressive role of IL-35 on the development and/or function of other cell types deserves further investigation.

Treg cells also use effector cell *cytolysis* as a way of regulating immune responses. Human Treg-mediated target-cell killing depends upon both perforin and granzyme A, whereas in mice cytotoxic activity requires granzyme B (Grossman et al., 2004; Gondek et al., 2005; Cao et al., 2007). Nevertheless, recent studies have identified additional cytotoxic mechanisms used by Tregs, such as expression of galectin-1 or induction of apoptosis through the TRAIL-DR5 (tumor necrosis factor-related apoptosis-inducing ligand-death receptor 5) pathway (Garin et al., 2007; Ren et al., 2007).

Metabolic disruption is another strategy used by Tregs to suppress other cells. A primary mechanism is consumption of local IL-2, a cytokine they need for proliferation and survival, like effector T lymphocytes, but are unable to produce. Tregs were shown to mediate IL-2-deprivation mediated apoptosis of effector T cells (Thornton and Shevach, 1998; de la Rosa et al., 2004; Pandiyan et al., 2007), although other studies suggest this is not a bona fide Treg cell mechanism (Fontenot et al., 2005; Duthoit et al., 2005; Oberle et al., 2007). Importantly, addition of exogenous IL-2 abrogates *in vitro* Treg-induced suppression (Thornton and Shevach, 1998). Furthermore, preferential expression in Tregs of the ectoenzymes CD39 and CD73, which convert, respectively, ATP to AMP and AMP to nucleosides, decreases local concentration of ATP, and suppresses effector T cell function through activation of the adenosine receptor 2A (Kobie et al., 2006; Deaglio et al., 2007; Borsellino et al., 2007).

Hence, surface receptors such as CTLA-4 and LAG-3 as well as membrane-bound TGF-β and granzyme B expression have been related with Treg suppressive function requiring close contact with target cells. A cell–cell interaction with effector T cells is also critical for production of cytokines by Tregs, such as IL-35, that can act on cells in the vicinity (Collison et al., 2009). This interaction requirement for adequate cytokine production by Treg cells has led to an initial dismissal of soluble factors for their function. However, secretion of antiinflammatory cytokines, like IL-10 and IL-35, or consumption of factors essential for the activation of conventional T cells, such as IL-2, are examples of suppression mechanisms that do not involve cell-to-cell contact.

6. UNCONVENTIONAL REGULATORY T CELL POPULATIONS

Besides conventional $CD4^{+}CD25^{+}Foxp3^{+}$ Tregs, other T cells can display a regulatory behavior.

6.1 Th3 cells

The so-called Th3 cells are CD4 T lymphocytes with a similar phenotype to conventional Tregs that secrete TGF-β and IL-10 and are distinctive for also expressing IL-4 (Peterson, 2012; Inobe et al., 1998). They are induced from naïve CD4 T cells by TGF-β and have an important role in oral tolerance to nonself antigens. Th3 cells are triggered in an antigen-specific manner but, because their suppression mechanism is through TGF-β secretion, they suppress many cells specific for other antigens in a process called bystander suppression (Weiner, 2001).

6.2 T follicular regulatory (Tfr) cells

Among specialized regulatory cells, Tfr cells are unique in having a genetic program allowing access to the B cell follicle and germinal centers in secondary lymphoid organs (Chung et al., 2011; Linterman et al., 2011; Wollenberg et al., 2011). Tfr cells express Foxp3 as well as Bcl-6, a transcription factor essential for T follicular helper cells (Johnston et al., 2009; Nurieva et al., 2009). Tfr cells derive from thymic tTregs and can regulate the magnitude of GC responses (Wollenberg et al., 2011).

6.3 Type 1 regulatory T (Tr1) cells

There are $Foxp3^{-}$ memory-like IL-10-producing T cells, named Tr1, that can be induced following activation in the presence of IL-10, and constitute a population of regulatory cells different from $Foxp3^{+}$ Tregs (Lloyd and Hawrylowicz, 2009; Levings and Roncarolo, 2000). These cells also produce small amounts of IL-4, IL-17, IL-2, IL-5, and IFN-γ, and can be identified by cell-surface expression of LAG-3 and the integrin alpha 2 subunit (CD49b) (Bacchetta et al., 1990; Fujio et al., 2010; Gagliani et al., 2013). Tr1 cells have been identified in mice and humans and are currently under clinical trials (Battaglia and Roncarolo, 2011; Wood et al., 2012).

6.4 Regulatory natural killer T (NKTreg) cells

NKT cells are unconventional T lymphocytes whose TCR responds to lipid antigens. Their cardinal role is the orchestration of immune responses through rapid and copious cytokine secretion, thereby promoting or suppressing the activation of other immune cells [reviewed in (Monteiro and Graca, 2014)]. Activation of murine or human NKT cells in the presence of TGF-β induces Foxp3 expression and acquisition of suppressive function (Monteiro et al., 2010). Of note, *in vivo* administration of α-galactosylceramide, an NKT-cell TCR agonist, prevents the onset of EAE, a mouse model of multiple sclerosis (MS), and correlates with the emergence of $Foxp3^+$ NKT cells in the draining lymph nodes (Singh et al., 2001; Monteiro et al., 2010; Mars et al., 2009).

6.5 Regulatory γδT cells

Upon TCR cognate interactions, together with TGF-β and IL-15 signaling, γδT cells can acquire a regulatory phenotype with upregulation of CD25, CTL-4, and Foxp3 (Casetti et al., 2009). In humans, small intestinal $CD8^+TCR\gamma\delta$ cells show a regulatory behavior in celiac disease, dependent on the TCR triggering as well as cross-linking of NKG2A, which in turn increases the levels on TGF-β (Bhagat et al., 2008).

6.6 Regulatory CD8 T cells

When activated by immature DCs, CD8 T cells can become regulatory, depending on IL-10 for their mechanism of action (Gilliet and Liu, 2002; Dhodapkar and Steinman, 2002). TCR and TGF-β signaling are pivotal for CD8 Treg function (Rich et al., 1995). The $CD8^+CD28^-$ subset recognizes specifically MHC class I antigens on APCs and prevents upregulation of B7 molecules on the target APC, interfering with the CD28-B7 interaction required for T helper activation (Liu et al., 1998). Foxp3 expression by $CD8^+CD28^-$ cells has not been observed to date. Recently, a $CD8^+CD28^{low}Foxp3^+$ population was identified, displaying reduced expression of GARP, GITR, Foxp3, CD62L, CD28, and CTLA-4, despite a highly suppressive role. Importantly, IL-2 antibody complexes conjugated with rapamycin seem to have an impact on the expansion of this population *in vivo* (Robb et al., 2012).

7. TOLERANCE INDUCTION

The mechanisms leading to tolerance achievement are complex and often work under positive feedback effects. For instance, when transferred into secondary recipients, Tregs are able to instruct the recipient naïve CD4 T cells to become regulatory, thus transferring a tolerant state from one organism to another. This phenomenon is known as *infectious tolerance* (Graca et al., 2000; Qin et al., 1993). In addition, if a tolerated antigen and a third-party antigen are coexpressed within the same tissue or APC, the organism becomes tolerant to that third-party antigen, a fact described as *linked suppression* (Davies et al., 1996). However, if it is not linked to the tolerated antigen, the animals remain fully competent to reject cells expressing this third-party antigen, which illustrates a key feature of tolerance conferred by Tregs: antigen specificity.

Hematopoietic chimerism is considered to generate robust allogeneic tolerance (Merino et al., 1993). Yet, albeit chimerism, it is possible for donor tissues to be rejected, an effect known as *split tolerance*, mostly observed in skin grafts (Al-Adra and Anderson, 2011). In split tolerance, mixed chimeras maintain donor hematopoietic cells but reject skin transplants, the cause of which is likely immunity toward polymorphic alloantigens expressed by the donor skin, but absent from donor bone marrow cells (Luo et al., 2007; Ildstad et al., 1985; Al-Adra and Anderson, 2011).

Over the years with the increasing knowledge on the induction, expansion, and function of Tregs, several protocols have been developed that take advantage of these cells to achieve immune tolerance. The typical *in vivo* approaches take into account that cognate TCR triggering increases Treg frequency and/or potency due to either expansion of tTreg or induction of pTreg (Wieckiewicz et al., 2010).

Generation of Treg can be achieved by attenuation of activating signals during antigen presentation (Oliveira et al., 2011). Such an effect can be achieved with the use of MAbs targeting molecules involved in the immune synapse established between T cells and APCs, where molecules involved in T cell costimulation localize. Almost 3 decades have passed since the initial demonstrations of long-term transplantation tolerance induced following a brief treatment with MAbs (Benjamin and Waldmann, 1986; Gutstein et al., 1986; Graca et al., 2003), and that tolerogenic MAbs can be used to treat EAE (Brostoff and Mason, 1984; Duarte et al., 2012). Rapamycin-mediated increase of Foxp3$^+$ Tregs is associated with its interference in T cell costimulation, reduction on cell division and ability to inhibit mTORC1, therefore having an impact on Ca2$^+$ influx (Daniel et al., 2010). Amino acid starvation has a similar impact in facilitating Treg induction and immune tolerance (Cobbold et al., 2009).

Another approach is the use of substances that have a direct impact on Treg signaling. A striking example is that of IVIg, frequently used in tolerizing regimens for high-risk transplants due to an expansion of Tregs (Kessel et al., 2007). In fact, Treg epitopes have been identified in the Fc fragment of IgG that are capable of specifically activating tTregs (De Groot et al., 2008). Treg epitopes alone can mimic the effect of IVIg, demonstrating their usefulness as immune modulators with possible applications in transplantation and autoimmunity (Cousens et al., 2013, 2014; Elyaman et al., 2011). In allergen-specific immunotherapy (SIT), it has been shown that Foxp3$^+$IL-10$^+$ Tregs can be induced during the course of the treatment (Jutel et al., 2003). This effect has been attributed to autocrine IL-10 and TGF-β secretion, in addition to TCR signals resulting from consecutive low doses of allergen administered (Akdis et al., 1998; Jutel et al., 2003; Francis et al., 2003).

Lessons learned from this diversity of tolerance-inducing protocols have been important in guiding therapeutic applications for Treg cells.

8. REGULATORY T CELLS IN THE CLINIC

Adoptive Treg therapy offers several advantages in comparison to conventional pharmacologic immune suppression; namely, lower toxicity and the potential ability to specifically suppress deleterious immune responses without hindering overall immune surveillance. The scarcity of clinical trials using adoptive Treg therapy in humans has been largely due to the difficulty in obtaining sufficient Treg numbers under GMP conditions. Due to the paucity of Tregs in peripheral blood, several groups are investigating the possibility of expanding these cells *in vitro* after selection. The ability to boost Treg numbers and function in humans may be relevant to a large number of patients to whom the lack of immune tolerance plays a central role in disease pathogenesis.

The safety and efficacy of adoptive Treg therapy has already been assessed by Phase I/II clinical trials in the context of allogeneic hematopoietic stem cell transplantation (allo-HSCT) (Brunstein et al., 2011; Trzonkowski et al., 2009; Di Ianni et al., 2011; Martelli et al., 2014) and type 1 diabetes (T1D) (Marek-Trzonkowska et al., 2012). Overall, the small-scale trials performed thus far indicate that Treg therapy is feasible, safe, and potentially effective, encouraging the application of Treg infusion in other clinical settings.

8.1 Regulatory T cell therapy in the context of allo-HSCT

In patients who have successfully engrafted donor hematopoietic progenitor and immune cells after allo-HSCT, the inability to establish immune tolerance results in development of graft versus host disease (GVHD). The severe form of chronic GVHD (cGVHD) is associated with abnormal low levels of circulating Treg cells (Zorn et al., 2005). In animal models, donor Treg infusion protects allo-HSCT recipients from GVHD without compromising graft versus leukemia (GVL) effect (Trenado et al., 2003; Edinger et al., 2003; Jones et al., 2003). Nevertheless, the translation of these findings to patients submitted to allo-HSCT has been difficult and the development of approaches to enhance Treg numbers and/or function *in vivo* is still ongoing.

8.1.1 Clinical results

The observation that deficient Treg reconstitution is associated with a high incidence of cGVHD (Matsuoka et al., 2010) set the stage for a Phase I trial of low-dose IL-2 in patients with steroid-refractory cGVHD as an approach to selectively expand Treg *in vivo* (Koreth et al., 2011). IL-2 treatment specifically increased the number of circulating Tregs, which was accompanied by a significant clinical improvement in approximately half of the patients with active cGVHD (Koreth et al., 2011). These initial studies demonstrated that *in vivo* manipulation of donor Treg homeostasis after allo-HSCT is safe and potentially effective in the treatment of cGVHD.

Another important strategy for enhancing Treg function involves purification of Treg cells *ex vivo* for subsequent adoptive therapy. Phase I clinical trials are currently ongoing to assess the safety and efficacy of infusing freshly isolated donor Treg in patients with steroid-refractory cGVHD, with or without additional low-dose IL-2. The rationale for these approaches hypothesizes that the inability to respond to IL-2 therapy observed in half of the cGVHD patients in the Phase I low-dose IL-2 trial (Koreth et al., 2011) may be due to insufficient Treg counts. It is currently unknown if adoptive transfer of donor-derived Treg cells alone is enough to induce a therapeutic response in patients with cGVHD and, if so, what is the minimal cell dose required. Alternatively, coadministration of IL-2 may be necessary to achieve the Treg levels needed to obtain a tangible therapeutic effect. The latter strategy would rely on IL-2-driven expansion *in vivo* of the infused Treg as an attempt to circumvent the limitations of current approaches to expand large numbers of Treg *in vitro*.

The first report of adoptive Treg therapy in humans described the impact of *ex vivo* expanded Treg in two patients who developed GVHD following HSCT (Trzonkowski et al., 2009). Although Treg infusion allowed a reduction of pharmacological immune suppression and associated with clinical improvement of the patient with cGVHD, it only transiently improved the condition of the patient with steroid-refractory grade IV acute GVHD, who eventually died of multiorgan dysfunction (Trzonkowski et al., 2009).

Since then, adoptive immunotherapy with donor Tregs has been reported to successfully prevent GVHD after umbilical cord blood unrelated (Brunstein et al., 2011) and haploidentical related (Di Ianni et al., 2011) allo-HSCT. Both these studies used Tregs purified by magnetic-activated cell sorting (MACS). The standard GMP protocol for Treg enrichment by MACS is a two-step procedure: first depleting $CD19^+$ B cells and CD8 T cells, and then positively selecting $CD25^{bright}$ cells with subsaturating levels of anti-CD25 antibody-coated magnetic beads. In contrast to adult peripheral blood, cord blood-derived Tregs can be isolated by MACS in a one-step procedure based on CD25 positive selection and their *in vitro* expansion does not require rapamycin to prevent effector T cell outgrowth. In the umbilical cord allo-HSCT report, patients received two unrelated cord blood units as a source of hematopoietic progenitors, plus Treg cells purified from a partially HLA-matched third-party cord blood unit (Brunstein et al., 2011). The administration of cord blood-derived Treg cells, expanded *in vitro* with anti-CD3/CD28-coated beads and IL-2 prior to infusion, associated with a reduced incidence of acute GVHD when compared to historical control subjects (Brunstein et al., 2011). However, a two-year patient follow-up has revealed a potential higher risk for viral infections in the first month following cord blood-derived Treg infusion, although no adverse effect on long-term outcomes was observed (Brunstein et al., 2013). The indication that Treg infusion may be associated with excessive suppression and, consequently, with an increased risk of infection post-HSCT, highlights the need to closely monitor immune competence in patients undergoing Treg-infusion protocols. In haploidentical allo-HSCT, administration of donor Treg prior to infusion of purified $CD34^+$ hematopoietic progenitors, plus conventional CD4 T cells, permitted a 100-fold increase in the number of donor T cells administered at the time of transplant, leading to a significantly faster recovery of posttransplant immunity against opportunistic infections, without GVHD, even in the absence of pharmacological prophylaxis (Di Ianni et al., 2011). In a subsequent Phase II clinical trial aiming to assess whether adoptive Treg-- conventional CD4 T cell therapy prevents leukemia relapse, the disease relapse rates reported were significantly lower than those observed in historical controls, suggesting that Treg + conventional CD4 T-cell therapy may provide an important GVL effect in the absence of GVHD (Martelli et al., 2014).

A preliminary Phase I safety and feasibility trial infused freshly isolated donor Treg after withdrawal of pharmacologic GVHD prophylaxis into HSCT recipients with high risk of leukemia relapse (Edinger and Hoffmann, 2011). Additional conventional T cells were administered to promote the GVL effect and no disease relapse was reported. Importantly, neither GVHD nor opportunistic infections were observed after Treg infusion, suggesting safety and feasibility of this therapeutic approach (Edinger and Hoffmann, 2011).

The application of Treg cells for the treatment of acute and chronic GVHD is currently being assessed by a European consortium (TREGeneration, J. F. Lacerda Coordinator) performing parallel clinical trials to assess the safety and preliminary efficacy of different Treg cell products in patients with steroid-refractory GVHD.

8.1.2 Regulatory T cell expansion in vitro *for clinical use*

Ideally, adoptive transfer protocols would employ Treg doses allowing a 1:1 infused Treg to target effector T cell ratio to be reached *in vivo*. However, one of the main limitations of such therapeutic approaches is the production of sufficiently high numbers of pure and functionally stable Treg cells for clinical usage.

The paucity of Treg cells in the peripheral blood suggests that *in vitro* expansion might be a viable strategy to obtain stable populations of clinical-grade pure Treg cells. In order to obtain higher yields of expanded Treg, artificial antigen-presenting cells (aAPC) loaded with anti-CD3 antibody and the CD28/CTLA-4 ligand CD86 have been used as an alternative to bead-based Treg expansion protocols (Hippen et al., 2011). The same group that performed the abovementioned clinical trial infusing cord blood-derived Treg expanded *in vitro* with anti-CD3/CD28 beads and IL-2 (Brunstein et al., 2011, 2013) is currently assessing the safety and efficacy of cord blood-derived Treg expanded with aAPC in a Phase I dose-escalation trial [Clinicaltrials.gov identifier NCT00602693] (Hanley et al., 2015).

In a mouse model of HSCT, infusion of recipient-specific Treg expanded *ex vivo* prevented GVHD through alloreactive-specific immune suppression, which was associated with improved and accelerated immune reconstitution (Gaidot et al., 2011). Thus, the development of recipient-specific donor Treg may have significant advantages relative to polyclonal Treg by avoiding generalized immune suppression. Importantly, mouse models have also shown that Treg suppression of GVHD was not associated with loss of the GVL effect (Trenado et al., 2003; Edinger et al., 2003; Jones et al., 2003). A Phase I clinical trial is currently evaluating the safety of sirolimus-based immune suppression and *ex vivo* expanded allo-specific donor Treg for the prevention of acute GVHD following HLA-matched sibling allo-HSCT [Clinicaltrials.gov identifier NCT01795573]. The allo-specific Treg, obtained by coculturing donor Treg with recipient-derived DCs, are infused prior to allo-HSCT.

Therefore, it is anticipated that antigen-specific Tregs in humans may be able to induce immunologic tolerance against normal recipient cells, while allowing the recognition of tumor cells as foreign by donor effector T cells. However, this hypothesis remains to be confirmed.

8.2 Other clinical settings

8.2.1 Solid organ transplantation

The first adoptive Treg therapy trials in the context of solid organ transplantation are currently ongoing, assessing the safety and possible efficacy of different Treg cell populations in kidney and liver transplant recipients (Edozie et al., 2014; Juvet et al., 2014).

In the setting of kidney transplantation, a multicenter study sponsored by the European Community is currently comparing the safety, feasibility, and potential efficacy of different regulatory cell therapy products: polyclonally expanded tTreg isolated either by magnetic- or fluorescence-activated cell sorting; alloantigen-specific tTreg; Tr1 cells; anergic Tregs; tolerogenic recipient DCs; and regulatory macrophages (Geissler, 2012). All centers will employ the same immune suppression protocol in order to compare the impact of the different regulatory populations on transplant outcome, with the ultimate aim of identifying which protocols have the potential to progress to large-scale trials assessing efficacy (The ONE Study, http://www.onestudy.org/).

A preliminary study infusing iTregs in patients undergoing living-donor liver transplantation suggested that adoptive Treg therapy is safe and may allow for early reduction and/or withdrawal of immune suppression (Juvet et al., 2014). Although promising, adequate control groups and long-term follow-up are required to ascertain the safety and efficacy of this strategy.

8.2.2 Autoimmunity

The therapeutic potential of manipulating Treg cells in the setting of autoimmune diseases has been extensively investigated. Nevertheless, the promising results obtained in preclinical studies have been difficult to translate into successful clinical trials in humans.

8.2.2.1 Type 1 diabetes

The association between type 1 diabetes (T1D) and peripheral blood Treg counts remains to be elucidated. Although T1D patients have been reported to have lower Treg numbers (Kukreja et al., 2002), other studies have shown similar Treg counts between T1D patients and age-matched healthy controls (Brusko et al., 2007; Putnam et al., 2009). As for Treg function, the apparent functional impairment of Treg from T1D patients, observed in suppression assays with autologous conventional T cells, appears to be attributable to a higher resistance to suppression of responder CD4 T cells from T1D patients when compared to healthy donors (Putnam et al., 2009; Battaglia et al., 2006).

Preclinical studies have reported that adoptive transfer of antigen-specific Tregs in nonobese diabetic mice (Tang et al., 2004; Tarbell et al., 2007), as well as of polyclonal Tregs in diabetes-prone BB rats (Lundsgaard et al., 2005), can prevent diabetes. Antigen-specific Tregs have been further shown to reverse diabetes after disease onset (Tang et al., 2004; Tarbell et al., 2007), suggesting that adoptive transfer of Treg cells may be used for the prevention and treatment of T1D.

The first in-human clinical trial infusing polyclonally expanded autologous Tregs in children with T1D has demonstrated that this approach is safe and associated with a dramatic increase of the frequency of circulating Treg cells, prolonging remission in comparison to patients not treated with Tregs (Marek-Trzonkowska et al., 2012). Long-term follow-up of these patients is ongoing in order to ascertain whether Treg-mediated remission is sustained (Marek-Trzonkowska et al., 2012).

8.2.2.2 Rheumatoid arthritis

Treg cells from patients with rheumatoid arthritis (RA) appear to be functionally defective, despite increased Treg numbers in the joints of patients (Sarkar and Fox, 2007). Promising preclinical studies have demonstrated that adoptive transfer of polyclonally activated Tregs (Kelchtermans et al., 2009) or TGFβ-induced iTreg (Kong et al., 2012) improves clinical symptoms of collagen-induced arthritis in mice, even in the presence of ongoing inflammation.

In RA patients, the extent to which the clinical efficacy of pharmacological therapy is due to an impact on Treg numbers and/or function remains to be elucidated (Esensten et al., 2009). Nevertheless, adoptive Treg therapy appears to have the potential to mediate long-term antigen-specific immune suppression, abrogating pathologic inflammation in RA patients without compromising overall immune competence (Esensten et al., 2009).

8.2.2.3 Inflammatory bowel disease

The association between IBD and either deficient Treg numbers or functionally impaired Treg cells remains to be clarified (Himmel et al., 2012).

Murine studies have demonstrated a vital role for IL-10 in maintaining Treg-suppressive function (Murai et al., 2009) and in Treg-mediated colitis prevention (Huber et al., 2011; Rubtsov et al., 2008). Although subcutaneous administration of recombinant human IL-10 produced disappointing results in patients with Crohn's disease (Fedorak et al., 2000; Schreiber et al., 2000), adoptive transfer of IL-10-producing Tr1 cells may prove a more effective IL-10 delivery strategy, with the added benefit of allowing antigen-specific suppression. Preclinical studies have shown that ovalbumin-specific Tr1 cells are able to prevent and control colitis in a mouse model of chronic IBD (Groux et al., 1997; Foussat et al., 2003). A Phase I/IIa clinical trial assessing the safety and efficacy of antigen-specific Treg cells in the treatment of refractory Crohn's disease has reported that administration of ovalbumin-specific Tr1-like cell clones was well tolerated and had dose-related efficacy (Desreumaux et al., 2012). Future adoptive Treg therapy approaches may aim to generate Treg cells specific for disease-driving pathogenic antigens in IBD.

8.2.2.4 Multiple sclerosis

The role of Treg in the pathogenesis of MS remains controversial. The frequency of circulating Treg cells in MS patients appears to be similar to that observed in healthy individuals (Haas et al., 2005), although there are conflicting reports (Praksova et al., 2012). However, the ability to suppress myelin-specific immune responses has been shown to be impaired in Tregs from MS patients (Haas et al., 2005; Kumar et al., 2006). Importantly, decreased expression of Foxp3 within the Treg pool have been observed in MS (Huan et al., 2005). In addition to decreased suppressive potency, Treg migration across the blood–brain barrier appears to be compromised in patients with relapsing–remitting MS (Schneider-Hohendorf et al., 2010).

Preclinical studies of adoptive Treg transfer in EAE have produced contradictory data. Administration of myelin antigen-specific Treg, but not polyclonal Treg, prior to disease onset has been shown to prevent EAE (Kohm et al., 2002; Stephens et al., 2009). The requirement of antigen-specific Tregs may compromise the production of suitable Treg cell products for adoptive therapy in MS patients, given that the relevant MS antigens are poorly defined (Buc, 2013). Importantly, Treg infusion during active disease, as presented by the vast majority of MS patients, has been demonstrated to be less effective in EAE treatment (Olivares-Villagomez et al., 1998; Van de Keere and Tonegawa, 1998). Furthermore, myelin-specific Treg adoptively transferred into EAE mice have been reported to accumulate in the central nervous system (CNS), but failed to prevent disease onset (Korn et al., 2007). These Treg cells were only unable to suppress the proliferation of conventional CD4 T cells isolated from the CNS of mice with active EAE, which secreted high levels of IL-6 and TGF-β, but not naïve myelin-specific T cells (Korn et al., 2007). Hence, defective inhibition of conventional CD4 T cell proliferation by Tregs from MS patients may not be due only to impaired Treg function, but also to conventional T cells being highly resistant to Treg-mediated suppression in MS patients. The relative contribution of Treg impairment and conventional CD4 T cell resistance needs to be clarified in order to understand whether Treg immunotherapy has the potential to benefit MS patients.

8.2.3 Allergy

Although the use of Treg therapy to treat allergic diseases appears promising, several issues remain to be clarified before Treg-based approaches can be successfully implemented. Treg cells, particularly Tr1 cells, have been found to play an important role in modulating allergic immune responses (Akdis et al., 2004). In murine allergy models, therapeutic Treg transfer suppresses allergic airway inflammation (Maazi et al., 2012), but it appears to be less effective in preventing IgE responses (Kearley et al., 2008). These preclinical studies suggest that therapeutic approaches to enhance Treg cell numbers and/or function during and after allergen-SIT may have some clinical benefits.

8.2.4 Cancer

In the field of cancer immunotherapy, Treg cells are actually targeted in an attempt to reduce the number and/or suppressive function of tumor-infiltrating Tregs, which inhibit tumor-specific effector T cell responses (Nishikawa and Sakaguchi, 2014).

In order to specifically target Treg-suppressing antitumor immunity, while avoiding overall Treg depletion and loss of self-tolerance, markers that identify tumor-infiltrating highly suppressive Treg, but not naïve Treg, such as CCR4 (Sugiyama et al., 2013), are being investigated as potential targets for cell-depleting antibody therapeutic approaches. Future cancer immunotherapy approaches are likely to combine targeted inhibition of Treg-suppressive function and specific stimulation of antitumor effector T cell responses (Nishikawa and Sakaguchi, 2014; Jacobs et al., 2012).

8.3 Future regulatory T cell immunotherapy trials: Challenges and strategies

The clinical application of Treg immunotherapy is not completely devoid of potential risks, as any therapeutic approach. In particular, the use of iTregs is associated with an underlying risk of the infused iTreg reverting to effector T cell phenotype *in vivo*. This may be particularly harmful when using antigen-specific iTreg cells, which could potentially increase the pool of disease-driving antigen-specific effector T cells and thus worsen the clinical condition.

Another potential drawback to consider is the possibility that Treg infusion may lead to excessive immune suppression, hindering not only the target effector responses that mediate the clinical symptoms, but also crucial immune responses required to confer protection against infectious agents or malignant diseases. Important decisions in managing this risk include the dose of Treg to be administered and the degree of TCR specificity of the infused Treg population.

Future Treg immunotherapy protocols must take into account the pros and cons of several alternatives in terms of Treg cell product manipulation (freshly isolated versus *in vitro* expanded Treg; in the latter scenario, polyclonal versus antigen-specific Treg), Treg dose (the required dose of antigen-specific Tregs is expected to be lower than that of freshly isolated or polyclonally expanded Tregs), differentiation state of the infused Tregs (total Tregs versus naïve/memory Tregs subsets), and migration potential (expression of homing receptors relevant for the target tissues where disease-driving effector responses are occurring, such as skin or gut). It is unlikely to find an unique Treg cell therapy ideal for multiple conditions. Instead, the type of Treg therapy will probably vary according to the clinical setting.

In addition to the clinical benefits of these different approaches, their cost-effectiveness also needs to be assessed, as it constitutes one of the major hurdles for the implementation of adoptive Treg therapy into current clinical practice. Importantly, Treg immunotherapy may prove to be financially feasible in the long run, despite high initial costs, if it succeeds in expediting immune suppression withdrawal and in reducing the hospitalization periods associated with the underlying disease and/or with the secondary effects of standard pharmacological therapy (Juvet et al., 2014).

Overall, although much remains to be elucidated in terms of the suitability of adoptive Treg therapy in different clinical settings, the trials performed thus far suggest this therapeutic approach is safe and has the potential to improve clinical outcomes in a variety of inflammatory diseases. Clinical trials that are currently ongoing will hopefully shed light on many of the unresolved issues and set the stage for larger-scale trials that may ascertain the efficacy of adoptive Treg therapy in the context of immune tolerance dysfunction.

REFERENCES

Akdis, C.A., Blesken, T., Akdis, M., Wuthrich, B., Blaser, K., 1998. Role of interleukin 10 in specific immunotherapy. J. Clin. Invest. 102, 98–106.

Akdis, M., Verhagen, J., Taylor, A., Karamloo, F., Karagiannidis, C., Crameri, R., Thunberg, S., Deniz, G., Valenta, R., Fiebig, H., Kegel, C., Disch, R., Schmidt-Weber, C.B., Blaser, K., Akdis, C.A., 2004. Immune responses in healthy and allergic individuals are characterized by a fine balance between allergen-specific T regulatory 1 and T helper 2 cells. J. Exp. Med. 199, 1567–1575.

Al-Adra, D.P., Anderson, C.C., 2011. Mixed chimerism and split tolerance: mechanisms and clinical correlations. Chimerism 2, 89–101.

Aluvihare, V.R., Kallikourdis, M., Betz, A.G., 2004. Regulatory T cells mediate maternal tolerance to the fetus. Nat. Immunol. 5, 266–271.

Annacker, O., Asseman, C., Read, S., Powrie, F., 2003. Interleukin-10 in the regulation of T cell-induced colitis. J. Autoimmun. 20, 277–279.

Asseman, C., Mauze, S., Leach, M.W., Coffman, R.L., Powrie, F., 1999. An essential role for interleukin 10 in the function of regulatory T cells that inhibit intestinal inflammation. J. Exp. Med. 190, 995–1004.

Au-Yeung, B.B., Levin, S.E., Zhang, C., Hsu, L.Y., Cheng, D.A., Killeen, N., Shokat, K.M., Weiss, A., 2010. A genetically selective inhibitor demonstrates a function for the kinase Zap70 in regulatory T cells independent of its catalytic activity. Nat. Immunol. 11, 1085–1092.

Awasthi, A., Carrier, Y., Peron, J.P., Bettelli, E., Kamanaka, M., Flavell, R.A., Kuchroo, V.K., Oukka, M., Weiner, H.L., 2007. A dominant function for interleukin 27 in generating interleukin 10-producing anti-inflammatory T cells. Nat. Immunol. 8, 1380–1389.

Bacchetta, R., De Waal Malefijt, R., Yssel, H., Abrams, J., De Vries, J.E., Spits, H., Roncarolo, M.G., 1990. Host-reactive CD4+ and CD8+ T cell clones isolated from a human chimera produce IL-5, IL-2, IFN-gamma and granulocyte/macrophage-colony-stimulating factor but not IL-4. J. Immunol. 144, 902–908.

Barnard, J.A., Beauchamp, R.D., Coffey, R.J., Moses, H.L., 1989. Regulation of intestinal epithelial cell growth by transforming growth factor type beta. Proc. Natl. Acad. Sci. U. S. A. 86, 1578–1582.

Barnard, J.A., Polk, W.H., Moses, H.L., Coffey, R.J., 1991. Production of transforming growth factor-alpha by normal rat small intestine. Am. J. Physiol. 261, C994–C1000.

Basu, S., Hubbard, B., Shevach, E.M., 2015. Foxp3-mediated inhibition of Akt inhibits Glut1 (glucose transporter 1) expression in human T regulatory cells. J. Leukoc. Biol. 97 (2), 279–283.

Battaglia, M., Roncarolo, M.G., 2011. Immune intervention with T regulatory cells: past lessons and future perspectives for type 1 diabetes. Semin. Immunol. 23, 182–194.

Battaglia, M., Stabilini, A., Migliavacca, B., Horejs-Hoeck, J., Kaupper, T., Roncarolo, M.G., 2006. Rapamycin promotes expansion of functional CD4+CD25+FOXP3+ regulatory T cells of both healthy subjects and type 1 diabetic patients. J. Immunol. 177, 8338–8347.

Benjamin, R.J., Waldmann, H., 1986. Induction of tolerance by monoclonal antibody therapy. Nature 320, 449–451.

Bennett, C.L., Christie, J., Ramsdell, F., Brunkow, M.E., Ferguson, P.J., Whitesell, L., Kelly, T.E., Saulsbury, F.T., Chance, P.F., Ochs, H.D., 2001. The immune dysregulation, polyendocrinopathy, enteropathy, X-linked syndrome (IPEX) is caused by mutations of FOXP3. Nat. Genet. 27, 20–21.

Beres, A., Komorowski, R., Mihara, M., Drobyski, W.R., 2011. Instability of Foxp3 expression limits the ability of induced regulatory T cells to mitigate graft versus host disease. Clin. Cancer Res. 17, 3969–3983.

Bergmann, C., Strauss, L., Zeidler, R., Lang, S., Whiteside, T.L., 2007. Expansion and characteristics of human T regulatory type 1 cells in co-cultures simulating tumor microenvironment. Cancer Immunol. Immunother. 56, 1429–1442.

Bettelli, E., Dastrange, M., Oukka, M., 2005. Foxp3 interacts with nuclear factor of activated T cells and NF-kappa B to repress cytokine gene expression and effector functions of T helper cells. Proc. Natl. Acad. Sci. U. S. A. 102, 5138–5143.

Bhagat, G., Naiyer, A.J., Shah, J.G., Harper, J., Jabri, B., Wang, T.C., Green, P.H., Manavalan, J.S., 2008. Small intestinal CD8+TCRgammadelta+NKG2A+ intraepithelial lymphocytes have attributes of regulatory cells in patients with celiac disease. J. Clin. Invest. 118, 281–293.

Bilate, A.M., Lafaille, J.J., 2012. Induced CD4+Foxp3+ regulatory T cells in immune tolerance. Annu. Rev. Immunol. 30, 733–758.

Borsellino, G., Kleinewietfeld, M., Di Mitri, D., Sternjak, A., Diamantini, A., Giometto, R., Hopner, S., Centonze, D., Bernardi, G., Dell'acqua, M.L., Rossini, P.M., Battistini, L., Rotzschke, O., Falk, K., 2007. Expression of ectonucleotidase CD39 by Foxp3+ Treg cells: hydrolysis of extracellular ATP and immune suppression. Blood 110, 1225–1232.

Brostoff, S.W., Mason, D.W., 1984. Experimental allergic encephalomyelitis: successful treatment in vivo with a monoclonal antibody that recognizes T helper cells. J. Immunol. 133, 1938–1942.

Brunkow, M.E., Jeffery, E.W., Hjerrild, K.A., Paeper, B., Clark, L.B., Yasayko, S.A., Wilkinson, J.E., Galas, D., Ziegler, S.F., Ramsdell, F., 2001. Disruption of a new forkhead/winged-helix protein, scurfin, results in the fatal lymphoproliferative disorder of the scurfy mouse. Nat. Genet. 27, 68–73.

Brunstein, C.G., Blazar, B.R., Miller, J.S., Cao, Q., Hippen, K.L., McKenna, D.H., Curtsinger, J., Mcglave, P.B., Wagner, J.E., 2013. Adoptive transfer of umbilical cord blood-derived regulatory T cells and early viral reactivation. Biol. Blood Marrow Transplant. 19, 1271–1273.

Brunstein, C.G., Miller, J.S., Cao, Q., McKenna, D.H., Hippen, K.L., Curtsinger, J., Defor, T., Levine, B.L., June, C.H., Rubinstein, P., Mcglave, P.B., Blazar, B.R., Wagner, J.E., 2011. Infusion of ex vivo expanded T regulatory cells in adults transplanted with umbilical cord blood: safety profile and detection kinetics. Blood 117, 1061–1070.

Brusko, T., Wasserfall, C., Mcgrail, K., Schatz, R., Viener, H.L., Schatz, D., Haller, M., Rockell, J., Gottlieb, P., Clare-Salzler, M., Atkinson, M., 2007. No alterations in the frequency of FOXP3+ regulatory T-cells in type 1 diabetes. Diabetes 56, 604–612.

Buc, M., 2013. Role of regulatory T cells in pathogenesis and biological therapy of multiple sclerosis. Mediators Inflammation 2013, 963748.

Burzyn, D., Benoist, C., Mathis, D., 2013. Regulatory T cells in nonlymphoid tissues. Nat. Immunol. 14, 1007–1013.

Campbell, D.J., Koch, M.A., 2011. Phenotypical and functional specialization of FOXP3+ regulatory T cells. Nat. Rev. Immunol. 11, 119–130.

Cao, X., Cai, S.F., Fehniger, T.A., Song, J., Collins, L.I., Piwnica-Worms, D.R., Ley, T.J., 2007. Granzyme B and perforin are important for regulatory T cell-mediated suppression of tumor clearance. Immunity 27, 635–646.

Casetti, R., Agrati, C., Wallace, M., Sacchi, A., Martini, F., Martino, A., Rinaldi, A., Malkovsky, M., 2009. Cutting edge: TGF-beta1 and IL-15 Induce FOXP3+ gammadelta regulatory T cells in the presence of antigen stimulation. J. Immunol. 183, 3574–3577.

Cederbom, L., Hall, H., Ivars, F., 2000. CD4+CD25+ regulatory T cells down-regulate co-stimulatory molecules on antigen-presenting cells. Eur. J. Immunol. 30, 1538–1543.

Chattopadhyay, G., Shevach, E.M., 2013. Antigen-specific induced T regulatory cells impair dendritic cell function via an IL-10/MARCH1-dependent mechanism. J. Immunol. 191, 5875–5884.

Chaudhry, A., Rudra, D., Treuting, P., Samstein, R.M., Liang, Y., Kas, A., Rudensky, A.Y., 2009. CD4+ regulatory T cells control TH17 responses in a Stat3-dependent manner. Science 326, 986–991.

Chaudhry, A., Samstein, R.M., Treuting, P., Liang, Y., Pils, M.C., Heinrich, J.M., Jack, R.S., Wunderlich, F.T., Bruning, J.C., Muller, W., Rudensky, A.Y., 2011. Interleukin-10 signaling in regulatory T cells is required for suppression of Th17 cell-mediated inflammation. Immunity 34, 566–578.

Chen, S., Ishii, N., Ine, S., Ikeda, S., Fujimura, T., Ndhlovu, L.C., Soroosh, P., Tada, K., Harigae, H., Kameoka, J., Kasai, N., Sasaki, T., Sugamura, K., 2006. Regulatory T cell-like activity of Foxp3+ adult T cell leukemia cells. Int. Immunol. 18, 269–277.

Chen, W., Jin, W., Hardegen, N., Lei, K.J., Li, L., Marinos, N., Mcgrady, G., Wahl, S.M., 2003. Conversion of peripheral CD4+CD25- naive T cells to CD4+CD25+ regulatory T cells by TGF-beta induction of transcription factor Foxp3. J. Exp. Med. 198, 1875–1886.

Chen, X., Oppenheim, J.J., 2011. The phenotypic and functional consequences of tumour necrosis factor receptor type 2 expression on CD4(+) FoxP3(+) regulatory T cells. Immunology 133, 426–433.

Chung, Y., Tanaka, S., Chu, F., Nurieva, R.I., Martinez, G.J., Rawal, S., Wang, Y.H., Lim, H., Reynolds, J.M., Zhou, X.H., Fan, H.M., Liu, Z.M., Neelapu, S.S., Dong, C., 2011. Follicular regulatory T cells expressing Foxp3 and Bcl-6 suppress germinal center reactions. Nat. Med. 17, 983–988.

Cobbold, S.P., Adams, E., Farquhar, C.A., Nolan, K.F., Howie, D., Lui, K.O., Fairchild, P.J., Mellor, A.L., Ron, D., Waldmann, H., 2009. Infectious tolerance via the consumption of essential amino acids and mTOR signaling. Proc. Natl. Acad. Sci. U. S. A. 106, 12055–12060.

Collison, L.W., Chaturvedi, V., Henderson, A.L., Giacomin, P.R., Guy, C., Bankoti, J., Finkelstein, D., Forbes, K., Workman, C.J., Brown, S.A., Rehg, J.E., Jones, M.L., Ni, H.T., Artis, D., Turk, M.J., Vignali, D.A., 2010. IL-35-mediated induction of a potent regulatory T cell population. Nat. Immunol. 11, 1093–1101.

Collison, L.W., Pillai, M.R., Chaturvedi, V., Vignali, D.A., 2009. Regulatory T cell suppression is potentiated by target T cells in a cell contact, IL-35- and IL-10-dependent manner. J. Immunol. 182, 6121–6128.

Collison, L.W., Workman, C.J., Kuo, T.T., Boyd, K., Wang, Y., Vignali, K.M., Cross, R., Sehy, D., Blumberg, R.S., Vignali, D.A., 2007. The inhibitory cytokine IL-35 contributes to regulatory T-cell function. Nature 450, 566–569.

Coombes, J.L., Siddiqui, K.R., Arancibia-Carcamo, C.V., Hall, J., Sun, C.M., Belkaid, Y., Powrie, F., 2007. A functionally specialized population of mucosal CD103+ DCs induces Foxp3+ regulatory T cells via a TGF-beta and retinoic acid-dependent mechanism. J. Exp. Med. 204, 1757–1764.

Cousens, L., Najafian, N., Martin, W.D., De Groot, A.S., 2014. Tregitope: immunomodulation powerhouse. Hum. Immunol. 75, 1139–1146.

Cousens, L.P., Su, Y., Mcclaine, E., Li, X., Terry, F., Smith, R., Lee, J., Martin, W., Scott, D.W., De Groot, A.S., 2013. Application of IgG-derived natural Treg epitopes (IgG Tregitopes) to antigen-specific tolerance induction in a murine model of type 1 diabetes. J. Diabetes Res. 2013, 621693.

Daniel, C., Wennhold, K., Kim, H.J., Von Boehmer, H., 2010. Enhancement of antigen-specific Treg vaccination in vivo. Proc. Natl. Acad. Sci. U. S. A. 107, 16246–16251.

Davidson, T.S., Dipaolo, R.J., Andersson, J., Shevach, E.M., 2007. Cutting Edge: IL-2 is essential for TGF-beta-mediated induction of Foxp3+ T regulatory cells. J. Immunol. 178, 4022–4026.

Davies, J.D., Leong, L.Y., Mellor, A., Cobbold, S.P., Waldmann, H., 1996. T cell suppression in transplantation tolerance through linked recognition. J. Immunol. 156, 3602–3607.

De Groot, A.S., Moise, L., Mcmurry, J.A., Wambre, E., Van Overtvelt, L., Moingeon, P., Scott, D.W., Martin, W., 2008. Activation of natural regulatory T cells by IgG Fc-derived peptide "Tregitopes" Blood 112, 3303–3311.

De La Rosa, M., Rutz, S., Dorninger, H., Scheffold, A., 2004. Interleukin-2 is essential for CD4+CD25+ regulatory T cell function. Eur. J. Immunol. 34, 2480–2488.

Deaglio, S., Dwyer, K.M., Gao, W., Friedman, D., Usheva, A., Erat, A., Chen, J.F., Enjyoji, K., Linden, J., Oukka, M., Kuchroo, V.K., Strom, T.B., Robson, S.C., 2007. Adenosine generation catalyzed by CD39 and CD73 expressed on regulatory T cells mediates immune suppression. J. Exp. Med. 204, 1257–1265.

Demengeot, J., Zelenay, S., Moraes-Fontes, M.F., Caramalho, I., Coutinho, A., 2006. Regulatory T cells in microbial infection. Springer Semin. Immunopathol. 28, 41–50.

Deng, G., Podack, E.R., 1993. Suppression of apoptosis in a cytotoxic T-cell line by interleukin 2-mediated gene transcription and deregulated expression of the protooncogene bcl-2. Proc. Natl. Acad. Sci. U. S. A. 90, 2189–2193.

Desreumaux, P., Foussat, A., Allez, M., Beaugerie, L., Hebuterne, X., Bouhnik, Y., Nachury, M., Brun, V., Bastian, H., Belmonte, N., Ticchioni, M., Duchange, A., Morel-Mandrino, P., Neveu, V., Clerget-Chossat, N., Forte, M., Colombel, J.F., 2012. Safety and efficacy of antigen-specific regulatory T-cell therapy for patients with refractory Crohn's disease. Gastroenterology 143 (1207–17), e1–e2.

Dhodapkar, M.V., Steinman, R.M., 2002. Antigen-bearing immature dendritic cells induce peptide-specific CD8(+) regulatory T cells in vivo in humans. Blood 100, 174–177.

Di Ianni, M., Falzetti, F., Carotti, A., Terenzi, A., Castellino, F., Bonifacio, E., Del Papa, B., Zei, T., Ostini, R.I., Cecchini, D., Aloisi, T., Perruccio, K., Ruggeri, L., Balucani, C., Pierini, A., Sportoletti, P., Aristei, C., Falini, B., Reisner, Y., Velardi, A., Aversa, F., Martelli, M.F., 2011. Tregs prevent GVHD and promote immune reconstitution in HLA-haploidentical transplantation. Blood 117, 3921–3928.

Dieckmann, D., Plottner, H., Berchtold, S., Berger, T., Schuler, G., 2001. Ex vivo isolation and characterization of CD4(+)CD25(+) T cells with regulatory properties from human blood. J. Exp. Med. 193, 1303–1310.

Dipaolo, R.J., Brinster, C., Davidson, T.S., Andersson, J., Glass, D., Shevach, E.M., 2007. Autoantigen-specific TGFbeta-induced Foxp3+ regulatory T cells prevent autoimmunity by inhibiting dendritic cells from activating autoreactive T cells. J. Immunol. 179, 4685–4693.

Duarte, J., Carrie, N., Oliveira, V.G., Almeida, C., Agua-Doce, A., Rodrigues, L., Simas, J.P., Mars, L.T., Graca, L., 2012. T cell apoptosis and induction of Foxp3+ regulatory T cells underlie the therapeutic efficacy of CD4 blockade in experimental autoimmune encephalomyelitis. J. Immunol. 189, 1680–1688.

Duthoit, C.T., Mekala, D.J., Alli, R.S., Geiger, T.L., 2005. Uncoupling of IL-2 signaling from cell cycle progression in naive CD4+ T cells by regulatory CD4+CD25+ T lymphocytes. J. Immunol. 174, 155–163.

Edinger, M., Hoffmann, P., 2011. Regulatory T cells in stem cell transplantation: strategies and first clinical experiences. Curr. Opin. Immunol. 23, 679–684.

Edinger, M., Hoffmann, P., Ermann, J., Drago, K., Fathman, C.G., Strober, S., Negrin, R.S., 2003. CD4+CD25+ regulatory T cells preserve graft-versus-tumor activity while inhibiting graft-versus-host disease after bone marrow transplantation. Nat. Med. 9, 1144–1150.

Edozie, F.C., Nova-Lamperti, E.A., Povoleri, G.A., Scotta, C., John, S., Lombardi, G., Afzali, B., 2014. Regulatory T-cell therapy in the induction of transplant tolerance: the issue of subpopulations. Transplantation 98, 370–379.

Edwards, J.P., Fujii, H., Zhou, A.X., Creemers, J., Unutmaz, D., Shevach, E.M., 2013. Regulation of the expression of GARP/latent TGF-beta1 complexes on mouse T cells and their role in regulatory T cell and Th17 differentiation. J. Immunol. 190, 5506–5515.

Elyaman, W., Khoury, S.J., Scott, D.W., De Groot, A.S., 2011. Potential application of tregitopes as immunomodulating agents in multiple sclerosis. Neurol. Res. Int. 2011, 256460.

Esensten, J.H., Wofsy, D., Bluestone, J.A., 2009. Regulatory T cells as therapeutic targets in rheumatoid arthritis. Nat. Rev. Rheumatol. 5, 560–565.

Fahlen, L., Read, S., Gorelik, L., Hurst, S.D., Coffman, R.L., Flavell, R.A., Powrie, F., 2005. T cells that cannot respond to TGF-beta escape control by CD4(+)CD25(+) regulatory T cells. J. Exp. Med. 201, 737–746.

Fallarino, F., Grohmann, U., Hwang, K.W., Orabona, C., Vacca, C., Bianchi, R., Belladonna, M.L., Fioretti, M.C., Alegre, M.L., Puccetti, P., 2003. Modulation of tryptophan catabolism by regulatory T cells. Nat. Immunol. 4, 1206–1212.

Fedorak, R.N., Gangl, A., Elson, C.O., Rutgeerts, P., Schreiber, S., Wild, G., Hanauer, S.B., Kilian, A., Cohard, M., Lebeaut, A., Feagan, B., 2000. Recombinant human interleukin 10 in the treatment of patients with mild to moderately active Crohn's disease. The interleukin 10 inflammatory bowel disease cooperative study group. Gastroenterology 119, 1473–1482.

Finlay, C.M., Walsh, K.P., Mills, K.H., 2014. Induction of regulatory cells by helminth parasites: exploitation for the treatment of inflammatory diseases. Immunol. Rev. 259, 206–230.

Floess, S., Freyer, J., Siewert, C., Baron, U., Olek, S., Polansky, J., Schlawe, K., Chang, H.D., Bopp, T., Schmitt, E., Klein-Hessling, S., Serfling, E., Hamann, A., Huehn, J., 2007. Epigenetic control of the foxp3 locus in regulatory T cells. PLoS Biol. 5, e38.

Fontenot, J.D., Gavin, M.A., Rudensky, A.Y., 2003. Foxp3 programs the development and function of CD4+CD25+ regulatory T cells. Nat. Immunol. 4, 330–336.

Fontenot, J.D., Rasmussen, J.P., Williams, L.M., Dooley, J.L., Farr, A.G., Rudensky, A.Y., 2005. Regulatory T cell lineage specification by the forkhead transcription factor foxp3. Immunity 22, 329–341.

Foussat, A., Cottrez, F., Brun, V., Fournier, N., Breittmayer, J.P., Groux, H., 2003. A comparative study between T regulatory type 1 and CD4+CD25+ T cells in the control of inflammation. J. Immunol. 171, 5018–5026.

Francis, J.N., Till, S.J., Durham, S.R., 2003. Induction of IL-10+CD4+CD25+ T cells by grass pollen immunotherapy. J. Allergy Clin. Immunol. 111, 1255–1261.

Fujio, K., Okamura, T., Yamamoto, K., 2010. The family of IL-10-secreting CD4+ T cells. Adv. Immunol. 105, 99–130.

Gagliani, N., Magnani, C.F., Huber, S., Gianolini, M.E., Pala, M., Licona-Limon, P., Guo, B., Herbert, D.R., Bulfone, A., Trentini, F., Di Serio, C., Bacchetta, R., Andreani, M., Brockmann, L., Gregori, S., Flavell, R.A., Roncarolo, M.G., 2013. Coexpression of CD49b and LAG-3 identifies human and mouse T regulatory type 1 cells. Nat. Med. 19, 739–746.

Gaidot, A., Landau, D.A., Martin, G.H., Bonduelle, O., Grinberg-Bleyer, Y., Matheoud, D., Gregoire, S., Baillou, C., Combadiere, B., Piaggio, E., Cohen, J.L., 2011. Immune reconstitution is preserved in hematopoietic stem cell transplantation coadministered with regulatory T cells for GVHD prevention. Blood 117, 2975–2983.

Garin, M.I., Chu, C.C., Golshayan, D., Cernuda-Morollon, E., Wait, R., Lechler, R.I., 2007. Galectin-1: a key effector of regulation mediated by CD4+CD25+ T cells. Blood 109, 2058–2065.

Gavin, M.A., Clarke, S.R., Negrou, E., Gallegos, A., Rudensky, A., 2002. Homeostasis and anergy of CD4 (+)CD25(+) suppressor T cells in vivo. Nat. Immunol. 3, 33–41.

Geissler, E.K., 2012. The ONE Study compares cell therapy products in organ transplantation: introduction to a review series on suppressive monocyte-derived cells. Transplant. Res. 1, 11.

Gilliet, M., Liu, Y.J., 2002. Generation of human CD8 T regulatory cells by CD40 ligand-activated plasmacytoid dendritic cells. J. Exp. Med. 195, 695–704.

Glinka, Y., Prud'homme, G.J., 2008. Neuropilin-1 is a receptor for transforming growth factor beta-1, activates its latent form, and promotes regulatory T cell activity. J. Leukoc. Biol. 84, 302–310.

Gomez De Aguero, M., Vocanson, M., Hacini-Rachinel, F., Taillardet, M., Sparwasser, T., Kissenpfennig, A., Malissen, B., Kaiserlian, D., Dubois, B., 2012. Langerhans cells protect from allergic contact dermatitis in mice by tolerizing CD8(+) T cells and activating Foxp3(+) regulatory T cells. J. Clin. Invest. 122, 1700–1711.

Gondek, D.C., Lu, L.F., Quezada, S.A., Sakaguchi, S., Noelle, R.J., 2005. Cutting edge: contact-mediated suppression by CD4 + CD25 + regulatory cells involves a granzyme B-dependent, perforin-independent mechanism. J. Immunol. 174, 1783–1786.

Graca, L., Chen, T.C., Le Moine, A., Cobbold, S.P., Howie, D., Waldmann, H., 2005. Dominant tolerance: activation thresholds for peripheral generation of regulatory T cells. Trends Immunol. 26, 130–135.

Graca, L., Honey, K., Adams, E., Cobbold, S.P., Waldmann, H., 2000. Cutting edge: anti-CD154 therapeutic antibodies induce infectious transplantation tolerance. J. Immunol. 165, 4783–4786.

Graca, L., Le Moine, A., Cobbold, S.P., Waldmann, H., 2003. Antibody-induced transplantation tolerance: the role of dominant regulation. Immunol. Res. 28, 181–191.

Grainger, J.R., Askenase, M.H., Guimont-Desrochers, F., Da Fonseca, D.M., Belkaid, Y., 2014. Contextual functions of antigen-presenting cells in the gastrointestinal tract. Immunol. Rev. 259, 75–87.

Grinberg-Bleyer, Y., Baeyens, A., You, S., Elhage, R., Fourcade, G., Gregoire, S., Cagnard, N., Carpentier, W., Tang, Q., Bluestone, J., Chatenoud, L., Klatzmann, D., Salomon, B.L., Piaggio, E., 2010. IL-2 reverses established type 1 diabetes in NOD mice by a local effect on pancreatic regulatory T cells. J. Exp. Med. 207, 1871–1878.

Grohmann, U., Orabona, C., Fallarino, F., Vacca, C., Calcinaro, F., Falorni, A., Candeloro, P., Belladonna, M.L., Bianchi, R., Fioretti, M.C., Puccetti, P., 2002. CTLA-4-Ig regulates tryptophan catabolism in vivo. Nat. Immunol. 3, 1097–1101.

Grossman, W.J., Verbsky, J.W., Tollefsen, B.L., Kemper, C., Atkinson, J.P., Ley, T.J., 2004. Differential expression of granzymes A and B in human cytotoxic lymphocyte subsets and T regulatory cells. Blood 104, 2840–2848.

Groux, H., O'Garra, A., Bigler, M., Rouleau, M., Antonenko, S., De Vries, J.E., Roncarolo, M.G., 1997. A CD4+ T-cell subset inhibits antigen-specific T-cell responses and prevents colitis. Nature 389, 737–742.

Gutstein, N.L., Seaman, W.E., Scott, J.H., Wofsy, D., 1986. Induction of immune tolerance by administration of monoclonal antibody to L3T4. J. Immunol. 137, 1127–1132.

Haas, J., Hug, A., Viehover, A., Fritzsching, B., Falk, C.S., Filser, A., Vetter, T., Milkova, L., Korporal, M., Fritz, B., Storch-Hagenlocher, B., Krammer, P.H., Suri-Payer, E., Wildemann, B., 2005. Reduced suppressive effect of CD4 + CD25high regulatory T cells on the T cell immune response against myelin oligodendrocyte glycoprotein in patients with multiple sclerosis. Eur. J. Immunol. 35, 3343–3352.

Hanley, P.J., Bollard, C.M., Brunstein, C.G., 2015. Adoptive immunotherapy with the use of regulatory T cells and virus-specific T cells derived from cord blood. Cytotherapy 17 (6), 749–755.

Haribhai, D., Williams, J.B., Jia, S., Nickerson, D., Schmitt, E.G., Edwards, B., Ziegelbauer, J., Yassai, M., Li, S.H., Relland, L.M., Wise, P.M., Chen, A., Zheng, Y.Q., Simpson, P.M., Gorski, J., Salzman, N.H., Hessner, M.J., Chatila, T.A., Williams, C.B., 2011. A requisite role for induced regulatory T cells in tolerance based on expanding antigen receptor diversity. Immunity 35, 109–122.

Hawrylowicz, C.M., O'Garra, A., 2005. Potential role of interleukin-10-secreting regulatory T cells in allergy and asthma. Nat. Rev. Immunol. 5, 271–283.

Hench, V.K., Su, L., 2011. Regulation of IL-2 gene expression by Siva and FOXP3 in human T cells. BMC Immunol. 12, 54.

Hilchey, S.P., De, A., Rimsza, L.M., Bankert, R.B., Bernstein, S.H., 2007. Follicular lymphoma intratumoral CD4 + CD25 + GITR + regulatory T cells potently suppress CD3/CD28-costimulated autologous and allogeneic CD8 + CD25- and CD4 + CD25- T cells. J. Immunol. 178, 4051–4061.

Hill, J.A., Hall, J.A., Sun, C.M., Cai, Q., Ghyselinck, N., Chambon, P., Belkaid, Y., Mathis, D., Benoist, C., 2008. Retinoic acid enhances Foxp3 induction indirectly by relieving inhibition from CD4 + CD44hi Cells. Immunity 29, 758–770.

Himmel, M.E., Yao, Y., Orban, P.C., Steiner, T.S., Levings, M.K., 2012. Regulatory T-cell therapy for inflammatory bowel disease: more questions than answers. Immunology 136, 115–122.

Hippen, K.L., Merkel, S.C., Schirm, D.K., Sieben, C.M., Sumstad, D., Kadidlo, D.M., McKenna, D.H., Bromberg, J.S., Levine, B.L., Riley, J.L., June, C.H., Scheinberg, P., Douek, D.C., Miller, J.S., Wagner, J.E., Blazar, B.R., 2011. Massive ex vivo expansion of human natural regulatory T cells (T(regs)) with minimal loss of in vivo functional activity. Sci. Transl. Med. 3, 83ra41.

Hori, S., Nomura, T., Sakaguchi, S., 2003. Control of regulatory T cell development by the transcription factor Foxp3. Science 299, 1057–1061.

Huan, J., Culbertson, N., Spencer, L., Bartholomew, R., Burrows, G.G., Chou, Y.K., Bourdette, D., Ziegler, S.F., Offner, H., Vandenbark, A.A., 2005. Decreased FOXP3 levels in multiple sclerosis patients. J. Neurosci. Res. 81, 45–52.

Huang, C.T., Workman, C.J., Flies, D., Pan, X., Marson, A.L., Zhou, G., Hipkiss, E.L., Ravi, S., Kowalski, J., Levitsky, H.I., Powell, J.D., Pardoll, D.M., Drake, C.G., Vignali, D.A., 2004. Role of LAG-3 in regulatory T cells. Immunity 21, 503–513.

Huber, S., Gagliani, N., Esplugues, E., O'Connor Jr., W., Huber, F.J., Chaudhry, A., Kamanaka, M., Kobayashi, Y., Booth, C.J., Rudensky, A.Y., Roncarolo, M.G., Battaglia, M., Flavell, R.A., 2011. Th17 cells express interleukin-10 receptor and are controlled by Foxp3(−) and Foxp3+ regulatory CD4+ T cells in an interleukin-10-dependent manner. Immunity 34, 554–565.

Huter, E.N., Punkosdy, G.A., Glass, D.D., Cheng, L.I., Ward, J.M., Shevach, E.M., 2008. TGF-beta-induced Foxp3+ regulatory T cells rescue scurfy mice. Eur. J. Immunol. 38, 1814–1821.

Ildstad, S.T., Wren, S.M., Bluestone, J.A., Barbieri, S.A., Sachs, D.H., 1985. Characterization of mixed allogeneic chimeras. Immunocompetence, in vitro reactivity, and genetic specificity of tolerance. J. Exp. Med. 162, 231–244.

Inobe, J., Slavin, A.J., Komagata, Y., Chen, Y., Liu, L., Weiner, H.L., 1998. IL-4 is a differentiation factor for transforming growth factor-beta secreting Th3 cells and oral administration of IL-4 enhances oral tolerance in experimental allergic encephalomyelitis. Eur. J. Immunol. 28, 2780–2790.

Itoh, M., Takahashi, T., Sakaguchi, N., Kuniyasu, Y., Shimizu, J., Otsuka, F., Sakaguchi, S., 1999. Thymus and autoimmunity: production of CD25+CD4+ naturally anergic and suppressive T cells as a key function of the thymus in maintaining immunologic self-tolerance. J. Immunol. 162, 5317–5326.

Izcue, A., Coombes, J.L., Powrie, F., 2009. Regulatory lymphocytes and intestinal inflammation. Annu. Rev. Immunol. 27, 313–338.

Jacobs, J.F., Nierkens, S., Figdor, C.G., De Vries, I.J., Adema, G.J., 2012. Regulatory T cells in melanoma: the final hurdle towards effective immunotherapy? Lancet Oncol. 13, e32–e42.

Joetham, A., Takeda, K., Taube, C., Miyahara, N., Matsubara, S., Koya, T., Rha, Y.H., Dakhama, A., Gelfand, E.W., 2007. Naturally occurring lung CD4(+)CD25(+) T cell regulation of airway allergic responses depends on IL-10 induction of TGF-beta. J. Immunol. 178, 1433–1442.

Johnston, R.J., Poholek, A.C., Ditoro, D., Yusuf, I., Eto, D., Barnett, B., Dent, A.L., Craft, J., Crotty, S., 2009. Bcl6 and Blimp-1 are reciprocal and antagonistic regulators of T follicular helper cell differentiation. Science 325, 1006–1010.

Jones, S.C., Murphy, G.F., Korngold, R., 2003. Post-hematopoietic cell transplantation control of graft-versus-host disease by donor CD425 T cells to allow an effective graft-versus-leukemia response. Biol. Blood Marrow Transplant. 9, 243–256.

Jonuleit, H., Schmitt, E., Stassen, M., Tuettenberg, A., Knop, J., Enk, A.H., 2001. Identification and functional characterization of human CD4(+)CD25(+) T cells with regulatory properties isolated from peripheral blood. J. Exp. Med. 193, 1285–1294.

Josefowicz, S.Z., Lu, L.F., Rudensky, A.Y., 2012. Regulatory T cells: mechanisms of differentiation and function. Annu. Rev. Immunol. 30, 531–564.

Jutel, M., Akdis, M., Budak, F., Aebischer-Casaulta, C., Wrzyszcz, M., Blaser, K., Akdis, C.A., 2003. IL-10 and TGF-beta cooperate in the regulatory T cell response to mucosal allergens in normal immunity and specific immunotherapy. Eur. J. Immunol. 33, 1205–1214.

Juvet, S.C., Whatcott, A.G., Bushell, A.R., Wood, K.J., 2014. Harnessing regulatory T cells for clinical use in transplantation: the end of the beginning. Am. J. Transplant. 14, 750–763.

Kearley, J., Robinson, D.S., Lloyd, C.M., 2008. CD4+CD25+ regulatory T cells reverse established allergic airway inflammation and prevent airway remodeling. J. Allergy Clin. Immunol. 122 (617–24), e6.

Kelchtermans, H., Geboes, L., Mitera, T., Huskens, D., Leclercq, G., Matthys, P., 2009. Activated CD4+CD25+ regulatory T cells inhibit osteoclastogenesis and collagen-induced arthritis. Ann. Rheum. Dis. 68, 744–750.

Kelley, C.M., Ikeda, T., Koipally, J., Avitahl, N., Wu, L., Georgopoulos, K., Morgan, B.A., 1998. Helios, a novel dimerization partner of Ikaros expressed in the earliest hematopoietic progenitors. Curr. Biol. 8, 508–515.

Kessel, A., Ammuri, H., Peri, R., Pavlotzky, E.R., Blank, M., Shoenfeld, Y., Toubi, E., 2007. Intravenous immunoglobulin therapy affects T regulatory cells by increasing their suppressive function. J. Immunol. 179, 5571–5575.

Khattri, R., Cox, T., Yasayko, S.A., Ramsdell, F., 2003. An essential role for Scurfin in CD4+CD25+ T regulatory cells. Nat. Immunol. 4, 337–342.

Khattri, R., Kasprowicz, D., Cox, T., Mortrud, M., Appleby, M.W., Brunkow, M.E., Ziegler, S.F., Ramsdell, F., 2001. The amount of scurfin protein determines peripheral T cell number and responsiveness. J. Immunol. 167, 6312–6320.

Killebrew, J.R., Perdue, N., Kwan, A., Thornton, A.M., Shevach, E.M., Campbell, D.J., 2011. A self-reactive TCR drives the development of Foxp3+ regulatory T cells that prevent autoimmune disease. J. Immunol. 187, 861–869.

Kim, H.P., Leonard, W.J., 2007. CREB/ATF-dependent T cell receptor-induced FoxP3 gene expression: a role for DNA methylation. J. Exp. Med. 204, 1543–1551.

Klein, L., Khazaie, K., Von Boehmer, H., 2003. In vivo dynamics of antigen-specific regulatory T cells not predicted from behavior in vitro. Proc. Natl. Acad. Sci. U. S. A. 100, 8886–8891.

Kobie, J.J., Shah, P.R., Yang, L., Rebhahn, J.A., Fowell, D.J., Mosmann, T.R., 2006. T regulatory and primed uncommitted CD4 T cells express CD73, which suppresses effector CD4 T cells by converting 5'-adenosine monophosphate to adenosine. J. Immunol. 177, 6780–6786.

Koch, M.A., Tucker-Heard, G., Perdue, N.R., Killebrew, J.R., Urdahl, K.B., Campbell, D.J., 2009. The transcription factor T-bet controls regulatory T cell homeostasis and function during type 1 inflammation. Nat. Immunol. 10, 595–602.

Kohm, A.P., Carpentier, P.A., Anger, H.A., Miller, S.D., 2002. Cutting edge: CD4+CD25+ regulatory T cells suppress antigen-specific autoreactive immune responses and central nervous system inflammation during active experimental autoimmune encephalomyelitis. J. Immunol. 169, 4712–4716.

Komatsu, N., Mariotti-Ferrandiz, M.E., Wang, Y., Malissen, B., Waldmann, H., Hori, S., 2009. Heterogeneity of natural Foxp3+ T cells: a committed regulatory T-cell lineage and an uncommitted minor population retaining plasticity. Proc. Natl. Acad. Sci. U. S. A. 106, 1903–1908.

Kong, N., Lan, Q., Chen, M., Wang, J., Shi, W., Horwitz, D.A., Quesniaux, V., Ryffel, B., Liu, Z., Brand, D., Zou, H., Zheng, S.G., 2012. Antigen-specific transforming growth factor beta-induced Treg cells, but not natural Treg cells, ameliorate autoimmune arthritis in mice by shifting the Th17/Treg cell balance from Th17 predominance to Treg cell predominance. Arthritis Rheum. 64, 2548–2558.

Koreth, J., Matsuoka, K., Kim, H.T., McDonough, S.M., Bindra, B., Alyea 3rd., E.P., Armand, P., Cutler, C., Ho, V.T., Treister, N.S., Bienfang, D.C., Prasad, S., Tzachanis, D., Joyce, R.M., Avigan, D.E., Antin, J.H., Ritz, J., Soiffer, R.J., 2011. Interleukin-2 and regulatory T cells in graft-versus-host disease. N. Engl. J. Med. 365, 2055–2066.

Korn, T., Reddy, J., Gao, W., Bettelli, E., Awasthi, A., Petersen, T.R., Backstrom, B.T., Sobel, R.A., Wucherpfennig, K.W., Strom, T.B., Oukka, M., Kuchroo, V.K., 2007. Myelin-specific regulatory T cells accumulate in the CNS but fail to control autoimmune inflammation. Nat. Med. 13, 423–431.

Kornete, M., Sgouroudis, E., Piccirillo, C.A., 2012. ICOS-dependent homeostasis and function of Foxp3+ regulatory T cells in islets of nonobese diabetic mice. J. Immunol. 188, 1064–1074.

Kukreja, A., Cost, G., Marker, J., Zhang, C., Sun, Z., Linsu, K., Ten, S., Sanz, M., Exley, M., Wilson, B., Porcelli, S., Maclaren, N., 2002. Multiple immuno-regulatory defects in type-1 diabetes. J. Clin. Invest. 109, 131–140.

Kumar, M., Putzki, N., Limmroth, V., Remus, R., Lindemann, M., Knop, D., Mueller, N., Hardt, C., Kreuzfelder, E., Grosse-Wilde, H., 2006. CD4+CD25+FoxP3+ T lymphocytes fail to suppress myelin basic protein-induced proliferation in patients with multiple sclerosis. J. Neuroimmunol. 180, 178–184.

Kuniyasu, Y., Takahashi, T., Itoh, M., Shimizu, J., Toda, G., Sakaguchi, S., 2000. Naturally anergic and suppressive CD25(+)CD4(+) T cells as a functionally and phenotypically distinct immunoregulatory T cell subpopulation. Int. Immunol. 12, 1145–1155.

Kursar, M., Koch, M., Mittrucker, H.W., Nouailles, G., Bonhagen, K., Kamradt, T., Kaufmann, S.H., 2007. Cutting edge: regulatory T cells prevent efficient clearance of Mycobacterium tuberculosis. J. Immunol. 178, 2661–2665.

Le Douarin, N., Corbel, C., Bandeira, A., Thomas-Vaslin, V., Modigliani, Y., Coutinho, A., Salaun, J., 1996. Evidence for a thymus-dependent form of tolerance that is not based on elimination or anergy of reactive T cells. Immunol. Rev. 149, 35–53.

Levings, M.K., Roncarolo, M.G., 2000. T-regulatory 1 cells: a novel subset of CD4 T cells with immunoregulatory properties. J. Allergy Clin. Immunol. 106, S109–S112.

Li, H., Yu, J.P., Cao, S., Wei, F., Zhang, P., An, X.M., Huang, Z.T., Ren, X.B., 2007a. CD4+CD25+ regulatory T cells decreased the antitumor activity of cytokine-induced killer (CIK) cells of lung cancer patients. J. Clin. Immunol. 27, 317–326.

Li, M.O., Sanjabi, S., Flavell, R.A., 2006. Transforming growth factor-beta controls development, homeostasis, and tolerance of T cells by regulatory T cell-dependent and -independent mechanisms. Immunity 25, 455–471.

Li, M.O., Wan, Y.Y., Flavell, R.A., 2007b. T cell-produced transforming growth factor-beta1 controls T cell tolerance and regulates Th1- and Th17-cell differentiation. Immunity 26, 579–591.

Liang, B., Workman, C., Lee, J., Chew, C., Dale, B.M., Colonna, L., Flores, M., Li, N., Schweighoffer, E., Greenberg, S., Tybulewicz, V., Vignali, D., Clynes, R., 2008. Regulatory T cells inhibit dendritic cells by lymphocyte activation gene-3 engagement of MHC class II. J. Immunol. 180, 5916–5926.

Liao, G., Nayak, S., Regueiro, J.R., Berger, S.B., Detre, C., Romero, X., De Waal Malefyt, R., Chatila, T.A., Herzog, R.W., Terhorst, C., 2010. GITR engagement preferentially enhances proliferation of functionally competent CD4+CD25+FoxP3+ regulatory T cells. Int. Immunol. 22, 259–270.

Linterman, M.A., Pierson, W., Lee, S.K., Kallies, A., Kawamoto, S., Rayner, T.F., Srivastava, M., Divekar, D.P., Beaton, L., Hogan, J.J., Fagarasan, S., Liston, A., Smith, K.G., Vinuesa, C.G., 2011. Foxp3+ follicular regulatory T cells control the germinal center response. Nat. Med. 17, 975–982.

Liu, Y., Zhang, P., Li, J., Kulkarni, A.B., Perruche, S., Chen, W., 2008. A critical function for TGF-beta signaling in the development of natural CD4+CD25+Foxp3+ regulatory T cells. Nat. Immunol. 9, 632–640.

Liu, Z., Tugulea, S., Cortesini, R., Suciu-Foca, N., 1998. Specific suppression of T helper alloreactivity by allo-MHC class I-restricted CD8+CD28- T cells. Int. Immunol. 10, 775–783.

Lloyd, C.M., Hawrylowicz, C.M., 2009. Regulatory T cells in asthma. Immunity 31, 438–449.

Lohning, M., Hutloff, A., Kallinich, T., Mages, H.W., Bonhagen, K., Radbruch, A., Hamelmann, E., Kroczek, R.A., 2003. Expression of ICOS in vivo defines CD4+ effector T cells with high inflammatory potential and a strong bias for secretion of interleukin 10. J. Exp. Med. 197, 181–193.

Long, S.A., Rieck, M., Tatum, M., Bollyky, P.L., Wu, R.P., Muller, I., Ho, J.C., Shilling, H.G., Buckner, J.H., 2011. Low-dose antigen promotes induction of FOXP3 in human CD4+ T cells. J. Immunol. 187, 3511–3520.

Loser, K., Apelt, J., Voskort, M., Mohaupt, M., Balkow, S., Schwarz, T., Grabbe, S., Beissert, S., 2007. IL-10 controls ultraviolet-induced carcinogenesis in mice. J. Immunol. 179, 365–371.

Lundsgaard, D., Holm, T.L., Hornum, L., Markholst, H., 2005. In vivo control of diabetogenic T-cells by regulatory CD4+CD25+ T-cells expressing Foxp3. Diabetes 54, 1040–1047.

Luo, B., Chan, W.F., Shapiro, A.M., Anderson, C.C., 2007. Non-myeloablative mixed chimerism approaches and tolerance, a split decision. Eur. J. Immunol. 37, 1233–1242.

Maazi, H., Shirinbak, S., Willart, M., Hammad, H.M., Cabanski, M., Boon, L., Ganesh, V., Baru, A.M., Hansen, G., Lambrecht, B.N., Sparwasser, T., Nawijn, M.C., Van Oosterhout, A.J., 2012. Contribution of regulatory T cells to alleviation of experimental allergic asthma after specific immunotherapy. Clin. Exp. Allergy 42, 1519–1528.

Mann, M.K., Maresz, K., Shriver, L.P., Tan, Y., Dittel, B.N., 2007. B cell regulation of CD4 + CD25 + T regulatory cells and IL-10 via B7 is essential for recovery from experimental autoimmune encephalomyelitis. J. Immunol. 178, 3447–3456.

Marek-Trzonkowska, N., Mysliwiec, M., Dobyszuk, A., Grabowska, M., Techmanska, I., Juscinska, J., Wujtewicz, M.A., Witkowski, P., Mlynarski, W., Balcerska, A., Mysliwska, J., Trzonkowski, P., 2012. Administration of CD4 + CD25highCD127- regulatory T cells preserves beta-cell function in type 1 diabetes in children. Diabetes Care 35, 1817–1820.

Marie, J.C., Letterio, J.J., Gavin, M., Rudensky, A.Y., 2005. TGF-beta1 maintains suppressor function and Foxp3 expression in CD4 + CD25 + regulatory T cells. J. Exp. Med. 201, 1061–1067.

Mars, L.T., Araujo, L., Kerschen, P., Diem, S., Bourgeois, E., Van, L.P., Carrie, N., Dy, M., Liblau, R.S., Herbelin, A., 2009. Invariant NKT cells inhibit development of the Th17 lineage. Proc. Natl. Acad. Sci. U. S. A. 106, 6238–6243.

Martelli, M.F., Di Ianni, M., Ruggeri, L., Falzetti, F., Carotti, A., Terenzi, A., Pierini, A., Massei, M.S., Amico, L., Urbani, E., Del Papa, B., Zei, T., Iacucci Ostini, R., Cecchini, D., Tognellini, R., Reisner, Y., Aversa, F., Falini, B., Velardi, A., 2014. HLA-haploidentical transplantation with regulatory and conventional T-cell adoptive immunotherapy prevents acute leukemia relapse. Blood 124, 638–644.

Matsuoka, K., Kim, H.T., McDonough, S., Bascug, G., Warshauer, B., Koreth, J., Cutler, C., Ho, V.T., Alyea, E.P., Antin, J.H., Soiffer, R.J., Ritz, J., 2010. Altered regulatory T cell homeostasis in patients with CD4+ lymphopenia following allogeneic hematopoietic stem cell transplantation. J. Clin. Invest. 120, 1479–1493.

Merino, A., Dror, Y., Benkerrou, M., Colombe, B.W., Cowan, M.J., 1993. Development of tolerance after haplocompatible T-depleted bone marrow transplantation. Bone Marrow Transplant. 12, 483–488.

Miyao, T., Floess, S., Setoguchi, R., Luche, H., Fehling, H.J., Waldmann, H., Huehn, J., Hori, S., 2012. Plasticity of Foxp3(+) T cells reflects promiscuous Foxp3 expression in conventional T cells but not reprogramming of regulatory T cells. Immunity 36, 262–275.

Miyara, M., Yoshioka, Y., Kitoh, A., Shima, T., Wing, K., Niwa, A., Parizot, C., Taflin, C., Heike, T., Valeyre, D., Mathian, A., Nakahata, T., Yamaguchi, T., Nomura, T., Ono, M., Amoura, Z., Gorochov, G., Sakaguchi, S., 2009. Functional delineation and differentiation dynamics of human CD4+ T cells expressing the FoxP3 transcription factor. Immunity 30, 899–911.

Molitor-Dart, M.L., Andrassy, J., Kwun, J., Kayaoglu, H.A., Roenneburg, D.A., Haynes, L.D., Torrealba, J.R., Bobadilla, J.L., Sollinger, H.W., Knechtle, S.J., Burlingham, W.J., 2007. Developmental exposure to noninherited maternal antigens induces CD4 + T regulatory cells: relevance to mechanism of heart allograft tolerance. J. Immunol. 179, 6749–6761.

Monteiro, M., Almeida, C.F., Caridade, M., Ribot, J.C., Duarte, J., Agua-Doce, A., Wollenberg, I., Silva-Santos, B., Graca, L., 2010. Identification of regulatory Foxp3+ invariant NKT cells induced by TGF-beta. J. Immunol. 185, 2157–2163.

Monteiro, M., Graca, L., 2014. iNKT cells: innate lymphocytes with a diverse response. Crit. Rev. Immunol. 34, 81–90.

Morikawa, H., Sakaguchi, S., 2014. Genetic and epigenetic basis of Treg cell development and function: from a FoxP3-centered view to an epigenome-defined view of natural Treg cells. Immunol. Rev. 259, 192–205.

Mosmann, T.R., Cherwinski, H., Bond, M.W., Giedlin, M.A., Coffman, R.L., 1986. Two types of murine helper T cell clone. I. Definition according to profiles of lymphokine activities and secreted proteins. J. Immunol. 136, 2348–2357.

Mucida, D., Kutchukhidze, N., Erazo, A., Russo, M., Lafaille, J.J., Curotto De Lafaille, M.A., 2005. Oral tolerance in the absence of naturally occurring Tregs. J. Clin. Invest. 115, 1923–1933.

Mucida, D., Park, Y., Kim, G., Turovskaya, O., Scott, I., Kronenberg, M., Cheroutre, H., 2007. Reciprocal TH17 and regulatory T cell differentiation mediated by retinoic acid. Science 317, 256–260.

Murai, M., Turovskaya, O., Kim, G., Madan, R., Karp, C.L., Cheroutre, H., Kronenberg, M., 2009. Interleukin 10 acts on regulatory T cells to maintain expression of the transcription factor Foxp3 and suppressive function in mice with colitis. Nat. Immunol. 10, 1178–1184.

Nagano, Y., Itoh, K., Honda, K., 2012. The induction of Treg cells by gut-indigenous Clostridium. Curr. Opin. Immunol. 24, 392–397.

Nausch, N., Midzi, N., Mduluza, T., Maizels, R.M., Mutapi, F., 2011. Regulatory and activated T cells in human Schistosoma haematobium infections. PLoS One 6, e16860.

Ng, W.F., Duggan, P.J., Ponchel, F., Matarese, G., Lombardi, G., Edwards, A.D., Isaacs, J.D., Lechler, R.I., 2001. Human CD4(+)CD25(+) cells: a naturally occurring population of regulatory T cells. Blood 98, 2736–2744.

Nishikawa, H., Sakaguchi, S., 2014. Regulatory T cells in cancer immunotherapy. Curr. Opin. Immunol. 27, 1–7.

Nurieva, R.I., Chung, Y., Martinez, G.J., Yang, X.O., Tanaka, S., Matskevitch, T.D., Wang, Y.H., Dong, C., 2009. Bcl6 mediates the development of T follicular helper cells. Science 325, 1001–1005.

Nutsch, K.M., Hsieh, C.S., 2012. T cell tolerance and immunity to commensal bacteria. Curr. Opin. Immunol. 24, 385–391.

Oberle, N., Eberhardt, N., Falk, C.S., Krammer, P.H., Suri-Payer, E., 2007. Rapid suppression of cytokine transcription in human CD4 + CD25 T cells by CD4 + Foxp3 + regulatory T cells: independence of IL-2 consumption, TGF-beta, and various inhibitors of TCR signaling. J. Immunol. 179, 3578–3587.

Oderup, C., Cederbom, L., Makowska, A., Cilio, C.M., Ivars, F., 2006. Cytotoxic T lymphocyte antigen-4-dependent down-modulation of costimulatory molecules on dendritic cells in CD4+ CD25+ regulatory T-cell-mediated suppression. Immunology 118, 240–249.

Ogawa, C., Tone, Y., Tsuda, M., Peter, C., Waldmann, H., Tone, M., 2014. TGF-beta-mediated Foxp3 gene expression is cooperatively regulated by Stat5, Creb, and AP-1 through CNS2. J. Immunol. 192, 475–483.

Olivares-Villagomez, D., Wang, Y., Lafaille, J.J., 1998. Regulatory CD4(+) T cells expressing endogenous T cell receptor chains protect myelin basic protein-specific transgenic mice from spontaneous autoimmune encephalomyelitis. J. Exp. Med. 188, 1883–1894.

Oliveira, V.G., Caridade, M., Paiva, R.S., Demengeot, J., Graca, L., 2011. Sub-optimal CD4+ T-cell activation triggers autonomous TGF-beta-dependent conversion to Foxp3+ regulatory T cells. Eur. J. Immunol. 41, 1249–1255.

Owen, C.J., Jennings, C.E., Imrie, H., Lachaux, A., Bridges, N.A., Cheetham, T.D., Pearce, S.H., 2003. Mutational analysis of the FOXP3 gene and evidence for genetic heterogeneity in the immunodysregulation, polyendocrinopathy, enteropathy syndrome. J. Clin. Endocrinol. Metab. 88, 6034–6039.

Pallotta, M.T., Orabona, C., Volpi, C., Vacca, C., Belladonna, M.L., Bianchi, R., Servillo, G., Brunacci, C., Calvitti, M., Bicciato, S., Mazza, E.M., Boon, L., Grassi, F., Fioretti, M.C., Fallarino, F., Puccetti, P., Grohmann, U., 2011. Indoleamine 2,3-dioxygenase is a signaling protein in long-term tolerance by dendritic cells. Nat. Immunol. 12, 870–878.

Pandiyan, P., Zheng, L., Ishihara, S., Reed, J., Lenardo, M.J., 2007. CD4 + CD25 + Foxp3 + regulatory T cells induce cytokine deprivation-mediated apoptosis of effector CD4+ T cells. Nat. Immunol. 8, 1353–1362.

Peters, J.H., Koenen, H.J., Fasse, E., Tijssen, H.J., Ijzermans, J.N., Groenen, P.J., Schaap, N.P., Kwekkeboom, J., Joosten, I., 2013. Human secondary lymphoid organs typically contain polyclonally-activated proliferating regulatory T cells. Blood 122, 2213–2223.

Peterson, R.A., 2012. Regulatory T-cells: diverse phenotypes integral to immune homeostasis and suppression. Toxicol. Pathol. 40, 186–204.

Pierson, W., Cauwe, B., Policheni, A., Schlenner, S.M., Franckaert, D., Berges, J., Humblet-Baron, S., Schonefeldt, S., Herold, M.J., Hildeman, D., Strasser, A., Bouillet, P., Lu, L.F., Matthys, P., Freitas, A.A., Luther, R.J., Weaver, C.T., Dooley, J., Gray, D.H., Liston, A., 2013. Antiapoptotic Mcl-1 is critical for the survival and niche-filling capacity of Foxp3(+) regulatory T cells. Nat. Immunol. 14, 959–965.

Polansky, J.K., Kretschmer, K., Freyer, J., Floess, S., Garbe, A., Baron, U., Olek, S., Hamann, A., Von Boehmer, H., Huehn, J., 2008. DNA methylation controls Foxp3 gene expression. Eur. J. Immunol. 38, 1654–1663.

Praksova, P., Stourac, P., Bednarik, J., Vlckova, E., Mikulkova, Z., Michalek, J., 2012. Immunoregulatory T cells in multiple sclerosis and the effect of interferon beta and glatiramer acetate treatment on T cell subpopulations. J. Neurol. Sci. 319, 18–23.

Putnam, A.L., Brusko, T.M., Lee, M.R., Liu, W., Szot, G.L., Ghosh, T., Atkinson, M.A., Bluestone, J.A., 2009. Expansion of human regulatory T-cells from patients with type 1 diabetes. Diabetes 58, 652–662.

Qin, S., Cobbold, S.P., Pope, H., Elliott, J., Kioussis, D., Davies, J., Waldmann, H., 1993. "Infectious" transplantation tolerance. Science 259, 974–977.

Ren, X., Ye, F., Jiang, Z., Chu, Y., Xiong, S., Wang, Y., 2007. Involvement of cellular death in TRAIL/DR5-dependent suppression induced by CD4(+)CD25(+) regulatory T cells. Cell Death Differ. 14, 2076–2084.

Rich, S., Seelig, M., Lee, H.M., Lin, J., 1995. Transforming growth factor beta 1 costimulated growth and regulatory function of staphylococcal enterotoxin B-responsive CD8+ T cells. J. Immunol. 155, 609–618.

Robb, R.J., Lineburg, K.E., Kuns, R.D., Wilson, Y.A., Raffelt, N.C., Olver, S.D., Varelias, A., Alexander, K.A., Teal, B.E., Sparwasser, T., Hammerling, G.J., Markey, K.A., Koyama, M., Clouston, A.D., Engwerda, C.R., Hill, G.R., MacDonald, K.P., 2012. Identification and expansion of highly suppressive CD8(+)FoxP3(+) regulatory T cells after experimental allogeneic bone marrow transplantation. Blood 119, 5898–5908.

Rossetti, M., Spreafico, R., Saidin, S., Chua, C., Moshref, M., Leong, J.Y., Tan, Y.K., Thumboo, J., Van Loosdregt, J., Albani, S., 2015. Ex Vivo-expanded but not in vitro-induced human regulatory T cells are candidates for cell therapy in autoimmune diseases thanks to stable demethylation of the FOXP3 regulatory T cell-specific demethylated region. J. Immunol. 194, 113–124.

Rowe, J.H., Ertelt, J.M., Xin, L., Way, S.S., 2012. Pregnancy imprints regulatory memory that sustains anergy to fetal antigen. Nature 490, 102–106.

Rubtsov, Y.P., Rasmussen, J.P., Chi, E.Y., Fontenot, J., Castelli, L., Ye, X., Treuting, P., Siewe, L., Roers, A., Henderson Jr., W.R., Muller, W., Rudensky, A.Y., 2008. Regulatory T cell-derived interleukin-10 limits inflammation at environmental interfaces. Immunity 28, 546–558.

Sakaguchi, S., Sakaguchi, N., Asano, M., Itoh, M., Toda, M., 1995. Immunologic self-tolerance maintained by activated T cells expressing IL-2 receptor alpha-chains (CD25). Breakdown of a single mechanism of self-tolerance causes various autoimmune diseases. J. Immunol. 155, 1151–1164.

Salomon, B., Lenschow, D.J., Rhee, L., Ashourian, N., Singh, B., Sharpe, A., Bluestone, J.A., 2000. B7/CD28 costimulation is essential for the homeostasis of the CD4+CD25+ immunoregulatory T cells that control autoimmune diabetes. Immunity 12, 431–440.

Samstein, R.M., Josefowicz, S.Z., Arvey, A., Treuting, P.M., Rudensky, A.Y., 2012. Extrathymic generation of regulatory T cells in placental mammals mitigates maternal-fetal conflict. Cell 150, 29–38.

Sarkar, S., Fox, D.A., 2007. Regulatory T cell defects in rheumatoid arthritis. Arthritis Rheum. 56, 710–713.

Sarris, M., Andersen, K.G., Randow, F., Mayr, L., Betz, A.G., 2008. Neuropilin-1 expression on regulatory T cells enhances their interactions with dendritic cells during antigen recognition. Immunity 28, 402–413.

Sauer, S., Bruno, L., Hertweck, A., Finlay, D., Leleu, M., Spivakov, M., Knight, Z.A., Cobb, B.S., Cantrell, D., O'Connor, E., Shokat, K.M., Fisher, A.G., Merkenschlager, M., 2008. T cell receptor signaling controls Foxp3 expression via PI3K, Akt, and mTOR. Proc. Natl. Acad. Sci. U. S. A. 105, 7797–7802.

Schneider-Hohendorf, T., Stenner, M.P., Weidenfeller, C., Zozulya, A.L., Simon, O.J., Schwab, N., Wiendl, H., 2010. Regulatory T cells exhibit enhanced migratory characteristics, a feature impaired in patients with multiple sclerosis. Eur. J. Immunol. 40, 3581–3590.

Schoenbrunn, A., Frentsch, M., Kohler, S., Keye, J., Dooms, H., Moewes, B., Dong, J., Loddenkemper, C., Sieper, J., Wu, P., Romagnani, C., Matzmohr, N., Thiel, A., 2012. A converse 4-1BB and CD40 ligand expression pattern delineates activated regulatory T cells (Treg) and conventional T cells enabling direct isolation of alloantigen-reactive natural Foxp3+ Treg. J. Immunol. 189, 5985–5994.

Schreiber, S., Fedorak, R.N., Nielsen, O.H., Wild, G., Williams, C.N., Nikolaus, S., Jacyna, M., Lashner, B.A., Gangl, A., Rutgeerts, P., Isaacs, K., Van Deventer, S.J., Koningsberger, J.C., Cohard, M., Lebeaut, A., Hanauer, S.B., 2000. Safety and efficacy of recombinant human interleukin 10 in chronic active Crohn's disease. Crohn's disease IL-10 cooperative study group. Gastroenterology 119, 1461–1472.

Schumacher, A., Wafula, P.O., Bertoja, A.Z., Sollwedel, A., Thuere, C., Wollenberg, I., Yagita, H., Volk, H.D., Zenclussen, A.C., 2007. Mechanisms of action of regulatory T cells specific for paternal antigens during pregnancy. Obstet. Gynecol. 110, 1137–1145.

Seddon, B., Mason, D., 2000. The third function of the thymus. Immunol. Today 21, 95–99.

Selvaraj, R.K., Geiger, T.L., 2008. Mitigation of experimental allergic encephalomyelitis by TGF-beta induced Foxp3+ regulatory T lymphocytes through the induction of anergy and infectious tolerance. J. Immunol. 180, 2830–2838.

Setoguchi, R., Hori, S., Takahashi, T., Sakaguchi, S., 2005. Homeostatic maintenance of natural Foxp3(+) CD25(+) CD4(+) regulatory T cells by interleukin (IL)-2 and induction of autoimmune disease by IL-2 neutralization. J. Exp. Med. 201, 723–735.

Shevach, E.M., Thornton, A.M., 2014. tTregs, pTregs, and iTregs: similarities and differences. Immunol. Rev. 259, 88–102.

Shull, M.M., Ormsby, I., Kier, A.B., Pawlowski, S., Diebold, R.J., Yin, M., Allen, R., Sidman, C., Proetzel, G., Calvin, D., 1992. Targeted disruption of the mouse transforming growth factor-beta 1 gene results in multifocal inflammatory disease. Nature 359, 693–699.

Singh, A.K., Wilson, M.T., Hong, S., Olivares-Villagomez, D., Du, C., Stanic, A.K., Joyce, S., Sriram, S., Koezuka, Y., Van Kaer, L., 2001. Natural killer T cell activation protects mice against experimental autoimmune encephalomyelitis. J. Exp. Med. 194, 1801–1811.

Sledzinska, A., Hemmers, S., Mair, F., Gorka, O., Ruland, J., Fairbairn, L., Nissler, A., Muller, W., Waisman, A., Becher, B., Buch, T., 2013. TGF-beta signalling is required for CD4(+) T cell homeostasis but dispensable for regulatory T cell function. PLoS Biol. 11, e1001674.

Smigiel, K.S., Richards, E., Srivastava, S., Thomas, K.R., Dudda, J.C., Klonowski, K.D., Campbell, D.J., 2014. CCR7 provides localized access to IL-2 and defines homeostatically distinct regulatory T cell subsets. J. Exp. Med. 211, 121–136.

Steinbrink, K., Wolfl, M., Jonuleit, H., Knop, J., Enk, A.H., 1997. Induction of tolerance by IL-10-treated dendritic cells. J. Immunol. 159, 4772–4780.

Stephens, L.A., Malpass, K.H., Anderton, S.M., 2009. Curing CNS autoimmune disease with myelin-reactive Foxp3+ Treg. Eur. J. Immunol. 39, 1108–1117.

Stoop, J.N., Woltman, A.M., Biesta, P.J., Kusters, J.G., Kuipers, E.J., Janssen, H.L., Van Der Molen, R.G., 2007. Tumor necrosis factor alpha inhibits the suppressive effect of regulatory T cells on the hepatitis B virus-specific immune response. Hepatology 46, 699–705.

Strauss, L., Bergmann, C., Szczepanski, M., Gooding, W., Johnson, J.T., Whiteside, T.L., 2007. A unique subset of CD4+CD25highFoxp3+ T cells secreting interleukin-10 and transforming growth factor-beta1 mediates suppression in the tumor microenvironment. Clin. Cancer Res. 13, 4345–4354.

Sugiyama, D., Nishikawa, H., Maeda, Y., Nishioka, M., Tanemura, A., Katayama, I., Ezoe, S., Kanakura, Y., Sato, E., Fukumori, Y., Karbach, J., Jager, E., Sakaguchi, S., 2013. Anti-CCR4 mAb selectively depletes effector-type FoxP3+CD4+ regulatory T cells, evoking antitumor immune responses in humans. Proc. Natl. Acad. Sci. U. S. A. 110, 17945–17950.

Sun, C.M., Hall, J.A., Blank, R.B., Bouladoux, N., Oukka, M., Mora, J.R., Belkaid, Y., 2007. Small intestine lamina propria dendritic cells promote de novo generation of Foxp3 T reg cells via retinoic acid. J. Exp. Med. 204, 1775–1785.

Taams, L.S., Smith, J., Rustin, M.H., Salmon, M., Poulter, L.W., Akbar, A.N., 2001. Human anergic/suppressive CD4(+)CD25(+) T cells: a highly differentiated and apoptosis-prone population. Eur. J. Immunol. 31, 1122–1131.

Taams, L.S., Van Amelsfort, J.M., Tiemessen, M.M., Jacobs, K.M., De Jong, E.C., Akbar, A.N., Bijlsma, J.W., Lafeber, F.P., 2005. Modulation of monocyte/macrophage function by human CD4 +CD25+ regulatory T cells. Hum. Immunol. 66, 222–230.

Takahashi, T., Kuniyasu, Y., Toda, M., Sakaguchi, N., Itoh, M., Iwata, M., Shimizu, J., Sakaguchi, S., 1998. Immunologic self-tolerance maintained by CD25+CD4+ naturally anergic and suppressive T cells: induction of autoimmune disease by breaking their anergic/suppressive state. Int. Immunol. 10, 1969–1980.

Tang, Q., Adams, J.Y., Penaranda, C., Melli, K., Piaggio, E., Sgouroudis, E., Piccirillo, C.A., Salomon, B.L., Bluestone, J.A., 2008. Central role of defective interleukin-2 production in the triggering of islet autoimmune destruction. Immunity 28, 687–697.

Tang, Q., Henriksen, K.J., Bi, M., Finger, E.B., Szot, G., Ye, J., Masteller, E.L., Mcdevitt, H., Bonyhadi, M., Bluestone, J.A., 2004. In vitro-expanded antigen-specific regulatory T cells suppress autoimmune diabetes. J. Exp. Med. 199, 1455–1465.

Tang, Q., Henriksen, K.J., Boden, E.K., Tooley, A.J., Ye, J., Subudhi, S.K., Zheng, X.X., Strom, T.B., Bluestone, J.A., 2003. Cutting edge: CD28 controls peripheral homeostasis of CD4 + CD25 + regulatory T cells. J. Immunol. 171, 3348–3352.

Tarbell, K.V., Petit, L., Zuo, X., Toy, P., Luo, X., Mqadmi, A., Yang, H., Suthanthiran, M., Mojsov, S., Steinman, R.M., 2007. Dendritic cell-expanded, islet-specific CD4+ CD25+ CD62L+ regulatory T cells restore normoglycemia in diabetic NOD mice. J. Exp. Med. 204, 191–201.

Taylor, M.D., Van Der Werf, N., Harris, A., Graham, A.L., Bain, O., Allen, J.E., Maizels, R.M., 2009. Early recruitment of natural CD4+ Foxp3+ Treg cells by infective larvae determines the outcome of filarial infection. Eur. J. Immunol. 39, 192–206.

Thornton, A.M., Korty, P.E., Tran, D.Q., Wohlfert, E.A., Murray, P.E., Belkaid, Y., Shevach, E.M., 2010. Expression of Helios, an Ikaros transcription factor family member, differentiates thymic-derived from peripherally induced Foxp3+ T regulatory cells. J. Immunol. 184, 3433–3441.

Thornton, A.M., Shevach, E.M., 1998. CD4 + CD25 + immunoregulatory T cells suppress polyclonal T cell activation in vitro by inhibiting interleukin 2 production. J. Exp. Med. 188, 287–296.

Tiemessen, M.M., Jagger, A.L., Evans, H.G., Van Herwijnen, M.J., John, S., Taams, L.S., 2007. CD4 + CD25 + Foxp3 + regulatory T cells induce alternative activation of human monocytes/macrophages. Proc. Natl. Acad. Sci. U. S. A. 104, 19446–19451.

Tommasini, A., Ferrari, S., Moratto, D., Badolato, R., Boniotto, M., Pirulli, D., Notarangelo, L.D., Andolina, M., 2002. X-chromosome inactivation analysis in a female carrier of FOXP3 mutation. Clin. Exp. Immunol. 130, 127–130.

Tone, Y., Furuuchi, K., Kojima, Y., Tykocinski, M.L., Greene, M.I., Tone, M., 2008. Smad3 and NFAT cooperate to induce Foxp3 expression through its enhancer. Nat. Immunol. 9, 194–202.

Tran, D.Q., Andersson, J., Wang, R., Ramsey, H., Unutmaz, D., Shevach, E.M., 2009. GARP (LRRC32) is essential for the surface expression of latent TGF-beta on platelets and activated FOXP3+ regulatory T cells. Proc. Natl. Acad. Sci. U. S. A. 106, 13445–13450.

Tran, D.Q., Ramsey, H., Shevach, E.M., 2007. Induction of FOXP3 expression in naive human CD4 + FOXP3 T cells by T-cell receptor stimulation is transforming growth factor-beta dependent but does not confer a regulatory phenotype. Blood 110, 2983–2990.

Trenado, A., Charlotte, F., Fisson, S., Yagello, M., Klatzmann, D., Salomon, B.L., Cohen, J.L., 2003. Recipient-type specific CD4 + CD25 + regulatory T cells favor immune reconstitution and control graft-versus-host disease while maintaining graft-versus-leukemia. J. Clin. Invest. 112, 1688–1696.

Trzonkowski, P., Bieniaszewska, M., Juscinska, J., Dobyszuk, A., Krzystyniak, A., Marek, N., Mysliwska, J., Hellmann, A., 2009. First-in-man clinical results of the treatment of patients with graft versus host disease with human ex vivo expanded CD4 + CD25 + CD127- T regulatory cells. Clin. Immunol. 133, 22–26.

Tsuji, M., Komatsu, N., Kawamoto, S., Suzuki, K., Kanagawa, O., Honjo, T., Hori, S., Fagarasan, S., 2009. Preferential generation of follicular B helper T cells from Foxp3+ T cells in gut Peyer's patches. Science 323, 1488–1492.

Turner, M.S., Isse, K., Fischer, D.K., Turnquist, H.R., Morel, P.A., 2014. Low TCR signal strength induces combined expansion of Th2 and regulatory T cell populations that protect mice from the development of type 1 diabetes. Diabetologia 57, 1428–1436.

Turner, M.S., Kane, L.P., Morel, P.A., 2009. Dominant role of antigen dose in CD4 + Foxp3 + regulatory T cell induction and expansion. J. Immunol. 183, 4895–4903.

Van De Keere, F., Tonegawa, S., 1998. CD4(+) T cells prevent spontaneous experimental autoimmune encephalomyelitis in anti-myelin basic protein T cell receptor transgenic mice. J. Exp. Med. 188, 1875–1882.

Vang, K.B., Yang, J., Mahmud, S.A., Burchill, M.A., Vegoe, A.L., Farrar, M.A., 2008. IL-2, -7, and -15, but not thymic stromal lymphopoeitin, redundantly govern CD4 + Foxp3 + regulatory T cell development. J. Immunol. 181, 3285–3290.

Vukmanovic-Stejic, M., Agius, E., Booth, N., Dunne, P.J., Lacy, K.E., Reed, J.R., Sobande, T.O., Kissane, S., Salmon, M., Rustin, M.H., Akbar, A.N., 2008. The kinetics of CD4 + Foxp3 + T cell accumulation during a human cutaneous antigen-specific memory response in vivo. J. Clin. Invest. 118, 3639–3650.

Waldmann, H., Adams, E., Fairchild, P., Cobbold, S., 2006. Infectious tolerance and the long-term acceptance of transplanted tissue. Immunol. Rev. 212, 301–313.

Walker, L.S., Chodos, A., Eggena, M., Dooms, H., Abbas, A.K., 2003. Antigen-dependent proliferation of CD4+ CD25+ regulatory T cells in vivo. J. Exp. Med. 198, 249–258.

Warnatz, K., Bossaller, L., Salzer, U., Skrabl-Baumgartner, A., Schwinger, W., Van Der Burg, M., Van Dongen, J.J., Orlowska-Volk, M., Knoth, R., Durandy, A., Draeger, R., Schlesier, M., Peter, H.H., Grimbacher, B., 2006. Human ICOS deficiency abrogates the germinal center reaction and provides a monogenic model for common variable immunodeficiency. Blood 107, 3045–3052.

Weber, S.E., Harbertson, J., Godebu, E., Mros, G.A., Padrick, R.C., Carson, B.D., Ziegler, S.F., Bradley, L.M., 2006. Adaptive islet-specific regulatory CD4 T cells control autoimmune diabetes and mediate the disappearance of pathogenic Th1 cells in vivo. J. Immunol. 176, 4730–4739.

Webster, K.E., Walters, S., Kohler, R.E., Mrkvan, T., Boyman, O., Surh, C.D., Grey, S.T., Sprent, J., 2009. In vivo expansion of T reg cells with IL-2-mAb complexes: induction of resistance to EAE and long-term acceptance of islet allografts without immunosuppression. J. Exp. Med. 206, 751–760.

Weiner, H.L., 2001. Induction and mechanism of action of transforming growth factor-beta-secreting Th3 regulatory cells. Immunol. Rev. 182, 207–214.

Weiss, J.M., Bilate, A.M., Gobert, M., Ding, Y., Curotto De Lafaille, M.A., Parkhurst, C.N., Xiong, H., Dolpady, J., Frey, A.B., Ruocco, M.G., Yang, Y., Floess, S., Huehn, J., Oh, S., Li, M.O., Niec, R.E., Rudensky, A.Y., Dustin, M.L., Littman, D.R., Lafaille, J.J., 2012. Neuropilin 1 is expressed on thymus-derived natural regulatory T cells, but not mucosa-generated induced Foxp3+ T reg cells. J. Exp. Med. 209 (1723–42), S1.

Weissler, K.A., Caton, A.J., 2014. The role of T-cell receptor recognition of peptide:MHC complexes in the formation and activity of Foxp3(+) regulatory T cells. Immunol. Rev. 259, 11–22.

Wieckiewicz, J., Goto, R., Wood, K.J., 2010. T regulatory cells and the control of alloimmunity: from characterisation to clinical application. Curr. Opin. Immunol. 22, 662–668.

Wildin, R.S., Smyk-Pearson, S., Filipovich, A.H., 2002. Clinical and molecular features of the immunodysregulation, polyendocrinopathy, enteropathy, X linked (IPEX) syndrome. J. Med. Genet. 39, 537–545.

Wing, K., Onishi, Y., Prieto-Martin, P., Yamaguchi, T., Miyara, M., Fehervari, Z., Nomura, T., Sakaguchi, S., 2008. CTLA-4 control over Foxp3+ regulatory T cell function. Science 322, 271–275.

Wollenberg, I., Agua-Doce, A., Hernandez, A., Almeida, C., Oliveira, V.G., Faro, J., Graca, L., 2011. Regulation of the germinal center reaction by Foxp3+ follicular regulatory T cells. J. Immunol. 187, 4553–4560.

Wood, K.J., Bushell, A., Hester, J., 2012. Regulatory immune cells in transplantation. Nat. Rev. Immunol. 12, 417–430.

Workman, C.J., Cauley, L.S., Kim, I.J., Blackman, M.A., Woodland, D.L., Vignali, D.A., 2004. Lymphocyte activation gene-3 (CD223) regulates the size of the expanding T cell population following antigen activation in vivo. J. Immunol. 172, 5450–5455.

Wu, Y., Borde, M., Heissmeyer, V., Feuerer, M., Lapan, A.D., Stroud, J.C., Bates, D.L., Guo, L., Han, A., Ziegler, S.F., Mathis, D., Benoist, C., Chen, L., Rao, A., 2006. FOXP3 controls regulatory T cell function through cooperation with NFAT. Cell 126, 375–387.

Xiao, X., Gong, W., Demirci, G., Liu, W., Spoerl, S., Chu, X., Bishop, D.K., Turka, L.A., Li, X.C., 2012. New insights on OX40 in the control of T cell immunity and immune tolerance in vivo. J. Immunol. 188, 892–901.

Xu, L., Kitani, A., Stuelten, C., Mcgrady, G., Fuss, I., Strober, W., 2010. Positive and negative transcriptional regulation of the Foxp3 gene is mediated by access and binding of the Smad3 protein to enhancer I. Immunity 33, 313–325.

Yadav, M., Louvet, C., Davini, D., Gardner, J.M., Martinez-Llordella, M., Bailey-Bucktrout, S., Anthony, B.A., Sverdrup, F.M., Head, R., Kuster, D.J., Ruminski, P., Weiss, D., Von Schack, D., Bluestone, J.A., 2012. Neuropilin-1 distinguishes natural and inducible regulatory T cells among regulatory T cell subsets in vivo. J. Exp. Med. 209 (1713–22), S1–S19.

Yamaguchi, T., Sakaguchi, S., 2006. Regulatory T cells in immune surveillance and treatment of cancer. Semin. Cancer Biol. 16, 115–123.

Yamazaki, S., Iyoda, T., Tarbell, K., Olson, K., Velinzon, K., Inaba, K., Steinman, R.M., 2003. Direct expansion of functional CD25+ CD4+ regulatory T cells by antigen-processing dendritic cells. J. Exp. Med. 198, 235–247.

Yokosuka, T., Kobayashi, W., Takamatsu, M., Sakata-Sogawa, K., Zeng, H., Hashimoto-Tane, A., Yagita, H., Tokunaga, M., Saito, T., 2010. Spatiotemporal basis of CTLA-4 costimulatory molecule-mediated negative regulation of T cell activation. Immunity 33, 326–339.

Yuan, X., Malek, T.R., 2012. Cellular and molecular determinants for the development of natural and induced regulatory T cells. Hum. Immunol. 73, 773–782.

Zheng, Y., Chaudhry, A., Kas, A., Deroos, P., Kim, J.M., Chu, T.T., Corcoran, L., Treuting, P., Klein, U., Rudensky, A.Y., 2009. Regulatory T-cell suppressor program co-opts transcription factor IRF4 to control T(H)2 responses. Nature 458, 351–356.

Zheng, Y., Josefowicz, S., Chaudhry, A., Peng, X.P., Forbush, K., Rudensky, A.Y., 2010. Role of conserved non-coding DNA elements in the Foxp3 gene in regulatory T-cell fate. Nature 463, 808–812.

Zorn, E., Kim, H.T., Lee, S.J., Floyd, B.H., Litsa, D., Arumugarajah, S., Bellucci, R., Alyea, E.P., Antin, J.H., Soiffer, R.J., Ritz, J., 2005. Reduced frequency of FOXP3+ CD4+CD25+ regulatory T cells in patients with chronic graft-versus-host disease. Blood 106, 2903–2911.

Zorn, E., Nelson, E.A., Mohseni, M., Porcheray, F., Kim, H., Litsa, D., Bellucci, R., Raderschall, E., Canning, C., Soiffer, R.J., Frank, D.A., Ritz, J., 2006. IL-2 regulates FOXP3 expression in human CD4+CD25+ regulatory T cells through a STAT-dependent mechanism and induces the expansion of these cells in vivo. Blood 108, 1571–1579.

CHAPTER 9

Regulatory B Cells

Q. Simon, S. Hillion
Université de Brest, and LabEx IGO, Brest, France
Laboratory of Immunology, Brest University Medical School Hospital, Brest, France

Contents

1. HISTORY OF REGULATORY B CELLS

1.1 Regulatory B cells in mice

Suppressive or regulatory properties of B cells was first suggested in the 1970s when several groups made the observation that B cell-depleted splenocytes from guinea pigs sensitized to ovalbumin in Freund's incomplete adjuvant failed to ameliorate hypersensitivity response upon passive transfer into normal guinea pigs (Katz et al., 1974; Neta and Salvin, 1974). Twenty years later, the regulatory capacity of B cells was revisited in the experimental autoimmune encephalomyelitis (EAE) model, a mouse model for multiple sclerosis. In this model, wild-type C57BL/6 mice developed spontaneous remission of EAE, which is induced with immunization with myelin oligodendocyte glyprotein (MOG) (Wolf et al., 1996). In contrast, B cell-deficient (μMT) C57BL/6 mice developed a severe nonremitting form of the disease in this model.

Subsequent studies demonstrated EAE disease was exacerbated in chimeric mice in which IL-10 deficiency was restricted to B cells (Fillatreau et al., 2002). Importantly, adoptive transfer of wild-type B cells, but not IL-10-deficient B cells, normalized EAE severity in μMT mice, suggesting B cell-derived IL-10 is critical for diminishing the clinical manifestations in this model. This subset of IL-10-producing B cells, which were found in the spleen, exhibited a $CD43^-$ B2 phenotype, and produced IL-10 upon BCR and anti-CD40 stimulation, and were thus coined "B10."

Translational Immunology
http://dx.doi.org/10.1016/B978-0-12-801577-3.00017-4

The existence of B10 was extended to numerous pathology models. Mizoguchi et al. examined the role of B cells in a mouse model of inflammatory bowel disease (IBD) in which genetic deficiency in T cell receptor alpha (TCRα) spontaneously developed chronic colitis. They reported a subset of $CD5^{+}$ $CD1d^{+}$ B cells located in the gut-associated lymphoid tissues suppressed the progression of the disease through downregulation of the IL-1/STAT3 activation pathway (Mizoguchi et al., 2002). In the dextran sulfate sodium (DSS)-induced colitis, B cell deficiency led to exacerbated disease (Yanaba et al., 2011). Others have confirmed that B cells are capable of secreting a high quantity of IL-10 during the acute inflammation period. From these early observations quickly came the question of the phenotypic identity of such regulatory B cells (Bregs), which to date remains a major debate in the field (Maseda et al., 2013).

In the collagen-induced arthritis mice models, Breg cells have been identified with a $CD21^{high}$ $CD23^{+}$ IgM^{high} T2/marginal zone precursor phenotype, which is associated with IL-10 production (Evans et al., 2007). Subsequent studies with several mouse models have expanded the Breg surface markers to include CD1d, CD19, CD5, CD24, CD27, CD38, IgM, and CD21 (Iwata et al., 2011). T cell domain and mucin domain protein-1 (TIM1) was described on a subset of B cells with regulatory function. After TIM-1 ligation, $TIM\text{-}1^{+}$ B cells could transfer donor-specific long-term graft survival in a model of islet allograft. TIM-1 expression was expressed mostly on marginal zone B cells, B-1 ($CD5^{+}$) and immature/transitional B cells (Ding et al., 2011).

Recent data suggested that B10 could rapidly convert into plasmablast after *in vivo* or *in vitro* activation. Shen et al. (2014) have described a novel Breg population within $CD138^{+}$ $CXCR4^{+}$ plasmablast subset capable of expressing IL-35 and IL-10 and suppressing EAE. In the same year, Matsumoto et al. (2014) utilized IL-10 reporter transgenic mice to show that $CD44^{high}$ $CD138^{+}$ plasmablasts were the major source of IL-10 production *in vivo* (Matsumoto et al., 2014). Furthermore, they demonstrated that during the course of EAE, IL-10-producing plasmablasts were generated in an IRF-4-dependent manner. Human B cells could also differentiate into IL-10-producing plasmablasts with a $CD27^{high}$ $CD38^{high}$ phenotype, suggesting the existence of a human regulatory plasmablast subset counterpart.

1.2 Regulatory B cells in humans

Despite more than 30 years since the first appreciation for Breg cells in animal model studies, reliable phenotypic markers and transcription factors defining human Bregs subsets have remained elusive. A common feature of all described Breg subsets is their ability to produce IL-10 in a variety of pathological conditions. Blair et al. (2010) reported that $CD19^{+}$ $CD24^{high}$ $CD38^{high}$ transitional B cells purified from peripheral blood comprised the highest fraction of IL-10-producing B cells following CD40 stimulation in healthy individuals (Blair et al., 2010). As in mice, additional stimuli are required to enhance IL-10 production. For example, toll-like receptor 9 (TLR9) agonist significantly increased IL-10 production in B cells but mostly in $CD27^+$ $CD24^+$ subset (Iwata et al., 2011; Candando et al., 2014). Controversies exist regarding the precise identification of human B10. It has been reported that $CD20^+$ $CD27^+$ $CD43^+$ $CD70^-$ human B1 cells may also secrete a high quantity of IL-10 (Griffin et al., 2011; Lundy and Boros, 2002). In an elegant study, van de Veen et al. (2013) performed a whole genome microarray expression analysis on sorted IL-10 positive B cells comparing with the IL-10 negative counterpart. They demonstrated that IL-10 positive B cells showed increased expression of CD25, CD71, and PD-L1 and a decrease of CD73 (van de Veen et al., 2013). Subsequently, the same group transfected IL-10 gene into peripheral human B cells to analyze gene signature associated with IL-10. Interestingly, they demonstrated that IL-10-overexpressing B cells acquired an immunoregulatory phenotype characterized by CD25, GARP, and PDL-1. CD25 and PDL-1 have been also described to be upregulated on regulatory T cells (Tregs) (see Chapter 8) (Stanic et al., 2015).

The findings by Stanic et al. (2015) are in line with the notion of coexistence of different progenitor B10 cells, which are inherently not competent to express IL-10, but they require additional stimuli such as CD40 and TLR9 signals (Tedder, 2015). In this regard, Masumoto et al. (2014) have analyzed differentiation of different sorted human B cell subsets following CpG, IL-2, IL-6, and IFN-α activation and found transitional B cells differentiate into IL-10-secreting $CD27^{int}$ $CD38^+$ plasmablasts. These data suggest there might exist a developmental link between previously reported human Bregs and $IL\text{-}10^+$ plasmablasts (Matsumoto et al., 2014).

In addition to IL-10-mediated immune suppression, Bregs also possess additional immunosuppressive mechanisms (Klinker and Lundy, 2012; Rincon-Arevalo et al., 2015). Several groups reported that Bregs may act as killer B cells as described for NK or $CD8^+$ T cells. Expression of FasL was reported on CD5-positive B cells that have the ability to kill antigen-specific T helper cells (Lundy et al., 2001). Furthermore, B cells isolated from tumor-draining lymphocytes nodes were able to induce apoptosis of tumor cells *in vivo* in an IL-10-independent manner in a mouse model of breast cancer (Tao et al., 2014). Another group found B cells may be influenced by IL-21 to produce granzyme B leading to T cell apoptosis (Lindner et al., 2013; Chesneau et al., 2015). The same authors showed that IL-21 together with BCR stimulation induced indoleamine 2–3 dioxygenase (IDO) in peripheral blood B cells. Finally, TGF-β-producing B cells are regarded as another subset of Breg cells, although there is no evidence demonstrating that IL-10 and TGF-β production by Bregs are mutually exclusive. Recently, we showed that B cells are involved in the generation of Tregs *in vitro* through the TGF-β/IDO pathway (Nouel et al., 2015).

Given the complexity of Breg characterization and its various assigned functions, a nomenclature for classifying Bregs, similar to what was proposed for Tregs, was suggested: B10 or Br1 for IL-10-producing B cells, Br3 for TGF-β producing B cells, and Breg for B cells with undefined characteristics (Noh and Lee, 2011).

2. PLASTICITY OF REGULATORY B CELLS

2.1 Regulatory B cells in infection and cancer

The adaptive and innate immune systems are designed to protect us from pathogens but also from autoimmune manifestation and tumors development. Regulatory cells are the key to the control of immune balance leading to specific and efficient immune response without harming the host. For example, mice deficient in MALT1, a key protein in NFκB signaling, revealed a profound defect in Tregs and IL-10-producing B cells, which led to a spontaneous multiorgan pathology (Bornancin et al., 2015).

Several mouse models demonstrated that B cell deficiency correlated with enhanced resistance to infections, suggesting that B cells could suppress protective immune response (Goenka et al., 2011; Neves et al., 2010). Neves et al. (2010) demonstrated an accumulation of IL-10-producing $CD19^{+}$ $CD38^{+}$ plasmablast cells in the spleen during *Salmonella* infection, suggesting that the pathogen could manipulate B cells to control protective immune response (Nothelfer et al., 2015). *Leishmania major* is another pathogen reported to induce Bregs to control allergen response in mice (Ronet et al., 2010). IL-10-producing B cells were also induced during HIV-1 infection, which correlated with disease activity (Liu et al., 2014; Siewe et al., 2013).

Studies utilizing μMT mice also revealed that absence of B cells can enhance $CD4^{+}$ T cell priming and $CD8^{+}$ T cell-dependent cytotoxicity (Shah et al., 2005). Other studies have described the possibility that the tumor might convert B cells into Bregs to inhibit antitumor immune response (Wejksza et al., 2013). It was also suggested that lymphoma could abrogate anti-CD20 antibody therapeutic efficacy through induction of B10 (Horikawa et al., 2011). Altogether, these data underline the extreme plasticity of B cells that could move from precursors of antibody-secreting cells to Bregs depending on the specific signal.

2.2 Regulatory B cells in autoimmunes diseases

B cells can play positive and negative roles during the course of disease. For example, in the EAE model, B cell depletion using an anti-CD20 mAb during the early phase of the disease exacerbated the disease (Matsushita et al., 2008). In contrast, depletion of B cells during the late phase of the EAE disease reduced the severity and the disease symptoms. It is possible that IL-10-producing Breg cells are the early responders in an inflammatory response in the EAE model. And that anti-CD20-mediated depletion is effective in established EAE disease because it depletes the antigen-presenting function of B cells. Interestingly, in nonobese diabetic (NOD) mice, B cell depletion delayed diabetes by increasing $Foxp3^{+}$ Treg, while repeated transfer of activated B cells into 6-week-old NOD mice reduced the severity of diabetes (Marino et al., 2009; Hussain and Delovitch, 2007).

In humans, $CD24^{hi}$ $CD38^{hi}$ transitional B cells and $CD24^{hi}$ $CD27^{+}$ B cells are two major peripheral blood B cell subsets. Both subsets have been functionally studied following *ex vivo* separation. Interestingly, in SLE patients, $CD24^{hi}$ $CD38^{hi}$ B cell lacked their suppressive capacity in a model of Th1 differentiation (Blair et al., 2010) or in a model of T cell proliferation (Lemoine et al., 2011). We thus desperately need biomarkers to monitor Bregs during disease course or during therapeutic treatment. This will require the development of better tools to separate, characterize, and understand Breg function *in vivo*.

3. MULTIPARAMETRIC FLOW CYTOMETRY ANALYSIS OF REGULATORY B CELLS SUBSETS

Tracking the heterogeneity of different and rare Bregs subsets *in vivo* remains challenging. For example, in order to run a 10-color flow cytometry data set, experimenters must choose one or two markers at the beginning of the analysis (Fig. 1A). As the number of different biaxial plots is represented by $m*(m-1)/2$, where m designates the marker used for the analysis, the number of combinations stands at $(10*9)/2=45$ (Fig. 1B). In this way, to study one cell population, experimenters are forced to create successive gates and have to multiply biaxial plots to quantify more than one cell population.

To replace such tedious manual analyses, algorithms have been developed to represent all the possible biaxial combinations in an automatic way. Their ability to analyze multiple single-cell parameters helps avoid misinterpretation among sample analyses, and enables lead to more rigorous conclusions when quantification and comparisons of cell populations are performed between patients and controls. In addition, an

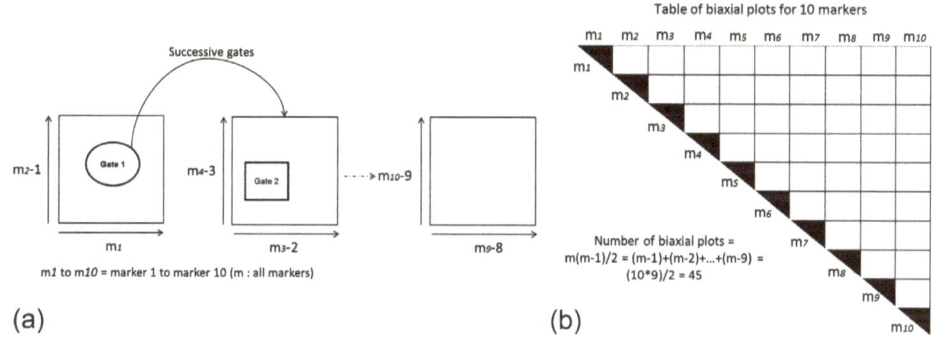

Figure 1 Manual gating on a 10-color analysis data.

automated flow cytometry method allows the visualization of both abundant and rare populations. Because Bregs are detectable in rare cell populations, we believe that bioinformatic analysis of flow cytometry data is the most promising approach to identify and track Bregs in disease settings.

FLOCK (flow clustering without K) is a very powerful algorithm developed to compare flow cytometry data of patients with those of healthy volunteers. FLOCK representation of $m^{\star}(m-1)/2$ biaxial plots allows us to visualize all the identified population on a same plot (Fig. 2). Cross sample comparisons can be run to obtain quantitative

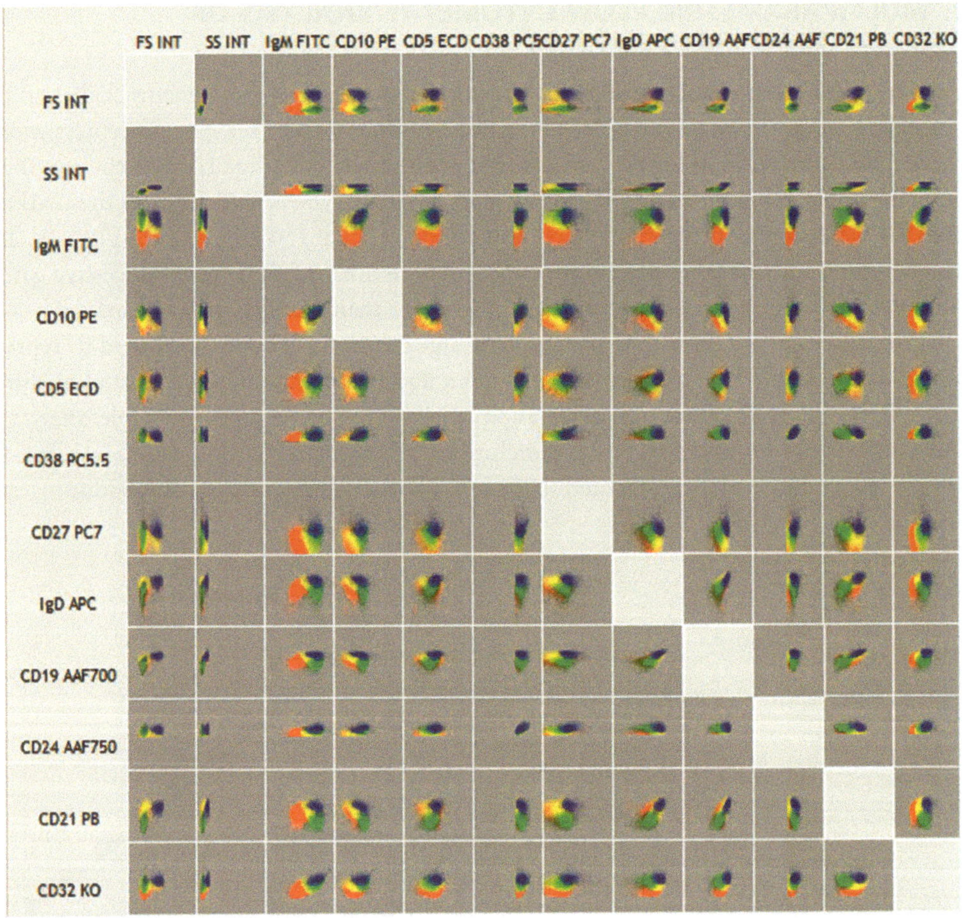

Figure 2 Event clusters identified by FLOCK analysis. FLOCK version 1.0 (Qian et al., 2010) was run unsupervised on human-enriched B cells from one healthy control (HC), stained with the 10-color B cell panel of Abs (in table) pregated on $CD19^{+}$ lymphoid events. Overlay of the 15 identified clusters, indicated in colors, are shown as two-dimensional plots.

results for each detected cell population in comparative, prospective, and retrospective studies. In addition, FLOCK analyses can help in the adjustment of flow cytometry cell-sorting protocols to perform further genomic, transcriptomic, or *in vitro* functional experiments.

A computational approach for multiparameters flow cytometry data analysis is a powerful tool to study *in vivo* rare cell populations. In 2010, Qian and colleagues used the FLOCK approach to study human peripheral blood B cells (Qian et al., 2010). They elucidated and quantified 17 B cell subsets. They also ran a cross-sample comparison between pre-vaccinated (day 0) and post-vaccinated subjects (days 5, 6, 7, 8, and 15). The time course study of plasmablast frequencies led to the establishment of an *in vivo* cell-differentiation scheme (Qian et al., 2010). As plasmablasts have been described to exhibit regulatory properties, this study serves as a basis for the identification of *in vivo*-induced Bregs (Matsumoto et al., 2014).

SPADE (spanning-tree progression analysis of density-normalized events) is a complementary algorithm for the analyses of flow cytometry data. SPADE is a hierarchical tree enabling multiple cell populations to be visualized in a branched tree structure according to a combination of marker intensities. This method allows experimenters to prioritize the cells with known populations and sometimes undescribed new populations, without quantification. As with the FLOCK algorithm, the matrix complexity obtained with SPADE depends on the number of included markers.

Also, SPADE is a strong helpful approach to study the expression of one molecule in all populations defined in a previously validated tree. For example, we performed a 10-color flow cytometry analysis of peripheral blood B cells using SPADE to study abundant and rare B cell populations in a branched tree based on maturational markers. Interestingly, a rare $CD27^+$ transitional B cell population could be detected that was highly positive for CD10. We also identified transitional type 3 B cells exhibiting low expression of CD10 (unpublished data and Fig. 3).

4. SUMMARY AND CONCLUDING REMARKS

Bregs are distinct functional populations in the B cell lineage. Beyond IL-10 production, there is growing evidence that supports the existence of other regulatory mechanisms, such as the production of TGFβ, induced cell death of effector T cells, and the induction of $CD4^+CD25^-Foxp3^+$ Treg. Bregs may differ from one pathology to another, in terms of phenotype, origin, and response to the stimulatory signals that activate their diverse functions (Rosser and Mauri, 2015). Finally, Bregs are rare and hard to detect in human.

Thus the ability to detect and monitor Bregs *in vivo* as well as increased understanding of the regulatory mechanisms governing Breg differentiation and function will no doubt help guide therapeutic intervention strategies.

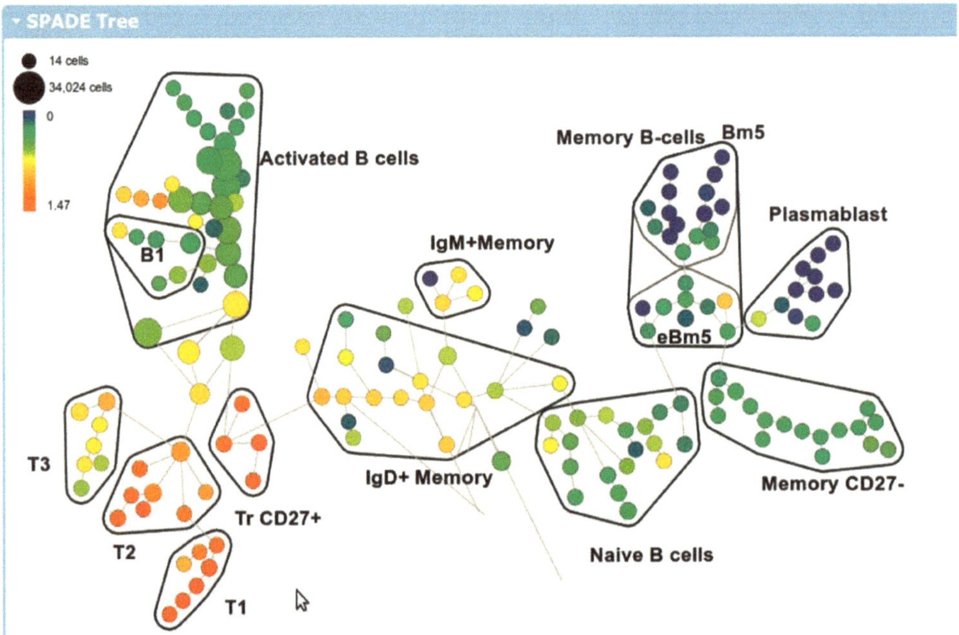

Figure 3 The SPADE bioinformatic analysis was applied to the 10-color flow cytometry analysis. To interpret the SPADE analysis we derived annotations according to the differential pattern of each marker previously defined. The SPADE software built a hierarchical tree with bubble according to MFI density of each marker. To interpret the tree, we have realized functional nodes that can be colored according to the median intensity of each evaluated marker.

REFERENCES

Blair, P.A., Norena, L.Y., Flores-Borja, F., Rawlings, D.J., Isenberg, D.A., Ehrenstein, M.R., Mauri, C., 2010. CD19(+)CD24(hi)CD38(hi) B cells exhibit regulatory capacity in healthy individuals but are functionally impaired in systemic Lupus Erythematosus patients. Immunity 32, 129–140.

Bornancin, F., Renner, F., Touil, R., Sic, H., Kolb, Y., Touil-Allaoui, I., Rush, J.S., Smith, P.A., Bigaud, M., Junker-Walker, U., Burkhart, C., Dawson, J., Niwa, S., Katopodis, A., Bornancin, F., Renner, F., Touil, R., Sic, H., Kolb, Y., Touil-Allaoui, I., Rush, J.S., Smith, P.A., Bigaud, M., Junker-Walker, U., Burkhart, C., Dawson, J., Niwa, S., Katopodis, A., Nuesslein-Hildesheim, B., Weckbecker, G., Zenke, G., Kinzel, B., Traggiai, E., Brenner, D., Brustle, A., St Paul, M., Zamurovic, N., Mccoy, K.D., Rolink, A., Regnier, C.H., Mak, T.W., Ohashi, P.S., Patel, D.D., Calzascia, T., 2015. Deficiency of MALT1 paracaspase activity results in unbalanced regulatory and effector T and B cell responses leading to multiorgan inflammation. J. Immunol. 194, 3723–3734.

Candando, K.M., Lykken, J.M., Tedder, T.F., 2014. B10 cell regulation of health and disease. Immunol. Rev. 259, 259–272.

Chesneau, M., Michel, L., Dugast, E., Chenouard, A., Baron, D., Pallier, A., Durand, J., Braza, F., Guerif, P., Laplaud, D.A., Soulillou, J.P., Giral, M., Degauque, N., Chiffoleau, E., Brouard, S., 2015. Tolerant kidney transplant patients produce B cells with regulatory properties. J. Am. Soc. Nephrol. Feb 2. pii: JASN.2014040404.

Ding, Q., Yeung, M., Camirand, G., Zeng, Q., Akiba, H., Yagita, H., Chalasani, G., Sayegh, M.H., Najafian, N., Rothstein, D.M., 2011. Regulatory B cells are identified by expression of TIM-1 and can be induced through TIM-1 ligation to promote tolerance in mice. J. Clin. Invest. 121, 3645–3656.

Evans, J.G., Chavez-Rueda, K.A., Eddaoudi, A., Meyer-Bahlburg, A., Rawlings, D.J., Ehrenstein, M.R., Mauri, C., 2007. Novel suppressive function of transitional 2 B cells in experimental arthritis. J. Immunol. 178, 7868–7878.

Fillatreau, S., Sweenie, C.H., Mcgeachy, M.J., Gray, D., Anderton, S.M., 2002. B cells regulate autoimmunity by provision of IL-10. Nat. Immunol. 3, 944–950.

Goenka, R., Parent, M.A., Elzer, P.H., Baldwin, C.L., 2011. B cell-deficient mice display markedly enhanced resistance to the intracellular bacterium Brucella abortus. J. Infect. Dis. 203, 1136–1146.

Griffin, D.O., Holodick, N.E., Rothstein, T.L., 2011. Human B1 cells in umbilical cord and adult peripheral blood express the novel phenotype CD20+ CD27+ CD43+ CD70. J. Exp. Med. 208, 67–80.

Horikawa, M., Minard-Colin, V., Matsushita, T., Tedder, T.F., 2011. Regulatory B cell production of IL-10 inhibits lymphoma depletion during CD20 immunotherapy in mice. J. Clin. Invest. 121, 4268–4280.

Hussain, S., Delovitch, T.L., 2007. Intravenous transfusion of BCR-activated B cells protects NOD mice from type 1 diabetes in an IL-10-dependent manner. J. Immunol. 179, 7225–7232.

Iwata, Y., Matsushita, T., Horikawa, M., Dilillo, D.J., Yanaba, K., Venturi, G.M., Szabolcs, P.M., Bernstein, S.H., Magro, C.M., Williams, A.D., Hall, R.P., St Clair, E.W., Tedder, T.F., 2011. Characterization of a rare IL-10-competent B-cell subset in humans that parallels mouse regulatory B10 cells. Blood 117, 530–541.

Katz, S.I., Parker, D., Turk, J.L., 1974. B-cell suppression of delayed hypersensitivity reactions. Nature 251, 550–551.

Klinker, M.W., Lundy, S.K., 2012. Multiple mechanisms of immune suppression by B lymphocytes. Mol. Med. 18, 123–137.

Lemoine, S., Morva, A., Youinou, P., Jamin, C., 2011. Human T cells induce their own regulation through activation of B cells. J. Autoimmun. 36, 228–238.

Lindner, S., Dahlke, K., Sontheimer, K., Hagn, M., Kaltenmeier, C., Barth, T.F., Beyer, T., Reister, F., Fabricius, D., Lotfi, R., Lunov, O., Nienhaus, G.U., Simmet, T., Kreienberg, R., Moller, P., Schrezenmeier, H., Jahrsdorfer, B., 2013. Interleukin 21-induced granzyme B-expressing B cells infiltrate tumors and regulate T cells. Cancer Res. 73, 2468–2479.

Liu, J., Zhan, W., Kim, C.J., Clayton, K., Zhao, H., Lee, E., Cao, J.C., Ziegler, B., Gregor, A., Yue, F.Y., Huibner, S., Macparland, S., Schwartz, J., Song, H.H., Benko, E., Gyenes, G., Kovacs, C., Kaul, R., Ostrowski, M., 2014. IL-10-producing B cells are induced early in HIV-1 infection and suppress HIV-1-specific T cell responses. PLoS One 9. e89236.

Lundy, S.K., Boros, D.L., 2002. Fas ligand-expressing B-1a lymphocytes mediate CD4(+)-T-cell apoptosis during schistosomal infection: induction by interleukin 4 (IL-4) and IL-10. Infect. Immun. 70, 812–819.

Lundy, S.K., Lerman, S.P., Boros, D.L., 2001. Soluble egg antigen-stimulated T helper lymphocyte apoptosis and evidence for cell death mediated by FasL(+) T and B cells during murine Schistosoma mansoni infection. Infect. Immun. 69, 271–280.

Marino, E., Villanueva, J., Walters, S., Liuwantara, D., Mackay, F., Grey, S.T., 2009. CD4(+)CD25(+) T-cells control autoimmunity in the absence of B-cells. Diabetes 58, 1568–1577.

Maseda, D., Candando, K.M., Smith, S.H., Kalampokis, I., Weaver, C.T., Plevy, S.E., Poe, J.C., Tedder, T.F., 2013. Peritoneal cavity regulatory B cells (B10 cells) modulate IFN-gamma+CD4+ T cell numbers during colitis development in mice. J. Immunol. 191, 2780–2795.

Matsumoto, M., Baba, A., Yokota, T., Nishikawa, H., Ohkawa, Y., Kayama, H., Kallies, A., Nutt, S.L., Sakaguchi, S., Takeda, K., Kurosaki, T., Baba, Y., 2014. Interleukin-10-producing plasmablasts exert regulatory function in autoimmune inflammation. Immunity 41, 1040–1051.

Matsushita, T., Yanaba, K., Bouaziz, J.D., Fujimoto, M., Tedder, T.F., 2008. Regulatory B cells inhibit EAE initiation in mice while other B cells promote disease progression. J. Clin. Invest. 118, 3420–3430.

Mizoguchi, A., Mizoguchi, E., Takedatsu, H., Blumberg, R.S., Bhan, A.K., 2002. Chronic intestinal inflammatory condition generates IL-10-producing regulatory B cell subset characterized by CD1d upregulation. Immunity 16, 219–230.

Neta, R., Salvin, S.B., 1974. Specific suppression of delayed hypersensitivity: the possible presence of a suppressor B cell in the regulation of delayed hypersensitivity. J. Immunol. 113, 1716–1725.

Neves, P., Lampropoulou, V., Calderon-Gomez, E., Roch, T., Stervbo, U., Shen, P., Kuhl, A.A., Loddenkemper, C., Haury, M., Nedospasov, S.A., Kaufmann, S.H., Steinhoff, U., Calado, D.P.,

Fillatreau, S., 2010. Signaling via the MyD88 adaptor protein in B cells suppresses protective immunity during Salmonella typhimurium infection. Immunity 33, 777–790.
Noh, G., Lee, J.H., 2011. Regulatory B cells and allergic diseases. Allergy Asthma Immunol. Res. 3, 168–177.
Nothelfer, K., Sansonetti, P.J., Phalipon, A., 2015. Pathogen manipulation of B cells: the best defence is a good offence. Nat. Rev. Microbiol. 13, 173–184.
Nouel, A., Pochard, P., Simon, Q., Segalen, I., Le Meur, Y., Pers, J.O., Hillion, S., 2015. B-Cells induce regulatory T cells through TGF-beta/IDO production in A CTLA-4 dependent manner. J. Autoimmun. 59, 53–60.
Qian, Y., Wei, C., Eun-Hyung Lee, F., Campbell, J., Halliley, J., Lee, J.A., Cai, J., Kong, Y.M., Sadat, E., Thomson, E., Dunn, P., Seegmiller, A.C., Karandikar, N.J., Tipton, C.M., Mosmann, T., Sanz, I., Scheuermann, R.H., 2010. Elucidation of seventeen human peripheral blood B-cell subsets and quantification of the tetanus response using a density-based method for the automated identification of cell populations in multidimensional flow cytometry data. Cytometry B Clin. Cytom. 78 (Suppl 1), S69–82.
Rincon-Arevalo, H., Sanchez-Parra, C.C., Castano, D., Yassin, L., Vasquez, G., 2015. Regulatory B cells and mechanisms. Int. Rev. Immunol. Early Online 1–21.
Ronet, C., Hauyon-La Torre, Y., Revaz-Breton, M., Mastelic, B., Tacchini-Cottier, F., Louis, J., Launois, P., 2010. Regulatory B cells shape the development of Th2 immune responses in BALB/c mice infected with Leishmania major through IL-10 production. J. Immunol. 184, 886–894.
Rosser, E.C., Mauri, C., 2015. Regulatory B cells: origin, phenotype, and function. Immunity 42, 607–612.
Shah, S., Divekar, A.A., Hilchey, S.P., Cho, H.M., Newman, C.L., Shin, S.U., Nechustan, H., Challita-Eid, P.M., Segal, B.M., Yi, K.H., Rosenblatt, J.D., 2005. Increased rejection of primary tumors in mice lacking B cells: inhibition of anti-tumor CTL and TH1 cytokine responses by B cells. Int. J. Cancer 117, 574–586.
Shen, P., Roch, T., Lampropoulou, V., O'connor, R.A., Stervbo, U., Hilgenberg, E., Ries, S., Dang, V.D., Jaimes, Y., Daridon, C., Li, R., Jouneau, L., Boudinot, P., Wilantri, S., Sakwa, I., Miyazaki, Y., Leech, M.D., Mcpherson, R.C., Wirtz, S., Neurath, M., Hoehlig, K., Meinl, E., Grutzkau, A., Grun, J.R., Horn, K., Kuhl, A.A., Dorner, T., Bar-Or, A., Kaufmann, S.H., Anderton, S.M., Fillatreau, S., 2014. IL-35-producing B cells are critical regulators of immunity during autoimmune and infectious diseases. Nature 507, 366–370.
Siewe, B., Stapleton, J.T., Martinson, J., Keshavarzian, A., Kazmi, N., Demarais, P.M., French, A.L., Landay, A., 2013. Regulatory B cell frequency correlates with markers of HIV disease progression and attenuates anti-HIV CD8(+) T cell function in vitro. J. Leukoc. Biol. 93, 811–818.
Stanic, B., Van De Veen, W., Wirz, O.F., Ruckert, B., Morita, H., Sollner, S., Akdis, C.A., Akdis, M., 2015. IL-10-overexpressing B cells regulate innate and adaptive immune responses. J. Allergy Clin. Immunol. 135, 771–780. e778.
Tao, H., Lu, L., Xia, Y., Dai, F., Wang, Y., Bao, Y., Lundy, S.K., Ito, F., Pan, Q., Zhang, X., Zheng, F., Shu, G., Fang, B., Jiang, J., Xia, J., Huang, S., Li, Q., Chang, A.E., 2014. Antitumor effector B cells directly kill tumor cells via the Fas/FasL pathway and are regulated by IL-10. Eur. J. Immunol. 45 (4), 999–1009.
Tedder, T.F., 2015. B10 cells: a functionally defined regulatory B cell subset. J. Immunol. 194, 1395–1401.
Van De Veen, W., Stanic, B., Yaman, G., Wawrzyniak, M., Sollner, S., Akdis, D.G., Ruckert, B., Akdis, C.A., Akdis, M., 2013. IgG4 production is confined to human IL-10-producing regulatory B cells that suppress antigen-specific immune responses. J. Allergy Clin. Immunol. 131, 1204–1212.
Wejksza, K., Lee-Chang, C., Bodogai, M., Bonzo, J., Gonzalez, F.J., Lehrmann, E., Becker, K., Biragyn, A., 2013. Cancer-produced metabolites of 5-lipoxygenase induce tumor-evoked regulatory B cells via peroxisome proliferator-activated receptor alpha. J. Immunol. 190, 2575–2584.
Wolf, S.D., Dittel, B.N., Hardardottir, F., Janeway Jr., C.A., 1996. Experimental autoimmune encephalomyelitis induction in genetically B cell-deficient mice. J. Exp. Med. 184, 2271–2278.
Yanaba, K., Yoshizaki, A., Asano, Y., Kadono, T., Tedder, T.F., Sato, S., 2011. IL-10-producing regulatory B10 cells inhibit intestinal injury in a mouse model. Am. J. Pathol. 178, 735–743.

SECTION C

New Approaches

CHAPTER 10

Therapeutic Immune Tolerance Approaches for the Treatment of Allergic Disease

C.B. Smarr, D.R. Getts, S.D. Miller
Department of Microbiology-Immunology and Interdepartmental Immunobiology Center, Feinberg School of Medicine, Northwestern University, Chicago, IL, United States

Contents

1. INTRODUCTION

As a group of disorders, autoimmunity, and allergy are increasingly prevalent in developed nations, resulting in heightened patient morbidity and excessive pressure on global health care systems. In the context of allergy, specific immunotherapy (SIT)

Translational Immunology
http://dx.doi.org/10.1016/B978-0-12-801577-3.00011-3

is the only specific treatment option that directly targets the Th2 bias underlying allergy. However, the most widespread clinical applications of SIT require a long period of dose escalation with soluble antigen and carry a significant risk of adverse reactions, particularly in highly sensitized patients who stand to benefit most from a curative treatment. Therefore, the development of safer, more efficient methods to induce antigen-specific immune tolerance is critical to advancing allergy treatment.

1.1 CD4$^+$ T cells in allergy

CD4$^+$ T helper (Th) cells can be divided into several distinct subsets with unique cytokine and transcription factor profiles, resulting in distinct immune responses. Seminal work by Mosmann and Coffman identified Th1 and Th2 subsets as mutually antagonistic populations with distinct cytokine profiles and effects on B cells among other responses (Mosmann and Coffman, 1989; Fiorentino et al., 1989; Mosmann et al., 1986). Th1 cells are associated with protective immunity to intracellular pathogens and, when unregulated, pathogenic autoimmunity (Zhu and Paul, 2008). In conjunction with TCR stimulation, cytokines such as IFN-γ activate STAT1, inducing the transcription factor T-bet, which drives expression of IL-12Rβ2 (Mullen et al., 2001; Afkarian et al., 2002). This allows for IL-12 signaling to activate STAT4, which further induces T-bet, resulting in Th1 differentiation and IFN-γ production (Thieu et al., 2008). Th1-derived IFN-γ, in turn, induces murine B cell class switching to the IgG2a isotype (Snapper et al., 1988). Th2 cells, on the other hand, are associated with protective immunity against extracellular parasites and, when unregulated, allergic disease (Zhu and Paul, 2008). IL-4 signaling through STAT6 induces the transcription factor GATA3 (Kurata et al., 1999; Zhu et al., 2001). GATA3 is necessary and sufficient for Th2 differentiation and cytokine production by binding to multiple sites, including the *Il4/Il13* gene locus (Zheng and Flavell, 1997; Zhu et al., 2004; Yagi et al., 2011). Th2-derived IL-4 induces B cell class switching to IgE and IgG1 (Mosmann et al., 1986). IL-4 and other hallmark Th2 cytokines such as IL-5 and IL-13 also act directly on epithelial cells and effector cells such as eosinophils, promoting tissue inflammation, hyperreactivity, and remodeling. GATA3 inhibits Th1 differentiation by suppressing IL-12-STAT4 signaling (Ouyang et al., 1998; Usui et al., 2003; Zhu et al., 2004). This action highlights the mutual antagonism between Th1 and Th2 responses, as IL-12 signaling and T-bet, in turn, inhibit GATA3 (Ouyang et al., 1998; Hwang et al., 2005). Continuing this pattern of mutual antagonism, Th1-associated STAT4 and Th2-associated STAT6 bind to many of the same genes with opposite outcomes (Said et al., 2010).

In addition to the classical Th1/Th2 dichotomy, several novel Th subsets have recently been identified. Th17, defined by the transcription factor RORγT and production of IL-17, is perhaps the most prominent of these new Th subsets (Zhu and Paul, 2008). Th17 responses are associated with protection against extracellular bacteria and fungi as well as pathogenic autoimmunity (Zhu and Paul, 2008). IL-9-producing Th9 cells are defined by expression of the transcription factors IRF4 and PU.1 and are associated with mast cell accumulation (Dardalhon et al., 2008; Veldhoen et al., 2008; Staudt et al., 2010; Chang et al., 2010). IL-22-producing Th22 cells protect against mucosal microbial infection and are defined by coexpression of T-bet and AhR (Basu et al., 2012). Finally, as described earlier, subsets of regulatory $CD4^+$ T cells such as IL-10-producing Tr1 cells and $Foxp3^+$ Tregs have been demonstrated to inhibit inflammation (Groux et al., 1997; Zhu and Paul, 2008).

1.2 B cells in allergy

B cells produce antibodies, making up the humoral arm of the adaptive immune response. Upon antigen encounter, mature B cells traffic to lymphoid tissues, enter germinal centers, and receive and provide help to T cells through TCR-MHC, ICOS-ICOS-L, CD28-CD80/CD86, and CD40-CD40L interactions (Kurosaki et al., 2010; Kawabe et al., 1994). Within germinal centers, B cells undergo affinity maturation, expanding B cells with higher antigen affinity via somatic hypermutation (Umar et al., 1991). This response leads to an expanded population of antibody-producing plasma cells and long-lived memory B cells. Additionally, activated B cells undergo class switching to produce antibodies of different isotypes. Class switch recombination requires T cell help in the form of CD40-CD40L signaling and cytokines (Kawabe et al., 1994). IL-4 induces production of the IgG1 and IgE isotypes while IFN-γ induces IgG2a (Hasbold et al., 1999). Furthermore, the human-specific antibody isotype, IgG4, upregulated by many immunotherapies for allergic disease, is induced by a combination of IL-4 and IL-10 (Jeannin et al., 1998). The absolute requirement for T cell help for the generation of allergy-associated class switched antibodies highlights the pivotal role of T cells in the induction of allergy and the potential for targeting T cells as a means to inhibit the B cell response.

In the case of allergies, IgE and IgG1 antibodies bind high-affinity FcRs on effector cells such as mast cells and basophils, lending these innate immune cells an antigen-specific reactivity that can result in anaphylaxis, tissue remodeling, and inflammation (Dombrowicz et al., 1993). Beyond antibody production, B cells have inflammatory and immunoregulatory functions including production of cytokines such as IL-4 and IL-10 and can serve as APCs to activate T cells (Crawford et al., 2006; Fillatreau et al., 2002). Notably, B cell production of IL-10, in particular by a regulatory population of B10 cells, is important for the regulation of inflammatory diseases including EAE and inflammatory bowel disease (Fillatreau et al., 2002; Yoshizaki et al., 2012; Dilillo et al., 2010). Given the role of B cells in initiating and regulating a diverse range of immune responses, regulation of B cell specificity and development is critical.

2. MECHANISMS OF IMMUNOLOGICAL TOLERANCE

2.1 Central tolerance

Central tolerance is a highly complex phenomenon that results in the deletion of self-reactive T cells in the thymus. Hematopoietic precursors enter the thymus and undergo rapid proliferation as they commit to the T cell lineage. These cells first progress through a $CD4^-CD8^-$ double negative stage, requiring successful TCRβ locus rearrangement before moving to the $CD4^+CD8^+$ double positive stage and rearrangement of the TCRα locus (Kyewski and Klein, 2006). Following successful TCR rearrangement, thymocytes undergo positive selection. T cells recognize peptide antigens presented on major histocompatibility molecules (MHC). More specifically, $CD8^+$ T cells are restricted to antigens presented in the context of MHC I and $CD4^+$ T cells are restricted to antigens loaded into MHC II. During positive selection requiring affinity for self-peptide presented on MHC by cortical thymic epithelial cells (cTECs) to avoid preprogrammed apoptosis is the fate of the vast majority of thymocytes (Klein et al., 2014; Surh and Sprent, 1994).

Following positive selection in the cortex, developing T cells migrate to the thymic medulla where they undergo negative selection. T cells with too high an affinity for self-peptide presented on MHC by medullary thymic epithelial cells (mTECs) undergo apoptosis, resulting in clonal deletion of highly self-reactive, autoimmune potentiating T cells (Surh and Sprent, 1994; Kyewski and Klein, 2006). This model of affinity-driven selection was supported by recent studies using Nur77 reporter mice, a gene upregulated in T cells immediately following TCR stimulation. In short, T cells undergoing positive selection exhibit low levels of TCR stimulation similar to that maintained in the periphery by tonic self-peptide exposure. T cells undergoing deletion by negative selection, however, exhibit strong TCR signals consistent with higher affinity for self (Moran et al., 2011). Therefore, thymic selection establishes a broad repertoire of T cells that are able to recognize antigen presented on MHC but do not have high affinity for self-antigens. Natural thymus-derived Tregs present an exception to this general rule and will be discussed in detail later in this chapter.

2.2 Peripheral tolerance

Central tolerance is a complex phenomenon that is essential for host survival. Interestingly, whether by design or mistake, not all self-reactive T cells are deleted during this process. As such, a number of mechanisms have evolved to regulate these T cells once they are migrate into the periphery.

2.2.1 Immunoregulatory molecules

In addition to the costimulatory molecules CD80/CD86 and their receptors, other B7 receptor family members play important roles in regulating T cell activation. The programmed death 1 (PD-1) receptor, originally identified as a gene upregulated in apoptotic T cells, is important for immune regulation as demonstrated by the autoimmune phenotype of PD-1 deficient mice (Nishimura et al., 1999, 2001; Ishida et al., 1992). PD-1 is rapidly upregulated by activated T cells and is particularly highly expressed in areas of rapid cell turnover such as the thymus and by exhausted T cells in the context of chronic viral infection (Keir et al., 2008). PD-1 engagement antagonizes signaling through the TCR and CD28, thereby inhibiting T cell activation (Keir et al., 2008).

PD-1 has two ligands, the B7 family members PD-L1 and PD-L2. These molecules are differentially induced by Th1 and Th2 responses and, in turn, differentially regulate those same Th phenotypes. For example, on macrophages, PD-L1 is upregulated by the Th1 cytokine IFN-γ while PD-L2 is upregulated in response to the Th2 cytokine IL-4 (Loke and Allison, 2003). Consequently, PD-L1 and PD-L2 are associated with regulation of Th1 and Th2 responses, respectively (Singh et al., 2011). For example, in a Th2-mediated model of allergic airway inflammation, PD-L1$^{-/-}$ mice have reduced pathology compared to wild-type animals while PD-L2$^{-/-}$ have exacerbated disease (Akbari et al., 2009).

IL-10 is a suppressive cytokine produced by a variety of cell types, including monocytes, DCs, B cells, and Treg cells (Moore et al., 2001; Dilillo et al., 2010; Groux et al., 1997; Foussat et al., 2003). Following an early observation that IL-10 is produced by LPS-activated monocytes and suppresses immune responses (De Waal Malefyt et al., 1991), IL-10 acts as a suppressive cytokine in response to inflammation. IL-10 acts on APCs by downregulating MHC class II and costimulatory molecules and inhibiting expression of proinflammatory cytokines and chemokines and their receptors (Mcbride et al., 2002; Moore et al., 2001; De Waal Malefyt et al., 1991). IL-10 also acts directly on T cells, inhibiting their activation by suppressing IL-2 production and costimulatory signaling via CD28 and ICOS, thereby raising the threshold for T cell activation and inducing anergy (De Waal Malefyt et al., 1993; Taylor et al., 2007; Akdis et al., 2001). Interestingly, IL-10 promotes the survival, proliferation, and differentiation of human B cells, inducing class switching to the suppressive IgG4 isotype (Satoguina et al., 2005). IL-10 has also been shown to promote regulatory feedback loops, maintaining Foxp3 expression by Tregs and inducing the differentiation of IL-10 producing DCs and Tr1 cells (Murai et al., 2009; Wakkach et al., 2003).

2.2.2 Regulatory T cells

Treg cells, which can be broadly categorized as CD25^{+}Foxp3^{+} Tregs and inducible IL-10 producing T regulatory 1 (Tr1) cells, comprise subsets of Th cells that have demonstrated importance in the regulation of inflammation, including Th2-mediated allergic inflammation. Supporting this, human studies have demonstrated relatively higher ratios of Tregs and Tr1 cells to Th2 cells in healthy and high-dose allergen-tolerized patients compared to allergic patients (Meiler et al., 2008; Akdis et al., 2004).

The importance of Tregs in suppressing immune responses was highlighted by studies demonstrating that mutations in Foxp3, the defining transcription factor required for Treg suppressive functions (Hori et al., 2003; Fontenot et al., 2005), result in the multiorgan inflammatory pathologies known as IPEX in humans and scurfy in mice (Bennett et al., 2001; Brunkow et al., 2001). Foxp3 deficiency is also characterized by significantly elevated levels of IgE and inflammatory eosinophilia, which is notable for the regulation of allergy (Ozcan et al., 2008). Many specific immunotherapies (SITs) for the treatment of allergic diseases have been shown to induce Tregs (Fujita et al., 2012). In murine models of allergic airway inflammation, transfer of Tregs inhibits and reverses airway hyperresponsiveness (AHR), lung inflammation, and Th2 responses (Kearley et al., 2005, 2008). Furthermore, antibody-mediated Treg inactivation results in enhanced allergic airway inflammation (Lewkowich et al., 2005).

Tregs suppress allergic immune responses through a variety of cell contact dependent and independent pathways. Tregs express CTLA-4, which inhibits costimulatory signals through CD28 and induces production of the immunosuppressive enzyme IDO (Wing et al., 2008; Sucher et al., 2012). CTLA-4 blockade enhances allergic airway inflammation in an OVA/alum model of allergic airway inflammation (Hellings et al., 2002). Tregs can directly inhibit mast cell degranulation via OX40-OX40L interactions (Gri et al., 2008). The pleiotropic molecules of the TGF-β family induce Foxp3 expression and Treg differentiation and are, in turn, produced by Tregs in a regulatory positive feedback loop (Chen et al., 2003). TGF-β-induced Tregs inhibit allergic airway inflammation, while TGF-β alone has been shown to directly inhibit immune responses (Chen et al., 2003; Green et al., 2003). IL-10 acts on Tregs to maintain Foxp3 expression and has also been demonstrated to be important for both Treg and Tr1 suppressive activity (Murai et al., 2009; Huber et al., 2011). Furthermore, through production of IL-10 and TGF-β, Tregs have the potential to induce production of IgA and IgG4 antibodies, which are protective in allergic models in part through competition with IgE (Coffman et al., 1989; Sonoda et al., 1989; Satoguina et al., 2005, 2008; Jeannin et al., 1998; Francis et al., 2008).

3. SYMPTOMATIC TREATMENTS FOR ALLERGY

The most common clinical approaches to allergic diseases consist of allergen avoidance and symptom control. Despite the lack of a curative treatment, this standard of care is quite effective for the control of acute reactions and general quality of life. These treatments include general immunosuppressants such as glucocorticoids as well as antagonists of allergic mediator molecules.

Corticosteroids are the "gold standard" treatment for management of asthma (Chauhan and Ducharme, 2012). Glucocorticoids effectively inhibit eosinophils, mast cells, and other elements of the allergic response (Rothenberg, 1998; Yoshikawa et al., 1999). Glucocorticoids also act on T cells, inhibiting their proliferation and inducing apoptosis (Webster et al., 2002). Furthermore, glucocorticoids broadly inhibit the expression of cytokines and chemokines, including IL-3, IL-4, IL-5, GM-CSF, TSLP, and eotaxin, with implications for most allergic effector cells (Kato et al., 2007; Stellato et al., 1999; Rothenberg and Hogan, 2006; Webster et al., 2002). However, seemingly paradoxical to their use as a treatment for allergy, glucocorticoids have been associated with skewing immune responses from Th1 toward Th2, primarily by modulation of IL-12 (Nieto et al., 1992; Webster et al., 2002).

Produced by mast cells and basophils during acute allergic reactions, histamine induces smooth muscle contraction and vasodilation, contributing to acute allergic responses such as bronchoconstriction and anaphylaxis (Wechsler et al., 2013). There is evidence that histamine acts directly on immune cells through four distinct receptors (H1R–H4R) to modulate multiple aspects of the allergic response including T cell activation and trafficking (Bryce et al., 2006; Dunford et al., 2006; Swartzendruber et al., 2012). Antihistamines targeting H1R have been used for the treatment of Th2-mediated diseases such as allergic rhinitis, but are not used as a therapy for asthmatic patients (Simons and Simons, 2011).

Various treatments have been developed to directly target IgE, which provides the antigen-specific trigger for type 1 hypersensitivity reactions when bound to FcεRI on innate effector cells such as mast cells and basophils. Foremost among these anti-IgE treatments is omalizumab, an IgE-specific IgG1 that neutralizes serum IgE, preventing binding to FcεR molecules. Omalizumab has been shown to successfully modulate allergic responses and has also been coadministered with SIT to prevent adverse reactions and improve efficacy in patients with severe allergies (Holgate et al., 2005; Kopp, 2011). However, the efficacy of omalizumab is variable, possibly relating to the ratio of Ag-specific to total IgE and the relative sensitivity of IgE-reactive cells such as basophils and mast cells (Macglashan et al., 2012). Work has been done to further refine anti-IgE treatments not only by increasing the specificity of antibody for IgE, but also by enhancing binding of the Fc portion of the antibody to "suppressive" receptors such as FcγRIIb (Chu et al., 2012). Another approach targeting IgE is lumiliximab, an antibody against the low-affinity IgE receptor FcεRII. In clinical trials, lumiliximab improved outcomes by reducing serum IgE and inhibiting allergen-specific T cell responses by acting on APCs (Poole et al., 2005; Rosenwasser et al., 2003).

In many cases symptom abatement provides short-lived disease relief. However, the underlying cause of disease is not addressed and patients will continue to suffer from disease unless complete avoidance of the causative antigen occurs. As such, there have been numerous attempts to develop therapies that completely inactivate the allergic response.

4. ANTIGEN-SPECIFIC IMMUNE THERAPIES

4.1 Specific immunotherapy

Although the standard clinical response to allergic disease is one of allergen avoidance and symptom control, SIT consisting of gradually increasing doses of soluble allergen has been used for over 100 years for the treatment of allergic disease (Noon, 1911; Freeman,

1911). Despite the long history of SIT and its promise of ultimately providing an antigen-specific cure for allergic disease rather than lifelong symptom control, advances in SIT have been slow to enter clinical practice. This has been in part due to concerns over the efficacy and safety of SIT in allergic patients, as well as a lack of understanding of the mechanisms underlying the action of SIT. Efforts to refine SIT have largely focussed on one or more of three key areas: the route of administration of antigen, modification of antigen to improve safety and efficacy, and finally the use of adjuvants to skew immune responses away from Th2 and toward Th1 and Treg-dominated phenotypes.

4.2 Route of administration

Immune responses are highly context-dependent, mediated by various innate and adaptive immune cells that are informed by the local environment. The presence of different APC populations can be critical to the success of SIT, while the distribution of effector cells such as mast cells can influence the development of adverse reactions upon treatment (Allam et al., 2008; Novak and Bieber, 2008; Novak et al., 2004). Therefore, the tissues targeted by various routes of SIT administration can have a considerable impact on the efficacy and safety of treatment. Following the pioneering work of Noon and Freeman, most SIT has been delivered subcutaneously (SCIT) (Noon, 1911; Freeman, 1911). Indeed, SCIT is the only route of administration currently approved by the FDA (Cox et al., 2011). Mucosal routes of administration have also been studied extensively, although their clinical adoption has been slow. Only sublingual immunotherapy (SLIT) is currently approved for clinical use, with this approval being restricted to Europe. Additionally, ultrasonography has enabled intralymphatic injection of antigen, which has the advantage of directly supplying antigen to immune cells. However, recent evidence suggests that issues with safety and efficacy may be directly related to route of administration.

4.3 Subcutaneous immunotherapy

SCIT has been demonstrated to reduce Th2 and increase Th1 cytokine production (Secrist et al., 1993). Additionally, SCIT skews human antibody responses from pathogenic IgE to protective IgA, IgG1, and IgG4 isotypes (Francis et al., 2008; Jutel et al., 1995). IL-10 is a critical mechanism of SCIT, inducing antigen-specific T cell anergy and inhibiting AHR, airway inflammation, Th2 cytokines, and antigen-specific IgE (Akdis et al., 1998; Vissers et al., 2004). The skin has a high proportion of Langerhans cells, which are considered tolerogenic but can also recruit inflammatory dendritic epidermal cells (IDECs) and tissue resident mast cells, which may account for some of the local and systemic adverse events associated with SCIT (Allam et al., 2008; Novak and Bieber, 2008; Novak et al., 2004). Interestingly, IDECs can produce Th1-skewing IL-12 and IL-18, which may improve the efficacy of SCIT by encouraging the switch to

Th1-mediated immune responses (Novak and Bieber, 2008). A recent clinical trial in patients with birch pollen allergies showed reduced symptom scores, medication use, and skin prick test (SPT) reactivity after SCIT (Möbs et al., 2010). Although birch pollen-specific Th2 cells producing IL-5 were increased early in treatment there was a concurrent, transient increase in IL-10-secreting Tr1 cells and decrease in symptoms, suggesting active suppression of Th2 responses as a major early mechanism of tolerance (Möbs et al., 2012). A shift from Th2 to Th1 responses was observed in both the T and B cell compartments in the maintenance phase of treatment with a particular increase in IgE-blocking IgG4 (Möbs et al., 2010).

Despite its relative success, SCIT requires frequent clinical visits and runs a significant risk of systemic adverse events. An interesting variation on traditional SCIT that addresses these issues is epicutaneous delivery of antigen by a patch. This provides a potentially more convenient alternative to traditional SCIT with improved safety due to the lack of epidermal vascularization. A clinical trial of epicutaneous immunotherapy in grass pollen allergy was modestly effective but well tolerated with only minor local adverse reactions in some subjects (Senti et al., 2009a).

SCIT has a long history of inducing tolerance/immune deviation for the treatment of multiple allergic diseases. However, the need for frequent injections inhibits patient compliance (Cox et al., 2011) while local and systemic adverse events including granulomas, fatal airway obstruction, and anaphylactic shock impair treatment in the most highly sensitized patients (Akdis et al., 1998; Vogelbruch et al., 2000). Therefore, alternative routes of antigen delivery have become increasingly well studied.

4.4 Mucosal immunotherapy

Mucosal surfaces are generally regarded as tolerogenic sites, encountering and tolerating food and benign aeroantigens in healthy individuals. Mucosal APCs such as oral Langerhans cells typically display an immature phenotype and produce tolerogenic cytokines such as IL-10 and TGF-β and induce regulatory cytokine production in T cells (Allam et al., 2010). However, mast cells are present in the mucosa at levels equivalent to the skin, resulting in similar risks for adverse events in sensitized patients (Allam et al., 2008). Sublingual and oral antigen administration are the primary mucosal routes that have been studied for SIT, although intranasal delivery of antigen is also known to be tolerogenic (Moldaver et al., 2014; Xiao et al., 2014).

SLIT is performed by administration of antigen drops or tablets that are held under the tongue for uptake by oral APCs, primarily Langerhans cells (Allam et al., 2008), prior to swallowing. Unlike SCIT, maintenance doses of SLIT can be easily self-administered. SLIT has entered clinical use in Europe as an alternative to SCIT, but has not yet been approved for use in the United States. Successful SLIT for the treatment of diseases such as food allergy and allergic rhinitis has demonstrated reduced symptom scores and medication use, reduced Th2 recall responses and increased IFN-γ, IL-10, Tregs, and IgG4 and typically only minor local adverse reactions (Radulovic et al., 2010; Fleischer et al., 2013; Bohle et al., 2007; Ciprandi et al., 2005; Scadding et al., 2010).

Comparisons of SLIT and SCIT have demonstrated similar reductions in symptom scores, antigen-specific IgE, and allergic reactions to antigen challenge (Yukselen et al., 2012; Eifan et al., 2010). However, the relative tolerability of each technique remains unclear due to conflicting data (Yukselen et al., 2012; Eifan et al., 2010; Pajno et al., 2005). A novel study of children with house dust mite allergy combined SCIT in the 4-month buildup phase of tolerance with SLIT in the maintenance phase over the next 14 months. Patients treated with this schedule exhibited a protective IL-10, TGF-β, and IgG4 response with reduced symptom scores and medication usage without any reported adverse events (Keles et al., 2011). This protocol combined the proven efficacy of SCIT for tolerance induction with the safety and compliance benefits of SLIT for maintenance.

4.5 Intralymphatic immunotherapy

Intralymphatic immunotherapy (ILIT) addresses two principal concerns with conventional SIT: safety and efficacy. By delivering antigen directly to lymphatic tissue, ILIT is proposed to induce a more robust immune response with less antigen; therefore, reducing adverse events. Indeed, rodent studies demonstrated significantly improved immune responses in vaccines delivered directly to lymph nodes rather than by other routes of administration (Newbould, 1964). This early observation has been expanded in further animal and human studies using whole-cell vaccines (Juillard et al., 1977, 1978), DNA (Maloy et al., 2001), peptides (Johansen et al., 2005), and proteins (Martínez-Gómez et al., 2009). These studies confirmed that intralymphatic injections induced significantly more robust immune responses, requiring considerably less antigen and adjuvant (Von Beust et al., 2005) than other routes of administration.

ILIT has only recently been investigated for use in allergy. A clinical trial found that patients receiving ILIT for grass pollen allergy experienced less pain than is induced by venous puncture and had fewer adverse reactions than patients undergoing SCIT (Senti et al., 2008). ILIT reduced symptoms in response to nasal challenge and SPT and decreased grass-specific IgE levels comparably to SCIT. Strikingly, ILIT required only 3 injections over 8 weeks as opposed to 54 injections over 3 years for SCIT, resulting in significantly improved compliance (Senti et al., 2008). The success of ILIT was replicated in a small-scale trial of patients with cat dander allergy (Senti et al., 2012). Patients receiving three treatments of ILIT showed improved nasal and skin tolerance to cat dander, increased dander-specific IgG4, but not IgE, and increased IL-10 production by dander-restimulated PBMCs (Senti et al., 2012). These successes underline the need for carefully targeted allergen administration for SIT.

4.6 Intravenous immunotherapy

Although the intravenous route of administration has recently been described by the FDA as safer than other routes for administration of immune modulating therapies, intravenous injection of antigen to treat disease has not been investigated in humans. Experimentally, we have shown in the EAE model of multiple sclerosis that the intravenous route is ideal for the induction of tolerance. When antigens associated with EAE are coupled to apoptotic splenocytes (Ag-SP) they induce tolerance only when administered intravenously (Tan et al., 1992; Getts et al., 2011). Antigen carriers administered intravenously localize primarily to the spleen and liver, with a concurrent accumulation of antigen-specific T cells in those organs. Indeed, the spleen was crucial for the induction of tolerance by antigen-coupled cells in EAE (Getts et al., 2011). Therefore, we contend that intravenous delivery of antigen carriers targets antigen to quiescent APCs in the spleen and liver for the tolerogenic representation of antigen.

5. NOVEL ANTIGEN DELIVERY STRATEGIES

5.1 Ag-SP tolerance in allergy

The use of Ag-SP has been extensively described and has been shown to be highly effective in rodent models of TH1 and TH17 disease(s) (Miller et al., 2007). Ag-SP have been used to prevent hapten-specific IgE responses in alum immunized mice, implying that Ag-SP could effectively induce tolerance in Th2-mediated models of allergy (Weber and Blaser, 1986).

Recently, we demonstrated that Ag-SP induced prophylactic tolerance for the inhibition of allergic airway inflammation (Smarr et al., 2011). Unlike soluble antigen, Ag-SP were well tolerated and nonanaphylactic in presensitized mice. This result is consistent with a previous report in EAE and is likely due to ECDI cross-linking antigens into allergoids with altered conformational epitopes (Smith et al., 2005). Mice treated postsensitization with Ag-SP demonstrated reduced proliferation and Th2 cytokine production in recall cultures. However, these mice had enhanced eosinophilic airway inflammation despite reduced levels of IL-5 in BALF. Although IL-5 is a potent inducer of eosinophilia, eotaxins are capable of inducing eosinophil recruitment in the absence of IL-5 (Dent et al., 1990; Webb et al., 2001). The presence of eotaxins in BALF was not assayed in these experiments, but should be considered in the future as it is possible that eotaxin-2 is unaffected or upregulated in Ag-SP tolerized recipients. Future studies would be well served by expanding cytokine panels to include other, primarily epithelial-derived Th2-promoting cytokines such as TSLP, IL-25, and IL-33 to examine their contribution to disease.

Ag-SP were also effective for the induction of tolerance in a murine model of food allergy to whole peanut extract (WPE) (Ganeshan et al., 2009). WPE-SP prophylactically inhibited allergic responses to peanut in this model while postsensitization treatment with WPE-SP was well tolerated, with no anaphylactic response observed (Smarr et al., 2011). Th2 cytokines were reduced in recall cultures as they were in the airway model. However, contrary to results in the airway model, WPE-SP treatment inhibited eosinophilia and symptom scores in response to oral challenge with WPE (Smarr et al., 2011). The reason for the differences in postsensitization efficacy in these models is unclear, but could be due to the different sensitization protocols employed, with only two intraperitoneal injections of OVA/alum employed in the airway model as opposed to a series of eight oral sensitizations with WPE with staphylococcal enterotoxin B as adjuvant in the food allergy model. It was also hypothesized that, because intravenously injected Ag-SP are known to traffic through the lungs, Ag-SP could induce eosinophilic airway inflammation directly in sensitized mice. However, intravenous administration of Ag-SP and other antigen carriers to sensitized mice did not directly promote influx of eosinophils into the airways.

5.2 PLG(Ag) tolerance against allergy

Poly(lactide-*co*-glycolide) (PLG) particles with encapsulated antigen have been primarily studied as antigen carriers to enhance immunization. Several studies used PLG carrying antigen and the potent Th1 adjuvant MPL to induce protective immune deviation away from Th2-mediated allergic responses (Lutsiak et al., 2006; Chong et al., 2005; Newman et al., 1998a,b). While MPL enhanced Th1 skewing, PLG(Ag) treatment has a significant potential for immune deviation on its own. Intraperitoneal immunization with PLG(Ag) induces a Th1 response characterized by antigen-specific production of IgG2a and IFN-γ (Batanero et al., 2003). Subcutaneously injected PLG(Ag) inhibit SPT reactivity and increase IFN-γ, IL-10, and IgG2a responses (Schöll et al., 2004). Oral administration of PLG particles with encapsulated milk allergen β-lactoglobulin (BLG) induced a striking reduction in BLG-IgE and T cell recall responses compared to soluble BLG alone (Pecquet et al., 2000).

Recently, in a murine model of allergic airway inflammation, we found that PLG(Ag) prophylactically inhibited allergic airway inflammation, without causing any anaphylaxis (Smarr et al., unpublished data). Unlike other antigen carriers assessed in the context of postsensitization treatment, PLG(Ag) inhibited not only recall responses and airway Th2 cytokines but also airway inflammation. Although the particles did not receive direct head-to-head comparisons within the same experiment, these studies identify PLG (Ag) as an improved treatment for established Th2 sensitization. The reasons for these differences are currently unclear, but may be related to increased antigen dose or more efficient uptake of PLG(Ag) than other carriers.

5.3 Virus-like particles

Virus-like particles (VLPs) are nanoparticles composed of multiple copies of recombinant viral structural proteins with diameters of 25–100 nm. Their immunogenicity stems from multiple factors, including their particulate structure, repetitive surface units that stimulate B cells, and in some cases the presence of PAMPs (Bachmann et al., 1993; Jennings and Bachmann, 2009). The efficacy of the antibody response generated by VLP vaccines is evident in the success of Gardasil and Cervarix in preventing human papilloma virus infection (Bessa et al., 2008). In addition to inducing immunity to the structural proteins from which they were derived, VLPs can be designed with encapsulated or surface-conjugated antigens, thereby inducing responses to these additional antigens.

VLPs made from bacteriophage Qβ and the cat allergen Fel d1 were highly immunogenic in mice, generating significant anti-Fel d1 IgG after a single immunization. Qβ-Fel d1 VLPs were well tolerated in sensitized mice, inducing neither local nor systemic adverse reactions. Furthermore, VLP treatment inhibited basophil and mast cell degranulation and, upon recall, abolished IgE memory responses (Schmitz et al., 2009). In a Phase I clinical trial, VLPs made from Qβ and house dust mite Der p1 peptide given either subcutaneously or intramuscularly to healthy adults were safe and generated significant anti-Der p1 antibodies, primarily of the IgG1 and IgG3 isotypes, after three injections (Kündig et al., 2006). Another trial with Qβ VLPs associated with house dust mite extract and A-type CpG adjuvant found VLPs to be well tolerated in allergic patients, ameliorating symptoms of rhinitis and allergic asthma after 10 weeks of treatment (Senti et al., 2009b).

The modular nature of VLPs allows for fine-tuning of the immune response. In one study, VLPs were made from Moloney murine leukemia virus core proteins gag and pol, mugwort pollen allergen Art v1 and HLA class II (Leb et al., 2009). VLP stimulation of antigen-specific T cells derived from allergic patients induced anergy in the absence of costimulation. VLPs coexpressing antigen and HLA class II with CD80 or CD86 induced proliferation, IFN-γ, IL-13, and IL-2 production, while VLPs coexpressing the adhesion molecule CD58 had a tolerogenic/Th1 skewed profile with the induction of IFN-γ and IL-10 and reduced proliferation and production of IL-2, IL-4, and IL-13 (Leb et al., 2009).

5.4 Polysaccharide particles

Polysaccharide-derived particles have been investigated as antigen carriers and adjuvants for the induction of tolerance (Smarr et al., 2013). Particulate formulations of chitin, a polymer of *N*-acetyl-D-glucosamine, and its deacetylated derivative, chitosan, have been extensively studied for use in mucosal SIT. Chitin particles are phagocytosed following binding to the mannose receptor (Shibata et al., 1997b) and subsequently induce production IL-12 that, in turn, induces Th1 differentiation (Shibata et al., 1997a). Oral administration of chitin particles increases antigen-specific IgG2a and decreases specific IgE and eosinophilia in sensitized mice (Shibata et al., 2000). In mice, therapeutic SLIT with positively charged chitosan nanoparticles enhances antigen uptake and processing by mucosal APCs, resulting in increased T cell activation and secretion of IFN-γ and IL-10 and inhibition of Th2 cytokines and airway inflammation (Saint-Lu et al., 2009).

Sepharose particles have been used as adjuvants to enhance SCIT in murine asthma models. Mice treated with sepharose particles show reduced airway inflammation and Th2 responses and enhanced Th1 responses (Grönlund et al., 2002; Neimert-Andersson et al., 2008). In a direct comparison to alum, subcutaneous injections of sepharose particles induced a greater Th1 response and did not induce the granulomatous tissue reactions associated with alum (Grönlund et al., 2002). Additionally, sepharose particles were reported to induce partial DC maturation, resulting in tolerance (Andersson et al., 2004). Overall, polysaccharide particles offer a promising alternative to current alum adjuvants by improved skewing toward tolerogenic Th1 responses and reduced adverse events.

SIT represents the primary curative approach to allergy. Standard SIT has a proven clinical track record but leaves considerable room for improvement in safety and efficiency of treatment. Innovations in the route, antigens, and adjuvants employed for SIT provide exciting potential solutions to these problems with the promise of improved efficacy and safety.

6. MECHANISMS OF ANTIGEN-SPECIFIC T REGULATION BY ANTIGEN ASSOCIATED WITH INERT CARRIERS

An interesting effect of treatment with several of the antigen carriers reviewed in the studies described above has been the observed induction of Th1-associated antigen-specific IgG2a. In murine models, this induction of IgG2a by Ag-SP and PLG(Ag) is partially mediated by IL-12, which operates upstream of IFN-γ to indirectly induce IgG2a (Smarr et al., unpublished data). We hypothesize that this induction of Ag-IgG2a is symptomatic of an initial, abortive activation event following intravenous administration of antigen carriers. Ag-specific T cells proliferate following Ag-SP and Ag-PLG infusion but are anergic upon secondary antigen encounter (Eagar et al., 2004; Getts et al., 2011; Bryant et al., 2014; Kheradmand et al., 2012). Ag-specific T cells upregulate IFN-γ shortly after Ag-SP and nanoparticle infusion (Z. N. Hunter, unpublished data; Kheradmand et al., 2012). Additionally, Ag-SP transiently upregulate CD40L on T cells, which provides costimulation for B cell class switching and induces IL-12 production by APCs (Kawabe et al., 1994; Lutsiak et al., 2006). Therefore, we propose a model where antigen carriers induce abortive activation of antigen-specific T cells. These T cells briefly proliferate and upregulate CD40L, inducing APCs to produce IL-12 that, in turn, stimulates T cell production of IFN-γ. T cell-derived IFN-γ and CD40L induce B cell class switching to IgG2a (Fig. 1). Notably, IL-12 and subsequent induction of IgG2a are dispensable in Ag-SP-induced tolerance against allergic airway inflammation, representing an artifact of this abortive activation. Therefore, although skewing toward competitive Th1 responses may contribute to some approaches to SIT, it may ultimately be less important than the induction of anergy or regulatory responses, particularly in the case of intravenously delivered antigen on apoptotic cells or carboxylated nanoparticles.

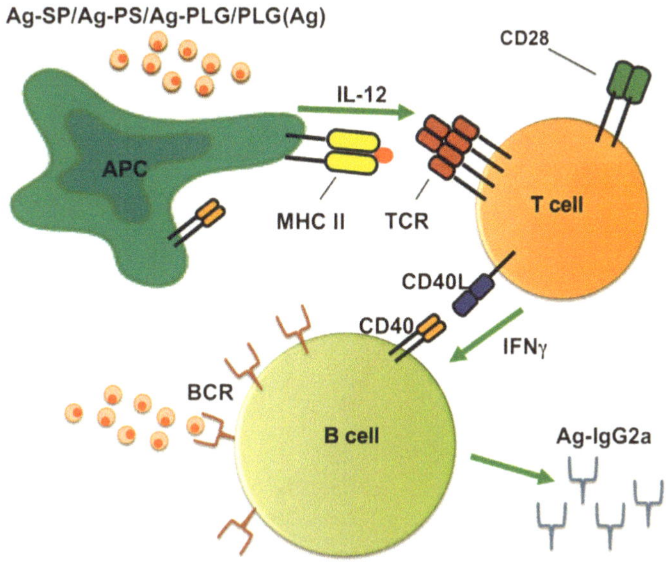

Figure 1 Abortive activation following antigen carrier-induced tolerance. Following intravenous administration of antigen-associated carriers, APCs process and present antigen without upregulating costimulatory molecules such as CD80 or CD86. In response to cognate antigen in the absence of costimulatory signals, antigen-specific T cells enter a state of abortive activation. These T cells briefly proliferate and transiently upregulate CD40L and, in response to IL-12, produce IFN-γ. IFN-γ and CD40 signaling induce B cell activation and class switching to IgG2a.

Finally, PLG(Ag) induced not only prophylactic tolerance, but also safe inhibition of airway inflammation postsensitization. Of the antigen carriers examined in these studies, PLG(Ag) are the most promising, not only for their postsensitization efficacy, but also because the flexible, modular nature of these biodegradable nanoparticles allows antigens or tolerogenic molecules to be encapsulated within the particle core or attached to the surface to provide multiple immunoregulatory signals. Ag-SP tolerance in this model does not require the activity of Tregs, IL-10, PD-L1, PD-L2, or IDO alone. Although the mechanisms of particle-induced tolerance have not been fully elucidated using PLG (Ag)-induced tolerance, we anticipate similar results as were found with Ag-SP. We hypothesize that intravenously delivered antigen-associated carriers are phagocytosed and processed by APCs in the spleen and liver, which deliver TCR stimulation (signal 1) in either the absence of costimulation (signal 2) or the presence of inhibitory signaling mediated by IL-10, PD-L1/PD-L2, or CTLA-4 that antagonizes stimulation (Fig. 2). This results in an abortive activation of Ag-specific T cells, which transiently proliferate and stimulate B cell class switching to IgG2a before becoming anergic. As highlighted by our study of immunosuppressive factors necessary for Ag-SP tolerance, this immune inhibition is robust and likely operates through multiple, redundant mechanisms including activation of Tregs (Hunter et al., 2014). These antigen carriers refine traditional

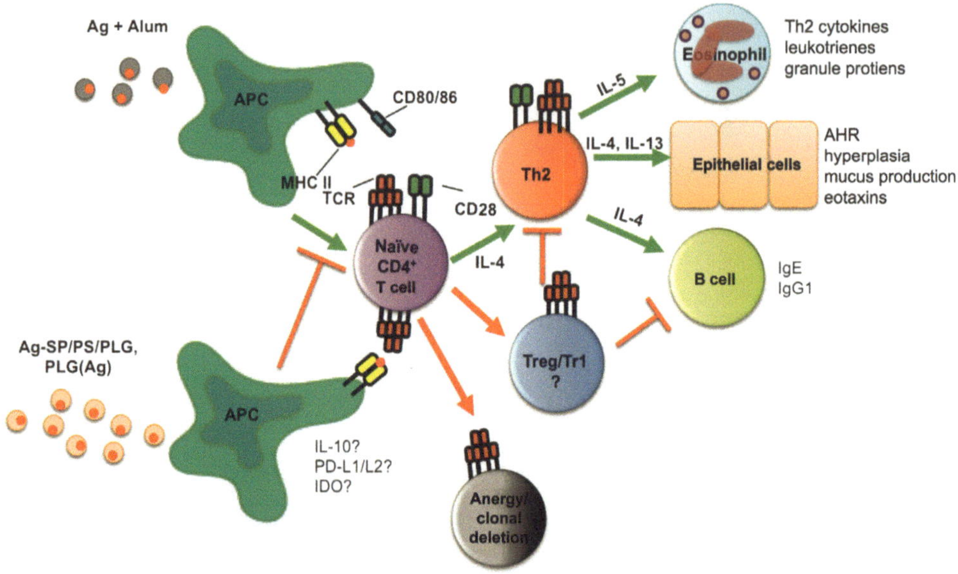

Figure 2 Antigen carriers inhibit Th2 priming and subsequent allergic airway inflammation via synergistic mechanisms. Immunization with antigen in alum adjuvant induces APCs to present antigen in the context of costimulation and Th2-promoting cytokines such as IL-4. Naïve $CD4^+$ T cells encounter antigen in this context and differentiate into Th2 cells. Th2 cytokines promote the allergic response by inducing eosinophilia and B cell class switching to IgE in addition to direct effects on epithelial cells. Prophylactic treatment with Ag-SP, Ag-PLG, and PLG(Ag) inhibit this sensitization. A proposed mechanism is the induction of anergy and clonal deletion of antigen-specific T cells as a result of antigen encounter in the absence of costimulation. Additional tolerogenic factors such as IL-10, IDO, PD-L1/L2, and Tregs have been implicated in other models of tolerance. However, these suppressive factors were found to be dispensable for induction of prophylactic Ag-SP tolerance and have not yet been examined with other carriers or time points in this model of allergic airway inflammation. Therefore, tolerance may operate by a network of redundant suppressive mechanisms or may be primarily due to antigen encounter (signal 1) in the absence of costimulation (signal 2).

approaches to SIT in three key areas: intravenously infused carriers localize to the spleen and liver where they are taken up by tolerogenic APCs, ECDI cross-linking and antigen encapsulation obscure allergenic conformational epitopes, and encounter with carriers induces anergy/clonal deletion and potentially regulatory populations of antigen-specific cells.

7. CONCLUSIONS

Significant advances in our understanding of immune tolerance are bringing its potential application in the treatment of allergic disease closer to reality. Multiple questions remain regarding the underlying molecular and cellular mechanisms that induce and maintain tolerance, which need to be examined in rodent models of allergic disease. However, translation of findings to human subjects remains the most important endeavor and hopefully will occur in the context of PLG(Ag) in the not too distant future.

Abbreviations

Ag antigen
Ag-PLG antigen-coupled poly(lactide-*co*-glycolide) particles
Ag-SP antigen-coupled splenocytes
APC antigen presenting cells
CTLA-4 cytotoxic T lymphocyte associated antigen-4
DC dendritic cell
ECDI 1-ethyl-3-(3-dimethylaminopropyl)-carbodiimide
IFN-γ interferon-gamma
Ig immunoglobulin
IL interleukin
ILIT intralymphatic immunotherapy
OIT oral immunotherapy
OVA ovalbumin
PD-1 programmed death receptor 1
PD-L1 programmed death receptor ligand 1
PD-L2 programmed death receptor ligand 2
PLG poly(lactide-*co*-glycolide)
PLG(Ag) antigen encapsulated poly(lactide-*co*-glycolide) particles
SCIT subcutaneous immunotherapy
SLIT sublingual immunotherapy
SPT skin prick test
TGF-β transforming growth factor beta
Th1 T helper type 1
Th2 T helper type 2
Th17 T helper type 17
Tr1 T regulatory 1 cell
Treg regulatory T cell
VLP virus-like particle

REFERENCES

Afkarian, M., Sedy, J.R., Yang, J., Jacobson, N.G., Cereb, N., Yang, S.Y., Murphy, T.L., Murphy, K.M., 2002. T-bet is a STAT1-induced regulator of IL-12R expression in naive CD4+ T cells. Nat. Immunol. 3, 549–557.

Akbari, O., Stock, P., Singh, A.K., Lombardi, V., Lee, W.L., Freeman, G.J., Sharpe, A.H., Umetsu, D.T., Dekruyff, R.H., 2009. PD-L1 and PD-L2 modulate airway inflammation and iNKT-cell-dependent airway hyperreactivity in opposing directions. Mucosal Immunol. 3, 81–91.

Akdis, C.A., Blesken, T., Akdis, M., Wuthrich, B., Blaser, K., 1998. Role of interleukin 10 in specific immunotherapy. J. Clin. Invest. 102, 98–106.

Akdis, C.A., Joss, A., Akdis, M., Blaser, K., 2001. Mechanism of IL-10-induced T cell inactivation in allergic inflammation and normal response to allergens. Int. Arch. Allergy Immunol. 124, 180–182.

Akdis, M., Verhagen, J., Taylor, A., Karamloo, F., Karagiannidis, C., Crameri, R., Thunberg, S., Deniz, G., Valenta, R., Fiebig, H., Kegel, C., Disch, R., Schmidt-Weber, C.B., Blaser, K., Akdis, C.A., 2004. Immune responses in healthy and allergic individuals are characterized by a fine balance between allergen-specific T regulatory 1 and T helper 2 cells. J. Exp. Med. 199, 1567–1575.

Allam, J.P., Stojanovski, G., Friedrichs, N., Peng, W., Bieber, T., Wenzel, J., Novak, N., 2008. Distribution of Langerhans cells and mast cells within the human oral mucosa: new application sites of allergens in sublingual immunotherapy? Allergy 63, 720–727.

Allam, J.P., Wurtzen, P.A., Reinartz, M., Winter, J., Vrtala, S., Chen, K.W., Valenta, R., Wenghoefer, M., Appel, T., Gros, E., Niederhagen, B., Bieber, T., Lund, K., Novak, N., 2010. Phl p 5 resorption in human oral mucosa leads to dose-dependent and time-dependent allergen binding by oral mucosal Langerhans cells, attenuates their maturation, and enhances their migratory and TGF-beta1 and IL-10-producing properties. J. Allergy Clin. Immunol. 126, 638–645, e631.

Andersson, T.N., Ekman, G.J., Grönlund, H., Buentke, E., Eriksson, T.L.J., Scheynius, A., Van Hage-Hamsten, M., Gafvelin, G., 2004. A novel adjuvant–allergen complex, CBP–rFel d 1, induces up-regulation of CD86 expression and enhances cytokine release by human dendritic cells in vitro. Immunol. 113, 253–259.

Bachmann, M.F., Rohrer, U.H., Kundig, T.M., Burki, K., Hengartner, H., Zinkernagel, R.M., 1993. The influence of antigen organization on B cell responsiveness. Science 262, 1448–1451.

Basu, R., O'quinn Darrell, B., Silberger, D.J., Schoeb, T.R., Fouser, L., Ouyang, W., Hatton, R.D., Weaver, C.T., 2012. Th22 cells are an important source of IL-22 for host protection against enteropathogenic bacteria. Immunity 37, 1061–1075.

Batanero, E., Barral, P., Villalba, M., Rodríguez, X., 2003. Encapsulation of Ole e 1 in biodegradable microparticles induces Th1 response in mice: a potential vaccine for allergy. J. Control. Release 92, 395–398.

Bennett, C.L., Christie, J., Ramsdell, F., Brunkow, M.E., Ferguson, P.J., Whitesell, L., Kelly, T.E., Saulsbury, F.T., Chance, P.F., Ochs, H.D., 2001. The immune dysregulation, polyendocrinopathy, enteropathy, X-linked syndrome (IPEX) is caused by mutations of FOXP3. Nat. Genet. 27, 20–21.

Bessa, J., Schmitz, N., Hinton, H.J., Schwarz, K., Jegerlehner, A., Bachmann, M.F., 2008. Efficient induction of mucosal and systemic immune responses by virus-like particles administered intranasally: implications for vaccine design. Eur. J. Immunol. 38, 114–126.

Bohle, B., Kinaciyan, T., Gerstmayr, M., Radakovics, A., Jahn-Schmid, B., Ebner, C., 2007. Sublingual immunotherapy induces IL-10-producing T regulatory cells, allergen-specific T-cell tolerance, and immune deviation. J. Allergy Clin. Immunol. 120, 707–713.

Brunkow, M.E., Jeffery, E.W., Hjerrild, K.A., Paeper, B., Clark, L.B., Yasayko, S.A., Wilkinson, J.E., Galas, D., Ziegler, S.F., Ramsdell, F., 2001. Disruption of a new forkhead/winged-helix protein, scurfin, results in the fatal lymphoproliferative disorder of the scurfy mouse. Nat. Genet. 27, 68–73.

Bryant, J., Hlavaty, K.A., Zhang, X., Yap, W.-T., Zhang, L., Shea, L.D., Luo, X., 2014. Nanoparticle delivery of donor antigens for transplant tolerance in allogeneic islet transplantation. Biomaterials 35, 8887–8894.

Bryce, P.J., Mathias, C.B., Harrison, K.L., Watanabe, T., Geha, R.S., Oettgen, H.C., 2006. The H1 histamine receptor regulates allergic lung responses. J. Clin. Invest. 116, 1624–1632.

Chang, H.C., Sehra, S., Goswami, R., Yao, W., Yu, Q., Stritesky, G.L., Jabeen, R., Mckinley, C., Ahyi, A.N., Han, L., Nguyen, E.T., Robertson, M.J., Perumal, N.B., Tepper, R.S., Nutt, S.L., Kaplan, M.H., 2010. The transcription factor PU.1 is required for the development of IL-9-producing T cells and allergic inflammation. Nat. Immunol. 11, 527–534.

Chauhan, B.F., Ducharme, F.M., 2012. Anti-leukotriene agents compared to inhaled corticosteroids in the management of recurrent and/or chronic asthma in adults and children. Cochrane Database Syst. Rev. 5, CD002314.

Chen, W., Jin, W., Hardegen, N., Lei, K.-J., Li, L., Marinos, N., Mcgrady, G., Wahl, S.M., 2003. Conversion of Peripheral CD4+CD25− Naive T Cells to CD4+CD25+ Regulatory T Cells by TGF-β Induction of Transcription Factor Foxp3. J. Exp. Med. 198, 1875–1886.

Chong, C.S., Cao, M., Wong, W.W., Fischer, K.P., Addison, W.R., Kwon, G.S., Tyrrell, D.L., Samuel, J., 2005. Enhancement of T helper type 1 immune responses against hepatitis B virus core antigen by PLGA nanoparticle vaccine delivery. J. Control. Release 102, 85–99.

Chu, S.Y., Horton, H.M., Pong, E., Leung, I.W.L., Chen, H., Nguyen, D.-H., Bautista, C., Muchhal, U.S., Bernett, M.J., Moore, G.L., Szymkowski, D.E., Desjarlais, J.R., 2012. Reduction of total IgE by targeted coengagement of IgE B-cell receptor and FcγRIIb with Fc-engineered antibody. J. Allergy Clin. Immunol. 129, 1102–1115.

Ciprandi, G., Fenoglio, D., Cirillo, I., Vizzaccaro, A., Ferrera, A., Tosca, M.A., Puppo, F., 2005. Induction of interleukin 10 by sublingual immunotherapy for house dust mites: a preliminary report. Ann. Allergy Asthma Immunol. 95, 38–44.

Coffman, R.L., Lebman, D.A., Shrader, B., 1989. Transforming growth factor beta specifically enhances IgA production by lipopolysaccharide-stimulated murine B lymphocytes. J. Exp. Med. 170, 1039–1044.

Cox, L., Nelson, H., Lockey, R., Calabria, C., Chacko, T., Finegold, I., Nelson, M., Weber, R., Bernstein, D.I., Blessing-Moore, J., Khan, D.A., Lang, D.M., Nicklas, R.A., Oppenheimer, J., Portnoy, J.M., Randolph, C., Schuller, D.E., Spector, S.L., Tilles, S., Wallace, D., 2011. Allergen immunotherapy: a practice parameter third update. J. Allergy Clin. Immunol. 127, S1–S55.

Crawford, A., Macleod, M., Schumacher, T., Corlett, L., Gray, D., 2006. Primary T cell expansion and differentiation in vivo requires antigen presentation by B cells. J. Immunol. 176, 3498–3506.

Dardalhon, V., Awasthi, A., Kwon, H., Galileos, G., Gao, W., Sobel, R.A., Mitsdoerffer, M., Strom, T.B., Elyaman, W., Ho, I.C., Khoury, S., Oukka, M., Kuchroo, V.K., 2008. IL-4 inhibits TGF-beta-induced Foxp3+ T cells, and together with TGF-beta, generates IL-9+ IL-10+ Foxp3(−) effector T cells. Nat. Immunol. 9, 1347–1355.

De Waal Malefyt, R., Abrams, J., Bennett, B., Figdor, C.G., De Vries, J.E., 1991. Interleukin 10(IL-10) inhibits cytokine synthesis by human monocytes: an autoregulatory role of IL-10 produced by monocytes. J. Exp. Med. 174, 1209–1220.

De Waal Malefyt, R., Yssel, H., De Vries, J.E., 1993. Direct effects of IL-10 on subsets of human CD4+ T cell clones and resting T cells. Specific inhibition of IL-2 production and proliferation. J. Immunol. 150, 4754–4765.

Dent, L.A., Strath, M., Mellor, A.L., Sanderson, C.J., 1990. Eosinophilia in transgenic mice expressing interleukin 5. J. Exp. Med. 172, 1425–1431.

Dilillo, D.J., Matsushita, T., Tedder, T.F., 2010. B10 cells and regulatory B cells balance immune responses during inflammation, autoimmunity, and cancer. Ann. N. Y. Acad. Sci. 1183, 38–57.

Dombrowicz, D., Flamand, V., Brigman, K.K., Koller, B.H., Kinet, J.-P., 1993. Abolition of anaphylaxis by targeted disruption of the high affinity immunoglobulin E receptor α chain gene. Cell 75, 969–976.

Dunford, P.J., O'donnell, N., Riley, J.P., Williams, K.N., Karlsson, L., Thurmond, R.L., 2006. The histamine H4 receptor mediates allergic airway inflammation by regulating the activation of CD4+ T cells. J. Immunol. 176, 7062–7070.

Eagar, T.N., Turley, D.M., Padilla, J., Karandikar, N.J., Tan, L., Bluestone, J.A., Miller, S.D., 2004. CTLA-4 regulates expansion and differentiation of Th1 cells following induction of peripheral T cell tolerance. J. Immunol. 172, 7442 7450.

Eifan, A.O., Akkoc, T., Yildiz, A., Keles, S., Ozdemir, C., Bahceciler, N.N., Barlan, I.B., 2010. Clinical efficacy and immunological mechanisms of sublingual and subcutaneous immunotherapy in asthmatic/rhinitis children sensitized to house dust mite: an open randomized controlled trial. Clin. Exp. Allergy 40, 922–932.

Fillatreau, S., Sweenie, C.H., Mcgeachy, M.J., Gray, D., Anderton, S.M., 2002. B cells regulate autoimmunity by provision of IL-10. Nat. Immunol. 3, 944–950.

Fiorentino, D.F., Bond, M.W., Mosmann, T.R., 1989. Two types of mouse T helper cell. IV. Th2 clones secrete a factor that inhibits cytokine production by Th1 clones. J. Exp. Med. 170, 2081–2095.

Fleischer, D.M., Burks, A.W., Vickery, B.P., Scurlock, A.M., Wood, R.A., Jones, S.M., Sicherer, S.H., Liu, A.H., Stablein, D., Henning, A.K., Mayer, L., Lindblad, R., Plaut, M., Sampson, H.A., 2013. Sublingual immunotherapy for peanut allergy: a randomized, double-blind, placebo-controlled multicenter trial. J. Allergy Clin. Immunol. 131, 119–127, e117.

Fontenot, J.D., Rasmussen, J.P., Williams, L.M., Dooley, J.L., Farr, A.G., Rudensky, A.Y., 2005. Regulatory T cell lineage specification by the forkhead transcription factor foxp3. Immunity 22, 329–341.

Foussat, A., Cottrez, F., Brun, V., Fournier, N., Breittmayer, J.-P., Groux, H., 2003. A comparative study between T regulatory type 1 and CD4+CD25+ T cells in the control of inflammation. J. Immunol. 171, 5018–5026.

Francis, J.N., James, L.K., Paraskevopoulos, G., Wong, C., Calderon, M.A., Durham, S.R., Till, S.J., 2008. Grass pollen immunotherapy: IL-10 induction and suppression of late responses precedes IgG4 inhibitory antibody activity. J. Allergy Clin. Immunol. 121, 1120–1125, e1122.

Freeman, J., 1911. Further observations on the treatment of hay fever by hypodermic inoculations of pollen vaccine. Lancet 178, 814–817.

Fujita, H., Soyka, M.B., Akdis, M., Akdis, C.A., 2012. Mechanisms of allergen-specific immunotherapy. Clin. Transl. Allergy 2, 2.

Ganeshan, K., Neilsen, C.V., Hadsaitong, A., Schleimer, R.P., Luo, X., Bryce, P.J., 2009. Impairing oral tolerance promotes allergy and anaphylaxis: a new murine food allergy model. J. Allergy Clin. Immunol. 123, 231–238, e234.

Getts, D.R., Turley, D.M., Smith, C.E., Harp, C.T., Mccarthy, D., Feeney, E.M., Getts, M.T., Martin, A.J., Luo, X., Terry, R.L., King, N.J., Miller, S.D., 2011. Tolerance induced by apoptotic antigen-coupled leukocytes is induced by PD-L1+ and IL-10-producing splenic macrophages and maintained by T regulatory cells. J. Immunol. 187, 2405–2417.

Green, E.A., Gorelik, L., Mcgregor, C.M., Tran, E.H., Flavell, R.A., 2003. CD4+CD25+ T regulatory cells control anti-islet CD8+ T cells through TGF-β–TGF-β receptor interactions in type 1 diabetes. Proc. Natl. Acad. Sci. U. S. A. 100, 10878–10883.

Gri, G., Piconese, S., Frossi, B., Manfroi, V., Merluzzi, S., Tripodo, C., Viola, A., Odom, S., Rivera, J., Colombo, M.P., Pucillo, C.E., 2008. CD4+CD25+ regulatory T cells suppress mast cell degranulation and allergic responses through OX40-OX40L interaction. Immunity 29, 771–781.

Grönlund, H., Vrtala, S., Wiedermann, U., Dekan, G., Kraft, D., Valenta, R., Van Hage-Hamsten, M., 2002. Carbohydrate-based particles: a new adjuvant for allergen-specific immunotherapy. Immunology 107, 523–529.

Groux, H., O'garra, A., Bigler, M., Rouleau, M., Antonenko, S., De Vries, J.E., Roncarolo, M.G., 1997. A CD4+ T-cell subset inhibits antigen-specific T-cell responses and prevents colitis. Nature 389, 737–742.

Hasbold, J., Hong, J.S.-Y., Kehry, M.R., Hodgkin, P.D., 1999. Integrating signals from IFN-γ and IL-4 by B Cells: positive and negative effects on CD40 ligand-induced proliferation, survival, and division-linked isotype switching to IgG1, IgE, and IgG2a. J. Immunol. 163, 4175–4181.

Hellings, P.W., Vandenberghe, P., Kasran, A., Coorevits, L., Overbergh, L., Mathieu, C., Ceuppens, J.L., 2002. Blockade of CTLA-4 enhances allergic sensitization and eosinophilic airway inflammation in genetically predisposed mice. Eur. J. Immunol. 32, 585–594.

Holgate, S.T., Djukanović, R., Casale, T., Bousquet, J., 2005. Anti-immunoglobulin E treatment with omalizumab in allergic diseases: an update on anti-inflammatory activity and clinical efficacy. Clin. Exp. Allergy 35, 408–416.

Hori, S., Nomura, T., Sakaguchi, S., 2003. Control of regulatory T cell development by the transcription factor Foxp3. Science 299, 1057–1061.

Huber, S., Gagliani, N., Esplugues, E., O'connor Jr., W., Huber, F.J., Chaudhry, A., Kamanaka, M., Kobayashi, Y., Booth, C.J., Rudensky, A.Y., Roncarolo, M.G., Battaglia, M., Flavell, R.A., 2011. Th17 cells express interleukin-10 receptor and are controlled by Foxp3− and Foxp3+ regulatory CD4+ T cells in an interleukin-10-dependent manner. Immunity 34, 554–565.

Hunter, Z., Mccarthy, D.P., Yap, W.T., Harp, C.T., Getts, D.R., Shea, L.D., Miller, S.D., 2014. A biodegradable nanoparticle platform for the induction of antigen-specific immune tolerance for treatment of autoimmune disease. ACS Nano 8, 2148–2160.

Hwang, E.S., Szabo, S.J., Schwartzberg, P.L., Glimcher, L.H., 2005. T helper cell fate specified by kinase-mediated interaction of T-bet with GATA-3. Science 307, 430–433.

Ishida, Y., Agata, Y., Shibahara, K., Honjo, T., 1992. Induced expression of PD-1, a novel member of the immunoglobulin gene superfamily, upon programmed cell death. EMBO J. 11, 3887–3895.

Jeannin, P., Lecoanet, S., Delneste, Y., Gauchat, J.-F., Bonnefoy, J.-Y., 1998. IgE versus IgG4 production can be differentially regulated by IL-10. J. Immunol. 160, 3555–3561.

Jennings, G.T., Bachmann, M.F., 2009. Immunodrugs: therapeutic VLP-based vaccines for chronic diseases. Annu. Rev. Pharmacol. Toxicol. 49, 303–326.
Johansen, P., Häffner, A.C., Koch, F., Zepter, K., Erdmann, I., Maloy, K., Simard, J.J., Storni, T., Senti, G., Bot, A., Wüthrich, B., Kündig, T.M., 2005. Direct intralymphatic injection of peptide vaccines enhances immunogenicity. Eur. J. Immunol. 35, 568–574.
Juillard, G.J., Boyer, P.J., Yamashiro, C.H., Snow, H.D., Weisenburger, T.H., Mccarthy, T., Miller, R.J., 1977. Regional intralymphatic infusion (ILI) of irradiated tumor cells with evidence of distant effects. Cancer 39, 126–130.
Juillard, G.J., Boyer, P.J., Yamashiro, C.H., 1978. A phase I study of active specific intralymphatic immunotherapy (ASILI). Cancer 41, 2215–2225.
Jutel, M., Pichler, W.J., Skrbic, D., Urwyler, A., Dahinden, C., Muller, U.R., 1995. Bee venom immunotherapy results in decrease of IL-4 and IL-5 and increase of IFN-gamma secretion in specific allergen-stimulated T cell cultures. J. Immunol. 154, 4187–4194.
Kato, A., Favoreto, S., Avila, P.C., Schleimer, R.P., 2007. TLR3- and Th2 cytokine-dependent production of thymic stromal lymphopoietin in human airway epithelial cells. J. Immunol. 179, 1080–1087.
Kawabe, T., Naka, T., Yoshida, K., Tanaka, T., Fujiwara, H., Suematsu, S., Yoshida, N., Kishimoto, T., Kikutani, H., 1994. The immune responses in CD40-deficient mice: impaired immunoglobulin class switching and germinal center formation. Immunity 1, 167–178.
Kearley, J., Barker, J.E., Robinson, D.S., Lloyd, C.M., 2005. Resolution of airway inflammation and hyperreactivity after in vivo transfer of CD4 + CD25 + regulatory T cells is interleukin 10 dependent. J. Exp. Med. 202, 1539–1547.
Kearley, J., Robinson, D.S., Lloyd, C.M., 2008. CD4 + CD25 + regulatory T cells reverse established allergic airway inflammation and prevent airway remodeling. J. Allergy Clin. Immunol. 122, 617–624, e616.
Keir, M.E., Butte, M.J., Freeman, G.J., Sharpe, A.H., 2008. PD-1 and its ligands in tolerance and immunity. Annu. Rev. Immunol. 26, 677–704.
Keles, S., Karakoc-Aydiner, E., Ozen, A., Izgi, A.G., Tevetoglu, A., Akkoc, T., Bahceciler, N.N., Barlan, I., 2011. A novel approach in allergen-specific immunotherapy: combination of sublingual and subcutaneous routes. J. Allergy Clin. Immunol. 128, 808–815, e807.
Kheradmand, T., Wang, S., Bryant, J., Tasch, J.J., Lerret, N., Pothoven, K.L., Houlihan, J.L., Miller, S.D., Zhang, Z.J., Luo, X., 2012. Ethylenecarbodiimide-fixed donor splenocyte infusions differentially target direct and indirect pathways of allorecognition for induction of transplant tolerance. J. Immunol. 189, 804–812.
Klein, L., Kyewski, B., Allen, P.M., Hogquist, K.A., 2014. Positive and negative selection of the T cell repertoire: what thymocytes see (and don't see). Nat. Rev. Immunol. 14, 377–391.
Kopp, M.V., 2011. Role of immunmodulators in allergen-specific immunotherapy. Allergy 66, 792–797.
Kündig, T.M., Senti, G., Schnetzler, G., Wolf, C., Prinz Vavricka, B.M., Fulurija, A., Hennecke, F., Sladko, K., Jennings, G.T., Bachmann, M.F., 2006. Der p 1 peptide on virus-like particles is safe and highly immunogenic in healthy adults. J. Allergy Clin. Immunol. 117, 1470–1476.
Kurata, H., Lee, H.J., O'garra, A., Arai, N., 1999. Ectopic expression of activated Stat6 induces the expression of Th2-specific cytokines and transcription factors in developing Th1 cells. Immunity 11, 677–688.
Kurosaki, T., Shinohara, H., Baba, Y., 2010. B cell signaling and fate decision. Annu. Rev. Immunol. 28, 21–55.
Kyewski, B., Klein, L., 2006. A central role for central tolerance. Annu. Rev. Immunol. 24, 571–606.
Leb, V.M., Jahn-Schmid, B., Kueng, H.J., Schmetterer, K.G., Haiderer, D., Neunkirchner, A., Fischer, G.F., Hartl, A., Thalhamer, J., Steinberger, P., Bohle, B., Seed, B., Pickl, W.F., 2009. Modulation of allergen-specific T-lymphocyte function by virus-like particles decorated with HLA class II molecules. J. Allergy Clin. Immunol. 124, 121–128.
Lewkowich, I.P., Herman, N.S., Schleifer, K.W., Dance, M.P., Chen, B.L., Dienger, K.M., Sproles, A.A., Shah, J.S., Köhl, J., Belkaid, Y., Wills-Karp, M., 2005. CD4 + CD25 + T cells protect against experimentally induced asthma and alter pulmonary dendritic cell phenotype and function. J. Exp. Med. 202, 1549–1561.
Loke, P.N., Allison, J.P., 2003. PD-L1 and PD-L2 are differentially regulated by Th1 and Th2 cells. Proc. Natl. Acad. Sci. U. S. A. 100, 5336–5341.

Lutsiak, M.E., Kwon, G.S., Samuel, J., 2006. Biodegradable nanoparticle delivery of a Th2-biased peptide for induction of Th1 immune responses. J. Pharm. Pharmacol. 58, 739–747.
Macglashan, D.W., Savage, J.H., Wood, R.A., Saini, S.S., 2012. Suppression of the basophil response to allergen during treatment with omalizumab is dependent on 2 competing factors. J. Allergy Clin. Immunol. 130, 1130–1135, e1135.
Maloy, K.J., Erdmann, I., Basch, V., Sierro, S., Kramps, T.A., Zinkernagel, R.M., Oehen, S., Kündig, T.M., 2001. Intralymphatic immunization enhances DNA vaccination. Proc. Natl. Acad. Sci. U. S. A. 98, 3299–3303.
Martínez-Gómez, J.M., Johansen, P., Erdmann, I., Senti, G., Crameri, R., Kündig, T.M., 2009. Intralymphatic injections as a new administration route for allergen-specific immunotherapy. Int. Arch. Allergy Immunol. 150, 59–65.
Mcbride, J.M., Jung, T., De Vries, J.E., Aversa, G., 2002. IL-10 alters DC function via modulation of cell surface molecules resulting in impaired T-cell responses. Cell. Immunol. 215, 162–172.
Meiler, F., Zumkehr, J., Klunker, S., Rückert, B., Akdis, C.A., Akdis, M., 2008. In vivo switch to IL-10–secreting T regulatory cells in high dose allergen exposure. J. Exp. Med. 205, 2887–2898.
Miller, S.D., Turley, D.M., Podojil, J.R., 2007. Antigen-specific tolerance strategies for the prevention and treatment of autoimmune disease. Nat. Rev. Immunol. 7, 665–677.
Möbs, C., Slotosch, C., Löffler, H., Jakob, T., Hertl, M., Pfützner, W., 2010. Birch pollen immunotherapy leads to differential induction of regulatory T cells and delayed helper T cell immune deviation. J. Immunol. 184, 2194–2203.
Möbs, C., Ipsen, H., Mayer, L., Slotosch, C., Petersen, A., Würtzen, P.A., Hertl, M., Pfützner, W., 2012. Birch pollen immunotherapy results in long-term loss of Bet v 1–specific TH2 responses, transient TR1 activation, and synthesis of IgE-blocking antibodies. J. Allergy Clin. Immunol. 130, 1108–1116, e1106.
Moldaver, D.M., Bharhani, M.S., Wattie, J.N., Ellis, R., Neighbour, H., Lloyd, C.M., Inman, M.D., Larche, M., 2014. Amelioration of ovalbumin-induced allergic airway disease following Der p 1 peptide immunotherapy is not associated with induction of IL-35. Mucosal Immunol. 7, 379–390.
Moore, K.W., De Waal Malefyt, R., Coffman, R.L., O'garra, A., 2001. Interleukin-10 and the interleukin-10 receptor. Annu. Rev. Immunol. 19, 683–765.
Moran, A.E., Holzapfel, K.L., Xing, Y., Cunningham, N.R., Maltzman, J.S., Punt, J., Hogquist, K.A., 2011. T cell receptor signal strength in Treg and iNKT cell development demonstrated by a novel fluorescent reporter mouse. J. Exp. Med. 208, 1279–1289.
Mosmann, T.R., Coffman, R.L., 1989. TH1 and TH2 cells: different patterns of lymphokine secretion lead to different functional properties. Annu. Rev. Immunol. 7, 145–173.
Mosmann, T.R., Cherwinski, H., Bond, M.W., Giedlin, M.A., Coffman, R.L., 1986. Two types of murine helper T cell clone. I. Definition according to profiles of lymphokine activities and secreted proteins. J. Immunol. 136, 2348–2357.
Mullen, A.C., High, F.A., Hutchins, A.S., Lee, H.W., Villarino, A.V., Livingston, D.M., Kung, A.L., Cereb, N., Yao, T.P., Yang, S.Y., Reiner, S.L., 2001. Role of T-bet in commitment of TH1 cells before IL-12-dependent selection. Science 292, 1907–1910.
Murai, M., Turovskaya, O., Kim, G., Madan, R., Karp, C.L., Cheroutre, H., Kronenberg, M., 2009. Interleukin 10 acts on regulatory T cells to maintain expression of the transcription factor Foxp3 and suppressive function in mice with colitis. Nat. Immunol. 10, 1178–1184.
Neimert-Andersson, T., Thunberg, S., Swedin, L., Wiedermann, U., Jacobsson-Ekman, G., Dahlén, S.E., Scheynius, A., Grönlund, H., Hage, M.V., Gafvelin, G., 2008. Carbohydrate-based particles reduce allergic inflammation in a mouse model for cat allergy. Allergy 63, 518–526.
Newbould, B.B., 1964. Lymphatic drainage and adjuvant-induced arthritis in rats. Br. J. Exp. Pathol. 45, 375–383.
Newman, K.D., Samuel, J., Kwon, G., 1998a. Ovalbumin peptide encapsulated in poly(d, l lactic-co-glycolic acid) microspheres is capable of inducing a T helper type 1 immune response. J. Control. Release 54, 49–59.
Newman, K.D., Sosnowski, D.L., Kwon, G.S., Samuel, J., 1998b. Delivery of MUC1 mucin peptide by Poly(d, l-lactic-co-glycolic acid) microspheres induces type 1 T helper immune responses. J. Pharm. Sci. 87, 1421–1427.

Nieto, M.A., Gonzalez, A., Gambon, F., Diaz-Espada, F., Lopez-Rivas, A., 1992. Apoptosis in human thymocytes after treatment with glucocorticoids. Clin. Exp. Immunol. 88, 341–344.
Nishimura, H., Nose, M., Hiai, H., Minato, N., Honjo, T., 1999. Development of lupus-like autoimmune diseases by disruption of the PD-1 gene encoding an ITIM motif-carrying immunoreceptor. Immunity 11, 141–151.
Nishimura, H., Okazaki, T., Tanaka, Y., Nakatani, K., Hara, M., Matsumori, A., Sasayama, S., Mizoguchi, A., Hiai, H., Minato, N., Honjo, T., 2001. Autoimmune dilated cardiomyopathy in PD-1 receptor-deficient mice. Science 291, 319–322.
Noon, L., 1911. Prophylactic inoculation against hay fever. Lancet 177, 1572–1573.
Novak, N., Bieber, T., 2008. Dendritic cells as regulators of immunity and tolerance. J. Allergy Clin. Immunol. 121, S370–S374.
Novak, N., Allam, J.P., Betten, H., Haberstok, J., Bieber, T., 2004. The role of antigen presenting cells at distinct anatomic sites: they accelerate and they slow down allergies. Allergy 59, 5–14.
Ouyang, W., Ranganath, S.H., Weindel, K., Bhattacharya, D., Murphy, T.L., Sha, W.C., Murphy, K.M., 1998. Inhibition of Th1 development mediated by GATA-3 through an IL-4-independent mechanism. Immunity 9, 745–755.
Ozcan, E., Notarangelo, L.D., Geha, R.S., 2008. Primary immune deficiencies with aberrant IgE production. J. Allergy Clin. Immunol. 122, 1054–1062.
Pajno, G.B., Vita, D., Caminiti, L., Arrigo, T., Lombardo, F., Incorvaia, C., Barberio, G., 2005. Children's compliance with allergen immunotherapy according to administration routes. J. Allergy Clin. Immunol. 116, 1380–1381.
Pecquet, S., Leo, E., Fritsche, R., Pfeifer, A., Couvreur, P., Fattal, E., 2000. Oral tolerance elicited in mice by beta-lactoglobulin entrapped in biodegradable microspheres. Vaccine 18, 1196–1202.
Poole, J.A., Meng, J., Reff, M., Spellman, M.C., Rosenwasser, L.J., 2005. Anti-CD23 monoclonal antibody, lumiliximab, inhibited allergen-induced responses in antigen-presenting cells and T cells from atopic subjects. J. Allergy Clin. Immunol. 116, 780–788.
Radulovic, S., Calderon Moises, A., Wilson, D. & Durham, S., 2010. Sublingual immunotherapy for allergic rhinitis. Cochrane Database Syst. Rev., John Wiley & Sons, Ltd.
Rosenwasser, L.J., Busse, W.W., Lizambri, R.G., Olejnik, T.A., Totoritis, M.C., 2003. Allergic asthma and an anti-CD23 mAb (IDEC-152). J. Allergy Clin. Immunol. 112, 563–570.
Rothenberg, M.E., 1998. Eosinophilia. N. Engl. J. Med. 338, 1592–1600.
Rothenberg, M.E., Hogan, S.P., 2006. The eonsinophil. Annu. Rev. Immunol. 24, 147–174.
Said, E.A., Dupuy, F.P., Trautmann, L., Zhang, Y., Shi, Y., El-Far, M., Hill, B.J., Noto, A., Ancuta, P., Peretz, Y., Fonseca, S.G., Van Grevenynghe, J., Boulassel, M.R., Bruneau, J., Shoukry, N.H., Routy, J.-P., Douek, D.C., Haddad, E.K., Sekaly, R.-P., 2010. Programmed death-1-induced interleukin-10 production by monocytes impairs CD4+ T cell activation during HIV infection. Nat. Med. 16, 452–459.
Saint-Lu, N., Tourdot, S., Razafindratsita, A., Mascarell, L., Berjont, N., Chabre, H., Louise, A., Van Overtvelt, L., Moingeon, P., 2009. Targeting the allergen to oral dendritic cells with mucoadhesive chitosan particles enhances tolerance induction. Allergy 64, 1003–1013.
Satoguina, J.S., Weyand, E., Larbi, J., Hoerauf, A., 2005. T regulatory-1 cells induce IgG4 production by B cells: role of IL-10. J. Immunol. 174, 4718–4726.
Satoguina, J.S., Adjobimey, T., Arndts, K., Hoch, J., Oldenburg, J., Layland, L.E., Hoerauf, A., 2008. Tr1 and naturally occurring regulatory T cells induce IgG4 in B cells through GITR/GITR-L interaction, IL-10 and TGF-β. Eur. J. Immunol. 38, 3101–3113.
Scadding, G.W., Shamji, M.H., Jacobson, M.R., Lee, D.I., Wilson, D., Lima, M.T., Pitkin, L., Pilette, C., Nouri-Aria, K., Durham, S.R., 2010. Sublingual grass pollen immunotherapy is associated with increases in sublingual Foxp3-expressing cells and elevated allergen-specific immunoglobulin G4, immunoglobulin A and serum inhibitory activity for immunoglobulin E-facilitated allergen binding to B cells. Clin. Exp. Allergy 40, 598–606.
Schmitz, N., Dietmeier, K., Bauer, M., Maudrich, M., Utzinger, S., Muntwiler, S., Saudan, P., Bachmann, M.F., 2009. Displaying Fel d1 on virus-like particles prevents reactogenicity despite greatly enhanced immunogenicity: a novel therapy for cat allergy. J. Exp. Med. 206, 1941–1955.

Schöll, I., Weissenböck, A., Förster-Waldl, E., Untersmayr, E., Walter, F., Willheim, M., Boltz-Nitulescu, G., Scheiner, O., Gabor, F., Jensen-Jarolim, E., 2004. Allergen-loaded biodegradable poly (d, l-lactic-co-glycolic) acid nanoparticles down-regulate an ongoing Th2 response in the BALB/c mouse model. Clin. Exp. Allergy 34, 315–321.

Secrist, H., Chelen, C.J., Wen, Y., Marshall, J.D., Umetsu, D.T., 1993. Allergen immunotherapy decreases interleukin 4 production in CD4+ T cells from allergic individuals. J. Exp. Med. 178, 2123–2130.

Senti, G., Prinz Vavricka, B.M., Erdmann, I., Diaz, M.I., Markus, R., Mccormack, S.J., Simard, J.J., Wüthrich, B., Crameri, R., Graf, N., Johansen, P., Kündig, T.M., 2008. Intralymphatic allergen administration renders specific immunotherapy faster and safer: a randomized controlled trial. Proc. Natl. Acad. Sci. U. S. A. 105, 17908–17912.

Senti, G., Graf, N., Haug, S., Ruedi, N., Von Moos, S., Sonderegger, T., Johansen, P., Kundig, T.M., 2009a. Epicutaneous allergen administration as a novel method of allergen-specific immunotherapy. J. Allergy Clin. Immunol. 124, 997–1002.

Senti, G., Johansen, P., Haug, S., Bull, C., Gottschaller, C., Müller, P., Pfister, T., Maurer, P., Bachmann, M.F., Graf, N., Kündig, T.M., 2009b. Use of A-type CpG oligodeoxynucleotides as an adjuvant in allergen-specific immunotherapy in humans: a phase I/IIa clinical trial. Clin. Exp. Allergy 39, 562–570.

Senti, G., Crameri, R., Kuster, D., Johansen, P., Martinez-Gomez, J.M., Graf, N., Steiner, M., Hothorn, L.A., Gronlund, H., Tivig, C., Zaleska, A., Soyer, O., Van Hage, M., Akdis, C.A., Akdis, M., Rose, H., Kundig, T.M., 2012. Intralymphatic immunotherapy for cat allergy induces tolerance after only 3 injections. J. Allergy Clin. Immunol. 129, 1290–1296.

Shibata, Y., Foster, L.A., Metzger, W.J., Myrvik, Q.N., 1997a. Alveolar macrophage priming by intravenous administration of chitin particles, polymers of N-acetyl-D-glucosamine, in mice. Infect. Immun. 65, 1734–1741.

Shibata, Y., Metzger, W.J., Myrvik, Q.N., 1997b. Chitin particle-induced cell-mediated immunity is inhibited by soluble mannan: mannose receptor-mediated phagocytosis initiates IL-12 production. J. Immunol. 159, 2462–2467.

Shibata, Y., Foster, L.A., Bradfield, J.F., Myrvik, Q.N., 2000. Oral administration of chitin down-regulates serum IgE levels and lung eosinophilia in the allergic mouse. J. Immunol. 164, 1314–1321.

Simons, F.E.R., Simons, K.J., 2011. Histamine and H1-antihistamines: celebrating a century of progress. J. Allergy Clin. Immunol. 128, e1134–e1150.

Singh, A.K., Stock, P., Akbari, O., 2011. Role of PD-L1 and PD-L2 in allergic diseases and asthma. Allergy 66, 155–162.

Smarr, C.B., Hsu, C.L., Byrne, A.J., Miller, S.D., Bryce, P.J., 2011. Antigen-fixed leukocytes tolerize Th2 responses in mouse models of allergy. J. Immunol. 187, 5090–5098.

Smarr, C.B., Bryce, P.J., Miller, S.D., 2013. Antigen-specific tolerance in immunotherapy of Th2-associated allergic diseases. Crit. Rev. Immunol. 33 (5), 389–414. PMID 24099300.

Smith, C.E., Eagar, T.N., Strominger, J.L., Miller, S.D., 2005. Differential induction of IgE-mediated anaphylaxis after soluble vs. cell-bound tolerogenic peptide therapy of autoimmune encephalomyelitis. Proc. Natl. Acad. Sci. U. S. A. 102, 9595–9600.

Snapper, C.M., Peschel, C., Paul, W.E., 1988. IFN-gamma stimulates IgG2a secretion by murine B cells stimulated with bacterial lipopolysaccharide. J. Immunol. 140, 2121–2127.

Sonoda, E., Matsumoto, R., Hitoshi, Y., Ishii, T., Sugimoto, M., Araki, S., Tominaga, A., Yamaguchi, N., Takatsu, K., 1989. Transforming growth factor beta induces IgA production and acts additively with interleukin 5 for IgA production. J. Exp. Med. 170, 1415–1420.

Staudt, V., Bothur, E., Klein, M., Lingnau, K., Reuter, S., Grebe, N., Gerlitzki, B., Hoffmann, M., Ulges, A., Taube, C., Dehzad, N., Becker, M., Stassen, M., Steinborn, A., Lohoff, M., Schild, H., Schmitt, E., Bopp, T., 2010. Interferon-regulatory factor 4 is essential for the developmental program of T helper 9 cells. Immunity 33, 192–202.

Stellato, C., Matsukura, S., Fal, A., White, J., Beck, L.A., Proud, D., Schleimer, R.P., 1999. Differential regulation of epithelial-derived C-C chemokine expression by IL-4 and the glucocorticoid budesonide. J. Immunol. 163, 5624–5632.

Sucher, R., Fischler, K., Oberhuber, R., Kronberger, I., Margreiter, C., Ollinger, R., Schneeberger, S., Fuchs, D., Werner, E.R., Watschinger, K., Zelger, B., Tellides, G., Pilat, N., Pratschke, J., Margreiter, R., Wekerle, T., Brandacher, G., 2012. IDO and regulatory T cell support are critical for cytotoxic T lymphocyte-associated Ag-4 Ig-mediated long-term solid organ allograft survival. J. Immunol. 188, 37–46.

Surh, C.D., Sprent, J., 1994. T-cell apoptosis detected in situ during positive and negative selection in the thymus. Nature 372, 100–103.

Swartzendruber, J.A., Byrne, A.J., Bryce, P.J., 2012. Cutting edge: histamine is required for IL-4–driven eosinophilic allergic responses. J. Immunol. 188, 536–540.

Tan, L.J., Kennedy, M.K., Miller, S.D., 1992. Regulation of the effector stages of experimental autoimmune encephalomyelitis via neuroantigen-specific tolerance induction. II. Fine specificity of effector T cell inhibition. J. Immunol. 148, 2748–2755.

Taylor, A., Akdis, M., Joss, A., Akkoç, T., Wenig, R., Colonna, M., Daigle, I., Flory, E., Blaser, K., Akdis, C.A., 2007. IL-10 inhibits CD28 and ICOS costimulations of T cells via src homology 2 domain—containing protein tyrosine phosphatase 1. J. Allergy Clin. Immunol. 120, 76–83.

Thieu, V.T., Yu, Q., Chang, H.-C., Yeh, N., Nguyen, E.T., Sehra, S., Kaplan, M.H., 2008. Signal transducer and activator of transcription 4 is required for the transcription factor T-bet to promote T helper 1 cell-fate determination. Immunity 29, 679–690.

Umar, A., Schweitzer, P.A., Levy, N.S., Gearhart, J.D., Gearhart, P.J., 1991. Mutation in a reporter gene depends on proximity to and transcription of immunoglobulin variable transgenes. Proc. Natl. Acad. Sci. U. S. A. 88, 4902–4906.

Usui, T., Nishikomori, R., Kitani, A., Strober, W., 2003. GATA-3 suppresses Th1 development by downregulation of stat4 and not through effects on IL-12Rβ2 chain or T-bet. Immunity 18, 415–428.

Veldhoen, M., Uyttenhove, C., Van Snick, J., Helmby, H., Westendorf, A., Buer, J., Martin, B., Wilhelm, C., Stockinger, B., 2008. Transforming growth factor-beta 'reprograms' the differentiation of T helper 2 cells and promotes an interleukin 9-producing subset. Nat. Immunol. 9, 1341–1346.

Vissers, J.L., Van Esch, B.C., Hofman, G.A., Kapsenberg, M.L., Weller, F.R., Van Oosterhout, A.J., 2004. Allergen immunotherapy induces a suppressive memory response mediated by IL-10 in a mouse asthma model. J. Allergy Clin. Immunol. 113, 1204–1210.

Vogelbruch, M., Nuss, B., Körner, M., Kapp, A., Kiehl, P., Bohm, W., 2000. Aluminium-induced granulomas after inaccurate intradermal hyposensitization injections of aluminium-adsorbed depot preparations. Allergy 55, 883–887.

Von Beust, B.R., Johansen, P., Smith, K.A., Bot, A., Storni, T., Kündig, T.M., 2005. Improving the therapeutic index of CpG oligodeoxynucleotides by intralymphatic administration. Eur. J. Immunol. 35, 1869–1876.

Wakkach, A., Fournier, N., Brun, V., Breittmayer, J.P., Cottrez, F., Groux, H., 2003. Characterization of dendritic cells that induce tolerance and T regulatory 1 cell differentiation in vivo. Immunity 18, 605–617.

Webb, D.C., Mckenzie, A.N.J., Matthaei, K.I., Rothenberg, M.E., Foster, P.S., 2001. Distinct spatial requirement for eosinophil-induced airways hyperreactivity. Immunol. Cell Biol. 79, 165–169.

Weber, E.A., Blaser, K., 1986. Suppression of the anti-hapten IgE antibody response with hapten-modified spleen cells. Eur. J. Immunol. 16, 1527–1531.

Webster, J.I., Tonelli, L., Sternberg, E.M., 2002. Neuroendocrine regulation of immunity. Annu. Rev. Immunol. 20, 125–163.

Wechsler, J.B., Schroeder, H.A., Byrne, A.J., Chien, K.B., Bryce, P.J., 2013. Anaphylactic responses to histamine in mice utilize both histamine receptors 1 and 2. Allergy 68, 1338–1340.

Wing, K., Onishi, Y., Prieto-Martin, P., Yamaguchi, T., Miyara, M., Fehervari, Z., Nomura, T., Sakaguchi, S., 2008. CTLA-4 control over Foxp3+ regulatory T cell function. Science 322, 271–275.

Xiao, Y., Yu, S., Zhu, B., Bedoret, D., Bu, X., Francisco, L.M., Hua, P., Duke-Cohan, J.S., Umetsu, D.T., Sharpe, A.H., Dekruyff, R.H., Freeman, G.J., 2014. RGMb is a novel binding partner for PD-L2 and its engagement with PD-L2 promotes respiratory tolerance. J. Exp. Med. 211, 943–959.

Yagi, R., Zhu, J., Paul, W.E., 2011. An updated view on transcription factor GATA3-mediated regulation of Th1 and Th2 cell differentiation. Int. Immunol. 23, 415–420.

Yoshikawa, H., Nakajima, Y., Tasaka, K., 1999. Glucocorticoid suppresses autocrine survival of mast cells by inhibiting IL-4 production and ICAM-1 expression. J. Immunol. 162, 6162–6170.

Yoshizaki, A., Miyagaki, T., Dilillo, D.J., Matsushita, T., Horikawa, M., Kountikov, E.I., Spolski, R., Poe, J.C., Leonard, W.J., Tedder, T.F., 2012. Regulatory B cells control T-cell autoimmunity through IL-21-dependent cognate interactions. Nature 491, 264–268.

Yukselen, A., Kendirli, S.G., Yilmaz, M., Altintas, D.U., Karakoc, G.B., 2012. Effect of one-year subcutaneous and sublingual immunotherapy on clinical and laboratory parameters in children with rhinitis and asthma: a randomized, placebo-controlled, double-blind, double-dummy study. Int. Arch. Allergy Immunol. 157, 288–298.

Zheng, W.-P., Flavell, R.A., 1997. The transcription factor GATA-3 is necessary and sufficient for Th2 cytokine gene expression in CD4 T cells. Cell 89, 587–596.

Zhu, J., Paul, W.E., 2008. CD4 T cells: fates, functions, and faults. Blood 112, 1557–1569.

Zhu, J., Guo, L., Watson, C.J., Hu-Li, J., Paul, W.E., 2001. Stat6 is necessary and sufficient for IL-4's role in Th2 differentiation and cell expansion. J. Immunol. 166, 7276–7281.

Zhu, J., Min, B., Hu-Li, J., Watson, C.J., Grinberg, A., Wang, Q., Killeen, N., Urban Jr., J.F., Guo, L., Paul, W.E., 2004. Conditional deletion of Gata3 shows its essential function in T(H)1-T(H)2 responses. Nat. Immunol. 5, 1157–1165.

CHAPTER 11

Humanized Mice in Translational Immunology

M.A. Brehm[1], R. Bortell[1], M. Verma[2], L.D. Shultz[2], D.L. Greiner[1]
[1]University of Massachusetts Medical School, Diabetes Center of Excellence, Worcester, MA, United States
[2]The Jackson Laboratory, Bar Harbor, ME, United States

Contents

Translational Immunology
http://dx.doi.org/10.1016/B978-0-12-801577-3.00012-5

1. INTRODUCTION

Since the first description of using athymic "nude" mice for engraftment of xenogeneic tissues such as human tumor cell lines and solid tumors in the late 1960s (Rygaard and Povlsen, 1969), the development of CB17-*Prkdc*^{scid} (CB17-*scid*) mice in 1983 (Carroll and Bosma, 1988), and the subsequent engraftment of CB17-*scid* mice with human hematopoietic cells in 1988 (Kamel-Reid and Dick, 1988; McCune et al., 1988; Mosier et al., 1988), investigators have sought an immunodeficient mouse model that would demonstrate high-fidelity of human immune cell function following the engraftment of primary human cells and tissues. In this chapter, we review recent advances in attempts to achieve this goal, and the use of these "humanized mice" for translational immunology as well as their increasingly important role in accelerating the advancement of new therapies into the clinic.

1.1 Need for humanized mouse models

1.1.1 Differences in human and mouse biology

The study of human immune biology is limited by logistical and ethical restrictions of working with cells and tissue samples from human donors (Davis, 2012). To address this, many investigators have turned to animal models as surrogates of human biology. The overwhelming animal species of choice for these investigations are mice. Study of the immune system of mice has provided insights into many of the mechanisms underlying the development and regulation of the mammalian immune system. However, mouse and human immune systems diverged evolutionarily between 65 and 75 million years ago and many differences have developed and have been summarized (Mestas and Hughes, 2004). For example, there are fundamental differences in the blood cell populations of humans and mice with the innate immune cells such as neutrophils being the predominant leukocyte population in humans, comprising 50–70% of the circulating nucleated cells. Only 30–50% of the cells are lymphocytes (Langlois et al., 1997). In contrast, 75–90% of the circulating leukocytes in the blood of mice are lymphocytes (Doeing et al., 2003). Another example of a fundamental difference between immune systems of mice and humans extends to the observation that human endothelial cells can express both major histocompatibility complex (MHC) classes I and II molecules whereas mouse endothelial cells express only MHC class I (Choo et al., 1997). This differential expression of MHC molecules provides a uniquely human cell source of MHC class II-positive antigen-presenting cells (APC) capable of initiating immune responses in humans but not in mice. Moreover, additional differences in the immune systems of humans and mice are constantly being identified.

As noted above, there are many differences in human and mouse immune systems (Mestas and Hughes, 2004). A recent report extended this observation by noting that genomic mouse inflammatory responses do not mimic the genomic responses that are observed during human inflammation (Seok et al., 2013). However, a recent report analyzing the same data set calls this conclusion into question (Takao and Miyakawa, 2015). These authors reevaluated the same gene expression data sets as the original study that reported the genomic responses between mouse and human are highly different, but the reanalyzed data came to exactly the opposite conclusion. They concluded that the gene expression levels following induction of inflammatory responses in mice correlate well with those observed in humans (Takao and Miyakawa, 2015). The debate on whether mouse genomic inflammatory responses mimic human inflammatory responses is based on a 5.9–15.0% overlap between the genomic responses of the two species, and whether this represents significant overlap or poor overlap becomes a conceptual argument (Takao et al., 2015; Warren et al., 2014a). Notably, there are also a number of structural differences in innate immune molecules between mice and humans. So far, 10 and 12 functional toll-like receptors (TLRs) have been identified in humans and mice, respectively, with TLR1–TLR9 being conserved in both species. Mouse TLR10 is not functional because of a retrovirus insertion, and TLR11, TLR12, and TLR13 have been lost from the human genome (Kawai and Akira, 2010). These data suggest that there exist some fundamental differences in the molecular components used in innate immune responses between mice and humans.

While the answer to the similarity of mouse and human immune responses remains to be clarified, this chapter focuses on the use of humanized mice for the study of human immunity. The underlying premise using humanized mice is that they can act as a preclinical bridge for the study of human hematopoiesis, immunity, and autoimmunity, immune responses to infectious disease, as well as tumor and transplantation immunity (Fig. 1).

1.1.2 New categories of human-specific therapeutics

There is a rapidly developing class of new human-specific drugs. These are comprised of human-based cellular therapeutics and human-specific antibodies, particularly antibodies targeted to a group of molecules collectively termed "immune checkpoint proteins" (Weber, 2010). This rapidly developing field is based on a growing recognition that immune modulating drugs may be used to upregulate or suppress human immune responses in individuals. This has been highlighted by the recent publications of low-dose human IL2 therapy to induce regulatory T cells (Tregs) for the treatment of

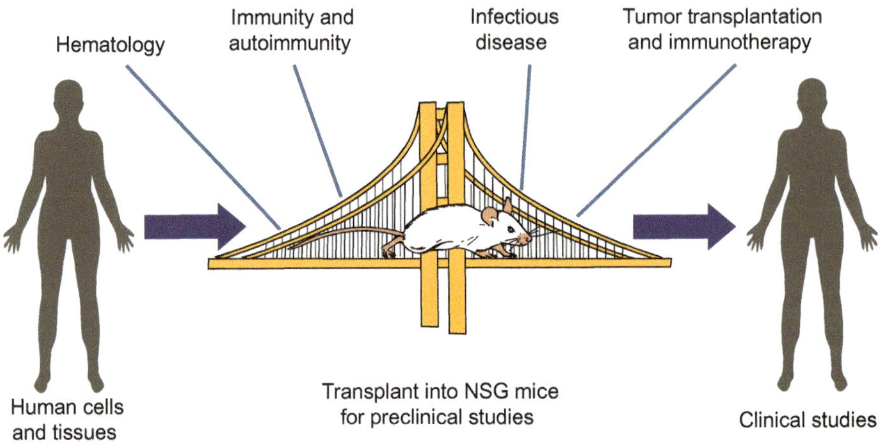

Figure 1 Biomedical areas in which humanized mice are being utilized for translational immunology research.

graft-versus-host disease (GVHD) (Koreth et al., 2011; Matsuoka et al., 2013) and for hepatitis C virus (HCV)-induced vasculitis (Saadoun et al., 2011). Cytokine treatment to induce *in vivo* the generation of Tregs is now being extended to the use of Treg cellular therapy for the treatment of transplantation rejection (Putnam et al., 2013; Tang and Bluestone, 2013). The availability of a humanized mouse model to evaluate the efficacy of the *in vivo* induction of Tregs (iTregs) and transplantation of *ex vivo*-generated human Tregs will likely provide a critical tool in accelerating translation of Treg cellular therapy to the clinic. Similarly, the evaluation of human-specific antibodies to modulate the immune system in humanized mice will become increasingly important based on the recent clinical trials using the checkpoint inhibitor, antiprogrammed death-1 (PD1) antibody, to inhibit the PD1/programmed death-1 ligand (PD-L1) pathway for the treatment of human melanoma, leading to spectacular results in some, but not all, patients (Ohaegbulam et al., 2015; Tumeh et al., 2014). PD1/PD-L1 blockade is also being tested clinically in a variety of other cancers, including non-small cell lung cancer (NSCLC), renal cell carcinoma (RCC), and bladder cancer (Ohaegbulam et al., 2015). The use of humanized mice will facilitate understanding the mechanism(s) underlying the variable response rates of patients to this class of checkpoint inhibitors and for the development of new approaches to target this pathway.

1.2 History of the development of immunodeficient mice for human immune system engraftment

There have been multiple reviews over the last few years on the development of immunodeficient mice for engraftment of functional human cells, tissues, and immune systems (Shultz et al., 2007, 2012; Brehm et al., 2014; Rongvaux et al., 2014; Ito et al., 2012;

Vuyyuru et al., 2011; Akkina, 2013b; Villaudy et al., 2014). These detail the progression from engraftment of athymic nude mice with human cells and tissues to the discovery and hematopoietic cell engraftment of CB17-*scid* mice. The first real breakthrough in the ability to engraft significant levels of human hematopoietic cells and immune cells into immunodeficient mice occurred with descriptions of NOD-*scid* mice in the early 2000s (Ito et al., 2002; Shultz et al., 2005). Although investigators achieved levels of ~10% human cells in the circulating hematopoietic system in NOD-*scid* mice, these mice still failed to develop a complete human immune system following transplantation of human hematopoietic stem cells (HSC) as human T cells failed to develop in this model (Shultz et al., 2012). Human immune cell engraftment was greatly enhanced with the discovery of the IL2 receptor common gamma chain (*IL2rg*) gene (Cao et al., 1993) and the development of immunodeficient mice bearing a null mutation in *IL2rg* ($IL2rg^{null}$) (reviewed in Shultz et al., 2012). There are multiple strains upon which immunodeficient mice with a mutated *IL2rg* gene have been generated, but the four most widely used and best characterized are those on two different inbred NOD strains as well as the BALB/c and C57BL6 strains (Fig. 2). These widely used strains have been rendered immunodeficient by the spontaneous protein kinase DNA activated, catalytic polypeptide mutation ($Prkdc^{scid}$ or *scid*) or by targeting the recombination-activating gene *(Rag)* 1 or 2. There are two different $IL2rg^{null}$ targeted mutations that have been widely employed for construction of these mice. One is a complete null ($IL2rg^{tm1Wjl}$) (Shultz et al., 2005) whereas the other binds to IL2 but is truncated and fails to signal ($IL2rg^{tm1Sug}$) (Ito et al., 2002). The most widely used strains are NOD.Cg-$Prkdc^{scid}Il2rg^{tm1Wjl}$ (NSG mice), NODShi.Cg-$Prkdc^{scid}Il2rg^{tm1Sug}$ (NOG mice), C;129S4- $Rag2^{tm1Flv}Il2rg^{tm1Flv.}$ stocks of mice (BRG mice), and recently, the B6.129S-$Rag2^{tm1Fwa}$ $Cd47^{tm1Fpl}$ $Il2rg^{tm1Wjl}$/J (B6RG-CD47) strain has been described. These differences in inbred strains and mutations that are used to induce immunodeficiency, as well as the type of mutated *IL2rg* gene used, lead to differences in the model systems that are important when considering the experimental question(s) to be addressed using humanized mice.

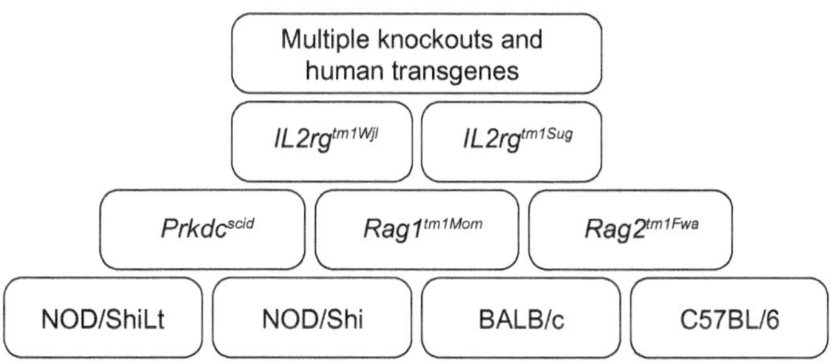

Figure 2 Various models of immunodeficient mice as platforms for engraftment of human immune systems.

2. APPROACHES FOR ESTABLISHMENT OF HUMAN IMMUNE SYSTEMS IN IMMUNODEFICIENT MICE

Using these different immunodeficient *IL2rg*^{null} mouse strains, a number of common approaches for engraftment of human immune systems have been developed.

2.1 Hu-PBL-SCID

The simplest approach to engraft a human immune system in immunodeficient mice is the intravenous (IV) or intraperitoneal (IP) injection of human peripheral blood mononuclear cells (PBMC) as first described in 1988 using CB17-*scid* mice (Mosier et al., 1988). This system has been coined the Human Peripheral Blood Lymphocyte SCID (Hu-PBL-SCID) model (Mosier et al., 1988). A similar model can be established following engraftment of cells obtained from any peripheral lymphoid tissue that contains mature T cells such as spleen, lymph nodes, and even bone marrow or cord blood samples that have not been depleted of human T cells. In the Hu-PBL-SCID models based on NSG or NOG mice, human lymphocytes engraft, rapidly expand, and the majority of the circulating blood cells are of human origin (Ito et al., 2009; King et al., 2009). However, the predominant human cell population that engrafts consists of activated $CD3^+$ T cells whereas human B cells and myeloid cells are lost from the mice within the first few days of engraftment (Ito et al., 2009; King et al., 2009). The majority of the T cells that engraft appear to be xenoreactive T cells that inevitably lead to a lethal GVHD-like syndrome, usually within 3–6 weeks.

Hu-PBL-SCID mice have been used as a preclinical model to study the immunosuppressive effects of human mesenchymal stem cells (MSC) that are purported to exhibit immunomodulatory properties. Introduction of human MSCs to the Hu-PBL-SCID model in two different systems delays the development of GVHD (Gregoire-Gauthier et al., 2012; Jang et al., 2014). The Hu-PBL-SCID model has also been used to investigate the ability of HLA-matched dendritic cells to enhance a T cell immune response (Harui et al., 2011) as well as a tool to evaluate human dendritic cell-based vaccine strategies *in vivo* (Spranger et al., 2012). The Hu-PBL-SCID model has also been used to evaluate the efficacy of an IL4 and IL13 antagonist, pitrakinra, that is being proposed as a clinical therapeutic for the treatment of atopic dermatitis. This drug works by the inhibition of human IgE secretion induced by IL4 (Zadeh-Khorasani et al., 2013). Of note is that the model was used within its limitations to address a mechanistic question, that of blocking the IL4-induction of IgE, rather than as a treatment of atopic dermatitis. Thus, humanized mice were used to identify the ability of the drug to target a pathway rather than a disease syndrome.

2.2 Hu-SRC-SCID

The implantation of human HSCs into immunodeficient mice was first reported in 1988 and led to partial engraftment of a hematopoietic system (Kamel-Reid and Dick, 1988). This system has been coined the Human SCID-Repopulating Cell SCID

(Hu-SRC-SCID) model (Kamel-Reid and Dick, 1988). However, Hu-SRC-SCID mice failed to develop human T cells from HSC until immunodeficient mice bearing a targeted mutation in the *IL2rg* gene were developed (Ito et al., 2002; Traggiai et al., 2004; Shultz et al., 2005). When engrafted with human HSC, immunodeficient *IL2rg*^{null} mice develop a full human immune system, including T cells, B cells, myeloid cells, and dendritic cells. Although the mice develop granulocyte, megakaryocyte, and red blood cell precursors in the bone marrow (Cheung et al., 2012), these myeloid cell populations fail to circulate in the blood, likely due to remaining host innate immune cells and lack of human-specific cytokines required for the development of these lineages (reviewed in Shultz et al., 2012).

The fidelity of the human immune cells that develop in Hu-SRC-SCID mice, that is, how closely these cell populations phenotypically and functionally resemble their counterparts that develop in humans, has been examined. The T cells that develop in NSG mice engrafted with human HSC generate a cell population with a human β chain T cell receptor that has V-J combinations equally distributed in the thymus and peripheral tissues and is comparable to that observed in humans (Pham et al., 2012) and exhibit a diverse repertoire (Shultz et al., 2005). Similarly, the antibody repertoire in HSC-engrafted humanized NSG mice also appears to have a human-like diversification and exhibits similar tolerance checkpoints as are observed in humans (Ippolito et al., 2012). However, impaired long-term maintenance of human CD8 T cells (Andre et al., 2010), first noted in the Bone marrow/Liver/Thymus (BLT) model described below (Biswas et al., 2011), as well as impaired maturation of human B cells are apparent in immunodeficient *IL2rg*^{null} recipients of human HSC. The natural killer (NK) cell compartment of humanized mice appears to be intact, but the NK cells require preactivation to acquire functional competence (Strowig et al., 2010). For example, administration of human IL15/IL15 receptor complexes enhances the functional maturation of human NK cells (Huntington et al., 2009) and simultaneously promotes human T cell reconstitution (Huntington et al., 2011).

In the myeloid compartment of humanized mice, human neutrophils, basophils, mast cells, monocytes, as well as conventional and plasmacytoid dendritic cells can be detected, and administration of granulocyte-colony stimulating factor (G-CSF) will lead to recruitment of low numbers of human granulocytes into the blood (Tanaka et al., 2012). Myelomonocytic lineage differentiation appears to be reduced and the monocytes that do develop are phenotypically immature (Gille et al., 2012). However, CD141^{+} dendritic cells can be stimulated with double stranded RNA to produce interferon-α, suggesting they can functionally respond to virus infection (Meixlsperger et al., 2013). Human granulocyte progenitors are present in the recipient mouse bone marrow, and when mobilized into the peripheral blood using G-CSF, the circulating human neutrophils appear to be functional as evidenced by an appropriate phenotypic upregulation of activation markers following *in vivo* lipopolysaccharide (LPS) stimulation and their sequestration in the lungs (Coughlan et al., 2012). Furthermore, they undergo a respiratory burst and degranulate in response to formyl-methionyl-leucyl-phenylalanine (fMLP) or *Escherichia coli* stimulation (Coughlan et al., 2012). Many of the noted deficiencies in human innate immune development are being overcome by transgenic expression of human-specific cytokines (see below). In summary, when testing drugs designed to target the adaptive and innate immune system in humanized mice, one must first confirm that the target of the therapy is present and functionally active and that the appropriate humanized mouse model for the study is chosen.

2.3 SCID-hu and BLT

The engraftment of human fetal thymus, liver, and HSCs into CB17-*scid* immunodeficient mice, first reported in 1988, leads to the development of a human thymus in the recipient (McCune et al., 1988). Although autologous HSC were also injected IV in this report, due to the inability of the CB17-*scid* mouse to engraft well with hematopoietic cells, human immune cell development was largely restricted to the implanted thymus fragment and was termed the SCID-hu model. More recently using the NOD-*scid* strain and subsequently the NSG strain, subrenal capsule implantation with fetal human liver and thymus fragments as in the SCID-hu model followed by IV injection of autologous HSC derived from the fetal liver leads to the development of a robust peripheral and mucosal human immune system (Melkus et al., 2006; Lan et al., 2006). This system is coined the BLT model as the IV-injected HSC repopulate the bone marrow of the recipient. As in the Hu-SRC-SCID model, all lineages of human immune cells develop. However, the engraftment of the human immune system in BLT mice is much more robust, likely due to the education of T cells in their autologous thymus leading to HLA-restricted human T cells that can interact productively with the engrafted human APCs. BLT mice develop both a peripheral and mucosal human immune system (for review see Shultz et al., 2012). One of the main caveats of the BLT system is the reported development of a wasting-like syndrome resembling a GVHD that limits the time window for experimentation in most (Greenblatt et al., 2012; Lockridge et al., 2013; Covassin et al., 2013) but not all (Onoe et al., 2011) laboratories.

2.4 Other immune system engraftment models

Fragments of human tonsils have been implanted into immunodeficient *IL2rg*^{null} mice, and in contrast to typical Hu-PBL-SCID mice implanted with single cell suspensions of blood, B cells persist in the tonsil fragment as well as T cell subsets, but the germinal center architecture is lost over time (Vallet et al., 2005). Furthermore, GVHD does not seem to develop in the recipients of tonsil fragments, likely due to the inability of the human immune cells in the fragments to repopulate the peripheral tissues of the CB17-*scid* mouse used as a recipient in this report (Vallet et al., 2005). Human fetal lymph node implantation into immunodeficient mice has also been performed (Shih et al., 2000). In this study, both CB17-*scid* and NOD-*scid* mice were used as recipients, and it was observed that implantation of the fetal lymph node into the subcutaneous pouches in the ears led to massive lymph node growth, and retention of the lymph node histologic architecture and cellular composition (Shih et al., 2000).

Human skin contains a diverse immune system that appears to be fundamentally different than that present in the peripheral lymphoid tissues (Nestle et al., 2009). For example, human epidermis and dermis are rich in Langerhans cells, a potent APC. There are also about twice as many T cells in the mucosal and skin tissues as compared to blood circulating cells and the majority of these express an effector/memory phenotype (Mueller et al., 2013). Recapitulation of this unique skin immune system has been accomplished by transplantation and long-term maintenance of human skin grafts on NSG mice (Soria et al., 2014; Racki et al., 2010). These models may be useful for studying human-specific therapeutics in the context of intact human structural tissue in immunodeficient mice.

3. HUMAN IMMUNE MODELS OF HUMANIZED MICE

3.1 Approaches for implantation of human PBMC and HSC for generation of an immune system

As varied as the platform strains and the model systems for humanization, there are also multiple technical approaches for engrafting human immune systems. In the Hu-PBL-SCID model, the standard approaches are IV or IP injection of single cell populations into young adult hosts. In the Hu-SRC-SCID mice, there are multiple variables for consideration. Human HSC can be obtained from bone marrow, cord blood, fetal liver, or G-CSF-mobilized peripheral blood mononuclear $CD34^+$ HSC. It has been shown that cord blood and fetal liver are most effective in reconstituting a human hematopoietic and immune system, whereas it requires higher numbers of human HSC and is more difficult to achieve high levels of human hematopoietic cell and immune system engraftment using bone marrow or mobilized HSC (Lepus et al., 2009; Shultz et al., 2005).

In most engraftment models described below, sublethal irradiation is commonly used to precondition the recipient, likely to create "niches" for human HSC engraftment and to induce bone marrow factors that enhance human HSC engraftment and differentiation. If an irradiator is not available, some investigators have found that conditioning with busulfan will facilitate human HSC engraftment in NSG mice (Hayakawa et al., 2009). Furthermore, it has been shown that human hematopoietic systems can be engrafted in young adult NSG mice without any preconditioning, but human T cells develop only poorly in unirradiated mice (Brehm et al., 2012b). Intrafemoral injection of human HSC into NSG mice can also lead to human hematopoietic cell engraftment in the absence of irradiation but chimerism is low (Bueno et al., 2010). Recently, the development of NSG and BRG mice with mutations in *Kit* have been described, and these mice support high levels of human hematopoietic cell engraftment, including myeloid cells, B cells, and intrathymic T cells following engraftment of human HSC, even in the absence of irradiation preconditioning (Cosgun et al., 2014). However, the development of peripheral T cells was not reported.

Mice at a range of ages of engraftment have been used, including newborns, 3- to 4-week-olds, and young adult mice that are 6 weeks of age or older. For newborn engraftment, four routes of HSC injection have been employed: IV via the facial vein, IV via intracardiac injection, intrahepatic injection, and IP injection (Pearson et al., 2008). The IV and intrahepatic injections into newborn mice lead to robust human HSC engraftment, but human HSC fail to engraft following IP injection. The IV injection via the facial vein can be technically difficult as can the intracardiac IV injection. Although the intrahepatic injection is relatively simple as the liver is readily visible through the newborn skin, if the injection is missed, the HSC are implanted in the peritoneal cavity and fail to engraft. If young adult recipients 6 weeks of age or older are used, good human hematopoietic system engraftment is observed following IV injection of HSC, but T cell development is poor. This is likely due to the cysts that develop with age in the thymus of NSG mice, resulting in failure to provide a nurturing environment for developing human T cells (Shultz et al., 2005). Young adult recipients can also be injected intrafemorally with human HSC, and this approach has shown more efficient engraftment in NSG mice with human HSC than in NOG mice (McDermott et al., 2010). Many investigators now routinely use 3- to 4-week-old recipients as they are technically easier to inject IV with the caveat that delayed, but good, T cell development is observed following engraftment of human HSC (Brehm et al., 2014).

3.2 Modifications of immunodeficient *IL2rg*^{null} mice that enhance human immune system engraftment

There remain a number of limitations of immunodeficient *IL2rg*^{null} mice that impede full human cell immune system engraftment and that prevent long-term study of humanized mice. Although the *IL2rg*^{null} mutation severely reduces innate immunity in mice that lack adaptive immunity (Cao et al., 1995), there remain host innate immune cell populations and factors that impede human immune cell engraftment. The lack of species-specific factors such as HLA molecules and cytokines further impede human immune system development and function. Moreover, the development of a GVHD like-syndrome in humanized mice limits the time window available for experimental use.

3.2.1 Reduction of host innate immunity

Multiple approaches have been used to further reduce host innate immunity. Anti-Ly6G (Gr1) antibody has been used to deplete host granulocytes and has been shown to facilitate human skin allograft engraftment in NSG mice. The skin xenografts can be rejected following injection of allogeneic PBMC in the Hu-PBL-SCID model (Racki et al., 2010). This system can now be used to test therapeutics targeting the prevention of human allograft rejection. Complement is an important component of the innate immune system, but NOD strain mice lack functional hemolytic complement due to a mutation in the *Hc* gene encoding the C5 complement component (Shultz et al., 1995). Two approaches to address this have been used. First, the development of BRG mice transgenically expressing human signal regulatory protein α (Sirpα) engraft at similar levels as NSG and NOG mice with human immune systems, and in contrast to NSG mice, have an intact complement system (Yamauchi et al., 2013; Strowig et al., 2011). Second, the crossing of an intact *Hc* gene onto NSG mice has been completed and is currently being characterized in the laboratory of LDS. These mice will be important for analyses of the complement-mediated effects of new human-specific antibodies such as the anti-CD20 mAb ofatumumab, which appears to have an effect in the clinic mediated in part by complement fixation (Pawluczkowycz et al., 2009).

Type 1 interferon (IFN) is a potent inhibitor of virus replication and is highly conserved across species. Knocking out innate immune genes such as the type 1 interferon receptor (type 1 IFNR) in NSG mice permitted the use of very low doses of Dengue virus to induce a productive infection for the development of a model system for the study of immunity to Dengue and as a platform for the evaluation of Dengue therapeutics (Jaiswal et al., 2015).

Human granulocytes, red blood cells (RBC), and platelets circulate poorly in NSG mice (Tanaka et al., 2012; Coughlan et al., 2012). Although progenitors of these cell lineages develop normally in the bone marrow of humanized mice engrafted with HSC, few mature cells circulate in the blood. A number of approaches have been used to enhance blood circulation of human RBCs, including expression of the human Sirpα gene in BRG mice, which improves survival of injected human RBCs (Strowig et al., 2011). The host macrophages appear to be a limiting factor for circulation of both RBCs and platelets as injection of liposome-encapsulated clodronate to deplete host macrophages leads to increased circulating levels of RBCs (Hu et al., 2011) and platelets (Hu and Yang, 2012; Rongvaux et al., 2011). Another approach is to repeatedly inject human RBCs into NSG mice, which leads to high circulating levels of human RBCs. This model has been used for the study of antimalarial drugs being developed for the clinic (Jimenez-Diaz et al., 2009). These approaches highlight novel new humanized mouse models for the study of therapeutics that may be targeted against RBCs or platelets or require these cell populations for survival of infectious agents. The potential role of macrophages in preventing the circulation of granulocytes has not been reported.

3.2.2 Provision of human-specific cytokines and HLA molecules in humanized mice

There are a number of species-specific cytokines that are needed for full development of a functional human immune system. These have been reviewed recently (Rongvaux et al.,

2013; Brehm et al., 2014; Shultz et al., 2012), and will not be exhaustively reviewed here. Instead, the multiple approaches for supplying these human cytokines will be described. First and simplest is the injection of human recombinant protein such as human IL7 to improve human T cell development and function (Shultz et al., 2005), B lymphocyte stimulating (BLyS or BAFF) factor to improve human B cell engraftment (Schmidt et al., 2008), IL15/IL15R complexes to improve human NK and T cell engraftment and function (Huntington et al., 2009, 2011), and Fms-related tyrosine kinase 3 ligand (FLT3L) to improve human dendritic cell (DC) generation (Ding et al., 2014) as a few examples. However, this approach is costly and significant variation may be observed between experiments among different laboratories. A second approach is the hydrodynamic injection of plasmids containing human cytokine genes. For example, hydrodynamic injection of plasmids containing granulocyte macrophage-CSF (GM-CSF) and IL4 have been shown to stimulate human antibody responses (Chen et al., 2012), injection of plasmids containing macrophage-CSF (M-CSF) have been shown to enhance human macrophage development (Li et al., 2013), and injection of IL10 plasmids into the Hu-PBL-SCID model has been shown to induce Treg cells and modulate the development of GVHD (Abraham et al., 2015). Surprisingly, it has recently been shown that IL10, long thought to be a regulatory cytokine, will exacerbate xenogeneic GVHD in the Hu-PBL-SCID model (Abraham et al., 2015). The caveat with the hydrodynamic approach is that plasmid expression can be variable and is not likely to be long lasting. Cytokines can also be provided by vectors such as adeno-associated virus (AAV) vectors containing human cDNA. For example, a recent study used AAV vectors to transgenically express human HLA-A2, and human GM-CSF, IL3, IL4, IL7, and IL15 in humanized mice (Huang et al., 2014). Hu-SRC-SCID NSG mice treated with the AAV-expressing vectors generated high levels of protein expression for up to 10 weeks. Although levels diminished by 16 weeks, the generation of A2-restricted human CD8 T cell responses following vaccination was observed. Based on these results, it appears that replacement of human cytokines and HLA molecules, even transiently, can enhance human immune responses and may be useful for preclinical evaluation of vaccine candidates.

An alternative approach that leads to more permanent protein expression is transgenic expression of human cytokines via cDNA transgenic expression, BAC transgenic expression, or via knock-in technology (Brehm et al., 2014; Rongvaux et al., 2013). The simplest approach is the transgenic expression of cDNA, but gene expression is commonly controlled by a constitutive promoter that results in nonregulated but long-term cytokine expression. This has been useful in the generation of mice for enhanced engraftment and development of, for example, human mast cells by expression of human membrane-bound stem cell factor (mSCF) (Takagi et al., 2012), and human myeloid cells (Miller et al., 2013), as well as human Treg cells (Billerbeck et al., 2011) by transgenic expression of GM-CSF, IL3, and soluble SCF in NSG mice. However, expression of these cytokines is not regulated by their natural promoters, and host cytokine expression remains intact. The presence of host cytokines can be problematic as transgenic expression of human BLyS fails to mediate the biological effects that are observed when high pharmacological levels of recombinant BLyS are injected, perhaps due to the competitive effects of mouse BLyS production, which can bind to human BLyS receptors on B cells but does not lead to productive signaling (Schmidt et al., 2008). For BLyS, and similar cytokines such as IL7, knock-in technology may be needed to enhance human cell growth and differentiation.

Generation of transgenic mice using human BAC constructs brings the same caveat as cDNA transgenic expression in that the murine gene is still expressed. However, the BAC construct will likely have its endogenous promoters expressed, suggesting that in many cases gene expression will be appropriately regulated leading to physiological levels of cytokine expression.

Finally, knock-in technology has been used extensively, particularly in the BRG strain of mice (Rongvaux et al., 2013). The advantage of this approach is that the murine gene is replaced by the human gene, so that the appropriate regulation of gene expression remains intact and there is no competitive expression of the murine gene. This has been a highly successful approach for the generation of multiple human cytokine transgenic mice. However, unanticipated adverse events, as in transgenic expression, can occur. When BRG-TPO knock-in mice were analyzed, the levels of human thrombopoietin (TPO) were ~10-fold lower than physiological levels of mice, leading to a decreased number of mouse platelets and thrombocytopenia because human platelets do not circulate in humanized mice (Rongvaux et al., 2011). Similarly, BRG-IL3/GM-CSF knock-in mice resulted in enhanced engraftment of human alveolar macrophages, but nonengrafted mice developed pulmonary alveolar proteinosis caused by the absence of mouse GM-CSF (Willinger et al., 2011). These models demonstrate unanticipated results using knock-in technology that may occur. More recently, BRG mice expressing human Sirpα and a number of other human genes, including TPO, IL3, GM-CSF, or M-CSF, developed robust innate immune cell populations, particularly cells of the myeloid lineage (Rongvaux et al., 2014). However, the development of human T cells in these mice was not described, and adaptive human immune responses remained poor.

For the generation of human HLA-restricted human T cell responses, two model systems can be used. First, human T cells developing in HSC engrafted immunodeficient *IL2rg*^{null} mice are educated on mouse MHC and are H2-restricted (Watanabe et al., 2009). This permits the human T cells to interact with mouse APCs, but not with human APCs during the generation of an immune response. The transgenic expression of HLA-DR4 in immunodeficient *IL2rg*^{null} mice has been shown to enhance human CD4 T cell development and antibody production after engraftment with DR4-positive HSC

(Suzuki et al., 2012; Danner et al., 2011). Using a different approach, transgenic expression of human HLA molecules such as HLA-A2 can lead to HLA-restricted human CD8 T cell responses following human HLA-matched HSC engraftment (Shultz et al., 2010; Strowig et al., 2009; Jaiswal et al., 2009, 2012). Furthermore, the use of the BLT model in which the human T cells are educated on their autologous HLA-matched thymus will lead to robust human HLA-restricted CD8 T cell responses (Rongvaux et al., 2013; Shultz et al., 2012).

3.2.3 Approaches for ameliorating the GVHD-like syndrome in humanized mice

The primary targets of human xenoreactive T cells in humanized mice are the murine MHC classes I and II antigens, and engrafting human PBMC into NSG mice that are deficient in either MHC class I or class II delays the development of GVHD (King et al., 2009). Furthermore, engrafting purified $CD4^+$ T cells into NSG mice deficient in MHC class II leads to a significant delay in the development of GVHD (Covassin et al., 2011). This approach has been extended to establish a model of HLA class II allogeneic GVHD by engraftment of HLA-DR4-negative PBMC into NSG-Ab^{null} (H2 class II deficient) mice transgenically expressing HLA-DR4 (Covassin et al., 2011). It will be important to determine the development of GVHD in humanized mice lacking both MHC classes I and II and whether this recipient will provide a GVHD-free Hu-PBL-SCID model for experimental studies.

Of additional potential interest for preventing the development of GVHD in BLT mice is the description of a new recipient, the B6RG-CD47 strain of mice (Lavender et al., 2013). CD47 is involved in a critical pathway for innate immunity. The CD47-SIRPα ligand-receptor pathway is responsible for recognition by macrophages of CD47 expressed on almost all cells. This recognition is a negative "do not eat me" signal, and in the absence of self-CD47 expression, macrophages will phagocytose the cells. C57BL/6-SIRPα does not recognize human CD47 as self, and knocking out the mouse CD47 incapacitates this ligand-receptor pathway, leading to the lack of phagocytosis of the engrafted human HSCs. These mice surprisingly failed to develop GVHD-like syndromes by 29 weeks after engraftment, a time point at which GVHD is observed in most BLT mice generated in other laboratories (Covassin et al., 2013; Greenblatt et al., 2012; Lockridge et al., 2013). Detailed description of the methodology of engrafting B6RG-CD47 mice has recently been published (Lavender et al., 2014), which should accelerate confirmation by other laboratories that this strain fails to develop GVHD. It is clear, however, that the SIRPα/CD47 axis is critical in determining human hematopoietic cell engraftment in immunodeficient $IL2rg^{null}$ mice. Transgenic expression of human SIRPα in C57BL/6 immunodeficient $IL2rg^{null}$ mice (Iwamoto et al., 2014) and BRG mice (Yamauchi et al., 2013; Strowig et al., 2011) greatly enhances the engraftment of human HSC.

4. MODELS OF HUMANIZED MICE FOR EVALUATION OF IMMUNOMODULATORY DRUGS

As described above, there are multiple platforms and approaches for engraftment of human immune systems to generate humanized mice. These models are used to establish humanized mouse models of infection, tumor immunity, transplantation, and autoimmunity that are available for study of human immune function and evaluation of drugs that modulate immune responses.

4.1 Humanized mouse models for study of infectious diseases

There are a number of viral and bacterial infectious diseases in which humans are the only known reservoir, including some that cannot be investigated in nonhuman primates because of biological or ethical constraints, such as human immunodeficiency virus (HIV) and *Salmonella enteric serovar* Typhi (*S.* Typhi) (Wolfe et al., 2007; Baumler and Fang, 2013). The development of humanized mice engrafted with human cells, tissues, and immune systems has provided a small animal model for the study of these human-specific infectious agents (Brehm et al., 2013, 2014; Leung et al., 2013; Rongvaux et al., 2013; Shultz et al., 2012)

4.1.1 Humanized mouse models for the study of HIV

Humanized mice are the most used small animal model for the study of HIV (reviewed in Sliva, 2014; Bennett and Akkina, 2013; Gonzalez et al., 2013; Hofer et al., 2013; Munz, 2014; Leung et al., 2013). The BLT model has been widely utilized due to the engraftment of a mucosal human immune system and provides a critical tool for studying oral, rectal, and vaginal transmission of HIV as well as evaluation of drugs to prevent mucosal transmission (Chateau et al., 2013a,b; Deruaz and Luster, 2013; Wheeler et al., 2013; Denton and Garcia, 2012; Hur et al., 2012; Wahl et al., 2012; Neff et al., 2011; Stoddart et al., 2011, 2012). This model also supports studies to determine the efficacy of broadly neutralizing antibodies for HIV treatment (Balazs et al., 2012; Hur et al., 2012), to investigate gene therapy approaches for the prevention and treatment of HIV (Bennett and Akkina, 2013; Didigu et al., 2013; Hofer et al., 2013; Hur et al., 2012; McNeer et al., 2012; Schleifman et al., 2011, 2013), to evaluate new long-acting antiretroviral drugs for HIV (Nischang et al., 2012), and for evaluation of a novel CD4 aptamer-siRNA chimeric model for HIV treatment (Wheeler et al., 2013).

One of the biggest hurdles in the treatment of HIV in patients is the resurgence of the virus after extensive therapy when no virus particles can be detected in the blood and the therapy has been discontinued, a process termed HIV latency. The reservoir for the latent HIV in humans is poorly understood and has been hypothesized to be in the brain, gastrointestinal tract, and/or in monocytes/macrophages (Kumar et al., 2014; Siliciano and Siliciano, 2014; Brown and Mattapallil, 2014; Taube and Peterlin, 2013).

Understanding the molecular mechanisms underlying HIV latency represents a major goal for identifying approaches to achieve long-term cure of HIV-infected individuals (Taube and Peterlin, 2013). To address this, humanized mice have been used to establish HIV latency models for the identification of the tissue and cell reservoirs and mechanisms underlying HIV latency (Honeycutt et al., 2013; Choudhary et al., 2012; Denton et al., 2012; Marsden et al., 2012). Recently, using humanized mice, a critical mechanism of latency was discovered. It was shown that the vast majority of latent viruses carry CTL escape mutations, and that unless therapy is started early, these escape mutants develop and are extremely difficult to clear (Deng et al., 2015).

4.1.2 Humanized mouse models for the study of filoviruses

The Ebola outbreak of 2014 represents one of the most challenging infectious disease crises that has occurred in recent history, and at the present time there are no proven drugs, vaccines, or antibodies that are available for Ebola infection, prevention, or treatment (Whaley et al., 2014; Marzi and Feldmann, 2014; Wong et al., 2014; Chowell and Nishiura, 2014; Burd, 2015; Beeching et al., 2014; Tseng and Chan, 2015). Mouse-adapted Ebola virus has recently been used to model host genetic diversity in the response to virus infection in mice (Rasmussen et al., 2014), but mouse-adapted Ebola virus is very different from primary clinical isolates of Ebola. Nonhuman primates (De et al., 2011; Warren et al., 2014b; Choi et al., 2015) and humanized mice are the only animal models that are available for the study of the pathogenesis of clinical isolates of Ebola and other filoviruses and for the evaluation of the efficacy of potential drugs.

4.1.3 Humanized mouse models for the study of human-specific pathogens

In addition to HIV and filoviruses, humanized mouse models have been established for many other human-specific viruses. These include modeling HBV and HVC infection, first described in 2001 (Mercer et al., 2001), and these models have been used extensively to investigate the pathogenesis and response of the virus to drugs (reviewed in Billerbeck et al., 2013; Bility et al., 2013; Yoshizato and Tateno, 2013; Von et al., 2014). Humanized mouse models for Epstein-Barr virus (EBV) and Dengue, two human-specific viruses, have also been developed. The infection, pathogenesis, vaccine development, and drug therapy have been studied in humanized mice infected with EBV (Fujiwara et al., 2013; Fujiwara, 2014; Chatterjee et al., 2014; Akkina, 2013a). The critical role of human CD8 T cells in controlling EBV infection was demonstrated directly by adoptive transfer of EBV-specific CD8 T cell clones into EBV-infected humanized mice (Antsiferova et al., 2014). Interestingly, EBV causes B cell lymphoma in Africa, and humanized mice have been used to investigate a potential molecular basis of this lymphoma. It was observed that a mutant EBV virus was able to infect humanized mice and induce human B cell lymphomas (Ma et al., 2012). More recently, NSG mice were engrafted with human cord blood HSC that was infected with wild-type EBV or EBV deficient in latent membrane protein-1 (LMP1) (Ma et al., 2015). LMP1 is an EBV oncoprotein that mimics a constitutively active CD40 receptor. HSC infected with LMP1-deficient EBV required human $CD4^{+}$ T cells for human lymphoma growth, demonstrating the key role of human immune cells in the development of EBV-induced lymphomas. This report shows the utility of humanized mice for investigating the interactions of virus infection, human immunity, and cancer (Ma et al., 2015). Humanized mice infected with Dengue virus have been used to study transmission via mosquito bites (Cox et al., 2012), investigate how clinical symptoms develop (Mota and Rico-Hesse, 2009), and to generate broadly cross-reactive human antibodies to Dengue (Jaiswal et al., 2015).

Humanized mice have also been used to establish models for the study of bacterial infections. Humanized NSG-BLT or NSG Hu-SRC-SCID mouse models of tuberculosis have been established (Calderon et al., 2013; Lee et al., 2013; Heuts et al., 2013). Surprisingly, granuloma formation was enhanced by human $CD4^{+}$ T cells (Heuts et al., 2013). Using HLA-A2 NSG-BLT mice, development of adaptive HLA-A2-restricted human immune responses were observed (Lee et al., 2013). However, this reactivity did not translate into the control of BCG growth. The first animal models of *S.* Typhi have been described (Libby et al., 2010; Song et al., 2010). These models were used to screen transposon pools that revealed both known and previously unknown virulence determinants (Libby et al., 2010), and to document that a gene mutation that is required for virulence in humans is also required for replication in humanized mice (Song et al., 2010). These recently developed models for the first time will allow animal model investigation of *S.* Typhi and human immune responses to the agent in the laboratory.

Sepsis is a leading cause of death in critically ill patients in the United States due to cytokine storms and lymphocyte apoptosis (Bone et al., 2009). Humanized mice have been used to model sepsis, and to investigate drug efficacy and side effects on human immune systems. For example, Hu-SRC-SCID NSG mice in the cecal ligation puncture (CLP) model were used to document that there were marked elevations of human inflammatory cytokines as well as extensive lymphocyte apoptosis (Unsinger et al., 2009). In the NSG-BLT model of CLP-induced sepsis, targeted delivery of high mobility group protein B1 (HMGB1) siRNA to human macrophages and dendritic cells using a short acetylcholine receptor-binding peptide suppressed the secretion of HMGB1, reduced the human cytokine storm, decreased human lymphocyte apoptosis, and rescued the mice from death (Ye et al., 2012). In the group B streptococcus model of neonatal sepsis using Hu-SRC-SCID NSG mice harboring naïve human immune systems resembling that of neonates, sepsis was not reduced by the administration of betamethasone and indomethacin, drugs commonly used in neonates, and in fact, sepsis induced the reduction of human leukocytes in the spleen and increased the bacterial load in all organs analyzed, including the brain (Ernst et al., 2013).

4.1.4 Humanized mouse models for the study of malaria

Plasmodium falciparum infection causes the most lethal form of malaria and requires the liver for replication. It causes more than ~200 million cases annually, and ~600,000 deaths (WHO, 2014). There are a number of models of humanized mice that have been developed to study malaria (Kaushansky et al., 2014). To investigate the pathogenesis of *P. falciparum*, there are four main models of humanized immunodeficient mice engrafted with human hepatocytes that are available (Grompe and Strom, 2013). These are the urokinase-type plasminogen activator (uPA) transgenic mouse (Rhim et al., 1994), the fumarylacetoacetate hydrolase null (Fah^{null}) mouse (Azuma et al., 2007), the herpes simplex virus type 1 thymidine kinase (HSVtk) transgenic mouse (Hasegawa et al., 2011), and the transgenic mouse expressing a fusion protein of the FK506 binding protein (FKBP) and caspase 8 under the control of the albumin promoter (AFC8) (Washburn et al., 2011). The human liver engrafted mice have been used to investigate the complete liver stage life cycle in humanized mice, providing a potentially critical model for the study of immune-based drugs to block this stage of the life cycle of *P. falciparum* (Vaughan et al., 2012).

Three of these models have now been coengrafted with human liver and human HSCs that generate human immune systems permitting the investigation of the immune response to infectious agents such as HCV and *P. falciparum* (Bility et al., 2012; Wilson et al., 2014; Gutti et al., 2014). A variation of a model of human liver-immune system engraftment has been described that sustains the complete liver and red blood cell life cycle of *P. falciparum* and its transmission to *Anopheles stephensi* mosquitoes and will be available for analyses of approaches to interrupt or block this life cycle at various stages (Wijayalath et al., 2014). Another variation is a human immune system engrafted Hu-SRC-SCID NSG mouse model for study of *P. falciparum* that was generated by newborn injection of HSCs and supplemented with daily RBC injections and hydrodynamic injection of plasmids expressing IL15 and Flt3 ligand. These mice could support productive infection with *P. falciparum* and were used to demonstrate that human NK cells have a critical role in controlling infection (Chen et al., 2014). These humanized mouse models, along with the RBC engrafted NSG mouse model previously described (Jimenez-Diaz et al., 2009), have only recently been developed and will likely have an increasingly important role in studies of the pathogenesis of malaria and evaluation of the efficacy of therapies and vaccines.

5. HUMANIZED MICE FOR THE STUDY OF CANCER

Since the 1960s using athymic mice, investigators have attempted to model human patient-derived xenograft (PDX) tumors in immunodeficient mice (Shultz et al., 2014). With the development of immunodeficient $IL2rg^{null}$ mice (for review see Shultz et al., 2012), many human tumors, particularly hematological tumors, can now

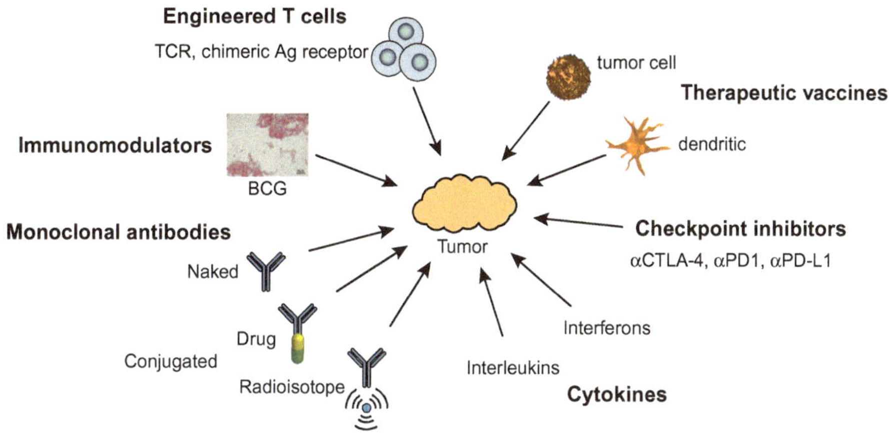

Figure 3 Emerging areas of cancer immunotherapy that utilize humanized mice as preclinical platforms for evaluation of drug safety and efficacy.

be grown *in vivo* in small animal models. Furthermore, for the first time, human tumor-immune interactions can now be studied in immunodeficient $IL2rg^{null}$ mice engrafted with the PDX tumor and a human immune system (Fig. 3). The development of these tumor-immune interaction humanized mouse models will be particularly important for enhancing the advancement of checkpoint inhibitors and chimeric antigen receptors (CAR) that have recently enjoyed remarkable success in the clinic.

5.1 Engineered T cells

CAR engineered T cells been used in over 100 clinical trials for hematological malignances and have shown remarkable efficacy (reviewed in Gill and June, 2015). These successful initial trials have led to an FDA approval for CARs as a "breakthrough therapy" and was initially piloted using a chimeric anti-CD19 T cell receptor for the treatment of B cell tumors such as chronic lymphocyte leukemia or lymphomas (Porter et al., 2011; Brentjens et al., 2011; Kochenderfer et al., 2012).

CAR therapy is based on the construction of a T cell receptor (TCR) with specificity for an antigen linked to molecules with the signaling features of a TCR mediated by a single polypeptide chain, typically the CD3 zeta (ζ) chain of the TCR. This permits the TCR to be redirected to an antigen of choice independent of MHC restrictions. For tumor immunotherapy, the antigen of choice is expressed on the tumor cells; for example, anti-CD19 directing T cells to B cell malignancies being in the forefront of tumor targets in the clinical trials. Tumor targeting by TCR has been enhanced by coexpression of CD28 and other costimulatory molecules (Savoldo et al., 2011), which enhance the activation of the CAR-expressing T cell upon encounter with the target cell. Although in the clinic for the treatment of B cell tumors, there are a number of questions remaining regarding the potential of CAR therapy for the treatment of other tumors, including solid tumors. Moreover, many fundamental questions regarding the mechanism of action of CAR therapy, including how the CAR T cell is constructed, the optimal costimulatory molecule for incorporation into the CAR, how the CAR is expressed in the T cells, or what the optimal *in vitro* expansion protocol for CAR T cells is, remain unanswered. Furthermore, basic questions such as the mechanisms by which CAR T cells mediate target cell death are not known.

Human PDX tumor-bearing immunodeficient *IL2rg*^{null} mice are being used as preclinical models to address these unanswered questions, and to pilot out the potential for CAR therapy to tumors other than B cell malignancies. The first report using matched patient tumor and CAR lymphocytes in NSG mice documented the feasibility of this personalized therapy for a tumor in humanized mice (Zhao et al., 2010). NSG mice have also been used to investigate the efficacy of various costimulatory molecules such as CD137 (Milone et al., 2009; Song et al., 2011), CD27 (Song et al., 2012), 4-1BB (Kloss et al., 2013), and ICOS (Guedan et al., 2014). A number of tumors other than B cell malignancies have been evaluated in PDX models of humanized mice. For example, mesothelin-specific SS1-based CARs have been tested in NSG mice bearing mesothelioma cells or NSCLC cells that express the SS1 antigen (Guedan et al., 2014). Although CD44 is expressed by multiple cells and tissues, a CD44 isoform variant 6 (CD44v6) is expressed in acute myeloid leukemia (AML) and multiple myeloma, and has been used to target CAR T cells to test the efficacy of CD44v6-directed CAR therapy to these tumors in NSG mice (Casucci et al., 2013). Receptor tyrosine kinase-like orphan receptor 1 (ROR1) is expressed on B-lymphoid and epithelial cells, and ROR1 CAR T cells have been used in NSG mice bearing human mantle cell lymphoma xenografts (Hudecek et al., 2013). NSG mice bearing prostate-specific membrane antigen-expressing (PSMA) tumors were used to demonstrate the *in vivo* efficacy of PMSA-CAR T cells coexpressing CD28 and 4-1BB costimulatory molecules against PSMA+ solid tumors (Kloss et al., 2013). These are a few of the examples of PDX-bearing NSG mouse models being used as preclinical models for the evaluation of CAR therapy.

CAR therapy in patients does come with the potential for adverse side effects (recently reviewed in Casucci et al., 2015). The selection of the antigen-specificity of the TCR used is critical, and should be as tumor-specific as possible. For example, MART-1 CAR therapy for the treatment of melanoma has led to toxicity against melanocyte-rich tissues such as skin, inner ear, and retina (Morgan et al., 2006). Adverse reactions such as the elevation of serum IFNγ and tumor necrosis factor have been observed (Porter et al., 2011; Brentjens et al., 2011; Kochenderfer et al., 2012), potentially leading to a pathology termed cytokine-release syndrome. There has also been one case report of the induction of anaphylaxis in humans following CAR therapy (Maus et al., 2013). The use of PDX humanized mouse models will be important for evaluating potential adverse reactions such as anaphylaxis, and a humanized mouse model of passive cutaneous anaphylaxis has recently been described (Ito et al., 2013).

5.2 Monoclonal antibodies directed against human tumor antigens

Monoclonal antibodies (mAb) directed against preferentially expressed antigens on tumors have been used as tumor immunotherapies. One of the first antibodies that was developed and patented in 1998 was the anti-CD20 mAb rituximab. This antibody was found to be an effective therapy against multiple tumors such as $CD20^{+}$ B cell non-Hodgkin lymphomas and other B cell leukemias (Scott, 1998). Although effective, even today the precise mechanisms by which it mediates efficacy remain unknown, and may include direct apoptosis, complement-dependent cytotoxicity (CDC), or antibody-dependent cellular cytotoxicity (ADCC). NSG mice are being used to investigate the mechanism of action of rituximab (Chu et al., 2015; Wong et al., 2012). However, NSG mice lack hemolytic complement (Shultz et al., 2005), and we are developing a complement-sufficient NSG strain that will permit the role of hemolytic complement to be determined. Another high-profile potential mAb therapy is anti-CD47 mAb (Chao et al., 2012). NSG mice have been used to demonstrate that one mechanism of action is via anti-CD47 promotion of phagocytosis of targeted $CD47^{+}$ tumor cells (Chao et al., 2010). Numerous other examples of antitumor antibodies being tested preclinically in NSG mice have been reported. Antibodies against chromosome maintenance protein 1, which is overexpressed in cancer cells, were shown to be efficacious against acute myeloid leukemia in NSG mice (Ranganathan et al., 2012). Similarly, an antibody against 4-1BB, a costimulatory molecule important in stimulating T cells, has been shown to mediate antitumor activity in the Hu-PBL-SCID model using NSG mice engrafted with human tumors (Fisher et al., 2012). The NSG tumor engrafted mouse will be a valuable preclinical model for the evaluation of efficacy and investigation into mechanisms of action of mAbs directed against human tumors.

5.3 Modeling human tumor immune interactions in humanized mice

One of the exciting emerging areas of tumor biology is the use of immunomodulatory agents targeting the immune system to enhance antitumor immunity. "Checkpoint inhibitors" have recently achieved spectacular success in a subset of patients with malignant melanoma. One of the first checkpoint inhibitors approved for treatment of melanoma was ipilimumab (Yervoy®) (Fellner, 2012; Hodi et al., 2010). This mAb blocks the cytotoxic T-lymphocyte antigen 4 (CTLA-4) molecule which downregulates T cell activation (Melero et al., 2007). A second checkpoint inhibitor therapy that has generated a lot of excitement for its efficacy against melanoma are anti-PD1 mAbs, produced by Bristol Meyers Squib and Merck, that block the interaction of PD1 with its ligand, PD-L1 (Mullard, 2013). These antibodies have been shown to induce durable remission of malignant melanoma (Hamid et al., 2013), even in metastatic melanoma (Hodi et al., 2010). mAbs blocking the PD1/PD-L1 pathways have also been used to treat NSCLC, RCC, and bladder cancer (for review, see Ohaegbulam et al., 2015).

However, not all patients respond to therapies with checkpoint inhibitors, and animal models for studying these novel therapeutics are urgently needed for investigation of the mechanisms by which they mediate their effects.

To address this, researchers are establishing humanized mice in which human tumor interactions with human immune systems can be modeled and used to evaluate human immunomodulatory drugs such as ipilimumab and mAbs that block PD1/PD-L1 interactions. Conceptually, this can be accomplished using one of the human immune system models described in Section 2 that are subsequently engrafted with primary human tumors. Early reports attempting to develop humanized mouse models for evaluating the efficacy and adverse effects of immunotherapeutic agents are now emerging. In many patients, administration of anti-CTLA-4 mAb for the treatment of tumors also induces a variety of immune-mediated adverse effects such as dermatitis, colitis, hepatitis, pancreatitis, hypothysitis, and uveitis (Kaehler et al., 2010). Humanized mice have been used to model this adverse effect. Hu-SRC-SCID NSG mice injected with ipilimumab anti-CTLA-4 mAb were observed to develop autoimmune syndromes characterized by the development of hepatitis, adrenalitis, sialitis, antinuclear antibodies, and weight loss (Vudattu et al., 2014). Moreover, treatment with tepilizumab (antihuman CD3) reversed this ipilimumab-induced disease, suggesting a role for human T cells in the disease progression. Humanized mice may provide a model for understanding the mechanisms underlying these adverse effects and as a preclinical tool for testing approaches to ameliorate them.

The most widely used humanized tumor-immune interaction model is a variant of the Hu-PBL-SCID, in which CAR T cells are adoptively transferred into tumor bearing immunodeficient $IL2rg^{null}$ mice (described above in Section 5.1). Variants of the CAR model include forced cytokine expression in primary human T cells to prolong their survival following adoptive transfer into NSG mice (Markley and Sadelain, 2010), and expansion of tumor reactive cytotoxic T cells (Decker et al., 2012; Distler et al., 2008) or expansion of human gamma delta T cells (Distler et al., 2008) prior to their adoptive transfer into NSG mice. One caveat of the Hu-PBL-SCID model is that this represents an effector T cell model, and does not permit the evaluation of other immune cells such as macrophages or NK cells for antitumor activity.

To address the lack of functional NK cells in humanized mice, investigators have established a variant of the Hu-PBL-SCID model by *ex vivo* expanding NK cells and transferring them into NSG mice bearing human leukemia cells to evaluate the efficacy of NK-mediated antitumor activity (Cany et al., 2013). Furthermore, a major mechanism by which NK cells mediate antitumor activity is via ADCC. However, although human NK cells develop in HSC-engrafted immunodeficient $IL2rg^{null}$ mice, they require additional signals for licensing to mediate their cytotoxic activity (Shultz et al., 2012). To establish a human NK cell ADCC humanized model, human NK cells were recovered from the blood of donors, and injected into NOG mice engrafted with the human

Burkitt lymphoma cell line (Daudi) along with rituximab (anti-CD20). The primary human NK cells engrafted in the NOG mice were able to retain their killing activity and suppress the growth of the tumor (Shiokawa et al., 2010).

A more sophisticated model is the Hu-SRC-SCID mouse in which a complete human immune system develops. In one report, human HSC and human breast cancer cells were cotransplanted into NSG mice. Tumor growth was accompanied by tumor cell-specific T cell activation and NK cell accumulation in the tumor and the production of tumor-specific antibodies (Wege et al., 2011, 2014). In a recent report, investigators used a BRG strain mouse expressing knocked-in human M-CSF, IL3, GM-CSF, and TPO genes and transgenically expressing a BAC encoding human SIRPα (Rongvaux et al., 2014). These human genes promoted the development of human macrophages following engraftment with human fetal liver HSCs. After immune system development, the mice were injected subcutaneously with the human melanoma cell line Me290. Eleven days later, the solid tumor was heavily infiltrated with human $CD163^{+}$ HLA-DR^{low} $CD206^{+}$ macrophages, with enhanced tumor growth as compared to similarly engrafted NSG mice, suggesting that the macrophages promoted growth of the tumor (Rongvaux et al., 2014). However, in these models the human immune system was allogeneic to the engrafted human tumor. To overcome this HLA-mismatch, investigators recently recovered bone marrow HSC from patients with carcinomas and transplanted each patient's tumor into NSG mice bearing the patient's own hematopoietic and immune system, permitting study of the patients' immune system interaction with their own tumor (Werner-Klein et al., 2014). This elegant model will provide an excellent system for the testing of human immunomodulators such as the checkpoint reagents in a completely autologous tumor/immune system model.

5.4 Humanized mice for the development of cancer vaccines

As noted in Section 5.3, human immune engrafted mice are now being used to study human immune/tumor interactions (Spranger et al., 2012). It has been proposed that this model will be useful for the evaluation of human dendritic cell-based vaccine strategies, a form of cancer therapy that is being applied to the clinic (Palucka and Banchereau, 2013). The use of humanized mice for this translational purpose is only now being tested and will likely be important in accelerating this approach to the clinic.

6. HUMANIZED MICE FOR THE STUDY OF TRANSPLANTATION IMMUNOLOGY

We have recently reviewed the use of humanized mice for the study of transplantation immunology, and refer the reader to this review (Brehm and Shultz, 2012).

7. HUMANIZED MOUSE MODELS OF HUMAN INNATE IMMUNE FUNCTION AND AUTOIMMUNITY

Although most studies of humanized mice have focussed on adaptive immune responses, innate immune responses are also critical components of the human immune system in mounting effective responses to infectious agents, tumors, or in autoimmunity. Most of these model are at early stages of development.

7.1 Models of autoimmune type 1 diabetes and multiple sclerosis

Type 1 diabetes (T1D) is a T cell-mediated autoimmune disorder, but the role of innate immunity is increasingly being recognized (Greenbaum et al., 2012; Todd et al., 2011). A number of humanized mouse models of diabetes have been developed to study T1D (Brehm et al., 2012a). Using the Hu-PBL-SCID model, lymphocytes from T1D donors have been used to induce inflammation in the islets of HLA-matched NSG recipients (Whitfield-Larry et al., 2011; Viehmann Milam et al., 2014). However, in both reports, inflammation was also observed in recipients of non-T1D lymphocytes and in neither report did the recipients progress to overt diabetes. Transfer of an HLA-A2-restricted human T cell clone with a TCR specificity against the islet autoantigen islet-specific glucose-6-phosphatase catalytic-subunit related protein (IGRP) into NSG-HLA-2 transgenic mice resulted in some islet infiltration and beta cell death, but again the mice did not progress to overt hyperglycemia (Unger et al., 2012). A recent report using human HLA-A2 CD8 T cells transduced with a human TCR isolated from T cell clones with a HLA-A2-restricted specificity against IGRP showed that adoptive transfer into NSG-A2 mice again led to infiltration of the islets, but not diabetes (Babad et al., 2014).

In a potential model of multiple sclerosis, PBMC from healthy donors were injected into NSG mice that were then immunized with myelin antigens in complete Freund's adjuvant plus autologous antigen-pulsed dendritic cells. These mice developed subclinical central nervous system inflammation with infiltrating human T cells (Zayoud et al., 2013).

7.2 Models of allergic asthma

Allergic asthma and anaphylaxis are debilitating diseases that are characterized by leukocyte infiltrations into the tissues and lung. Preclinical models are urgently needed for evaluation of new human-specific therapeutics for these diseases. To address this, investigators have attempted to develop humanized mouse models of these inflammatory diseases. Using the Hu-PBL-SCID NSG model, investigators injected PBMCs from donors allergic to birch pollen, and found pulmonary inflammation upon airway challenge with antigen (Martin et al., 2012). Similarly, in the Hu-PBL-SCID CB17-*scid* model, antibodies to T cell immunoglobulin-1 (TIM-1) were able to block experimental asthma (Sonar et al., 2010). However, Hu-PBL-SCID mice engraft poorly with myeloid cells, and HSC-engrafted humanized mice also have poorly developed myeloid cell populations and limited mast cell engraftment (Shultz et al., 2012). To address this, a NOG-IL3/GM-CSF human transgenic mouse has been developed, and has been shown to exhibit a human passive cutaneous anaphylaxis reaction upon challenge (Ito et al., 2013).

7.3 Models of atopic dermatitis, systemic vasculitis, colitis, and arthritis

A humanized Hu-PBL-SCID NSG model of atopic dermatitis was generated by treatment with oxazolone, and symptoms including keratosis, epithelial hyperplasia, and inflammatory cell infiltration were observed (Nolte et al., 2013b). A similar approach was used to establish a model of colitis using oxazolone or ethanol rectal challenge (Nolte et al., 2013a). Using the Hu-SRC-SCID NSG model, arthritis was induced by injection of complete Freund's adjuvant or thioglycolate into the joints, leading to infiltration with immune cells (Misharin et al., 2012). In this study, inflammation was markedly reduced following treatment with the TNF inhibitor etanercept. Finally, antiproteinase 3 antineutrophil cytoplasm autoantibodies recovered from patients with disease and injected into Hu-SRC-SCID NSG mice induced lung vasculitis and hemorrhage (Little et al., 2012). An interesting virus-induced model of arthritis was described in HSC-engrafted NOG mice infected with Epstein-Barr virus (Kuwana et al., 2011). The infection induced a dramatic erosive arthritis with many features resembling rheumatoid arthritis, establishing a model of virus-induced arthritis in humanized mice.

7.4 Models of systemic lupus erythematosus

A humanized mouse model of lupus would permit rapid evaluation of therapeutics that are desperately needed for this disease. Two preliminary reports have attempted to develop this model. In the Hu-PBL-SCID model using immunodeficient $IL2rg^{null}$ recipients of PBMC from patients with lupus, the mice were observed to develop proteinuria and exhibited human IgG deposits in the kidneys (Andrade et al., 2011). In a second model of lupus, immunodeficient mice were engrafted with PBMC from lupus patients, and the subsequent development of lupus-like symptoms were ameliorated using a complement receptor type 1 antibody, documenting the important role of complement in the pathogenesis of the disease (Kerekov et al., 2011).

Clearly, humanized mouse models of inflammation and autoimmunity are at their early stages of development and represent an important area for further development.

8. CONCLUSIONS AND THE FUTURE OF HUMANIZED MICE IN TRANSLATIONAL IMMUNOLOGY

Humanized mice are rapidly becoming the "go to" preclinical animal model for investigation of human immune responses and immune diseases. The key is to have the clinical

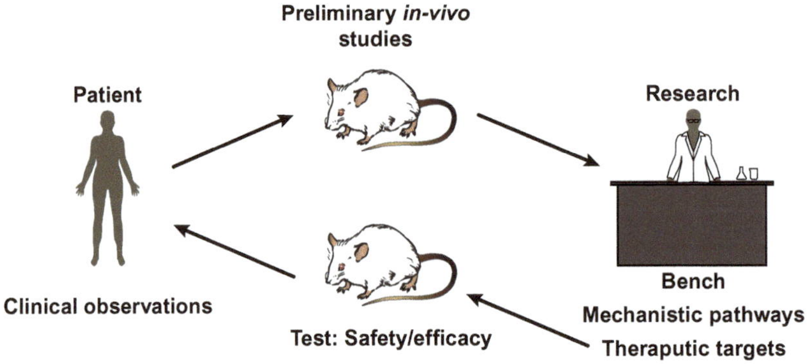

Figure 4 The future of humanized mice and their role in bedside-to-bench-to-bedside translational immunology research.

observations drive the questions being addressed in humanized mice. Cells, tissues, and organs from human donors can be engrafted in multiple humanized mice permitting robust numbers of "subjects" being available for experimental designs. Components of the human immune system can be manipulated at the bench level in multiple mice without the ethical constraints that are associated with performing experiments in humans. The laboratory findings can be used to identify new potential therapeutic pathways, and develop novel drugs to target these pathways that can, in turn, be tested for safety and efficacy in humanized mice. Ultimately, the research and evaluation of new drugs in humanized mice can be translated back into the clinic for the treatment of patients (Fig. 4).

A note of caution: Although many of the aspects of human immunity can be faithfully recapitulated in humanized mice, there are also many caveats. One of the best uses of humanized mice is to study pathways of human immune responses. These pathways can be specifically targeted with the new therapeutic mAbs that are becoming available. Also, investigators using humanized mice need to choose carefully the model that will be used, which is highly dependent on the question being addressed and should be based on clinical observations. However, the utility of humanized mice as preclinical models in translational immunology is already evident and has provided many insights into fundamental mechanisms of human immunity. Humanized mice will facilitate the preclinical evaluation of drugs on human immune responses, and allow human-specific reagents to be tested directly on human cells and tissues *in vivo*.

ACKNOWLEDGMENTS

This work was supported by National Institutes of Health grants U01 DK089572, P01 AI46629, R24 OD018259, UC4DK104218, CA034196, and R21 AI112321, The Leonard M. and Harry B. Helmsley Charitable Trust grants 2012PG-T1D018 and 2015PG-T1D057, and a Juvenile Diabetes Research Foundation grant 2-2011-416.

Abbreviations

ADCC antibody-dependent cellular cytotoxicity
AFC8 albumin promoter FKBP-caspase 8 fusion protein
AML acute myeloid leukemia
APC antigen-presenting cells
B6RG-CD47 B6.129S-$Rag2^{tm1Fwa}$ $Cd47^{tm1Fpl}$ $Il2rg^{tm1Wjl}$/J
BLT Bone marrow/Liver/Thymus
BLyS B lymphocyte stimulatin
BRG C;129S4- $Rag2^{tm1Flv}Il2rg^{tm1Flv}$
CAR chimeric antigen receptors
CDC complement-dependent cytotoxicity
CTLA-4 cytotoxic T-lymphocyte antigen
DC dendritic cell
EBV Epstein Barr virus
Fah^{null} fumarylacetoacetate hydrolase null
FKBP FK506 binding protein
FLT3L Fms-related tyrosine kinase 3 ligand
fMLP formyl-methionyl-leucyl-phenylal
G-CSF granulocyte-colony stimulating factor
GM-CSF granulocyte macrophage-colony stimulating factor
GVHD graft-versus-host disease
HCV hepatitis C virus
HIV human immunodeficiency virus
HMGB1 high mobility group protein B1
HSC hematopoietic stem cells
HSVtk herpes simplex virus type 1 thymidine kinase
Hu-PBL-SCID human peripheral blood lymphocyte SCID
Hu-SRC-SCID human SCID-repopulating cell SCID, $IL2rg^{null}$, IFN, interferon
IFNR interferon receptor
IGRP islet-specific glucose-6-phosphatase catalytic-subunit related protein
IL2 receptor common gamma chain null
IP intraperitoneal
IV intravenous
LMP1 latent membrane protein-1
mAb monoclonal antibody
M-CSF macrophage-colony stimulating factor
MHC major histocompatibility complex
MSC mesenchymal stem cells
mSCF membrane bound stem cell factor
NK natural killer
NOG NODShi.Cg-$Prkdc^{scid}Il2rg^{tm1Sug}$
NSCLC non-small cell lung cancer
NSG NOD.Cg-$Prkdc^{scid}Il2rg^{tm1Wjl}$
PBMC peripheral blood mononuclear cells
PD1 programmed death-1
PD-L1 programmed death-1 ligand
PDX patient-derived xenografts

***Prkdc**^scid* protein kinase DNA activated, catalytic polypeptide null mutation
PSMA prostate-specific membrane antigen-expressing
Rag recombination-activating gene
RBC red blood cells
RCC renal cell carcinoma
ROR Receptor tyrosine kinase-like orphan receptor
Sirpα signal regulatory protein alpha
***S.* Typhi** *Salmonella enteric serovar* Typhi
T1D type 1 diabetes
TCR T cell receptor
TIM-1 T cell immunoglobulin-1
TLR toll-like receptor
TPO thrombopoietin
Treg regulatory T cells
UPA urokinase-type plasminogen activator

REFERENCES

Abraham, S., Choi, J.G., Ye, C., Manjunath, N., Shankar, P., 2015. IL-10 exacerbates xenogeneic GVHD by inducing massive human T cell expansion. Clin. Immunol. 156, 58–64.

Akkina, R., 2013a. Human immune responses and potential for vaccine assessment in humanized mice. Curr. Opin. Immunol. 25, 403–409.

Akkina, R., 2013b. New generation humanized mice for virus research: comparative aspects and future prospects. Virology 435, 14–28.

Andrade, D., Redecha, P.B., Vukelic, M., Qing, X., Perino, G., Salmon, J.E., Koo, G.C., 2011. Engraftment of peripheral blood mononuclear cells from systemic lupus erythematosus and antiphospholipid syndrome patient donors into BALB-RAG-2-/- IL-2Rgamma-/- mice: a promising model for studying human disease. Arthritis Rheum. 63, 2764–2773.

Andre, M.C., Erbacher, A., Gille, C., Schmauke, V., Goecke, B., Hohberger, A., Mang, P., Wilhelm, A., Mueller, I., Herr, W., Lang, P., Handgretinger, R., Hartwig, U.F., 2010. Long-term human CD34+ stem cell-engrafted nonobese diabetic/SCID/IL-2R gamma(null) mice show impaired CD8+ T cell maintenance and a functional arrest of immature NK cells. J. Immunol. 185, 2710–2720.

Antsiferova, O., Muller, A., Ramer, P.C., Chijioke, O., Chatterjee, B., Raykova, A., Planas, R., Sospedra, M., Shumilov, A., Tsai, M.H., Delecluse, H.J., Munz, C., 2014. Adoptive transfer of EBV specific CD8+ T cell clones can transiently control EBV infection in humanized mice. PLoS Pathog. 10, e1004333.

Azuma, H., Paulk, N., Ranade, A., Dorrell, C., Al-Dhalimy, M., Ellis, E., Strom, S., Kay, M.A., Finegold, M., Grompe, M., 2007. Robust expansion of human hepatocytes in Fah-/-/Rag2-/-/Il2rg-/- mice. Nat. Biotechnol. 25, 903–910.

Babad, J., Mukherjee, G., Follenzi, A., Ali, R., Roep, B.O., Shultz, L.D., Santamaria, P., Yang, O.O., Goldstein, H., Greiner, D.L., Dilorenzo, T.P., 2014. Generation of beta cell-specific human cytotoxic T cells by lentiviral transduction and their survival in immunodeficient HLA-transgenic mice. Clin. Exp. Immunol. 131, 459–465.

Balazs, A.B., Chen, J., Hong, C.M., Rao, D.S., Yang, L., Baltimore, D., 2012. Antibody-based protection against HIV infection by vectored immunoprophylaxis. Nature 481, 81–84.

Baumler, A., Fang, F.C., 2013. Host specificity of bacterial pathogens. Cold Spring Harb. Perspect. Med. 3, a010041.

Beeching, N.J., Fenech, M., Houlihan, C.F., 2014. Ebola virus disease. BMJ 349, g7348.

Bennett, M.S., Akkina, R., 2013. Gene therapy strategies for HIV/AIDS: preclinical modeling in humanized mice. Viruses 5, 3119–3141.

Bility, M.T., Zhang, L., Washburn, M.L., Curtis, T.A., Kovalev, G.I., Su, L., 2012. Generation of a humanized mouse model with both human immune system and liver cells to model hepatitis C virus infection and liver immunopathogenesis. Nat. Protoc. 7, 1608–1617.
Bility, M.T., Li, F., Cheng, L., Su, L., 2013. Liver immune-pathogenesis and therapy of human liver tropic virus infection in humanized mouse models. J. Gastroenterol. Hepatol. 28 (Suppl. 1), 120–124.
Billerbeck, E., Barry, W.T., Mu, K., Dorner, M., Rice, C.M., Ploss, A., 2011. Development of human CD4 + FoxP3 + regulatory T cells in human stem cell factor-, granulocyte-macrophage colony-stimulating factor-, and interleukin-3-expressing NOD-SCID IL2Rgamma(null) humanized mice. Blood 117, 3076–3086.
Billerbeck, E., De, J.Y., Dorner, M., De La, F.C., Ploss, A., 2013. Animal models for hepatitis C. Curr. Top. Microbiol. Immunol. 369, 49–86.
Biswas, S., Chang, H., Sarkis, P.T., Fikrig, E., Zhu, Q., Marasco, W.A., 2011. Humoral immune responses in humanized BLT mice immunized with West Nile virus and HIV-1 envelope proteins are largely mediated via human CD5 + B cells. Immunology 134, 419–433.
Bone, R.C., Balk, R.A., Cerra, F.B., Dellinger, R.P., Fein, A.M., Knaus, W.A., Schein, R.M., Sibbald, W.J., 2009. Definitions for sepsis and organ failure and guidelines for the use of innovative therapies in sepsis. The ACCP/SCCM Consensus Conference Committee. American College of Chest Physicians/Society of Critical Care Medicine. 1992. Chest 136, e28.
Brehm, M.A., Shultz, L.D., 2012. Human allograft rejection in humanized mice: a historical perspective. Cell. Mol. Immunol. 3, 225–231.
Brehm, M.A., Powers, A.C., Shultz, L.D., Greiner, D.L., 2012a. Advancing animal models of human type 1 diabetes by engraftment of functional human tissues in immunodeficient mice. Cold Spring Harb. Perspect. Med. 2, a007757.
Brehm, M.A., Racki, W.J., Leif, J., Burzenski, L., Hosur, V., Wetmore, A., Gott, B., Herlihy, M., Ignotz, R., Dunn, R., Shultz, L.D., Greiner, D.L., 2012b. Engraftment of human HSC in non-irradiated newborn NOD-scid IL2rgammanull mice is enhanced by transgenic expression of membrane-bound human SCF. Blood 119, 2778–2788.
Brehm, M.A., Jouvet, N., Greiner, D.L., Shultz, L.D., 2013. Humanized mice for the study of infectious diseases. Curr. Opin. Immunol. 25, 428–435.
Brehm, M.A., Wiles, M.V., Greiner, D.L., Shultz, L.D., 2014. Generation of improved humanized mouse models for human infectious diseases. J. Immunol. Methods 410C, 3–17.
Brentjens, R.J., Riviere, I., Park, J.H., Davila, M.L., Wang, X., Stefanski, J., Taylor, C., Yeh, R., Bartido, S., Borquez-Ojeda, O., Olszewska, M., Bernal, Y., Pegram, H., Przybylowski, M., Hollyman, D., Usachenko, Y., Pirraglia, D., Hosey, J., Santos, E., Halton, E., Maslak, P., Scheinberg, D., Jurcic, J., Heaney, M., Heller, G., Frattini, M., Sadelain, M., 2011. Safety and persistence of adoptively transferred autologous CD19-targeted T cells in patients with relapsed or chemotherapy refractory B-cell leukemias. Blood 118, 4817–4828.
Brown, D., Mattapallil, J.J., 2014. Gastrointestinal tract and the mucosal macrophage reservoir in HIV infection. Clin. Vaccine Immunol. 21, 1469–1473.
Bueno, C., Montes, R., De La, C.T., Gutierrez-Aranda, I., Menendez, P., 2010. Intra-bone marrow transplantation of human CD34(+) cells into NOD/LtSz-scid IL-2rgamma(null) mice permits multilineage engraftment without previous irradiation. Cytotherapy 12, 45–49.
Burd, E.M., 2015. Ebola virus: a clear and present danger. J. Clin. Microbiol. 53, 4–8.
Calderon, V.E., Valbuena, G., Goez, Y., Judy, B.M., Huante, M.B., Sutjita, P., Johnston, R.K., Estes, D.M., Hunter, R.L., Actor, J.K., Cirillo, J.D., Endsley, J.J., 2013. A humanized mouse model of tuberculosis. PLoS One 8, e63331.
Cany, J., Van Der Waart, A.B., Tordoir, M., Franssen, G.M., Hangalapura, B.N., De, V.J., Boerman, O., Schaap, N., Van, D.V., Spanholtz, J., Dolstra, H., 2013. Natural killer cells generated from cord blood hematopoietic progenitor cells efficiently target bone marrow-residing human leukemia cells in NOD/SCID/IL2Rg(null) mice. PLoS One 8, e64384.
Cao, X., Kozak, C.A., Liu, Y.J., Noguchi, M., O'connell, E., Leonard, W.J., 1993. Characterization of cDNAs encoding the murine interleukin 2 receptor (IL-2R) gamma chain: chromosomal mapping and tissue specificity of IL-2R gamma chain expression. Proc. Natl. Acad. Sci. U. S. A. 90, 8464–8468.

Cao, X., Shores, E.W., Hu-Li, J., Anver, M.R., Kelsall, B.L., Russell, S.M., Drago, J., Noguchi, M., Grinberg, A., Bloom, E.T., Paul, W.E., Katz, S.I., Love, P.E., Leonard, W.J., 1995. Defective lymphoid development in mice lacking expression of the common cytokine receptor gamma chain. Immunity 2, 223–238.

Carroll, A.M., Bosma, M.J., 1988. Detection and characterization of functional T cells in mice with severe combined immune deficiency. Eur. J. Immunol. 18, 1965–1971.

Casucci, M., Nicolis Di, R.B., Falcone, L., Camisa, B., Norelli, M., Genovese, P., Gentner, B., Gullotta, F., Ponzoni, M., Bernardi, M., Marcatti, M., Saudemont, A., Bordignon, C., Savoldo, B., Ciceri, F., Naldini, L., Dotti, G., Bonini, C., Bondanza, A., 2013. CD44v6-targeted T cells mediate potent antitumor effects against acute myeloid leukemia and multiple myeloma. Blood 122, 3461–3472.

Casucci, M., Hawkins, R.E., Dotti, G., Bondanza, A., 2015. Overcoming the toxicity hurdles of genetically targeted T cells. Cancer Immunol. Immunother. 64, 123–130.

Chao, M.P., Alizadeh, A.A., Tang, C., Myklebust, J.H., Varghese, B., Gill, S., Jan, M., Cha, A.C., Chan, C.K., Tan, B.T., Park, C.Y., Zhao, F., Kohrt, H.E., Malumbres, R., Briones, J., Gascoyne, R.D., Lossos, I.S., Levy, R., Weissman, I.L., Majeti, R., 2010. Anti-CD47 antibody synergizes with rituximab to promote phagocytosis and eradicate non-Hodgkin lymphoma. Cell 142, 699–713.

Chao, M.P., Weissman, I.L., Majeti, R., 2012. The CD47-SIRPalpha pathway in cancer immune evasion and potential therapeutic implications. Curr. Opin. Immunol. 24, 225–232.

Chateau, M., Swanson, M.D., Garcia, J.V., 2013a. Inefficient vaginal transmission of tenofovir-resistant HIV-1. J. Virol. 87, 1274–1277.

Chateau, M.L., Denton, P.W., Swanson, M.D., Mcgowan, I., Garcia, J.V., 2013b. Rectal transmission of transmitted/founder HIV-1 is efficiently prevented by topical 1% tenofovir in BLT humanized mice. PLoS One 8, e60024.

Chatterjee, B., Leung, C.S., Munz, C., 2014. Animal models of Epstein Barr virus infection. J. Immunol. Methods 410, 80–87.

Chen, Q., He, F., Kwang, J., Chan, J.K., Chen, J., 2012. GM-CSF and IL-4 stimulate antibody responses in humanized mice by promoting T, B, and dendritic cell maturation. J. Immunol. 189, 5223–5229.

Chen, Q., Amaladoss, A., Ye, W., Liu, M., Dummler, S., Kong, F., Wong, L.H., Loo, H.L., Loh, E., Tan, S.Q., Tan, T.C., Chang, K.T., Dao, M., Suresh, S., Preiser, P.R., Chen, J., 2014. Human natural killer cells control Plasmodium falciparum infection by eliminating infected red blood cells. Proc. Natl. Acad. Sci. U. S. A. 111, 1479–1484.

Cheung, A.M., Leung, D., Rostamirad, S., Dhillon, K., Miller, P.H., Droumeva, R., Brinkman, R.R., Hogge, D., Roy, D.C., Eaves, C.J., 2012. Distinct but phenotypically heterogeneous human cell populations produce rapid recovery of platelets and neutrophils after transplantation. Blood 119, 3431–3439.

Choi, J.H., Jonsson-Schmunk, K., Qiu, X., Shedlock, D.J., Strong, J., Xu, J.X., Michie, K.L., Audet, J., Fernando, L., Myers, M.J., Weiner, D., Bajrovic, I., Tran, L.Q., Wong, G., Bello, A., Kobinger, G.P., Schafer, S.C., Croyle, M.A., 2015. A single dose respiratory recombinant adenovirus-based vaccine provides long-term protection for non-human primates from lethal ebola infection. Mol. Pharm 12, 2712–2731.

Choo, J.K., Seebach, J.D., Nickeleit, V., Shimizu, A., Lei, H., Sachs, D.H., Madsen, J.C., 1997. Species differences in the expression of major histocompatibility complex class II antigens on coronary artery endothelium: implications for cell-mediated xenoreactivity. Transplantation 64, 1315–1322.

Choudhary, S.K., Archin, N.M., Cheema, M., Dahl, N.P., Garcia, J.V., Margolis, D.M., 2012. Latent HIV-1 infection of resting CD4 T cells in the humanized Rag2/gammac/mouse. J. Virol. 86, 114–120.

Chowell, G., Nishiura, H., 2014. Transmission dynamics and control of Ebola virus disease (EVD): a review. BMC Med. 12, 196.

Chu, Y., Hochberg, J., Yahr, A., Ayello, J., Van, D.V., Barth, M.J., Czuczman, M.S., Cairo, M.S., 2015. Targeting CD20+ aggressive B-cell non-hodgkin lymphoma by anti-CD20 CAR mRNA modified expanded natural killer cells in vitro and in NSG mice. Cancer Immunol. Res. 3, 333–344. Epub, Dec. 9.

Cosgun, K.N., Rahmig, S., Mende, N., Reinke, S., Hauber, I., Schafer, C., Petzold, A., Weisbach, H., Heidkamp, G., Purbojo, A., Cesnjevar, R., Platz, A., Bornhauser, M., Schmitz, M., Dudziak, D.,

Hauber, J., Kirberg, J., Waskow, C., 2014. Kit regulates HSC engraftment across the human-mouse species barrier. Cell Stem Cell 15, 227–238.

Coughlan, A.M., Freeley, S.J., Robson, M.G., 2012. Humanised mice have functional human neutrophils. J. Immunol. Methods 385, 96–104.

Covassin, L., Laning, J., Abdi, R., Langevin, D.L., Phillips, N.E., Shultz, L.D., Brehm, M.A., 2011. Human peripheral blood CD4 T cell-engrafted non-obese diabetic-scid IL2rgamma(null) H2-Ab1 (tm1Gru) Tg (human leucocyte antigen D-related 4) mice: a mouse model of human allogeneic graft-versus-host disease. Clin. Exp. Immunol. 166, 269–280.

Covassin, L., Jangalwe, S., Jouvet, N., Laning, J., Burzenski, L., Shultz, L.D., Brehm, M.A., 2013. Human immune system development and survival of non-obese diabetic (NOD)-scid IL2rgamma(null) (NSG) mice engrafted with human thymus and autologous haematopoietic stem cells. Clin. Exp. Immunol. 174, 372–388.

Cox, J., Mota, J., Sukupolvi-Petty, S., Diamond, M.S., Rico-Hesse, R., 2012. Mosquito bite delivery of dengue virus enhances immunogenicity and pathogenesis in humanized mice. J. Virol. 86, 7637–7649.

Danner, R., Chaudhari, S.N., Rosenberger, J., Surls, J., Richie, T.L., Brumeanu, T.D., Casares, S., 2011. Expression of HLA class II molecules in humanized NOD.Rag1KO.IL2RgcKO mice is critical for development and function of human T and B cells. PLoS One 6, e19826.

Davis, M.M., 2012. Immunology taught by humans. Sci. Transl. Med. 4, 117fs2.

De, W.E., Feldmann, H., Munster, V.J., 2011. Tackling Ebola: new insights into prophylactic and therapeutic intervention strategies. Genome Med. 3, 5.

Decker, W.K., Shah, N., Xing, D., Lapushin, R., Li, S., Robinson, S.N., Yang, H., Parmar, S., Halpert, M.M., Keating, M.J., Gribben, J.G., Molldrem, J.J., Shpall, E.J., Wierda, W.G., 2012. Generation of functional CLL-specific cord blood CTL using CD40-ligated CLL APC. PLoS One 7, e51390.

Deng, K., Pertea, M., Rongvaux, A., Wang, L., Durand, C.M., Ghiaur, G., Lai, J., Mchugh, H.L., Hao, H., Zhang, H., Margolick, J.B., Gurer, C., Murphy, A.J., Valenzuela, D.M., Yancopoulos, G.D., Deeks, S.G., Strowig, T., Kumar, P., Siliciano, J.D., Salzberg, S.L., Flavell, R.A., Shan, L., Siliciano, R.F., 2015. Broad CTL response is required to clear latent HIV-1 due to dominance of escape mutations. Nature 517, 381–385.

Denton, P.W., Garcia, J.V., 2012. Mucosal HIV-1 transmission and prevention strategies in BLT humanized mice. Trends Microbiol. 20, 268–274.

Denton, P.W., Olesen, R., Choudhary, S.K., Archin, N.M., Wahl, A., Swanson, M.D., Chateau, M., Nochi, T., Krisko, J.F., Spagnuolo, R.A., Margolis, D.M., Garcia, J.V., 2012. Generation of HIV latency in humanized BLT mice. J. Virol. 86, 630–634.

Deruaz, M., Luster, A.D., 2013. BLT humanized mice as model to study HIV vaginal transmission. J. Infect. Dis. 208 (Suppl. 2), S131–S136.

Didigu, C.A., Wilen, C.B., Wang, J., Duong, J., Secreto, A.J., Net-Desnoyers, G.A., Riley, J.L., Gregory, P.D., June, C.H., Holmes, M.C., Doms, R.W., 2013. Simultaneous zinc-finger nuclease editing of the HIV coreceptors ccr5 and cxcr4 protects CD4+ T cells from HIV-1 infection. Blood 123, 61–69.

Ding, Y., Wilkinson, A., Idris, A., Fancke, B., O'keeffe, M., Khalil, D., Ju, X., Lahoud, M.H., Caminschi, I., Shortman, K., Rodwell, R., Vuckovic, S., Radford, K.J., 2014. FLT3-ligand treatment of humanized mice results in the generation of large numbers of CD141+ and CD1c+ dendritic cells in vivo. J. Immunol. 192, 1982–1989.

Distler, E., Wolfel, C., Kohler, S., Nonn, M., Kaus, N., Schnurer, E., Meyer, R.G., Wehler, T.C., Huber, C., Wolfel, T., Hartwig, U.F., Herr, W., 2008. Acute myeloid leukemia (AML)-reactive cytotoxic T lymphocyte clones rapidly expanded from CD8(+) CD62L((high)+) T cells of healthy donors prevent AML engraftment in NOD/SCID IL2Rgamma(null) mice. Exp. Hematol. 36, 451–463.

Doeing, D.C., Borowicz, J.L., Crockett, E.T., 2003. Gender dimorphism in differential peripheral blood leukocyte counts in mice using cardiac, tail, foot, and saphenous vein puncture methods. BMC Clin. Pathol. 3, 3.

Ernst, W., Zimara, N., Hanses, F., Mannel, D.N., Seelbach-Gobel, B., Wege, A.K., 2013. Humanized mice, a new model to study the influence of drug treatment on neonatal sepsis. Infect. Immun. 81, 1520–1531.

Fellner, C., 2012. Ipilimumab (yervoy) prolongs survival in advanced melanoma: serious side effects and a hefty price tag may limit its use. Proc. Natl. Acad. Sci. U. S. A. 37, 503–530.

Fisher, T.S., Kamperschroer, C., Oliphant, T., Love, V.A., Lira, P.D., Doyonnas, R., Bergqvist, S., Baxi, S.M., Rohner, A., Shen, A.C., Huang, C., Sokolowski, S.A., Sharp, L.L., 2012. Targeting of 4-1BB by monoclonal antibody PF-05082566 enhances T-cell function and promotes anti-tumor activity. Cancer Immunol. Immunother. 61, 1721–1733.

Fujiwara, S., 2014. Reproduction of epstein-barr virus infection and pathogenesis in humanized mice. Immune Netw. 14, 1–6.

Fujiwara, S., Matsuda, G., Imadome, K., 2013. Humanized mouse models of epstein-barr virus infection and associated diseases. Pathogens 2, 153–176.

Gill, S., June, C.H., 2015. Going viral: chimeric antigen receptor T-cell therapy for hematological malignancies. Immunol. Rev. 263, 68–89.

Gille, C., Orlikowsky, T.W., Spring, B., Hartwig, U.F., Wilhelm, A., Wirth, A., Goecke, B., Handgretinger, R., Poets, C.F., Andre, M.C., 2012. Monocytes derived from humanized neonatal NOD/SCID/IL2Rgamma(null) mice are phenotypically immature and exhibit functional impairments. Hum. Immunol. 73, 346–354.

Gonzalez, L., Strbo, N., Podack, E.R., 2013. Humanized mice: novel model for studying mechanisms of human immune-based therapies. Immunol. Res. 57, 326–334.

Greenbaum, C.J., Schatz, D.A., Haller, M.J., Sanda, S., 2012. Through the fog: recent clinical trials to preserve beta-cell function in type 1 diabetes. Diabetes 61, 1323–1330.

Greenblatt, M.B., Vbranac, V., Tivey, T., Tsang, K., Tager, A.M., Aliprantis, A.O., 2012. Graft versus host disease in the bone marrow, liver and thymus humanized mouse model. PLoS One 7, e44664.

Gregoire-Gauthier, J., Selleri, S., Fontaine, F., Dieng, M.M., Patey, N., Despars, G., Beausejour, C.M., Haddad, E., 2012. Therapeutic efficacy of cord blood-derived mesenchymal stromal cells for the prevention of acute graft-versus-host disease in a xenogenic mouse model. Stem Cells Dev. 21, 1616–1626.

Grompe, M., Strom, S., 2013. Mice with human livers. Gastroenterology 145, 1209–1214.

Guedan, S., Chen, X., Madar, A., Carpenito, C., Mcgettigan, S.E., Frigault, M.J., Lee, J., Posey Jr., A.D., Scholler, J., Scholler, N., Bonneau, R., June, C.H., 2014. ICOS-based chimeric antigen receptors program bipolar TH17/TH1 cells. Blood 124, 1070–1080.

Gutti, T.L., Knibbe, J.S., Makarov, E., Zhang, J., Yannam, G.R., Gorantla, S., Sun, Y., Mercer, D.F., Suemizu, H., Wisecarver, J.L., Osna, N.A., Bronich, T.K., Poluektova, L.Y., 2014. Human hepatocytes and hematolymphoid dual reconstitution in treosulfan-conditioned uPA-NOG mice. Am. J. Pathol. 184, 101–109.

Hamid, O., Robert, C., Daud, A., Hodi, F.S., Hwu, W.J., Kefford, R., Wolchok, J.D., Hersey, P., Joseph, R.W., Weber, J.S., Dronca, R., Gangadhar, T.C., Patnaik, A., Zarour, H., Joshua, A.M., Gergich, K., Elassaiss-Schaap, J., Algazi, A., Mateus, C., Boasberg, P., Tumeh, P.C., Chmielowski, B., Ebbinghaus, S.W., Li, X.N., Kang, S.P., Ribas, A., 2013. Safety and tumor responses with lambrolizumab (anti-PD-1) in melanoma. N. Engl. J. Med. 369, 134–144.

Harui, A., Kiertscher, S.M., Roth, M.D., 2011. Reconstitution of huPBL-NSG mice with donor-matched dendritic cells enables antigen-specific T-cell activation. J. Neuroimmune Pharmacol. 6, 148–157.

Hasegawa, M., Kawai, K., Mitsui, T., Taniguchi, K., Monnai, M., Wakui, M., Ito, M., Suematsu, M., Peltz, G., Nakamura, M., Suemizu, H., 2011. The reconstituted 'humanized liver' in TK-NOG mice is mature and functional. Biochem. Biophys. Res. Commun. 405, 405–410.

Hayakawa, J., Hsieh, M.M., Uchida, N., Phang, O., Tisdale, J.F., 2009. Busulfan produces efficient human cell engraftment in NOD/LtSz-Scid IL2Rgamma(null) mice. Stem Cells 27, 175–182.

Heuts, F., Gavier-Widen, D., Carow, B., Juarez, J., Wigzell, H., Rottenberg, M.E., 2013. CD4+ cell-dependent granuloma formation in humanized mice infected with mycobacteria. Proc. Natl. Acad. Sci. U. S. A. 110, 6482–6487.

Hodi, F.S., O'day, S.J., Mcdermott, D.F., Weber, R.W., Sosman, J.A., Haanen, J.B., Gonzalez, R., Robert, C., Schadendorf, D., Hassel, J.C., Akerley, W., Van Den Eertwegh, A.J., Lutzky, J., Lorigan, P., Vaubel, J.M., Linette, G.P., Hogg, D., Ottensmeier, C.H., Lebbe, C., Peschel, C., Quirt, I., Clark, J.I., Wolchok, J.D., Weber, J.S., Tian, J., Yellin, M.J., Nichol, G.M., Hoos, A., Urba, W.J., 2010. Improved survival with ipilimumab in patients with metastatic melanoma. N. Engl. J. Med. 363, 711–723.

Hofer, U., Henley, J.E., Exline, C.M., Mulhern, O., Lopez, E., Cannon, P.M., 2013. Pre-clinical modeling of CCR5 knockout in human hematopoietic stem cells by zinc finger nucleases using humanized mice. J. Infect. Dis. 208 (Suppl. 2), S160–S164.

Honeycutt, J.B., Wahl, A., Archin, N., Choudhary, S., Margolis, D., Garcia, J.V., 2013. HIV-1 infection, response to treatment and establishment of viral latency in a novel humanized T cell-only mouse (TOM) model. Retrovirology 10, 121.

Hu, Z., Yang, Y.G., 2012. Full reconstitution of human platelets in humanized mice after macrophage depletion. Blood 120, 1713–1716.

Hu, Z., Van, R.N., Yang, Y.G., 2011. Macrophages prevent human red blood cell reconstitution in immunodeficient mice. Blood 118, 5938–5946.

Huang, J., Li, X., Coelho-Dos-Reis,, J.G., Wilson, J.M., Tsuji, M., 2014. An AAV vector-mediated gene delivery approach facilitates reconstitution of functional human CD8+ T cells in mice. PLoS One 9, e88205.

Hudecek, M., Lupo-Stanghellini, M.T., Kosasih, P.L., Sommermeyer, D., Jensen, M.C., Rader, C., Riddell, S.R., 2013. Receptor affinity and extracellular domain modifications affect tumor recognition by ROR1-specific chimeric antigen receptor T cells. Clin. Cancer Res. 19, 3153–3164.

Huntington, N.D., Legrand, N., Alves, N.L., Jaron, B., Weijer, K., Plet, A., Corcuff, E., Mortier, E., Jacques, Y., Spits, H., Di Santo, J.P., 2009. IL-15 trans-presentation promotes human NK cell development and differentiation in vivo. J. Exp. Med. 206, 25–34.

Huntington, N.D., Alves, N.L., Legrand, N., Lim, A., Strick-Marchand, H., Mention, J.J., Plet, A., Weijer, K., Jacques, Y., Becker, P.D., Guzman, C., Soussan, P., Kremsdorf, D., Spits, H., Di Santo, J.P., 2011. IL-15 transpresentation promotes both human T-cell reconstitution and T-cell-dependent antibody responses in vivo. Proc. Natl. Acad. Sci. U. S. A. 108, 6217–6222.

Hur, E.M., Patel, S.N., Shimizu, S., Rao, D.S., Gnanapragasam, P.N., An, D.S., Yang, L., Baltimore, D., 2012. Inhibitory effect of HIV-specific neutralizing IgA on mucosal transmission of HIV in humanized mice. Blood 120, 4571–4582.

Ippolito, G.C., Hoi, K.H., Reddy, S.T., Carroll, S.M., Ge, X., Rogosch, T., Zemlin, M., Shultz, L.D., Ellington, A.D., Vandenberg, C.L., Georgiou, G., 2012. Antibody repertoires in humanized NOD-scid-IL2Rgamma(null) mice and human B cells reveals human-like diversification and tolerance checkpoints in the mouse. PLoS One 7, e35497.

Ito, M., Hiramatsu, H., Kobayashi, K., Suzue, K., Kawahata, M., Hioki, K., Ueyama, Y., Koyanagi, Y., Sugamura, K., Tsuji, K., Heike, T., Nakahata, T., 2002. NOD/SCID/gamma(c)(null) mouse: an excellent recipient mouse model for engraftment of human cells. Blood 100, 3175–3182.

Ito, R., Katano, I., Kawai, K., Hirata, H., Ogura, T., Kamisako, T., Eto, T., Ito, M., 2009. Highly sensitive model for xenogenic GVHD using severe immunodeficient NOG mice. Transplantation 87, 1654–1658.

Ito, R., Takahashi, T., Katano, I., Ito, M., 2012. Current advances in humanized mouse models. Cell. Mol. Immunol. 9, 208–214.

Ito, R., Takahashi, T., Katano, I., Kawai, K., Kamisako, T., Ogura, T., Ida-Tanaka, M., Suemizu, H., Nunomura, S., Ra, C., Mori, A., Aiso, S., Ito, M., 2013. Establishment of a human allergy model using human IL-3/GM-CSF-transgenic NOG mice. J. Immunol. 191, 2890–2899.

Iwamoto, C., Takenaka, K., Urata, S., Yamauchi, T., Shima, T., Kuriyama, T., Daitoku, S., Saito, Y., Miyamoto, T., Iwasaki, H., Kitabayashi, I., Itoh, K., Kishimoto, J., Kohda, D., Matozaki, T., Akashi, K., 2014. The BALB/c-specific polymorphic SIRPA enhances its affinity for human CD47, inhibiting phagocytosis against human cells to promote xenogeneic engraftment. Exp. Hematol. 42, 163–171.

Jaiswal, S., Pearson, T., Friberg, H., Shultz, L.D., Greiner, D.L., Rothman, A.L., Mathew, A., 2009. Dengue virus infection and virus-specific HLA-A2 restricted immune responses in humanized NOD-scid IL2rgammanull mice. PLoS One 4, e7251.

Jaiswal, S., Pazoles, P., Woda, M., Shultz, L.D., Greiner, D.L., Brehm, M.A., Mathew, A., 2012. Enhanced humoral and HLA-A2-restricted dengue virus-specific T-cell responses in humanized BLT NSG mice. Immunology 136, 334–343.

Jaiswal, S., Smith, K., Ramirez, A., Woda, M., Pazoles, P., Shultz, L.D., Greiner, D.L., Brehm, M.A., Mathew, A., 2015. Dengue virus infection induces broadly cross-reactive human IgM antibodies that recognize intact virions in humanized BLT-NSG mice. Exp. Biol. Med. (Maywood) 240, 67–78.

Jang, Y.K., Kim, M., Lee, Y.H., Oh, W., Yang, Y.S., Choi, S.J., 2014. Optimization of the therapeutic efficacy of human umbilical cord blood-mesenchymal stromal cells in an NSG mouse xenograft model of graft-versus-host disease. Cytotherapy 16, 298–308.

Jimenez-Diaz, M.B., Mulet, T., Viera, S., Gomez, V., Garuti, H., Ibanez, J., Varez-Doval, A., Shultz, L.D., Martinez, A., Gargallo-Viola, D., Ngulo-Barturen, I., 2009. Improved murine model of malaria using plasmodium falciparum competent strains and non-myelodepleted NOD-scid IL2Rgammanull mice engrafted with human erythrocytes. Antimicrob. Agents Chemother. 53, 4533–4536.

Kaehler, K.C., Piel, S., Livingstone, E., Schilling, B., Hauschild, A., Schadendorf, D., 2010. Update on immunologic therapy with anti-CTLA-4 antibodies in melanoma: identification of clinical and biological response patterns, immune-related adverse events, and their management. Semin. Oncol. 37, 485–498.

Kamel-Reid, S., Dick, J.E., 1988. Engraftment of immune-deficient mice with human hematopoietic stem cells. Science 242, 1706–1709.

Kaushansky, A., Mikolajczak, S.A., Vignali, M., Kappe, S.H., 2014. Of men in mice: the success and promise of humanized mouse models for human malaria parasite infections. Cell. Microbiol. 16, 602–611.

Kawai, T., Akira, S., 2010. The role of pattern-recognition receptors in innate immunity: update on Toll-like receptors. Nat. Immunol. 11, 373–384.

Kerekov, N.S., Mihaylova, N.M., Grozdev, I., Todorov, T.A., Nikolova, M., Baleva, M., Nikolova, M., Prechl, J., Erdei, A., Tchorbanov, A.I., 2011. Elimination of autoreactive B cells in humanized SCID mouse model of SLE. Eur. J. Immunol. 41, 3301–3311.

King, M.A., Covassin, L., Brehm, M.A., Racki, W., Pearson, T., Leif, J., Laning, J., Fodor, W., Foreman, O., Burzenski, L., Chase, T., Gott, B., Rossini, A.A., Bortell, R., Shultz, L.D., Greiner, D.L., 2009. Hu-PBL-NOD- scid IL2rg null mouse model of xenogeneic graft-versus-host-like disease and the role of host MHC. Clin. Exp. Immunol. 157, 104–118.

Kloss, C.C., Condomines, M., Cartellieri, M., Bachmann, M., Sadelain, M., 2013. Combinatorial antigen recognition with balanced signaling promotes selective tumor eradication by engineered T cells. Nat. Biotechnol. 31, 71–75.

Kochenderfer, J.N., Dudley, M.E., Feldman, S.A., Wilson, W.H., Spaner, D.E., Maric, I., Stetler-Stevenson, M., Phan, G.Q., Hughes, M.S., Sherry, R.M., Yang, J.C., Kammula, U.S., Devillier, L., Carpenter, R., Nathan, D.A., Morgan, R.A., Laurencot, C., Rosenberg, S.A., 2012. B-cell depletion and remissions of malignancy along with cytokine-associated toxicity in a clinical trial of anti-CD19 chimeric-antigen-receptor-transduced T cells. Blood 119, 2709–2720.

Koreth, J., Matsuoka, K., Kim, H.T., Mcdonough, S.M., Bindra, B., Alyea III, E.P., Armand, P., Cutler, C., Ho, V.T., Treister, N.S., Bienfang, D.C., Prasad, S., Tzachanis, D., Joyce, R.M., Avigan, D.E., Antin, J.H., Ritz, J., Soiffer, R.J., 2011. Interleukin-2 and regulatory T cells in graft-versus-host disease. N. Engl. J. Med. 365, 2055–2066.

Kumar, A., Abbas, W., Herbein, G., 2014. HIV-1 latency in monocytes/macrophages. Viruses 6, 1837–1860.

Kuwana, Y., Takei, M., Yajima, M., Imadome, K., Inomata, H., Shiozaki, M., Ikumi, N., Nozaki, T., Shiraiwa, H., Kitamura, N., Takeuchi, J., Sawada, S., Yamamoto, N., Shimizu, N., Ito, M., Fujiwara, S., 2011. Epstein-Barr virus induces erosive arthritis in humanized mice. PLoS One 6, e26630.

Lan, P., Tonomura, N., Shimizu, A., Wang, S., Yang, Y.G., 2006. Reconstitution of a functional human immune system in immunodeficient mice through combined human fetal thymus/liver and CD34+ cell transplantation. Blood 108, 487–492.

Langlois, M., Delanghe, J., Philippe, J., Ouyang, J., Bernard, D., De Buyzere, M., Van Nooten, G., Leroux-Roels, G., 1997. Distribution of lymphocyte subsets in bone marrow and peripheral blood is associated with haptoglobin type. Binding of haptoglobin to the B-cell lectin CD22. Eur. J. Clin. Chem. Clin. Biochem. 35, 199–205.

Lavender, K.J., Pang, W.W., Messer, R.J., Duley, A.K., Race, B., Phillips, K., Scott, D., Peterson, K.E., Chan, C.K., Dittmer, U., Dudek, T., Allen, T.M., Weissman, I.L., Hasenkrug, K.J., 2013. BLT-humanized C57BL/6 Rag2-/-gammac-/-CD47-/- mice are resistant to GVHD and develop B- and T-cell immunity to HIV infection. Blood 122, 4013–4020.

Lavender, K.J., Messer, R.J., Race, B., Hasenkrug, K.J., 2014. Production of bone marrow, liver, thymus (BLT) humanized mice on the C57BL/6 Rag2(-/-)gammac(-/-)CD47(-/-) background. J. Immunol. Methods 407, 127–134.

Lee, J., Brehm, M.A., Greiner, D., Shultz, L.D., Kornfeld, H., 2013. Engrafted human cells generate adaptive immune responses to Mycobacterium bovis BCG infection in humanized mice. BMC Immunol. 14, 53.

Lepus, C.M., Gibson, T.F., Gerber, S.A., Kawikova, I., Szczepanik, M., Hossain, J., Ablamunits, V., Kirkiles-Smith, N., Herold, K.C., Donis, R.O., Bothwell, A.L., Pober, J.S., Harding, M.J., 2009. Comparison of human fetal liver, umbilical cord blood, and adult blood hematopoietic stem cell engraftment in NOD-scid/gammac-/-, Balb/c-Rag1-/-gammac-/-, and C.B-17-scid/bg immunodeficient mice. Hum. Immunol. 70, 790–802.

Leung, C., Chijioke, O., Gujer, C., Chatterjee, B., Antsiferova, O., Landtwing, V., Mchugh, D., Raykova, A., Munz, C., 2013. Infectious diseases in humanized mice. Eur. J. Immunol. 43, 2246–2254.

Li, Y., Chen, Q., Zheng, D., Yin, L., Chionh, Y.H., Wong, L.H., Tan, S.Q., Tan, T.C., Chan, J.K., Alonso, S., Dedon, P.C., Lim, B., Chen, J., 2013. Induction of functional human macrophages from bone marrow promonocytes by M-CSF in humanized mice. J. Immunol. 191, 3192–3199.

Libby, S.J., Brehm, M.A., Greiner, D.L., Shultz, L.D., Mcclelland, M., Smith, K.D., Cookson, B.T., Karlinsey, J.E., Kinkel, T.L., Porwollik, S., Canals, R., Cummings, L.A., Fang, F.C., 2010. Humanized nonobese diabetic-scid IL2rgammanull mice are susceptible to lethal Salmonella Typhi infection. Proc. Natl. Acad. Sci. U. S. A. 107, 15589–15594.

Little, M.A., Al-Ani, B., Ren, S., Al-Nuaimi, H., Leite Jr., M., Alpers, C.E., Savage, C.O., Duffield, J.S., 2012. Anti-proteinase 3 anti-neutrophil cytoplasm autoantibodies recapitulate systemic vasculitis in mice with a humanized immune system. PLoS One 7, e28626.

Lockridge, J.L., Zhou, Y., Becker, Y.A., Ma, S., Kenney, S.C., Hematti, P., Capitini, C.M., Burlingham, W.J., Gendron-Fitzpatrick, A., Gumperz, J.E., 2013. Mice engrafted with human fetal thymic tissue and hematopoietic stem cells develop pathology resembling chronic graft-versus-host disease. Biol. Blood Marrow Transplant. 19, 1310–1322.

Ma, S.D., Yu, X., Mertz, J.E., Gumperz, J.E., Reinheim, E., Zhou, Y., Tang, W., Burlingham, W.J., Gulley, M.L., Kenney, S.C., 2012. An Epstein-Barr Virus (EBV) mutant with enhanced BZLF1 expression causes lymphomas with abortive lytic EBV infection in a humanized mouse model. J. Virol. 86, 7976–7987.

Ma, S.-D., Xu, X., Plowshay, J., Ranheim, E.A., Burlingham, W.J., Jensen, J.L., Asimakopoulos, F., Tang, W., Gulley, M.L., Cesarman, E., Gumperz, J.E., Kenney, S.C., 2015. LMP1-deficient Epstein-Barr virus mutant requires T cells for lymphomagenesis. J. Clin. Invest. 125, 304–315.

Markley, J.C., Sadelain, M., 2010. IL-7 and IL-21 are superior to IL-2 and IL-15 in promoting human T cell-mediated rejection of systemic lymphoma in immunodeficient mice. Blood 115, 3508–3519.

Marsden, M.D., Kovochich, M., Suree, N., Shimizu, S., Mehta, R., Cortado, R., Bristol, G., An, D.S., Zack, J.A., 2012. HIV latency in the humanized BLT mouse. J. Virol. 86, 339–347.

Martin, H., Reuter, S., Dehzad, N., Heinz, A., Bellinghausen, I., Saloga, J., Haasler, I., Korn, S., Jonuleit, H., Buhl, R., Becker, C., Taube, C., 2012. CD4-mediated regulatory T-cell activation inhibits the development of disease in a humanized mouse model of allergic airway disease. J. Allergy Clin. Immunol. 129 (521–8), 528.

Marzi, A., Feldmann, H., 2014. Ebola virus vaccines: an overview of current approaches. Expert Rev. Vaccines 13, 521–531.

Matsuoka, K., Koreth, J., Kim, H.T., Bascug, G., Mcdonough, S., Kawano, Y., Murase, K., Cutler, C., Ho, V.T., Alyea, E.P., Armand, P., Blazar, B.R., Antin, J.H., Soiffer, R.J., Ritz, J., 2013. Low-dose interleukin-2 therapy restores regulatory T cell homeostasis in patients with chronic graft-versus-host disease. Sci. Transl. Med. 5, 179ra43.

Maus, M.V., Haas, A.R., Beatty, G.L., Albelda, S.M., Levine, B.L., Liu, X., Zhao, Y., Kalos, M., June, C.H., 2013. T cells expressing chimeric antigen receptors can cause anaphylaxis in humans. Cancer Immunol. Res. 1, 26–31.

Mccune, J.M., Namikawa, R., Kaneshima, H., Shultz, L.D., Lieberman, M., Weissman, I.L., 1988. The SCID-hu mouse: murine model for the analysis of human hematolymphoid differentiation and function. Science 241, 1632–1639.

Mcdermott, S.P., Eppert, K., Lechman, E.R., Doedens, M., Dick, J.E., 2010. Comparison of human cord blood engraftment between immunocompromised mouse strains. Blood 116, 193–200.

Mcneer, N.A., Schleifman, E.B., Cuthbert, A., Brehm, M., Jackson, A., Cheng, C., Anandalingam, K., Kumar, P., Shultz, L.D., Greiner, D.L., Mark, S.W., Glazer, P.M., 2012. Systemic delivery of

triplex-forming PNA and donor DNA by nanoparticles mediates site-specific genome editing of human hematopoietic cells in vivo. Gene Ther. 20, 658–659.
Meixlsperger, S., Leung, C.S., Ramer, P.C., Pack, M., Vanoaica, L.D., Breton, G., Pascolo, S., Salazar, A.M., Dzionek, A., Schmitz, J., Steinman, R.M., Munz, C., 2013. CD141 + dendritic cells produce prominent amounts of IFN-alpha after dsRNA recognition and can be targeted via DEC-205 in humanized mice. Blood 121, 5034–5044.
Melero, I., Hervas-Stubbs, S., Glennie, M., Pardoll, D.M., Chen, L., 2007. Immunostimulatory monoclonal antibodies for cancer therapy. Nat. Rev. Cancer 7, 95–106.
Melkus, M.W., Estes, J.D., Padgett-Thomas, A., Gatlin, J., Denton, P.W., Othieno, F.A., Wege, A.K., Haase, A.T., Garcia, J.V., 2006. Humanized mice mount specific adaptive and innate immune responses to EBV and TSST-1. Nat. Med. 12, 1316–1322.
Mercer, D.F., Schiller, D.E., Elliott, J.F., Douglas, D.N., Hao, C., Rinfret, A., Addison, W.R., Fischer, K.P., Churchill, T.A., Lakey, J.R., Tyrrell, D.L., Kneteman, N.M., 2001. Hepatitis C virus replication in mice with chimeric human livers. Nat. Med. 7, 927–933.
Mestas, J., Hughes, C.C., 2004. Of mice and not men: differences between mouse and human immunology. J. Immunol. 172, 2731–2738.
Miller, P.H., Cheung, A.M., Beer, P.A., Knapp, D.J., Dhillon, K., Rabu, G., Rostamirad, S., Humphries, R.K., Eaves, C.J., 2013. Enhanced normal short-term human myelopoiesis in mice engineered to express human-specific myeloid growth factors. Blood 121, e1–e4.
Milone, M.C., Fish, J.D., Carpenito, C., Carroll, R.G., Binder, G.K., Teachey, D., Samanta, M., Lakhal, M., Gloss, B., Net-Desnoyers, G., Campana, D., Riley, J.L., Grupp, S.A., June, C.H., 2009. Chimeric receptors containing CD137 signal transduction domains mediate enhanced survival of T cells and increased antileukemic efficacy in vivo. Mol. Ther. 17, 1453–1464.
Misharin, A.V., Haines III, G.K., Rose, S., Gierut, A.K., Hotchkiss, R.S., Perlman, H., 2012. Development of a new humanized mouse model to study acute inflammatory arthritis. J. Transl. Med. 10, 190.
Morgan, R.A., Dudley, M.E., Wunderlich, J.R., Hughes, M.S., Yang, J.C., Sherry, R.M., Royal, R.E., Topalian, S.L., Kammula, U.S., Restifo, N.P., Zheng, Z., Nahvi, A., De Vries, C.R., Rogers-Freezer, L.J., Mavroukakis, S.A., Rosenberg, S.A., 2006. Cancer regression in patients after transfer of genetically engineered lymphocytes. Science 314, 126–129.
Mosier, D.E., Gulizia, R.J., Baird, S.M., Wilson, D.B., 1988. Transfer of a functional human immune system to mice with severe combined immunodeficiency. Nature 335, 256–259.
Mota, J., Rico-Hesse, R., 2009. Humanized mice show clinical signs of dengue fever according to infecting virus genotype. J. Virol. 83, 8638–8645.
Mueller, S.N., Gebhardt, T., Carbone, F.R., Heath, W.R., 2013. Memory T cell subsets, migration patterns, and tissue residence. Annu. Rev. Immunol. 31, 137–161.
Mullard, A., 2013. New checkpoint inhibitors ride the immunotherapy tsunami. Nat. Rev. Drug Discov. 12, 489–492.
Munz, C., 2014. Viral infections in mice with reconstituted human immune system components. Immunol. Lett. 161, 118–124.
Neff, C.P., Zhou, J., Remling, L., Kuruvilla, J., Zhang, J., Li, H., Smith, D.D., Swiderski, P., Rossi, J.J., Akkina, R., 2011. An aptamer-siRNA chimera suppresses HIV-1 viral loads and protects from helper CD4(+) T cell decline in humanized mice. Sci. Transl. Med. 3, 66ra6.
Nestle, F.O., Di, M.P., Qin, J.Z., Nickoloff, B.J., 2009. Skin immune sentinels in health and disease. Nat. Rev. Immunol. 9, 679–691.
Nischang, M., Sutmuller, R., Gers-Huber, G., Audige, A., Li, D., Rochat, M.A., Baenziger, S., Hofer, U., Schlaepfer, E., Regenass, S., Amssoms, K., Stoops, B., Van, C.A., Boden, D., Kraus, G., Speck, R.F., 2012. Humanized mice recapitulate key features of HIV-1 infection: a novel concept using long-acting anti-retroviral drugs for treating HIV-1. PLoS One 7, e38853.
Nolte, T., Zadeh-Khorasani, M., Safarov, O., Rueff, F., Gulberg, V., Herbach, N., Wollenberg, A., Mueller, T., Siebeck, M., Wolf, E., Gropp, R., 2013a. Oxazolone and ethanol induce colitis in non-obese diabetic-severe combined immunodeficiency interleukin-2Rgamma(null) mice engrafted with human peripheral blood mononuclear cells. Clin. Exp. Immunol. 172, 349–362.

Nolte, T., Zadeh-Khorasani, M., Safarov, O., Rueff, F., Varga, R., Herbach, N., Wanke, R., Wollenberg, A., Mueller, T., Gropp, R., Wolf, E., Siebeck, M., 2013b. Induction of oxazolone-mediated features of atopic dermatitis in NOD-scid IL2Rgamma(null) mice engrafted with human peripheral blood mononuclear cells. Dis. Model. Mech. 6, 125–134.
Ohaegbulam, K.C., Assal, A., Lazar-Molnar, E., Yao, Y., Zang, X., 2015. Human cancer immunotherapy with antibodies to the PD-1 and PD-L1 pathway. Trends Mol. Med. 21, 24–33.
Onoe, T., Kalscheuer, H., Danzl, N., Chittenden, M., Zhao, G., Yang, Y.G., Sykes, M., 2011. Human natural regulatory T cell development, suppressive function, and postthymic maturation in a humanized mouse model. J. Immunol. 187, 3895–3903.
Palucka, K., Banchereau, J., 2013. Dendritic-cell-based therapeutic cancer vaccines. Immunity 39, 38–48.
Pawluczkowycz, A.W., Beurskens, F.J., Beum, P.V., Lindorfer, M.A., Van De Winkel, J.G., Parren, P.W., Taylor, R.P., 2009. Binding of submaximal C1q promotes complement-dependent cytotoxicity (CDC) of B cells opsonized with anti-CD20 mAbs ofatumumab (OFA) or rituximab (RTX): considerably higher levels of CDC are induced by OFA than by RTX. J. Immunol. 183, 749–758.
Pearson, T., Greiner, D.L., Shultz, L.D., 2008. Creation of "humanized" mice to study human immunity. Supplement 81, Curr. Protoc. Immunol. Chapter 15, Unit–15.21. doi: 10.1002/0471142735.im1521s81.
Pham, H.P., Manuel, M., Petit, N., Klatzmann, D., Cohen-Kaminsky, S., Six, A., Marodon, G., 2012. Half of the T-cell repertoire combinatorial diversity is genetically determined in humans and humanized mice. Eur. J. Immunol. 42, 760–770.
Porter, D.L., Levine, B.L., Kalos, M., Bagg, A., June, C.H., 2011. Chimeric antigen receptor-modified T cells in chronic lymphoid leukemia. N. Engl. J. Med. 365, 725–733.
Putnam, A.L., Safinia, N., Medvec, A., Laszkowska, M., Wray, M., Mintz, M.A., Trotta, E., Szot, G.L., Liu, W., Lares, A., Lee, K., Laing, A., Lechler, R.I., Riley, J.L., Bluestone, J.A., Lombardi, G., Tang, Q., 2013. Clinical grade manufacturing of human alloantigen-reactive regulatory T cells for use in transplantation. Am. J. Transplant. 13, 3010–3020.
Racki, W.J., Covassin, L., Brehm, M., Pino, S., Ignotz, R., Dunn, R., Laning, J., Rossini, A.A., Shultz, L.D., Greiner, D.L., 2010. NOD- scid IL2rg null (NSG) mouse model of human skin transplantation and allograft rejection. Transplantation 89, 527–536.
Ranganathan, P., Yu, X., Na, C., Santhanam, R., Shacham, S., Kauffman, M., Walker, A., Klisovic, R., Blum, W., Caligiuri, M., Croce, C.M., Marcucci, G., Garzon, R., 2012. Preclinical activity of a novel CRM1 inhibitor in acute myeloid leukemia. Blood 120, 1765–1773.
Rasmussen, A.L., Okumura, A., Ferris, M.T., Green, R., Feldmann, F., Kelly, S.M., Scott, D.P., Safronetz, D., Haddock, E., Lacasse, R., Thomas, M.J., Sova, P., Carter, V.S., Weiss, J.M., Miller, D.R., Shaw, G.D., Korth, M.J., Heise, M.T., Baric, R.S., De Villena, F.P., Feldmann, H., Katze, M.G., 2014. Host genetic diversity enables Ebola hemorrhagic fever pathogenesis and resistance. Science 346, 987–991.
Rhim, J.A., Sandgren, E.P., Degen, J.L., Palmiter, R.D., Brinster, R.L., 1994. Replacement of diseased mouse liver by hepatic cell transplantation. Science 263, 1149–1152.
Rongvaux, A., Willinger, T., Takizawa, H., Rathinam, C., Auerbach, W., Murphy, A.J., Valenzuela, D.M., Yancopoulos, G.D., Eynon, E.E., Stevens, S., Manz, M.G., Flavell, R.A., 2011. Human thrombopoietin knockin mice efficiently support human hematopoiesis in vivo. Proc. Natl. Acad. Sci. U. S. A. 108, 2378–2383.
Rongvaux, A., Takizawa, H., Strowig, T., Willinger, T., Eynon, E.E., Flavell, R.A., Manz, M.G., 2013. Human hemato-lymphoid system mice: current use and future potential for medicine. Annu. Rev. Immunol. 31, 635–674.
Rongvaux, A., Willinger, T., Martinek, J., Strowig, T., Gearty, S.V., Teichmann, L.L., Saito, Y., Marches, F., Halene, S., Palucka, A.K., Manz, M.G., Flavell, R.A., 2014. Development and function of human innate immune cells in a humanized mouse model. Nat. Biotechnol. 32, 364–372.
Rygaard, J., Povlsen, C.O., 1969. Heterotransplantation of a human malignant tumour to "Nude" mice. Acta Pathol. Microbiol. Scand. 77, 758–760.
Saadoun, D., Rosenzwajg, M., Joly, F., Six, A., Carrat, F., Thibault, V., Sene, D., Cacoub, P., Klatzmann, D., 2011. Regulatory T-cell responses to low-dose interleukin-2 in HCV-induced vasculitis. N. Engl. J. Med. 365, 2067–2077.

Savoldo, B., Ramos, C.A., Liu, E., Mims, M.P., Keating, M.J., Carrum, G., Kamble, R.T., Bollard, C.M., Gee, A.P., Mei, Z., Liu, H., Grilley, B., Rooney, C.M., Heslop, H.E., Brenner, M.K., Dotti, G., 2011. CD28 costimulation improves expansion and persistence of chimeric antigen receptor-modified T cells in lymphoma patients. J. Clin. Invest. 121, 1822–1826.

Schleifman, E.B., Bindra, R., Leif, J., Del, C.J., Rogers, F.A., Uchil, P., Kutsch, O., Shultz, L.D., Kumar, P., Greiner, D.L., Glazer, P.M., 2011. Targeted disruption of the CCR5 gene in human hematopoietic stem cells stimulated by peptide nucleic acids. Chem. Biol. 18, 1189–1198.

Schleifman, E.B., Mcneer, N.A., Jackson, A., Yamtich, J., Brehm, M.A., Shultz, L.D., Greiner, D.L., Kumar, P., Saltzman, W.M., Glazer, P.M., 2013. Site-specific genome editing in PBMCs with PLGA nanoparticle-delivered PNAs confers HIV-1 resistance in humanized mice. Mol. Ther. Nucleic Acids. 2, e135.

Schmidt, M.R., Appel, M.C., Giassi, L.J., Greiner, D.L., Shultz, L.D., Woodland, R.T., 2008. Human BLyS facilitates engraftment of human PBL derived B cells in immunodeficient mice. PLoS One 3, e3192.

Scott, S.D., 1998. Rituximab: a new therapeutic monoclonal antibody for non-Hodgkin's lymphoma. Cancer Pract. 6, 195–197.

Seok, J., Warren, H.S., Cuenca, A.G., Mindrinos, M.N., Baker, H.V., Xu, W., Richards, D.R., Donald-Smith, G.P., Gao, H., Hennessy, L., Finnerty, C.C., Lopez, C.M., Honari, S., Moore, E.E., Minei, J.P., Cuschieri, J., Bankey, P.E., Johnson, J.L., Sperry, J., Nathens, A.B., Billiar, T.R., West, M.A., Jeschke, M.G., Klein, M.B., Gamelli, R.L., Gibran, N.S., Brownstein, B.H., Miller-Graziano, C., Calvano, S.E., Mason, P.H., Cobb, J.P., Rahme, L.G., Lowry, S.F., Maier, R.V., Moldawer, L.L., Herndon, D.N., Davis, R.W., Xiao, W., Tompkins, R.G., 2013. Genomic responses in mouse models poorly mimic human inflammatory diseases. Proc. Natl. Acad. Sci. U. S. A. 110, 3507–3512.

Shih, C.C., Hu, J., Arber, D., Lebon, T., Forman, S.J., 2000. Transplantation and growth characteristics of human fetal lymph node in immunodeficient mice. Exp. Hematol. 28, 1046–1053.

Shiokawa, M., Takahashi, T., Murakami, A., Kita, S., Ito, M., Sugamura, K., Ishii, N., 2010. In vivo assay of human NK-dependent ADCC using NOD/SCID/gammac(null) (NOG) mice. Biochem. Biophys. Res. Commun. 399, 733–737.

Shultz, L.D., Schweitzer, P.A., Christianson, S.W., Gott, B., Schweitzer, I.B., Mckenna, S., Mobraaten, L., Rajan, T.V., Greiner, D.L., Leiter, E.H., 1995. Multiple defects in innate and adaptive immunologic function in NOD/LtSz- scid mice. J. Immunol. 154, 180–191.

Shultz, L.D., Lyons, B.L., Burzenski, L.M., Gott, B., Chen, X., Chaleff, S., Gillies, S.D., King, M., Mangada, J., Greiner, D.L., Handgretinger, R., 2005. Human lymphoid and myeloid cell development in NOD/LtSz- scid IL2r g null mice engrafted with mobilized human hematopoietic stem cell. J. Immunol. 174, 6477–6489.

Shultz, L.D., Ishikawa, F., Greiner, D.L., 2007. Humanized mice in translational biomedical research. Nat. Rev. Immunol. 7, 118–130.

Shultz, L.D., Saito, Y., Najima, Y., Tanaka, S., Ochi, T., Tomizawa, M., Doi, T., Sone, A., Suzuki, N., Fujiwara, H., Yasukawa, M., Ishikawa, F., 2010. Generation of functional human T-cell subsets with HLA-restricted immune responses in HLA class I expressing NOD/SCID/IL2r gamma(null) humanized mice. Proc. Natl. Acad. Sci. U. S. A. 107, 13022–13027.

Shultz, L.D., Brehm, M.A., Garcia-Martinez, J.V., Greiner, D.L., 2012. Humanized mice for immune system investigation: progress, promise and challenges. Nat. Rev. Immunol. 12, 786–798.

Shultz, L.D., Goodwin, N., Ishikawa, F., Hosur, V., Lyons, B.L., Greiner, D.L., 2014. Human cancer growth and therapy in immunodeficient mouse models. Cold Spring Harb. Protoc. 2014, 694–708.

Siliciano, J.D., Siliciano, R.F., 2014. Recent developments in the search for a cure for HIV-1 infection: targeting the latent reservoir for HIV-1. J. Allergy Clin. Immunol. 134, 12–19.

Sliva, K., 2014. Latest animal models for anti-HIV drug discovery. Expert. Opin. Drug Discov. 10, 111–123.

Sonar, S.S., Hsu, Y.M., Conrad, M.L., Majeau, G.R., Kilic, A., Garber, E., Gao, Y., Nwankwo, C., Willer, G., Dudda, J.C., Kim, H., Bailly, V., Pagenstecher, A., Rennert, P.D., Renz, H., 2010. Antagonism of TIM-1 blocks the development of disease in a humanized mouse model of allergic asthma. J. Clin. Invest. 120, 2767–2781.

Song, J., Willinger, T., Rongvaux, A., Eynon, E.E., Stevens, S., Manz, M.G., Flavell, R.A., Galan, J.E., 2010. A mouse model for the human pathogen Salmonella typhi. Cell Host Microbe 8, 369–376.

Song, D.G., Ye, Q., Carpenito, C., Poussin, M., Wang, L.P., Ji, C., Figini, M., June, C.H., Coukos, G., Powell Jr., D.J., 2011. In vivo persistence, tumor localization, and antitumor activity of CAR-engineered T cells is enhanced by costimulatory signaling through CD137 (4-1BB). Cancer Res. 71, 4617–4627.

Song, D.G., Ye, Q., Poussin, M., Harms, G.M., Figini, M., Powell Jr., D.J., 2012. CD27 costimulation augments the survival and antitumor activity of redirected human T cells in vivo. Blood 119, 696–706.

Soria, A., Boccara, D., Chonco, L., Yahia, N., Dufossee, M., Cardinaud, S., Moris, A., Liard, C., Joulin-Giet, A., Julithe, M., Mimoun, M., Combadiere, B., Perrin, H., 2014. Long-term maintenance of skin immune system in a NOD-Scid IL2rgamma(null) mouse model transplanted with human skin. Exp. Dermatol. 23, 850–852.

Spranger, S., Frankenberger, B., Schendel, D.J., 2012. NOD/scid IL-2Rg(null) mice: a preclinical model system to evaluate human dendritic cell-based vaccine strategies in vivo. J. Transl. Med. 10, 30.

Stoddart, C.A., Maidji, E., Galkina, S.A., Kosikova, G., Rivera, J.M., Moreno, M.E., Sloan, B., Joshi, P., Long, B.R., 2011. Superior human leukocyte reconstitution and susceptibility to vaginal HIV transmission in humanized NOD-scid IL-2Rgamma(-/-) (NSG) BLT mice. Virology 417, 154–160.

Stoddart, C.A., Nault, G., Galkina, S.A., Bousquet-Gagnon, N., Bridon, D., Quraishi, O., 2012. Preexposure prophylaxis with albumin-conjugated C34 peptide HIV-1 fusion inhibitor in SCID-hu Thy/Liv mice. Antimicrob. Agents Chemother. 56, 2162–2165.

Strowig, T., Gurer, C., Ploss, A., Liu, Y.F., Arrey, F., Sashihara, J., Koo, G., Rice, C.M., Young, J.W., Chadburn, A., Cohen, J.I., Munz, C., 2009. Priming of protective T cell responses against virus-induced tumors in mice with human immune system components. J. Exp. Med. 206, 1423–1434.

Strowig, T., Chijioke, O., Carrega, P., Arrey, F., Meixlsperger, S., Ramer, P.C., Ferlazzo, G., Munz, C., 2010. Human NK cells of mice with reconstituted human immune system components require preactivation to acquire functional competence. Blood 116, 4158–4167.

Strowig, T., Rongvaux, A., Rathinam, C., Takizawa, H., Borsotti, C., Philbrick, W., Eynon, E.E., Manz, M.G., Flavell, R.A., 2011. Transgenic expression of human signal regulatory protein alpha in Rag2-/-{gamma}c-/- mice improves engraftment of human hematopoietic cells in humanized mice. Proc. Natl. Acad. Sci. U. S. A. 108, 13218–13223.

Suzuki, M., Takahashi, T., Katano, I., Ito, R., Ito, M., Harigae, H., Ishii, N., Sugamura, K., 2012. Induction of human humoral immune responses in a novel HLA-DR-expressing transgenic NOD/Shi-scid/gammacnull mouse. Int. Immunol. 24, 243–252.

Takagi, S., Saito, Y., Hijikata, A., Tanaka, S., Watanabe, T., Hasegawa, T., Mochizuki, S., Kunisawa, J., Kiyono, H., Koseki, H., Ohara, O., Saito, T., Taniguchi, S., Shultz, L.D., Ishikawa, F., 2012. Membrane-bound human SCF/KL promotes in vivo human hematopoietic engraftment and myeloid differentiation. Blood 119, 2768–2777.

Takao, K., Miyakawa, T., 2015. Genomic responses in mouse models greatly mimic human inflammatory diseases. Proc. Natl. Acad. Sci. U. S. A. 112, 1167–1172. Epub, Aug. 4.

Takao, K., Hagihara, H., Miyakawa, T., 2015. Reply to Warren et al. and Shay et al.: commonalities across species do exist and are potentially important. Proc. Natl. Acad. Sci. U. S. A. 112, E347–E348. Epub, Dec 24.

Tanaka, S., Saito, Y., Kunisawa, J., Kurashima, Y., Wake, T., Suzuki, N., Shultz, L.D., Kiyono, H., Ishikawa, F., 2012. Development of mature and functional human myeloid subsets in hematopoietic stem cell-engrafted NOD/SCID/IL2rgammaKO mice. J. Immunol. 188, 6145–6155.

Tang, Q., Bluestone, J.A., 2013. Regulatory T-cell therapy in transplantation: moving to the clinic. Cold Spring Harb. Perspect. Med. 3, 1–15.

Taube, R., Peterlin, M., 2013. Lost in transcription: molecular mechanisms that control HIV latency. Viruses 5, 902–927.

Todd, J., Knip, M., Mathieu, C., 2011. Towards disease mechanism-based strategies for the prevention of autoimmune Type 1 diabetes. Diabet. Med. 28, 1141–1143.

Traggiai, E., Chicha, L., Mazzucchelli, L., Bronz, L., Piffaretti, J.C., Lanzavecchia, A., Manz, M.G., 2004. Development of a human adaptive immune system in cord blood cell-transplanted mice. Science 304, 104–107.

Tseng, C., Chan, Y., 2015. Overview of Ebola virus disease in 2014. J. Chin. Med. Assoc. 78, 51–55.
Tumeh, P.C., Harview, C.L., Yearley, J.H., Shintaku, I.P., Taylor, E.J., Robert, L., Chmielowski, B., Spasic, M., Henry, G., Ciobanu, V., West, A.N., Carmona, M., Kivork, C., Seja, E., Cherry, G., Gutierrez, A.J., Grogan, T.R., Mateus, C., Tomasic, G., Glaspy, J.A., Emerson, R.O., Robins, H., Pierce, R.H., Elashoff, D.A., Robert, C., Ribas, A., 2014. PD-1 blockade induces responses by inhibiting adaptive immune resistance. Nature 515, 568–571.
Unger, W.W., Pearson, T., Abreu, J.R., Laban, S., Van Der Slik, A.R., Der Kracht, S.M., Kester, M.G., Serreze, D.V., Shultz, L.D., Griffioen, M., Drijfhout, J.W., Greiner, D.L., Roep, B.O., 2012. Islet-specific CTL Cloned from a Type 1 diabetes patient cause beta-cell destruction after engraftment into HLA-A2 Transgenic NOD/SCID/IL2RG Null Mice. PLoS One 7, e49213.
Unsinger, J., Mcdonough, J.S., Shultz, L.D., Ferguson, T.A., Hotchkiss, R.S., 2009. Sepsis-induced human lymphocyte apoptosis and cytokine production in "humanized" mice. J. Leukoc. Biol. 86, 219–227.
Vallet, V., Mauray, S., Kindler, V., Aubry, D., Ruegg, M., Cherpillod, J., Waridel, F., Schapira, M., Duchosal, M.A., 2005. Human tonsil implants xenotransplanted in SCID mice display broad lymphocytic diversity and cellular activation profile similar to those in the original lymphoid organ. Xenotransplantation 12, 38–48.
Vaughan, A.M., Mikolajczak, S.A., Wilson, E.M., Grompe, M., Kaushansky, A., Camargo, N., Bial, J., Ploss, A., Kappe, S.H., 2012. Complete Plasmodium falciparum liver-stage development in liver-chimeric mice. J. Clin. Invest. 122, 3618–3628.
Viehmann Milam, A.A., Maher, S.E., Gibson, J.A., Lebastchi, J., Wen, L., Ruddle, N.H., Herold, K.C., Bothwell, A.L., 2014. A humanized mouse model of autoimmune insulitis. Diabetes 63, 1712–1724.
Villaudy, J., Schotte, R., Legrand, N., Spits, H., 2014. Critical assessment of human antibody generation in humanized mouse models. J. Immunol. Methods 410C, 18–27.
Von, S.M., Ding, Q., Ploss, A., 2014. Visualizing hepatitis C virus infection in humanized mice. J. Immunol. Methods 410, 50–59.
Vudattu, N.K., Waldron-Lynch, F., Truman, L.A., Deng, S., Preston-Hurlburt, P., Torres, R., Raycroft, M.T., Mamula, M.J., Herold, K.C., 2014. Humanized mice as a model for aberrant responses in human T cell immunotherapy. J. Immunol. 193, 587–596.
Vuyyuru, R., Patton, J., Manser, T., 2011. Human immune system mice: current potential and limitations for translational research on human antibody responses. Immunol. Res. 51, 257–266.
Wahl, A., Swanson, M.D., Nochi, T., Olesen, R., Denton, P.W., Chateau, M., Garcia, J.V., 2012. Human breast milk and antiretrovirals dramatically reduce oral HIV-1 transmission in BLT humanized mice. PLoS Pathog. 8, e1002732.
Warren, H.S., Tompkins, R.G., Moldawer, L.L., Seok, J., Xu, W., Mindrinos, M.N., Maier, R.V., Xiao, W., Davis, R.W., 2014a. Mice are not men. Proc. Natl. Acad. Sci. U.S.A. 12, E345, Epub, Dec. 24.
Warren, T.K., Wells, J., Panchal, R.G., Stuthman, K.S., Garza, N.L., Van Tongeren, S.A., Dong, L., Retterer, C.J., Eaton, B.P., Pegoraro, G., Honnold, S., Bantia, S., Kotian, P., Chen, X., Taubenheim, B.R., Welch, L.S., Minning, D.M., Babu, Y.S., Sheridan, W.P., Bavari, S., 2014b. Protection against filovirus diseases by a novel broad-spectrum nucleoside analogue BCX4430. Nature 508, 402–405.
Washburn, M.L., Bility, M.T., Zhang, L., Kovalev, G.I., Buntzman, A., Frelinger, J.A., Barry, W., Ploss, A., Rice, C.M., Su, L., 2011. A humanized mouse model to study hepatitis C virus infection, immune response, and liver disease. Gastroenterology 140, 1334–1344.
Watanabe, Y., Takahashi, T., Okajima, A., Shiokawa, M., Ishii, N., Katano, I., Ito, R., Ito, M., Minegishi, M., Minegishi, N., Tsuchiya, S., Sugamura, K., 2009. The analysis of the functions of human B and T cells in humanized NOD/shi-scid/gammac(null) (NOG) mice (hu-HSC NOG mice). Int. Immunol. 21, 843–858.
Weber, J., 2010. Immune checkpoint proteins: a new therapeutic paradigm for cancer–preclinical background: CTLA-4 and PD-1 blockade. Semin. Oncol. 37, 430–439.
Wege, A.K., Ernst, W., Eckl, J., Frankenberger, B., Vollmann-Zwerenz, A., Mannel, D.N., Ortmann, O., Kroemer, A., Brockhoff, G., 2011. Humanized tumor mice-A new model to study and manipulate the immune response in advanced cancer therapy. Int. J. Cancer 129, 2194–2206.

Wege, A.K., Schmidt, M., Ueberham, E., Ponnath, M., Ortmann, O., Brockhoff, G., Lehmann, J., 2014. Co-transplantation of human hematopoietic stem cells and human breast cancer cells in NSG mice: a novel approach to generate tumor cell specific human antibodies. MAbs 6, 968–977.

Werner-Klein, M., Proske, J., Werno, C., Schneider, K., Hofmann, H.S., Rack, B., Buchholz, S., Ganzer, R., Blana, A., Seelbach-Gobel, B., Nitsche, U., Mannel, D.N., Klein, C.A., 2014. Immune humanization of immunodeficient mice using diagnostic bone marrow aspirates from carcinoma patients. PLoS One 9, e97860.

Whaley, K.J., Morton, J., Hume, S., Hiatt, E., Bratcher, B., Klimyuk, V., Hiatt, A., Pauly, M., Zeitlin, L., 2014. Emerging antibody-based products. Curr. Top. Microbiol. Immunol. 375, 107–126.

Wheeler, L.A., Vrbanac, V., Trifonova, R., Brehm, M.A., Gilboa-Geffen, A., Tanno, S., Greiner, D.L., Luster, A.D., Tager, A.M., Lieberman, J., 2013. Durable knockdown and protection from HIV transmission in humanized mice treated with gel-formulated CD4 aptamer-siRNA chimeras. Mol. Ther. 21, 1378–1389.

Whitfield-Larry, F., Young, E.F., Talmage, G., Fudge, E., Azam, A., Patel, S., Largay, J., Byrd, W., Buse, J., Calikoglu, A.S., Shultz, L.D., Frelinger, J.A., 2011. HLA-A2-matched peripheral blood mononuclear cells from type 1 diabetic patients, but not nondiabetic donors, transfer insulitis to NOD-scid/gammac(null)/HLA-A2 transgenic mice concurrent with the expansion of islet-specific CD8+ T cells. Diabetes 60, 1726–1733.

WHO, 2014. World Malaria Report. http://www.who.int/malaria/publications/world_malaria_report_2014/en/.

Wijayalath, W., Majji, S., Villasante, E.F., Brumeanu, T.D., Richie, T.L., Casares, S., 2014. Humanized HLA-DR4.RagKO.IL2RgammacKO.NOD (DRAG) mice sustain the complex vertebrate life cycle of Plasmodium falciparum malaria. Malar. J. 13, 386.

Willinger, T., Rongvaux, A., Takizawa, H., Yancopoulos, G.D., Valenzuela, D.M., Murphy, A.J., Auerbach, W., Eynon, E.E., Stevens, S., Manz, M.G., Flavell, R.A., 2011. Human IL-3/GM-CSF knock-in mice support human alveolar macrophage development and human immune responses in the lung. Proc. Natl. Acad. Sci. U. S. A. 108, 2390–2395.

Wilson, E.M., Bial, J., Tarlow, B., Bial, G., Jensen, B., Greiner, D.L., Brehm, M.A., Grompe, M., 2014. Extensive double humanization of both liver and hematopoiesis in FRGN mice. Stem Cell Res. 13, 404–412.

Wolfe, N.D., Dunavan, C.P., Diamond, J., 2007. Origins of major human infectious diseases. Nature 447, 279–283.

Wong, K.K., Brenneman, F., Chesney, A., Spaner, D.E., Gorczynski, R.M., 2012. Soluble CD200 is critical to engraft chronic lymphocytic leukemia cells in immunocompromised mice. Cancer Res. 72, 4931–4943.

Wong, G., Qiu, X., Olinger, G.G., Kobinger, G.P., 2014. Post-exposure therapy of filovirus infections. Trends Microbiol. 22, 456–463.

Yamauchi, T., Takenaka, K., Urata, S., Shima, T., Kikushige, Y., Tokuyama, T., Iwamoto, C., Nishihara, M., Iwasaki, H., Miyamoto, T., Honma, N., Nakao, M., Matozaki, T., Akashi, K., 2013. Polymorphic Sirpa is the genetic determinant for NOD-based mouse lines to achieve efficient human cell engraftment. Blood 121, 1316–1325.

Ye, C., Choi, J.G., Abraham, S., Wu, H., Diaz, D., Terreros, D., Shankar, P., Manjunath, N., 2012. Human macrophage and dendritic cell-specific silencing of high-mobility group protein B1 ameliorates sepsis in a humanized mouse model. Proc. Natl. Acad. Sci. U. S. A. 109, 21052–21057.

Yoshizato, K., Tateno, C., 2013. A mouse with humanized liver as an animal model for predicting drug effects and for studying hepatic viral infection: where to next? Expert Opin. Drug Metab. Toxicol. 9, 1419–1435.

Zadeh-Khorasani, M., Nolte, T., Mueller, T.D., Pechlivanis, M., Rueff, F., Wollenberg, A., Fricker, G., Wolf, E., Siebeck, M., Gropp, R., 2013. NOD-scid IL2R gammanull mice engrafted with human peripheral blood mononuclear cells as a model to test therapeutics targeting human signaling pathways. J. Transl. Med. 11, 4.

Zayoud, M., El, M.K., Frauenknecht, K., Trinschek, B., Kloos, L., Karram, K., Wanke, F., Georgescu, J., Hartwig, U.F., Sommer, C., Jonuleit, H., Waisman, A., Kurschus, F.C., 2013. Subclinical CNS inflammation as response to a myelin antigen in humanized mice. J. Neuroimmune Pharmacol. 8, 1037–1047.

Zhao, Y., Moon, E., Carpenito, C., Paulos, C.M., Liu, X., Brennan, A.L., Chew, A., Carroll, R.G., Scholler, J., Levine, B.L., Albelda, S.M., June, C.H., 2010. Multiple injections of electroporated autologous T cells expressing a chimeric antigen receptor mediate regression of human disseminated tumor. Cancer Res. 70, 9053–9061.

CHAPTER 12

Immunological Biomarkers for Patient Stratification

F. Ponchel, A.N. Burska, S.R. Harrison
University of Leeds, Leeds, United Kingdom

Contents

Translational Immunology
http://dx.doi.org/10.1016/B978-0-12-801577-3.00013-7

1. INTRODUCTION

The ultimate aim of stratified medicine is to "provide patients with the right treatment, for the right person, at the right time." This concept relies on the recently developed ability to classify patients into different groups according to their personal genetic makeup (disease heritability and susceptibility) and the impact that their lifestyle may have had on their health and disease risk associated with particular environmental influences. All these factors contribute to the molecular and cellular pathways that may or may not be used in a specific disease (disease heterogeneity) ultimately driving responsiveness to certain therapeutic approaches rather than others. Stratified medicine is nowadays recognized as a high-priority goal for health care providers, pharmaceutical and diagnostic industries, and patients.

Stratified medicine (also known as personalized or precision medicine) therefore relies on identifying subgroups of patients with distinct clinical characteristics and disease mechanisms that lead to better responses to certain treatments, allowing the delivery of the most effective and safe treatment for each patient. The approach to segregating patients between groups uses biological markers (biomarkers). To bring stratified medicine to its expectation, advances in technologies are required to reliably quantify such biomarkers. The use of biomarkers to stratify patients into disease subpopulations therefore represent a move away from empirical medicine, with "one size fits all" prescribing practice, toward identifying individuals most likely to respond to a certain medication, but also to those less likely to suffer adverse drug reactions. While stratified medicine is still a relatively recent concept, its aspirations are at the heart of new treatment developments for human disease. It is one step toward personalized medicine and may use many kinds of technology to achieve this goal.

Stratified medicine relies heavily on biomarkers. These are measurable indicators or surrogates of a specific feature of the disease. Any measureable physical or physiological traits (including by the use of imaging technologies such as ultrasound or MRI) or genetic factors complete with epigenetics and gene expression profiling, molecular or cellular, metabolomics, and kinase sequencing are all "biomarkers." In addition, there are many fields of personalized medicine where biomarkers are becoming essential tools for clinicians to decide on diagnosis, prognosis, to monitor disease activity, to predict therapeutic response, and to adapt drug dosage. For stratified medicine, the development of biomarkers of response to therapy follows the same pipeline as other biomarkers from discovery, validation, replication, clinical development, and adoption into clinical practice.

Stratified medicine is thought to be the key to the future of medicine, and as such is one of the most active areas of clinical research. The spectrum of diseases where stratified medicine biomarkers have been successfully developed is currently narrow. However, the need for future research and development has been internationally recognized and as such a "Workshop to clarify the scope for stratification biomarkers and to identify bottlenecks in the discovery and the use of such biomarkers" was recently run by the EU Commission. It defined the four major types of biomarker needed: biomarkers for (i) diagnostic, (ii) susceptibility and/or risk, (iii) prognostic, and (iv) predictive of treatment response. It defined stratification as the identification of a group of patients with shared "biological" characteristics enabling the selection of optimal management for these patients to achieve the best possible treatment outcome. The number of technologies allowing stratification has exploded in terms of the number and types of candidates to consider, and the list of potential biomarkers has also expanded exponentially to include any candidate from "omics" technologies, epigenetics, phenotyping, imaging, functional or clinical. In addition, biomarkers should be distinguished from their assays (ie, applicability of a qualified biomarker relies also on the development of a robust assay for its detection before it can be used in clinic). The fields for which stratified medicine is mostly needed were also discussed and ranked in priority with oncology first, followed by diabetes, cardiovascular diseases, and neurodegenerative diseases.

In this chapter, we will concentrate on immunological biomarkers detected/quantified by several methodologies that have the potential to be used in stratified medicine. To date, however, immunological biomarkers have mostly been validated for other purposes, mostly diagnostic, so we will also relate to success stories in stratifying biomarkers for cancer and review promising developments for immunological biomarkers, with a focus on autoimmune diseases (AID), notably.

2. GENETIC BIOMARKER

The completion of the Human Genome Project has made it possible to acquire precise information about the genetic makeup of populations and individuals. This has led to the identification of genes directly implicated in diseases and helped in diagnosing them. The likelihood that the genetic makeup of an individual is going to affect his/her ability to respond to the treatment more or less effectively is the fundamental basis of stratified medicine.

2.1 Success stories in cancer

Genetic profiling of patients with cancer is currently used to guide the best choice of therapy in several types of cancer, with the most advanced results in breast cancer. Tamoxifen is a highly effective drug for the treatment of breast cancer. It is metabolized by the cytochrome P450 2D6 (CYP2D6) enzyme to active two metabolites, 4-OH tamoxifen and endoxifen. Gene polymorphisms in the metabolism cascade used by several drugs are known to result in high and low metabolizers of tamoxifen since late 2000s (Dezentjé et al., 2009) allowing alternative treatments, such as aromatase inhibitors to be preferred (Schroth et al., 2007). Despite this, women receiving tamoxifen are not routinely tested for *CYP2D6* and *UGT1A1* polymorphism and debates are still ongoing since 2010 (Schilsky, 2010). Further classification of breast cancer using the estrogen receptor *HER2* gene allowed the identification of patients who are more likely to benefit from adjuvant paclitaxel treatment (Hayes et al., 2007). Other examples include activating mutations in the epidermal growth factor receptor gene (*EGFR*) in non-small cell lung cancer (NSCLC), which underlie responsiveness to gefitinib (Lynch et al., 2004); colorectal cancer with kirsten rat sarcoma viral oncogene homolog (*KRAS*) mutations, which correlates with panitumumab efficacy (Amado et al., 2008); and malignant gliomas with hypermethylation of the methyl guanine methyl transferase (*MGMT*) gene, which are responsive to temozomide (Hegi et al., 2005).

The Philadelphia chromosome or Philadelphia translocation is a specific chromosomal abnormality that is associated with chronic myelogenous leukemia (CML). It is the result of a translocation between chromosomes 9 and 22 [designated t(9;22)(q34; q11)] giving rise to a fusion gene, *bcr-ab*. The presence of this translocation is highly sensitive (95%) for CML however, the presence of the Philadelphia (Ph) chromosome is not sufficiently specific to diagnose CML as it is also found in acute lymphoblastic leukemia (Talpaz et al., 2006) (25–30% in adult and 2–10% in pediatric cases) and occasionally in acute myelogenous leukemia. Tyrosine kinase inhibitors STI-571 (imatinib, Gleevec/Glivec) were identified. Subsequent trials demonstrated that STI-571 inhibits proliferation of BCR-abl-expressing cells. Although it did not eradicate CML cells, it did greatly limit the growth of the tumor clone. The emerging Gleevec/Glivec-resistant BCR-abl clones in treated patients result from point mutations in the BCR-abl kinase. New inhibitors include dasatinib and nilotinib, which are significantly more potent than imatinib and may overcome resistance. These findings revolutionized the treatment of CML and allowed fully personalized treatment based on the presence of this genetic event.

2.2 Severe combined immunodeficiency

Severe combined immunodeficiency (SCID) is a rare primary immunodeficiency in which there is combined absence of T-lymphocyte and B-cells due to a number of different genetic defects (*X*-linked, *ADA*, *RGA1* or *2*, IL-7 signaling cascade, CD3 or CD45 deficiencies). These defects lead to extreme susceptibility to very serious infections. This condition is generally considered to be the most serious of the primary immunodeficiencies. Bone marrow transplantation is an effective treatment that can cure SCID. The diagnosis is usually first suspected in children because of an excessive number of infections, very strong reaction to chicken pox, herpes simplex, adenovirus, parainfluenza-3, Epstein-Barr virus, polioviruses, measles (rubella) and rotavirus, fungal infections, persistent diarrhea, as well as family history. The easiest diagnostic test is a blood cell count (even from cord blood) or an absolute lymphocyte count (average lymphocyte count falls to <1500 cell/mm^3 in a SCID child), confirmed by repeating tests over time and T-cell function done promptly to confirm or exclude the diagnosis. Ig levels are also very low in SCID patients and can be used as confirmation, although placental Ig may sometime confuse results.

Depending on the genetic cause of SCID, several available treatments can be selected: immunoglobulin replacement, modified form of the adenosine deaminase (ADA) enzyme PEG-ADA, or immune reconstitution by bone marrow transplantation from a healthy donor. Gene therapy has been explored with successful cases for X-linked and ADA-deficient SCID where a precise genetic defect can be corrected.

2.3 Warfarin dosing

Warfarin (also known as Coumadin, Jantoven, Marevan, or Uniwarfin) is an anticoagulant used to prevent the formation of blood clots and their migration in the body. Despite its effectiveness, warfarin treatment poses some issues as its dose–response relationship is unpredictable and its activity must be monitored weekly/monthly to ensure that an effective yet safe dose is taken (Ansell et al., 2008). Three single nucleotide polymorphisms in cytochrome P4502C9 (*CYP2C9*) and vitamin K epoxide reductase complex (*VKORC1*) genes were found to play key roles in determining the effect of warfarin therapy on coagulation. Warfarin directly inhibits VKORC1 while CYP2C9 is a very important drug metabolizing enzyme, directly responsible for warfarin bioavailability. Polymorphism in *CYP2C9* gene leads to warfarin hypersensitivity and a close relationship between CYP2C9 genotype, age, and warfarin dosing has been established (Linder et al., 2002). The prevalence of each polymorphism notably varies with ethnical background. The patient's genotype will therefore directly influence the speed of warfarin metabolism and the dose of warfarin needed to achieve anticoagulation will need to be adapted to his/her genotype. Polymorphisms in *VKORC1* lead to different levels of expression of the protein, hence lower/higher dose of warfarin can inhibit it. Again, the prevalence of these polymorphisms varies by race (Rieder et al., 2005).

2.4 Multiple myeloma risk groups and treatment stratification

Multiple myelomas (MM) are a frequent hematologic malignancy implicating plasma cells. They are staged by estimating the tumor cell mass based of the amount of monoclonal protein M in the serum and/or urine. The clonal nature of the plasma cells involved is very important for diagnosis on bone marrow examination. The stage of the disease is a strong determinant of survival chances, but it has little influence on the choice of therapy as the disease is generalized.

The repeat occurrence of certain genetic aberrations (deletion, translocations) observed in early stages of plasma cell disorders suggested that these could be used to classify risk in such patients (Fonseca et al., 2003; Avet-Loiseau et al., 2007). Translocations [t(14;16), t(4;14), or t(14;20)] and deletions in certain chromosomes (17p, notably the p53 locus) are now used to classify risk in MM based on retrospective cytogenetic findings. Therapy is then adapted according to the risk associated with these genetic events:

standard-risk patients can be treated with lenalidomide plus low-dose dexamethasone whereas intermediate and high-risk patients require bortezomib-cyclophosphamide-dexamethasone triple therapy (Rajkumar, 2014).

2.5 The major histocompatibility complex

The major histocompatibility complex (MHC) includes several cell surface receptors encoded by a gene family that are at the center of the immune system, the MHC molecules mediating the interactions between immune cells and other body cells. The MHC gene family, also known as the human leucocyte antigen (HLA) family, was identified in 1936 (Klein, 1986) and is divided into three classes: I, II, and III. MHC genes are highly polymorphic (Janeway et al., 2001). The most diverse loci, namely HLA-A, HLA-B (class I), and HLA-DRB1 (class II), have roughly 1000, 1600, and 870 known alleles, respectively. The MHC notably determines the compatibility between donor and recipient of organ transplant on one hand and the susceptibility to autoimmune disease (AID) on the other.

2.5.1 Transplantation

The transplantation of organs is one of the greatest medical achievements of the past century. The success of organ transplantation entirely depends on matching the recipient and donor MHC as the principal immune response responsible for accepting or rejecting the graft targets the MHC molecules on the surface of donor cells. Indeed a host recognizing the grafted tissues (or cells) as foreign will mount an immune response against it, a host versus graft disease, resulting in the rejection of the transplanted organ/cells. Immunosuppression has been used to limit such occurrence; however, if the host becomes too immunocompromised, T-cells included in the donor graft may become active and induce a graft versus host disease (GVHD), an event as fatal as graft rejection.

2.5.2 Rheumatoid arthritis as AID example

Strong genetic association between a specific allele of the HLA-DRB1 gene encoding a particular stretch of amino acids known as the shared epitope (SE) was first reported in rheumatoid arthritis in the 1980s (Gregersen et al., 1987). This association has provided diagnostic biomarker value for over 40 years and is still used today. The presence of SE in RA patients was further associated with poorer prognosis (Berglin et al., 2004; Van Gaalen et al., 2004; Mu et al., 1999; Gorman and Criswell, 2002), although to date it has not really been used in stratified medicine. More recent work associating SE and certain autoantibodies may prove more useful.

Response to tumor necrosis factor (TNF) inhibitor therapy was investigated with respect to the carriage of the SE sequence. Several studies reported no association (Martinez et al., 2004; Marotte et al., 2006; Miceli-Richard et al., 2008; Kang et al., 2005) although one suggested better response in the presence of two HLA-DRB1 alleles encoding the SE when using one particular drug (etanercept) (Criswell et al., 2004), while another study of response to adalimumab showed that an increased number of HLA-DRB1 SE copies was related to better response (Skapenko et al., 2010). This controversy was resolved using data from the British Society for Rheumatology Biologics Register. Having the statistical power to detect an effect, it showed no association between the SE motif and response to TNF inhibitor therapy (Potter et al., 2009). The conclusion of this work was that, overall, the presence of SE reflect best the susceptibility to RA (Emery and Dörner, 2011).

The remaining genetic risk associated with RA lies mostly in genes implicated in the immune system (Diogo et al., 2014; Bossini-Castillo et al., 2015). Response to TNF inhibitors was suggested to be different in patients bearing several single nucleotide polymorphisms (SNPs) in the genes of the p38 kinase cascade (Coulthard et al., 2011) however, much work remains to be done with respect to the other ~100 genes associated with RA. Contrasting viewpoints were reported with respect to the unresolved possible implication of the immunoglobulin receptor FcgRIIIA (Canete et al., 2009; Tutuncu et al., 2005; Kastbom et al., 2007) for response to TNF inhibitors, which may exert their effects in part via this receptor.

Therefore, in the context of a RA patient's response to biological therapies, there is no shortage of candidate genetic markers but rather limitations in the studies performed due to lack of power to detect what may be relatively small differences in treatment effects. In addition the three main anti-TNF agents used all have different mechanisms of action and this may contribute further to the difference in genes that may be relevant. A number of polymorphisms may certainly have good potential as prognostic markers (associated with disease severity or radiological damage) or diagnostic markers (like SE), but their use in stratified medicine remains a long way from clinical utility (Emery and Dörner, 2011).

3. GENE EXPRESSION SIGNATURES

Gene expression analysis has been one of the most successful approaches in translational research (Bullinger et al., 2004; Sotiriou and Piccart, 2007). It has been extensively used to investigate potential sources of biomarkers for diagnosis, prognosis, and prediction of treatment outcome. It has reached clinics with several clinical application tests already FDA/ISO approved and available on the market (Burska et al., 2014b), although mostly for cancer again. The successful translation of microarray data into clinical use provides a strong rationale for similar approaches to improve the care of patients with many diseases.

3.1 Success stories from oncology

The field of oncology has successfully used gene expression profiling to identify gene signatures that predict good or poor prognosis in patients with breast cancer (Colombo et al., 2011). This work led to the development of several gene expression-based products: mammaPrint® (Agendia, Amsterdam, the Netherlands) and Oncotype DX (Genomic Health, Redwood City, CA), THEROS Breast Cancer Index^{SM}, Molecular Grade Index (Aviara MGI^{SM}), Mammostrat™, BreastOncPx™, and PAM50 Breast Cancer Intrinsic Classifier tests. Although the change in breast cancer management and remission rate related to these products remains to be established, such successful translation of gene profiling to the clinics provides a strong rationale for similar approaches in other disciplines. Nonetheless, these tests are still not recommended by the American Society of Clinical Oncology and they are still considered investigational.

3.2 Type-I interferon signature

Immune gene profiling has been performed for several conditions, notably AID, although, lack of open data sharing policies in this field is delaying development. We and others recently reviewed progress in one of the most common AID, rheumatoid arthritis (RA), with the conclusion that gene expression profiling offers clear potential for understanding RA biology as well as for patient management and personalization of treatment decisions (Burska et al., 2014b; Van Baarsen et al., 2010a,b; Lindberg et al., 2010). There are, however, many technical (biological, material, platform, custom or commercial arrays), statistical (wide range of analytical procedures, reference databases, etc.), and clinical (mainly differences in patient characteristics and types of outcome used) reasons for the discordances reported so far. Future progress will depend on larger studies able to combine output and harmonize outcome measures.

Nonetheless, the interferon (IFN) gene pathway has been highlighted in several studies of different AID. IFNs are divided into three groups: type-I (including 13 IFN-α; and one each of IFN-β, -ε, -κ, and -ω), type-II (IFN-γ), and type-III (3 isoforms of IFN-λ: IFN-λ1, λ2, and λ3). Signatures implicate the type-I IFNs that regulate the global immune response (Biron, 2001), notably at antigen-presentation level and by mediating antiviral effects and tissue damage in response to pathogen recognition by immune cells. IFN-mediated responses can affect the initiation or amplification of autoimmunity and tissue damage through their diverse and broad actions on almost every cell type and by promoting T helper 1 (Th1) responses (Van Baarsen et al., 2009).

Type-I IFN responses were therefore implicated in a number of (auto)immune disorders such as systemic lupus erythematosus (SLE) (Baechler et al., 2003), systemic sclerosis (SSc) (Brkic et al., 2013), RA (Gordon et al., 2012; Lübbers et al., 2013), Sjogren's syndrome (SS) (Mavragani and Crow, 2010), multiple sclerosis (MS) (Verweij and Vosslamber, 2013), dermatomyositis (Baechler et al., 2007), type 1 diabetes mellitus (T1DM) (Reynier et al., 2010) and psoriatic arthritis (PsA) (Yao et al., 2008). Activation of an IFN-gene expression program therefore appears a common denominator in chronic inflammatory diseases (Rönnblom and Eloranta, 2013; Niewold, 2014).

Studies have focussed on IFN-β in RA (Lübbers et al., 2013), while those in SLE place greater emphasis on IFN-α (Crow, 2010, 2014; Obermoser and Pascual, 2010) with much better consistency in SLE than in other diseases thus far (Feng et al., 2006, 2014; Lauwerys et al., 2013). A type-I IFN signature was recently included in a clinical trial design as pharmacodynamic biomarkers for anti-IFN-α monoclonal antibody treatment in SLE (Yao et al., 2009a,b). IFN-β is released from fibroblast-like synoviocytes (FLS), macrophages, and dendritic cells (DCs), which play important roles in the initiation and persistence of synovial inflammation in RA (Roelofs et al., 2009; Van Holten et al., 2005). A predictive signature in RA was also suggested for the response to rituximab (B-cells depleting therapy) (Thurlings et al., 2010). Both the data in SLE and RA are promising of a future role for such signatures in personalizing medicine for stratifying patients to the correct drug (Häupl et al., 2011; Baechler et al., 2003).

3.3 MicroRNAs

MicroRNAs (miRNAs) are small noncoding RNAs that, upon base pairing to a messenger RNA (mRNA), mediate its cleavage, resulting in mRNA destabilization. They play a crucial role in the regulation of gene expression by repressing protein production. Given their impressive stability in serum or plasma, the limited number of miRNA allowing complete profiling, their simple chemical composition, and the availability of advanced and highly sensitive screening and quantification techniques, miRNAs are ideal biomarker candidates. The aberrant expression of miRNA can also reflect chromosomal abnormalities, mutations, SNPs, transcriptional deregulation, defects in the miRNA biogenesis machinery, and epigenetic changes.

The modulation of miRNA expression was shown to be characteristic of some diseases, allowing the identification of specific miRNA signatures for diagnosis (Ammari et al., 2013). Furthermore, evidence that miRNAs themselves might be involved in diseases was suggested by the detection of autoantibodies against certain proteins and other components of the RNAi machinery (Bhanji et al., 2007). However, while the involvement of miRNAs appears consensual in many diseases, a precise description of their cellular origin and the identification of their physiologically relevant targets are still lacking; yet this is a critical point, as miRNAs can exert opposite activities depending on the mRNA (and consequently the cell type) they are targeting. Therefore, the pathogenic role of miRNA remains to be elucidated in most diseases, although it appears that their disrupted function may be related to diseases, either caused by or causing the disruption; for example, miRNA involved in bone metabolic disease were shown to regulate osteogenesis and chondrogenesis (Dong et al., 2012). In RA functional dysregulation of miRNA revealed a role for cytokines in upregulating their expression (Pauley et al., 2008; Murata et al., 2010; Duroux-Richard et al., 2012, 2014).

To date, the use of miRNA for predicting response to therapies has been reported in many studies, so far mostly in cancer (Fu et al., 2011; Kuner et al., 2013; Selth et al., 2014; Hur et al., 2014). miRNA targeting immunological processes with respect to patient stratification has not been reported yet, although a miRNA that predicts response to a particular type of therapy (B-cell depletion with rituximab) across diseases (B-cell lymphoma and RA) has been reported (Duroux-Richard et al., 2014) suggesting that common processes can be targeted by miRNA. Altogether, miRNA have promising biomarker values but have not yet reached the point of clinical use with the exception of cancer where most advances have been made.

4. PROTEIN BIOMARKERS

4.1 Cytokines and receptors of cytokines

Cytokines have a pivotal role in many diseases and, notably, in inflammatory and AID. Cytokines usually circulate at very low levels (picomolar 10^{-12}); however, their concentration can increase up to 1000-fold when required. Despite sharing sequence homology and the promiscuity of their receptor, cytokines are highly specific in their function, notably, with opposing effects for different members of the same family. Methods for cytokines detection have considerably evolved, although ELISAs remain considered the "gold standard" in many cases, due to interferences from heterophillic antibodies in some other solid phase assays (Prince et al., 1973; Hunter and Budd, 1980; Howanitz et al., 1982; Zweig et al., 1987; Benoist et al., 1998; Boscato and Stuart, 1988; Nahm and Hoffmann, 1990), in particular rheumatoid factor (RF) in AID (Martins, 2002; De Jager et al., 2005; De Jager and Rijkers, 2006; Hueber et al., 2007; Churchman et al., 2012). We recently reviewed the value of cytokines as biomarkers in RA and the issue and concerns raised by their measurement (Burska et al., 2014a). These concerns apply to many other diseases but cytokines and chemokines (also growth factors) remain important classes of possible biomarkers notably for diagnosis (Dinan et al., 2006; Chun et al., 2007; Othman et al., 2008; Prince, 2005; Lembo et al., 2009; Rhodus et al., 2005; Goëb et al., 2013) and response to therapy (Das et al., 2014).

With respect to predicting response to treatment, many studies have proposed profiles of up to 15 cytokines as being predictive (Wright et al., 2012; Lindberg et al., 2006; Van Der Pouw Kraan et al., 2008; Marotte et al., 2005; Koczan et al., 2008; Smith et al., 2001; Fabre et al., 2008). A 24-biomarker signature combining autoantibodies and cytokines allowed the prediction of clinical response to one of the three anti-TNF agents across three RA cohorts (Hueber et al., 2009). However, a multivariate logistic regression analysis of cytokines also showed that expression at baseline could only explain ~10–15% of the variance in response to TNF-blockade in RA (Wijbrandts et al., 2008), suggesting that profiling itself would have a limited role in relation to personalized medicine. ELISA being costly, many groups resorted to use gene expression profiling of cytokines (using custom-based array including up to 100 candidates) with similar issues of nonreproducibility (Häupl et al., 2010; Stuhlmüller et al., 2005; Lequerré et al., 2006; Julià et al., 2009; Zivojinovic et al., 2012).

Similarly, many soluble receptors of cytokines have been reported to have biomarker value mostly in inflammatory disease severity and/or mortality. Chronic kidney disease is associated with higher levels of inflammatory biomarkers. Higher soluble TNF-receptor is associated with faster rates of kidney function deterioration (Tonelli et al., 2005). Elevated plasma levels of soluble TNF receptors were also associated with morbidity and mortality in patients with acute lung injury (Parsons et al., 2005). The soluble form of the interleukin-1 receptor (ST2 gene) is detectable in the serum of patients with severe chronic heart failure, is increased in those with neurohormonal activation (Weinberg et al., 2003) and is an independent predictor of subsequent mortality. Cytokines contribute to the development and progression of heart failure, are implicated in depressive disorders and circulating levels of inflammatory cytokines were directly associated with comorbid depression (Moorman et al., 2007). Receptor antagonist such as the IL-2RA has been shown to effectively discriminate patients with and without GVHD and to predict survival independently of GVHD grade (Paczesny et al., 2009).

Altogether, the use of soluble protein markers such as cytokines, chemokines, growth factors, and their receptors has been proposed on many occasions and it is possible that with time and more studies showing reproducibility, some of these may develop into clinically relevant markers.

4.2 Total immunoglobulin levels (IgM, IgG, IgE, IgA)

Patients with persistently low levels of one of the Ig subclasses may have a selective Ig-deficiency. IgG subclass deficiency is notably related to many diseases causing recurrent bacterial and viral infections (often respiratory). It is therefore critical to distinguish recurrent infections caused by viruses from those due to antibody deficiency. Often additional Ig-specificities need to be determined for precise diagnosis and treatment initiation. Furthermore, IgG-subclass (IgG1, IgG2, IgG3, IgG4) deficiencies must be separated from total IgG deficiency. Measurement of IgG subclass levels is not universally recommended for the evaluation of antibody-mediated immunity (due to cost and the need for repeated assessment as IgG subclass levels fluctuate over time).

Infection observed in immunodeficiencies are typically upper and lower respiratory tract infections (sinusitis, bronchitis, pneumonia) and gastroenteritis, and sometimes serious bacterial infections (meningitis, sepsis) leading to chronic diarrhea and failure to thrive, especially when caused by unusual viruses (adenovirus) or fungi (*Cryptosporidium*). Other signs include skin lesions (eczema, warts, abscesses, pyoderma, alopecia), oral or esophageal thrush, oral ulcers, and periodontitis. Such deficiency is also characteristic of primary immunodeficiency diseases, such as Wiskott-Aldrich syndrome and ataxia-telangiectasia as well as being associated with other Ig-subclass deficiencies (notably IgA). More significant antibody and immunoglobulin deficiencies, such as agammaglobulinemia or common variable immune deficiency (CVID) are also associated with characteristic serum IgG changes. Recently, a number of inflammatory diseases, including some forms of pancreatitis, were found to be associated with an elevated IgG4 level (Kamisawa and Okamoto, 2006). The causes for this elevation are unclear at this point.

Selective IgA deficiency is a primary immunodeficiency characterized by an undetectable level of IgA without other Ig deficiencies. Most IgA is present in secretions (at mucosal surfaces, including tears, saliva, colostrum, genital, respiratory, and gastrointestinal) playing a major role in protecting from infections in these areas. IgA deficiency is one of the most common primary immunodeficiency diseases, with 1/500 people affected, although with differences in rate associated with ethnic origins. IgA deficiency produces only mild symptoms of recurrent infection, therefore is often undiagnosed, with a very variable rate of progressing to a more serious condition. Associated IgG2 and/or IgG4 deficiency is thought to be relevant to the development of complications. IgA deficiencies are also often associated with AID (RA, SLE, immune thrombocytopenic purpura, and gastrointestinal AID). Allergies may also be more common among individuals with selective IgA deficiency, notably food allergies. The diagnosis of selective IgA deficiency is established when blood tests demonstrate undetectable levels of IgA (reported usually as <5–7 mg/dl), with normal levels of the other major classes of immunoglobulins (IgG and IgM). It is not currently possible to replace IgA in patients and it remains to be seen if replacement of IgA will be beneficial, in part because IgA in the serum does not remain in the circulation for very long.

Patients with hyperimmunoglobulin M (HIgM) syndrome have an inability to switch from the production of antibodies of the IgM type to antibodies of the IgG, IgA, or IgE types. As a result, patients with this disease have decreased levels of IgG and IgA but normal or elevated levels of IgM in their blood. Normally, B-cells produce IgM after activation by an antigen, but they need help from T cells to switch to IgG, IgA, or IgE. HIgM results from a variety of genetic defects (X-linked, CD40 deficiency, CD40Ligand deficiency, NEMO deficiency syndrome) that affect this interaction between T and B-cells. High levels of IgM are therefore used to diagnose HIgM syndrome, which is confirmed with further genetic testing.

Recurrent or chronic infections of the upper airways need comprehensive treatment to prevent permanent damage. Management includes the use of antibiotics to treat or prevent infections. IgG therapy is an option in the most severe cases that will use IgG-measurement as part of the clinical indication for this therapy when the more conservative treatments have failed. Additional tests such as failure to respond to a vaccine challenge are also mandatory with documented lack of response to antibiotics and sometimes chest X-rays. IgG subclass deficiencies also need to be monitored in children as some outgrow the disease, although testing usually requires a temporary discontinuation of IgG-replacement therapy.

4.3 AGE and RAGE, proteoglycan

Glycosylation is an important posttranslational modification that has a significant influence on the biological functioning of proteins. Glycan processing pathways are complex and reflect the environment both within and outside cells. These pathways are frequently disrupted in diseases such as cancer, congenital disorders of glycosylation, and inflammatory diseases, giving rise to the aberrant glycosylation of disease-related proteins (Rudd et al., 2001b; Marino et al., 2011). Glycoproteins are mixtures of glycosylated variants in which a protein is modified by the attachment of a heterogeneous collection of sugars at each glycosylation site. Advanced glycation end products (AGEs) interact with specific receptors (RAGE), inducing proinflammatory states involved in several diseases. The soluble forms of RAGE (sRAGE) also interact with AGE and are anti-inflammatory.

Many chronic inflammatory diseases are characterized by reduced levels of sRAGE (Maillard-Lefebvre et al., 2009). Many glycoproteins present in human serum are key components of the native and adaptive immune system (Rudd et al., 2001a). Immunoglobulins are important products of the humoral immune response and are heavily glycosylated with N-linked glycosylation sites located in the Fc and Fab region of the molecules (Arnold et al., 2007). Changes in serum protein glycosylation during disease have been extensively studied and present an interesting and promising basis for diagnosis, etiopathology, and therapy (Albrecht et al., 2014).

Glycated hemoglobin (*hemoglobin A1c, HbA_{1c}, A1C*, or Hb_{1c} HbA1c) is a form of hemoglobin that is measured primarily to identify the average plasma glucose concentration over prolonged periods of time. As the average amount of plasma glucose increases, the fraction of glycated hemoglobin increases in a predictable way. This serves as a marker for average blood glucose levels over the previous 2–3 months (ie, half-life of red blood cells). Monitoring HbA_{1c} has been widely used for the diagnosis of diabetes, although ambiguity remains regarding the use of HbA1c for the identification of prediabetes (Larsen et al., 1990). HbA1c is used for risk-stratification approaches for diabetes prevention (Gregg et al., 2013). Because HbA1c predicts diabetes and related outcomes across a wide range of HbA1c values the choice of optimal thresholds is currently a trade-off, wherein selecting a lower HbA1c cut-off point will lead to a higher rate of eligibility and health benefits for more people, while a higher HbA1c cut-off point will lead to fewer cases of diabetes prevented but greater "economic efficiency" in terms of cases prevented per intervention participant.

Altogether, the use of most protein biomarkers, AGEs/RAGEs, and other proteoglycans for stratified medicine represent potentially interesting future developments but are still at the development stage.

5. AUTOANTIBODIES

5.1 Diagnosis

Autoantibodies are the result of a failure of the immune system to discriminate between "self" and "nonself," which target a person's own antigen. Autoantibodies react with self-protein, cells, tissues, and/or organs, causing inflammation, damage, and/or dysfunction of organs, resulting in autoimmune disorders. Therefore, autoantibodies are prime candidates for diagnostic tests as illustrated in Table 1. Furthermore, some of these antibodies can be directly implicated in the pathogenesis of these diseases (Graves disease, thyroiditis), whereas others are thought to be secondary to the overall immune response (celiac disease and DMT1). High prevalence of various autoimmune conditions in families also suggests a genetic predisposition to autoantibody development. Testing for the presence of autoantibodies is often central to the diagnosis of an AID (Niewold et al., 2007; Avouac et al., 2006). For some, the levels and/or the diversity of autoantibodies may help classify the severity of the condition and disease progression.

Examples of using autoantibodies to monitor or predict response to treatment remain rare. Clinically significant autoantibodies are mostly of the IgG class, suggesting a fully developed immune response with T–B cells interactions. Although some autoreactivities can be observed in the IgM class, these are not always associated with disease. For example, IgM anticitrullinated peptide antibody (ACPA) are observed in up to 30% of the healthy population (Vincent et al., 1989), whereas IgG-ACPA, which are disease-specific, are present in only 1-2% and are associated with a 50% increased risk of progressing to RA (Rakieh et al., 2014). Plasma cells producing these antibodies are relatively insensitive to regulation (residing in protected environmental niches); therefore, levels of autoantibodies rarely normalize. For example, monitoring levels and specificities of ACPA following therapeutic B-cell depletion have showed only modest reductions in titers (reflecting the depletion of memory and short-lived plasma B-cells) (Vital et al., 2014; Vis et al., 2008), in contrast to the reduction in IgM-RF, another autoantibody commonly observed in several AID. With respect to stratification, autoantibody levels are mostly associated with severity and more rapid disease progression; ACPA, for example, has been shown to highly correlate with a rapid radiologic progression of RA (Van Der Woude et al., 2010; Mustila et al., 2010).

5.2 Antibodies against HLA

Hyperacute rejection of a transplanted organ has been clearly associated with the presence of anti-HLA antibodies (Terasaki et al., 1971; Terasaki and Ozawa, 2005; Terasaki and Cai, 2005). The role of anti-HLA antibodies in transplant rejection has been linked to immune-complex deposition in the graft, resulting in organ ischemia (Hanf et al., 2014; Legendre, 2014). Therefore, the presence of donor anti-HLA antibodies indicates an increased risk of acute rejection and reduced graft survival (Kim et al., 2014). The detection of anti-HLA antibodies prior to transplantation has also been shown to be

Table 1 Autoantibodies currently used for diagnosing a number of conditions

Autoantibody	Antibody target	Condition
Antinuclear antibodies	Ribonucleoproteins	Systemic lupus erythematosus, neonatal heart block
		Primary Sjögren's syndrome
	Centromere	Calcinosis, Reynaud's phenomenon, esophageal dysmotility, sclerodactyly and telangiectasia (CREST) syndrome
	Double-stranded DNA	Systemic lupus erythematosus
	Histidine-tRNA ligase	Inflammatory myopathy
	Ribonucleoprotein	Mixed connective tissue disease
	snRNP core proteins	Systemic lupus erythematosus
	Type I topoisomerase	Systemic sclerosis (anti-Scl-70 antibodies)
	Histones	Systemic lupus erythematosus and drug-induced LE
	Nucleoporin 62	Primary biliary cirrhosis
	Sp100 nuclear antigen	
	Nucleoporin 210 kDa	
Antitransglutaminase antibodies	Transglutaminase	Celiac disease, dermatitis herpetiformis
Anti-ganglioside antibodies	Ganglioside GQ1B	Miller-Fisher syndrome
	Ganglioside GD3	Acute motor axonal neuropathy
	Ganglioside GM1	Multifocal motor neuropathy
Antiactin antibodies	Actin	Celiac disease
Anti-CCP	Cyclic citrullinated peptide	Rheumatoid arthritis
Liver kidney microsomal type 1 antibody		Autoimmune hepatitis
Antithrombin	Thrombin	Systemic lupus erythematosus
Antiphospholipid antibodies	Phospholipid	Antiphospholipid syndrome
Antineutrophil cytoplasmic antibody	Proteins in neutrophil cytoplasm	Wegener's granulomatosis
	Neutrophil perinuclear	Microscopic polyangiitis Churg-Strauss syndrome Systemic vasculitides
Rheumatoid factor	IgG	Rheumatoid arthritis
Antismooth muscle antibody	Smooth muscle	Chronic autoimmune hepatitis
Antimitochondrial antibody	Mitochondria	Primary biliary cirrhosis

Continued

Table 1 Autoantibodies currently used for diagnosing a number of conditions—Cont'd

Autoantibody	Antibody target	Condition
Antisignal recognition particle	Signal recognition particle	Polymyositis
	Exosome complex	Scleromyositis
Antiacetyl choline receptor	Nicotinic acetylcholine receptor	Myasthenia gravis
Anti-MuSK	Muscle-specific kinase (MUSK)	Myasthenia gravis
Antivoltage-gated calcium channels	Voltage-gated calcium channel (P/Q-type)	Lambert-Eaton myasthenic syndrome
Antithyroid autoantibodies	Hashimoto's thyroiditis	Graves' disease
	Thyroglobulin	Hashimoto's thyroiditis
	TSH receptor	Graves' disease
Anti-Hu (ANNA-1)	Neuronal nuclear proteins	Paraneoplastic cerebellar degeneration, limbic encephalitis, encephalomyelitis Subacute sensory neuronopathy, choreathetosis
Anti-Yo	Cerebellar Purkinje cells	Paraneoplastic cerebellar degeneration
Anti-Ma		Encephalomyelitis, limbic encephalitis
Anti-Ri (ANNA-2)	Neuronal nuclear proteins	Opsoclonus myoclonus syndrome
Anti-Tr	Glutamate receptor	Paraneoplastic cerebellar syndrome
Antiamphiphysin	Amphiphysin	Stiff person syndrome, paraneoplastic cerebellar degeneration
Antiglutamic acid decarboxylase	Glutamate decarboxylase	Stiff Person Syndrome, type 1 diabetes mellitus (T1DM)
Antivoltage-gated potassium channels	Voltage-gated potassium channel (VGKC)	Limbic encephalitis, Isaac's syndrome
Anticollapsin response mediator protein-5	Collapsin response mediator protein-5	Optic neuropathy, chorea
	Basal Ganglia neurons	Sydenham's chorea, pediatric autoimmune neuropsychiatric disease associated with *Streptococcus*
Anti-*N*-methyl-D-aspartate receptor	*N*-methyl-D-aspartate receptor (NMDA)	Anti-NMDA receptor encephalitis
Neuromyelitis optica antibody	Aquaporin-4	Neuromyelitis Optica (Devic's syndrome)

predictive of graft rejection (Smith et al., 2014) and reducing these antibodies before transplantation improves outcomes (Gergis et al., 2014). Posttransplant, de novo development of donor anti-HLA antibodies is especially deleterious (Gerlach et al., 2014). Maintaining low antibody levels posttransplantation or to treat rejection, for example, using B cell depletion (Vieira et al., 2004), is also essential and is a measure of therapeutic efficacy. The detection of these antibodies in histocompatibility laboratories has therefore been instrumental in reducing the rate of hyperacute rejection. Complement dependent test, enzyme-linked immunosorbent assays (ELISAs) and flow cytometry have been successfully used to detect anti-HLA antibodies and are now routinely followed by an immune-beads detection system (Luminex).

5.3 Antidrug antibodies and other idiotypic antibodies

Antibodies (with other therapeutic proteins) are at the heart of the most recent therapies developed for several types of diseases, due to their high specificity for their target. As successful as antibody-mediated therapies are, they lose their efficacy over time due to the neutralization of the therapeutic molecule by the development of antibodies neutralizing therapeutic agents has been an important drawback of recent therapies using proteins as therapeutic agents (Sorensen et al., 2003; Satoh et al., 2006). As such, authorities (like the FDA or the EDA) have released guidance (Guidance for Industry-Immunogenicity Assessment for Therapeutic Protein Products, August 2014) on how to assess and limit the immunogenicity of protein products used as therapeutics and recommend approaches to evaluate and mitigate immune responses to or adverse immunologically related events associated with therapeutic protein products that may affect their safety and efficacy. Primary protein sequence (despite conservation between species or due to nucleotide polymorphisms), higher-order structure (fusion or bioengineered proteins may create neoepitopes), species of origin (xenogenic response), posttranscriptional modification (oxidation, deamidation, aldehyde modification, deamination, glycosylation), and the molecular weight of therapeutic proteins are all important factors that may contribute to their immunogenicity (Hudson and Souriau, 2003). Antibodies against drugs have therefore become biomarkers of non-response or loss of response to the initial agent (Van Schouwenburg et al., 2012). They are measured to determine the cause of loss of response and adjust treatment (Polman et al., 2010; Hegen et al., 2014; Radstake et al., 2009). As most therapeutic antibodies are derived from human or humanized antibodies, the immunogenic epitopes for the induction of antidrug antibodies lie within the regions of the protein that recognized the antigen.

6. CELL-BASED BIOMARKERS

Flow cytometry is now a well-adopted technology in hospital routine services allowing for an increasing number of clinical applications. Flow cytometry is a powerful tool for detailed analysis of complex populations of cells in a short period of time, both qualitatively and quantitatively. Immunophenotyping of cell subsets including up to 13 parameters can be achieved from any body fluid (blood, fluids from different compartments, urine, bone marrow) as well as from solid tissues following enzymatic digestion. DNA and RNA content analysis are also possible in addition to cell membrane-bound and intracellular proteins.

6.1 $CD4^+$ T-cell monitoring

HIV-infected patients need constant monitoring of their $CD4^+$ T-cell numbers. Flow cytometry offers the best way to achieve this safely. Absolute CD4 count provides a powerful and rapid tool for adapting treatment strategies. Quantifying viral load (most often using qPCR) remains an important complementary test that is inversely correlated with CD4 counts (Brown and Wittwer, 2000; Saag et al., 1996; Mellors et al., 1996). Both tests are essential for the management of HIV-infected patients, with CD4 counts reflecting more directly the patient's immune status. CD4 counts of a healthy adult range from 500–1200 cells/mm^3. Once infected by HIV, a patient's $CD4^+$ T-cells are attacked and killed by the virus, which uses the $CD4^+$ T-cells as a "self-replicating factory."

Residual CD4 counts are often the best way to measure a patient's remaining immune competence. In an asymptomatic infected person, CD4 count tests are performed every 3-6 months. CD4 counts of below 500–600 cells/mm^3 indicate the beginning of the AIDS process; hence, regular CD4 counts track virus progression. Once on therapy, drugs are intended to prevent further virus development and increasing weekly CD4 counts represent the best indicator of how efficient therapy is. Treatment guidelines have been produced and in the United Kingdom the British HIV Association recommends to start HIV treatment in people with a CD4 T-cell count $\leq$350 cells/mm^3. Similar guidelines were published for the NIH (http://aidsinfo.nih.gov/guidelines, December 2014) and other health authorities worldwide.

6.2 Multiple parameter flow cytometry (MPFC)

The ability to analyze multiple cellular characteristics, along with the development of new dyes allowing multistep gating strategies, has magnified the utility of flow cytometry in the diagnosis of several hematological disorders such as leukemia and lymphoma. These present subtle differences in their antigen profiles that make flow cytometry an ideal tool differentiating between the two. Over the past 20 years, combinations of signals for several cell surface markers/side scatter patterns have been established (Table 2) and diagnostic interpretation achieved through this, which also established lineage assignment. Cell immunophenotyping is therefore a key test approach to apply risk-adapted therapeutic protocols. Furthermore, the expression of certain phenotypes such as multidrug resistant leukemia can also be identified by the expression of the MDR-1 protein using flow cytometry (Hegewisch-Becker et al., 1996).

Table 2 Antibodies to define leukemia and lymphomas

Leukemia and lymphomas	Markers
B-cell acute lymphoblastic leukemia	CD19, CD79a, CD34 Terminal deoxynucleotidyl transferase
T-cell acute lymphoblastic leukemia	CD3, CD7, CD34 Terminal deoxynucleotidyl transferase
Acute myeloid leukemia	CD13, CD33, CD34, CD15, HLA-DR Cytoplasmic myeloperoxidase
B-cell lymphoproliferative syndrome	CD19/CD20, CD5, CD22, CD23, CD11c, CD25, CD103
T-cell lymphoproliferative syndrome	CD3/CD4/CD8, TCR
NK cell lymphoproliferative syndrome	CD3/CD16/CD56, CD2, CD5, CD8

This is a nonexhaustive list of the most common markers used in MPFC.

6.3 Immune deficiencies

Immunodeficiency (see previous section) need to be distinguished from recurrent infections due to inadequate antibiotic treatment (see also the section on Ig measurements). Frequent use of antibiotics may mask many of the common symptoms; therefore, immune function testing is the most accurate diagnostic tool. Prenatal testing is available for many disorders and is indicated if there is a family history of immunodeficiency with a known genetic cause, allowing gene therapy in some cases. To determine whether or not recurrent infections could be due to primary immunodeficiency, several tests are used.

Treatments for primary immunodeficiency involve preventing and treating infections, boosting the immune system, and treating the underlying cause of the immune problem. Infections are typically treated with antibiotics. Additional medications may be needed to relieve symptoms caused by infections such as pain and fever, congestion, and airways blocks. Immunoglobulin replacement therapy by injection can be a lifesaver for people with this condition. Monitoring of Ig levels is therefore critical to adjusting treatment. Gamma interferon therapy can treat chronic granulomatous disease. Growth factors, such as granulocyte-macrophage colony-stimulating factor (GMCSF) and granulocyte colony-stimulating factor (GCSF) can strengthen immune white blood cell functions.

6.4 Regulatory T-cells

The immune system aims to discriminate between self and nonself, although it is not always successful and autoreactive T-cells are released in the circulation. Regulatory T cells (Tregs), also known as suppressor T cells, are a subpopulation of T cells that can inhibit the activation and proliferation of T cells in order to maintain peripheral tolerance to self-antigens. This critical role that Tregs play within the immune system is evidenced in immunodysregulation polyendocrinopathy enteropathy X-linked (IPEX) syndrome, a rare disease linked to the dysfunction of the transcription factor FOXP3, the master regulator of the Treg lineage (Yong et al., 2008). Many models (both animal and human diseases) have implicated Tregs in infections, organ transplantation, AID, and cancer. While suppression by Treg may prevent the development of AID, it is not desirable during immune responses to infectious microorganisms or cancer cells. Current hypotheses suggest that several pathogens and cancer cells have developed means of evading the immune system by manipulating Tregs to suppress the host immune system and so potentiate their own survival. For example, Treg activity is increased in several retroviral infections (the most dangerous being HIV) but also mycobacterial infections (tuberculosis) and various parasitic infections (*Leishmania* and malaria). $CD4^+$ Treg are also increased in numbers in solid tumors and number of Tregs (notably, in breast, colorectal, and ovarian cancers) often indicates a poor prognosis (Dranoff, 2005). The use of flow cytometry to monitor Treg frequency in the blood of patients has therefore became an important tool for the management of these diseases.

Flow cytometry remains the method of choice for rapid quantification of the Treg. A phenotypic consensus ($CD3^+$ $CD4^+$ $CD25^{high}$, $FOXp3^+$, and $CD127^{low}$) took over 10 years to be established and the initial discrepancies in Treg quantification hampered the field for some more years. Unique combinations of markers are indeed required to distinguish cell populations by flow. Several markers have been proposed for human Treg, but so far the only reproducible human markers are CD25, CD127, and Foxp3. The continuum of CD25 expression from none to high levels complicated gating strategies as only cells exhibiting the highest levels of CD25 ($CD25^{high}$) have regulatory functions (Baecher-Allan et al., 2002). This posed a challenge for several years until the development of an accurate strategy for the quantification of Treg in health and disease was facilitated by the discovery of Foxp3 and CD127 as additional marker till the combinations giving the unique Treg phenotype (Baecher-Allan et al., 2002; Hori et al., 2003; Liu et al., 2006; Seddiki et al., 2006).

Therefore a number of studies report conflicting data, the frequency of human Treg in healthy controls (HC) varying from below 1% to above 10% and increasing with age (for review see Ponchel et al., 2014). Similarly, Treg frequencies in human conditions have been reported as being higher or lower than HC for several diseases. For example, we reported reduced frequency of Treg in RA patients (Lawson et al., 2006), whereas others reported higher (Van Amelsfort et al., 2004) or no difference (Cao et al., 2003, 2004). Another factor contributing to this was the use of several different commercially available antibody clones (not all recognizing the same epitope on their target) as well as frozen and fresh cells and different gating strategies (Ponchel et al., 2014).

In cancer two main strategies have been developed that either use (monitoring and stratification) or target Treg (with anti-Treg drugs). Monitoring Treg is therefore an important tool in clinical trials (in lung, renal, pancreas, colon, head and neck, breast, ovary, and prostate cancers as well as melanoma, multiple myeloma, leukemia, lymphoma, sarcoma, etc.) (Table 3) where it is considered a measure of therapeutic success. On the other hand, several innovative drugs have been recently developed (cell-based therapies, tumor antigen vaccines, monoclonal antibodies) that target Treg themselves trying to eradicate them (Table 3). These are mostly ongoing but are very promising with respect to the use of Treg in stratified medicine in the near future.

6.5 Other T cell subsets

Over the past 10 years, our group has focussed on demonstrating the value of phenotyping T-cells in the blood of RA patients. After the initial discovery of the loss of naïve and regulatory $CD4^{+}$ T-cells and the appearance of IRC (an abnormal T-cell subset expressing both naïve and memory cell differentiation markers) (Ponchel et al., 2002; Lawson et al., 2006), the role and relevance of these defects was further investigated (Ponchel et al., 2005; Burgoyne et al., 2008; Verburg et al., 2005). The potential biomarker value of T-cell subsets was then demonstrated for the prediction of relapse in patients achieving

Table 3 Use of Tregs as a tool in clinical trials

Tregs are used for	Intervention/drug target	Tissue origin/cancer	Trial ref number
To monitor response to treatment	Allogenic tumor cell vaccine (K562) and antiinflammatory (Celecoxib)	Sarcoma, Melanoma	NCT01313429
	Aldesleukin (interleukin-2) and kinase inhibitor (Sorafenib)	Renal cancer, Melanoma	NCT00418496
	Aldesleukin (interleukin-2) and Ipilimumab (antibody targeting CTLA-4)	Recurrent melanoma	NCT02203604
	Angiogenesis inhibitor (Bevacizumab)	Glioblastoma multiform	NCT01091792
	CD54-positive PA2024-loaded antigen presenting cells (Sipuleucel-T)	Prostate cancer	NCT02237170
	CT-011 monoclonal antibody, with/without dendritic cell fusion vaccine	Multiple myeloma	NCT01067287
	CT-011 monoclonal antibody, dendritic cell fusion vaccine	Renal cell carcinoma	NCT01441765

Continued

Table 3 Use of Tregs as a tool in clinical trials—Cont'd

Tregs are used for	Intervention/drug target	Tissue origin/cancer	Trial ref number
	Cyclophosphamide and ZYC300 (plasmid DNA encoding an inactivated form of the carcinogen activator cytochrome P450 with potential antineoplastic activity)	Breast, ovarian, prostate, colon, and renal cancer	NCT00381173
	Cyclophosphamide and antibody targeting CTLA-4 (Ipilimumab)	Malignant melanoma	NCT01740401
	Cytidine analog (Decitabine) and NY-ESO-1 (cancer antigen) peptide vaccine	Ovarian, peritoneal cavity cancer	NCT01673217
	Interleukin-18 and B cell depletion (Rituximab)	B cell non-Hodgkin's lymphoma	NCT00500058
	LMB-2 immunotoxin and MART-1 antigens (cancer antigens), peptide of 27–35 amino acids, bound by MHC and presented to T cells	Melanoma/non-melanomatous skin cancer	NCT00295958
	Melanoma antigen peptide therapy	Melanoma	NCT01425749
	Natural killer cells	Metastatic nasopharyngeal	NCT00717184
	Phosphodiesterase inhibitor (Tadalafil)	Head and neck squamous cell carcinoma	NCT0169780
	Therapeutic cancer vaccine against the NGcGM3 neoantigen on cancer cells (Racotumomab)	Advanced lung cancer	NCT01460472
	Stem cell transplant, macrolide (Tacrolimus)	Graft vs. host disease	NCT00639717
	Therapeutic cancer vaccine against the NGcGM3 neoantigen on cancer cells (Racotumomab)	Advanced non-small cell lung cancer	NCT01240447
	VEGFR1-peptide VEGFR2-peptide and ribonucleotide reductase inhibitors (Gemcitabine)	Pancreatic cancer	NCT00655785

Table 3 Use of Tregs as a tool in clinical trials—Cont'd

Tregs are used for	Intervention/drug target	Tissue origin/cancer	Trial ref number
To predict response to treatment	Angiogensis inhibitor (Bevacizumab)	Glioblastoma, glioma	NCT01836536
	Angiogenesis inhibitor (Bevacizumab) and topoisomerase inhibitor (Irinotecan)	Metastatic colorectal cancer	NCT01533740
	Antineoplastic agent, combining interleukin-2 and diphtheria toxin (Ontak)	Ovarian, peritoneal cancer	NCT00880360
	Neuroblastoma vaccine, cyclophosphamide	High-risk neuroblastoma	NCT01192555
	Stem cell transplant	Breast cancer, chronic myeloproliferative disorder, gestational trophoblastic tumor, leukemia, lymphoma, multiple myeloma and plasma cell neoplasm, myelodysplastic syndromes, myelodysplastic/myeloproliferative neoplasms, neuroblastoma, ovarian cancer, testicular germ cell tumor	NCT00651716
Whether therapy reduce Tregs as proof of concept	4-Peptide melanoma vaccine and anti-neoplastic agent, combining interleukin-2 and diphtheria toxin (Ontak)	Melanoma	NCT00515528
	Allogenic tumor cell vaccine (K562) 7 anti-inflammatory (Celecoxib)	Lung, esophageal, mesotheliom, sarcoma, thymic carcinoma	NCT01143545
	Antineoplastic agent, combining interleukin-2 and diphtheria toxin (Ontak)	Melanoma	NCT00313235

Continued

Table 3 Use of Tregs as a tool in clinical trials—Cont'd

Tregs are used for	Intervention/drug target	Tissue origin/cancer	Trial ref number
	Antineoplastic agent, combining interleukin-2 and diphtheria toxin (Ontak) and dendritic cell vaccine	Ovarian cancer	NCT00703105
	Autologous cytokine-induced killer cells	Solid tumors	NCT01868490
	Cytidine analog (Decitabine)	Recurrent adult acute myeloid leukemia	NCT01758367
	Inhibitor of mTOR (Everolimus)	Metastatic renal cell cancer	NCT01462214
	Nephrectomy—to verify whether nephrectomy will lower peripheral Tregs in early stage renal cancer	Renal cell carcinoma	NCT00717743
	Phosphodiesterase inhibitor (Tadalafil)	Metastatic melanoma	NCT00314093
	Radiofrequency ablation	Hepatocellular carcinoma	NCT01668381
	RNA-loaded dendritic cell vaccine and antibody to CD25 (interleukin-2 receptor) on T cells (Basiliximab)	Glioblastoma, lymphopenia	NCT00626483
	Stem cell transplant from umbilical cord and total lymphoid irradiation	Hematological malignancies	NCT00763490
Safety of depleting Tregs	Peptide blocking the activity of URLC10, CDCA1, VEGFR1, and VEGFR2	Non-small cell lung cancer	NCT00874588/ NCT00633724
	Stem cell transplantation; antiinterleukin-2 (CD25) on T cells (Basiliximab)	Multiple myeloma	NCT01526096

remission after administering classic disease modifying antirheumatic drugs (Burgoyne et al., 2008) and biologics (Saleem et al., 2010) and recently for the prediction of MTX-induced remission in early RA (Ponchel et al., 2014). Over the years, data accumulated suggest a model where the thymus is affected in RA and produces fewer new T-cells (Ponchel et al., 2002) but also responds to lymphopenia much slower than in cancer (Ponchel et al., 2005). These defects are associated with a lack of IL-7 being expressed in RA bone marrow (Ponchel et al., 2005) and, by extrapolation, in the thymic epithelium. Naïve $CD4^{+}$ T-cells released in the circulation are therefore less numerous but are also subjected to an abnormal drive for differentiation under the pressure of circulating high levels of IL-6 and TNF resulting in the appearance of IRC (Ponchel et al., 2002). These IRCs also express chemokine receptors (CXCR3, CXCR4, and CCR5) (Burgoyne et al., 2008) that direct them toward inflamed tissue while the disease is active. They are hyperresponsive to stimuli (PHA, IL-2, CD3/CD28, but not recall antigen). In clinical remission such expression and hyperreactivity decreased, IRC then recirculated, and their persistence in the blood predicted relapse (Burgoyne et al., 2008). We also showed that regulatory T-cell frequency is reduced in early RA but can be reversed to healthy levels in clinical remission (Lawson et al., 2006).

These data lead us to investigate whether these cell subsets could have biomarker value. We first investigated whether they could predict safe discontinuation of biologics once clinical remission had been achieved for 6 months (Saleem et al., 2010). Data showed that the recovery of normal naïve $CD4^{+}$ T-cell frequency and low levels of IRC were associated with sustained remission upon stopping anti-TNF. More recently, we established that the presence of normal (age corrected) frequencies of naïve $CD4^{+}$ T-cells in early RA at baseline first treatment with MTX was predictive of the ability of these patients to achieve remission with 79% specificity and 62% (Ponchel et al., 2014). Finally, we showed that the progression toward RA from preclinical stages ($ACPA^{+}$ arthralgia) could be predicted using a multiple T-cell subset signature (manuscript submitted for publication). These data were sufficiently encouraging for the British NHS-routine Immunology Services of the Leeds NHS Trust teaching hospitals to initiate a transfer of technology project a year ago. We first established protocols under NHS-Good Laboratory Practice and compared parallel results obtained in both research and routine settings. If reproducible under NHS setup, these biomarkers could soon be used in clinical practice. This is a promising and to our knowledge unique recent case of transfer of technology, but is exemplary of the time (15 years) needed to take a discovery to clinical utility.

7. CONCLUSION

The road to biomarker development (for diagnosis, prognosis, or stratification) is a long and winding one. It usually takes 1–2 decades starting with discovery and basic research, to validation, clinical utility evaluation, manufacturing, development, and finally approval by regulatory authorities (further complicated by the difference in legislation between the European Union, the United States, and other parts of the world) (Neumaier, 2005). In many cases for novel technology-based tests there is also a need for the development of good laboratory practice guidelines to establish the limitation of its usage in routine clinical labs.

One of the most difficult challenges still facing stratified medicine is that findings obtained from large groups of patients that predict response to treatments at a population level are not always easy to translate to the individual patient level. This aspect of personalized medicine, despite much interest from patients and their families as well as interest groups, remains delicate to explain. The concept of "risk" and "odds" that are used to describe population features and behaviors in response to a treatment are difficult to convey to patients, and much work remains to be done in this area.

The most difficult hurdle to overcome remains the need for pooling together the necessary resources and to share already gathered information to reach appropriate conclusions and proceed with the final validation steps necessary to translate research findings into clinical practice. To date, the main problem in biomarker research remains being able to sufficiently power studies to detect differences among genetic variants, protein biomarkers, and/or the function of cell subsets between groups of patients. This is the challenge that the medical community faces if it wants to use translational research to develop personalized medicine in our modern society. Regulatory authorities, patient organizations, and other stakeholders may need leverage to overcome this challenge. However, the successful translation of novel technologies into clinical use in cancer is a promising example of the successes and provide strong rationale for the use of similar approaches in all medical disciplines.

ACKNOWLEDGMENTS

We would like to thank to Dr. Ruth Chisman, member of the staff of routine NHS Immunology Services at St. James University Hospital for her advice.

This work was supported by a European Union-funded FP7-integrated project Masterswitch No. 223404 and the IMI-funded project BeTheCure No. 115142–2.

FP is part-funded by the National Institute for Health Research (NIHR) through the Leeds Musculoskeletal Biomedical Research Unit.

REFERENCES

Albrecht, S., Unwin, L., Muniyappa, M., Rudd, P.M., 2014. Glycosylation as a marker for inflammatory arthritis. Cancer Biomark. 14, 17–28.

Amado, R.G., Wolf, M., Peeters, M., Van Cutsem, E., Siena, S., Freeman, D.J., Juan, T., Sikorski, R., Suggs, S., Radinsky, R., 2008. Wild-type KRAS is required for panitumumab efficacy in patients with metastatic colorectal cancer. J. Clin. Oncol. 26, 1626–1634.

Ammari, M., Jorgensen, C., Apparailly, F., 2013. Impact of microRNAs on the understanding and treatment of rheumatoid arthritis. Curr. Opin. Rheumatol. 25, 225–233.

Ansell, J., Hirsh, J., Hylek, E., Jacobson, A., Crowther, M., Palareti, G., 2008. Pharmacology and Management of the Vitamin k Antagonists*: American College of Chest Physicians Evidence-Based Clinical Practice Guidelines (8th ed.). Chest 133, 160S–198S.

Arnold, J.N., Wormald, M.R., Sim, R.B., Rudd, P.M., Dwek, R.A., 2007. The impact of glycosylation on the biological function and structure of human immunoglobulins. Annu. Rev. Immunol. 25, 21–50.

Avet-Loiseau, H., Attal, M., Moreau, P., Charbonnel, C., Garban, F., Hulin, C., Leyvraz, S., Michallet, M., Yakoub-Agha, I., Garderet, L., 2007. Genetic abnormalities and survival in multiple myeloma: the experience of the Intergroupe Francophone du Myelome. Blood 109, 3489–3495.

Avouac, J., Gossec, L., Dougados, M., 2006. Diagnostic and predictive value of anti-cyclic citrullinated protein antibodies in rheumatoid arthritis: a systematic literature review. Ann. Rheum. Dis. 65, 845–851.

Baecher-Allan, C., Viglietta, V., Hafler, D.A., 2002. Inhibition of human CD4(+)CD25(+ high) regulatory T cell function. J. Immunol. 169, 6210–6217.

Baechler, E.C., Batliwalla, F.M., Karypis, G., Gaffney, P.M., Ortmann, W.A., Espe, K.J., Shark, K.B., Grande, W.J., Hughes, K.M., Kapur, V., 2003. Interferon-inducible gene expression signature in peripheral blood cells of patients with severe lupus. Proc. Natl. Acad. Sci. U. S. A. 100, 2610–2615.

Baechler, E.C., Bauer, J.W., Slattery, C.A., Ortmann, W.A., Espe, K.J., Novitzke, J., Ytterberg, S.R., Gregersen, P.K., Behrens, T.W., Reed, A.M., 2007. An interferon signature in the peripheral blood of dermatomyositis patients is associated with disease activity. Mol. Med. 13, 59.

Benoist, J.F., Orbach, D., Biou, D., 1998. False increase in C-reactive protein attributable to heterophilic antibodies in two renal transplant patients treated with rabbit antilymphocyte globulin. Clin. Chem. 44, 1980–1985.

Berglin, E., Padyukov, L., Sundin, U., Hallmans, G., Stenlund, H., Van Venrooij, W.J., Klareskog, L., Dahlqvist, S.R., 2004. A combination of autoantibodies to cyclic citrullinated peptide (CCP) and HLA-DRB1 locus antigens is strongly associated with future onset of rheumatoid arthritis. Arthritis Res. Ther. 6, R303.

Bhanji, R.A., Eystathioy, T., Chan, E.K., Bloch, D.B., Fritzler, M.J., 2007. Clinical and serological features of patients with autoantibodies to GW/P bodies. Clin. Immunol. 125, 247–256.

Biron, C.A., 2001. Interferons α and β as immune regulators—a new look. Immunity 14, 661–664.

Boscato, L.M., Stuart, M.C., 1988. Heterophilic antibodies—a problem for all immunoassays. Clin. Chem. 34, 27–33.

Bossini-Castillo, L., De Kovel, C., Kallberg, H., Van'T Slot, R., Italiaander, A., Coenen, M., Tak, P., Posthumus, M., Wijmenga, C., Huizinga, T., 2015. A genome-wide association study of rheumatoid arthritis without antibodies against citrullinated peptides. Ann. Rheum. Dis. 74, e15.

Brkic, Z., van Bon, L., van Helden-Meeuwsen, C.G., Vonk, M.C., Knaapen, H., van Den Berg, W., Dalm, V.A., van Daele, P.L., Maria, N.I., Guillen, S., 2013. Systemic sclerosis patients with the interferon type I signature show faster disease development and high BAFF gene expression and collagen synthesis. In: Brkic, Z. (Ed.), Interferon Type I Driven Immune Activation in Generalized Autoimmune Diseases, p. 85 (Chapter 4).

Brown, M., Wittwer, C., 2000. Flow cytometry: principles and clinical applications in hematology. Clin. Chem. 46, 1221–1229.

Bullinger, L., Dohner, K., Bair, E., Frohling, S., Schlenk, R.F., Tibshirani, R., Dohner, H., Pollack, J.R., 2004. Use of gene-expression profiling to identify prognostic subclasses in adult acute myeloid leukemia. N. Engl. J. Med. 350, 1605–1616.

Burgoyne, C.H., Field, S.L., Brown, A.K., Hensor, E.M., English, A., Bingham, S.L., Verburg, R., Fearon, U., Lawson, C.A., Hamlin, P., 2008. Abnormal T cell differentiation persists in patients with rheumatoid arthritis in clinical remission and predicts relapse. Ann. Rheum. Dis. 67, 750–757.

Burska, A., Boissinot, M., Ponchel, F., 2014a. Cytokines as biomarkers in rheumatoid arthritis. Mediat. Inflamm. 2014, 24. Article ID 545493.

Burska, A., Roget, K., Blits, M., Gomez, L.S., Van De Loo, F., Hazelwood, L., Verweij, C., Rowe, A., Goulielmos, G., Van Baarsen, L., 2014b. Gene expression analysis in RA: towards personalized medicine. Pharmacogenomics J. 14, 93–106.

Canete, J., Suarez, B., Hernandez, M., Sanmarti, R., Rego, I., Celis, R., Moll, C., Pinto, J., Blanco, F., Lozano, F., 2009. Influence of variants of Fcγ receptors IIA and IIIA on the American College of Rheumatology and European League Against Rheumatism responses to anti-tumour necrosis factor α therapy in rheumatoid arthritis. Ann. Rheum. Dis. 68, 1547–1552.

Cao, D., Malmström, V., Baecher-Allan, C., Hafler, D., Klareskog, L., Trollmo, C., 2003. Isolation and functional characterization of regulatory CD25brightCD4+ T cells from the target organ of patients with rheumatoid arthritis. Eur. J. Immunol. 33, 215–223.

Cao, D.J., Van Vollenhoven, R., Klareskog, L., Trollmo, C., Malmstrom, V., 2004. CD25(bright)CD4(+) regulatory T cells are enriched in inflamed joints of patients with chronic rheumatic disease. Arthritis Res. Ther. 6, 335–346.

Chun, H.-Y., Chung, J.-W., Kim, H.-A., Yun, J.-M., Jeon, J.-Y., Ye, Y.-M., Kim, S.-H., Park, H.-S., Suh, C.-H., 2007. Cytokine IL-6 and IL-10 as biomarkers in systemic lupus erythematosus. J. Clin. Immunol. 27, 461–466.

Churchman, S., Geiler, J., Parmar, R., Horner, E., Church, L., Emery, P., Buch, M., Mcdermott, M., Ponchel, F., 2012. Multiplexing immunoassays for cytokine detection in the serum of patients with rheumatoid arthritis: lack of sensitivity and interference by rheumatoid factor. Clin. Exp. Rheumatol. 30, 534–542.

Colombo, P.-E., Milanezi, F., Weigelt, B., Reis-Filho, J.S., 2011. Microarrays in the 2010s: the contribution of microarray-based gene expression profiling to breast cancer classification, prognostication and prediction. Breast Cancer Res. 13, 212.

Coulthard, L.R., Taylor, J.C., Eyre, S., Robinson, J.I., Wilson, A.G., Isaacs, J.D., Hyrich, K., Emery, P., Barton, A., Barrett, J.H., 2011. Genetic variants within the MAP kinase signalling network and anti-TNF treatment response in rheumatoid arthritis patients. Ann. Rheum. Dis. 70, 98–103.

Criswell, L.A., Lum, R.F., Turner, K.N., Woehl, B., Zhu, Y., Wang, J., Tiwari, H.K., Edberg, J.C., Kimberly, R.P., Moreland, L.W., 2004. The influence of genetic variation in the HLA–DRB1 and LTA–TNF regions on the response to treatment of early rheumatoid arthritis with methotrexate or etanercept. Arthritis Rheum. 50, 2750–2756.

Crow, M.K., 2010. Type I interferon in organ-targeted autoimmune and inflammatory diseases. Arthritis Res. Ther. 12, S5.

Crow, M.K., 2014. Type I interferon in the pathogenesis of lupus. J. Immunol. 192, 5459–5468.

Das, S., Vital, E.M., Horton, S., Bryer, D., El-Sherbiny, Y., Rawstron, A.C., Ponchel, F., Emery, P., Buch, M.H., 2014. Abatacept or tocilizumab after rituximab in rheumatoid arthritis? An exploratory study suggests non-response to rituximab is associated with persistently high IL-6 and better clinical response to IL-6 blocking therapy. Ann. Rheum. Dis. 73, 909–912, annrheumdis-2013-204417.

De Jager, W., Rijkers, G.T., 2006. Solid-phase and bead-based cytokine immunoassay: a comparison. Methods 38, 294–303.

De Jager, W., Prakken, B.J., Bijlsma, J.W.J., Kuis, W., Rijkers, G.T., 2005. Improved multiplex immunoassay performance in human plasma and synovial fluid following removal of interfering heterophilic antibodies. J. Immunol. Methods 300, 124–135.

Dezentjé, V.O., Guchelaar, H.-J., Nortier, J.W., Van De Velde, C.J., Gelderblom, H., 2009. Clinical implications of CYP2D6 genotyping in tamoxifen treatment for breast cancer. Clin. Cancer Res. 15, 15–21.

Dinan, T.G., Quigley, E.M., Ahmed, S.M., Scully, P., O'brien, S., O'mahony, L., O'mahony, S., Shanahan, F., Keeling, P., 2006. Hypothalamic-pituitary-gut axis dysregulation in irritable bowel syndrome: plasma cytokines as a potential biomarker? Gastroenterology 130, 304–311.

Diogo, D., Okada, Y., Plenge, R.M., 2014. Genome-wide association studies to advance our understanding of critical cell types and pathways in rheumatoid arthritis: recent findings and challenges. Curr. Opin. Rheumatol. 26, 85–92.

Dong, S., Yang, B., Guo, H., Kang, F., 2012. MicroRNAs regulate osteogenesis and chondrogenesis. Biochem. Biophys. Res. Commun. 418, 587–591.

Dranoff, G., 2005. The therapeutic implications of intratumoral regulatory T cells. Clin. Cancer Res. 11, 8226–8229.

Duroux-Richard, I., Pers, Y.-M., Fabre, S., Ammari, M., Baeten, D., Cartron, G., Touitou, I., Jorgensen, C., Apparailly, F., 2014. Circulating miRNA-125b is a potential biomarker predicting response to rituximab in rheumatoid arthritis. Mediat. Inflamm. 2014, 9. Article ID 342524.

Duroux-Richard, I., Jorgensen, C., Apparailly, F., 2012. What do microRNAs mean for rheumatoid arthritis? Arthritis Rheum. 64, 11–20.

Emery, P., Dörner, T., 2011. Optimising treatment in rheumatoid arthritis: a review of potential biological markers of response. Ann. Rheum. Dis. 70, 2063–2070.

Fabre, S., Dupuy, A.M., Dossat, N., Guisset, C., Cohen, J.D., Cristol, J.P., Daures, J.P., Jorgensen, C., 2008. Protein biochip array technology for cytokine profiling predicts etanercept responsiveness in rheumatoid arthritis. Clin. Exp. Immunol. 153, 188–195.

Feng, X., Wu, H., Grossman, J.M., Hanvivadhanakul, P., Fitzgerald, J.D., Park, G.S., Dong, X., Chen, W., Kim, M.H., Weng, H.H., Furst, D.E., Gorn, A., Mcmahon, M., Taylor, M., Brahn, E., Hahn, B.H., Tsao, B.P., 2006. Association of increased interferon-inducible gene expression with disease activity and lupus nephritis in patients with systemic lupus erythematosus. Arthritis Rheum. 54, 2951–2962.

Feng, X., Huang, J., Liu, Y., Xiao, L., Wang, D., Hua, B., Tsao, B.P., Sun, L., 2014. Identification of interferon-inducible genes as diagnostic biomarker for systemic lupus erythematosus. Clin. Rheumatol., 1–9.

Fonseca, R., Blood, E., Rue, M., Harrington, D., Oken, M.M., Kyle, R.A., Dewald, G.W., Van Ness, B., Van Wier, S.A., Henderson, K.J., 2003. Clinical and biologic implications of recurrent genomic aberrations in myeloma. Blood 101, 4569–4575.

Fu, S.W., Chen, L., Man, Y.-G., 2011. miRNA biomarkers in breast cancer detection and management. J. Cancer 2, 116.

Gergis, U., Mayer, S., Gordon, B., Mark, T., Pearse, R., Shore, T., Van Besien, K., 2014. A strategy to reduce donor-specific HLA Abs before allogeneic transplantation. Bone Marrow Transplant. 49, 722–724.

Gerlach, U.A., Lachmann, N., Sawitzki, B., Arsenic, R., Neuhaus, P., Schoenemann, C., Pascher, A., 2014. Clinical relevance of the de novo production of anti-HLA antibodies following intestinal and multivisceral transplantation. Transpl. Int. 27, 280–289.

Goëb, V., Aegerter, P., Parmar, R., Fardellone, P., Vittecoq, O., Conaghan, P.G., Emery, P., Le Loët, X., Ponchel, F., 2013. Progression to rheumatoid arthritis in early inflammatory arthritis is associated with low IL-7 serum levels. Ann. Rheum. Dis. 72, 1032–1036.

Gordon, R.A., Grigoriev, G., Lee, A., Kalliolias, G.D., Ivashkiv, L.B., 2012. The interferon signature and STAT1 expression in rheumatoid arthritis synovial fluid macrophages are induced by tumor necrosis factor α and counter-regulated by the synovial fluid microenvironment. Arthritis Rheum. 64, 3119–3128.

Gorman, J.D., Criswell, L.A., 2002. The shared epitope and severity of rheumatoid arthritis. Rheum. Dis. Clin. N. Am. 28, 59–78.

Gregersen, P.K., Silver, J., Winchester, R.J., 1987. The shared epitope hypothesis. An approach to understanding the molecular genetics of susceptibility to rheumatoid arthritis. Arthritis Rheum. 30, 1205–1213.

Gregg, E.W., Geiss, L., Zhang, P., Zhuo, X., Williamson, D.F., Albright, A.L., 2013. Implications of risk stratification for diabetes prevention: the case of hemoglobin A1c. Am. J. Prev. Med. 44, S375–S380.

Hanf, W., Bonder, C.S., Coates, P.T.H., 2014. Transplant glomerulopathy: the interaction of HLA antibodies and endothelium. J. Immunol. Res. 549315, 11.

Häupl, T., Stuhlmüller, B., Grützkau, A., Radbruch, A., Burmester, G.-R., 2010. Does gene expression analysis inform us in rheumatoid arthritis? Ann. Rheum. Dis. 69, i37–i42.

Häupl, T., Biesen, R., Smiljanovic, B., Grün, J.R., Weix, J., Stuhlmüller, B., Villiger, P.M., Burmester, G.-R., Radbruch, A., Grützkau, A., 2011. The type 1 interferon signature: facts, fads and fallacies. Ann. Rheum. Dis. 70, A24.

Hayes, D.F., Thor, A.D., Dressler, L.G., Weaver, D., Edgerton, S., Cowan, D., Broadwater, G., Goldstein, L.J., Martino, S., Ingle, J.N., 2007. HER2 and response to paclitaxel in node-positive breast cancer. N. Engl. J. Med. 357, 1496–1506.

Hegen, H., Millonig, A., Bertolotto, A., Comabella, M., Giovanonni, G., Guger, M., Hoelzl, M., Khalil, M., Killestein, J., Lindberg, R., 2014. Early detection of neutralizing antibodies to interferon-beta in multiple sclerosis patients: binding antibodies predict neutralizing antibody development. Mult. Scler. J. 20, 577–587.

Hegewisch-Becker, S., Faltz, C., Hossfeld, D., 1996. Prolongation of medium exchange is associated with a decrease in function but not expression of the P-glycoprotein pump in leukaemic cells. Eur. J. Haematol. 56, 12–22.

Hegi, M.E., Diserens, A.-C., Gorlia, T., Hamou, M.-F., De Tribolet, N., Weller, M., Kros, J.M., Hainfellner, J.A., Mason, W., Mariani, L., 2005. MGMT gene silencing and benefit from temozolomide in glioblastoma. N. Engl. J. Med. 352, 997–1003.

Hori, S., Nomura, T., Sakaguchi, S., 2003. Control of regulatory T cell development by the transcription factor Foxp3. Science 299, 1057–1061.

Howanitz, P.J., Howanitz, J.H., Lamberson, H.V., Ennis, K.M., 1982. Incidence and mechanism of spurious increases in serum thyrotropin. Clin. Chem. 28, 427–431.

Hudson, P.J., Souriau, C., 2003. Engineered antibodies. Nat. Med. 9, 129–134.

Hueber, W., Tomooka, B.H., Zhao, X.Y., Kidd, B.A., Drijfhout, J.W., Fries, J.F., Van Venrooij, W.J., Metzger, A.L., Genovese, M.C., Robinson, W.H., 2007. Proteomic analysis of secreted proteins in early rheumatoid arthritis: anti-citrulline autoreactivity is associated with up regulation of proinflammatory cytokines. Ann. Rheum. Dis. 66, 712–719.

Hueber, W., Tomooka, B.H., Batliwalla, F., Li, W., Monach, P.A., Tibshirani, R.J., Van Vollenhoven, R.F., Lampa, J., Saito, K., Tanaka, Y., 2009. Blood autoantibody and cytokine profiles predict response to anti-tumor necrosis factor therapy in rheumatoid arthritis. Arthritis Res. Ther. 11, R76.

Hunter, W.M., Budd, P.S., 1980. Circulating antibodies to ovine and bovine immunoglobulin in healthy-subjects—a hazard for immunoassays. Lancet 2, 1136.

Hur, K., Xu, G., Okugawa, Y., Toiyama, Y., Chang, A.N., Boland, C.R., Goel, A., 2014. Sa1898 next generation sequencing (NGS)-based transcriptomic approaches for the identification of novel colorectal cancer (CRC)-specific miRNA biomarkers. Gastroenterology 146, S-323.

Janeway, C.A., Travers, P., Walport, M., Shlomchik, M.J., 2001. The major histocompatibility complex and its functions in immunobiology: the immune system in health and disease, fifth ed. Garland Science, New York. Available from: http://www.ncbi.nlm.nih.gov/books/NBK27156.

Julià, A., Erra, A., Palacio, C., Tomas, C., Sans, X., Barceló, P., Marsal, S., 2009. An eight-gene blood expression profile predicts the response to infliximab in rheumatoid arthritis. PLoS One. 4, e7556.

Kang, C.P., Lee, K.-W., Yoo, D.-H., Kang, C., Bae, S.-C., 2005. The influence of a polymorphism at position − 857 of the tumour necrosis factor α gene on clinical response to etanercept therapy in rheumatoid arthritis. Rheumatology 44, 547–552.

Kastbom, A., Bratt, J., Ernestam, S., Lampa, J., Padyukov, L., Söderkvist, P., Skogh, T., 2007. Fcγ receptor type IIIA genotype and response to tumor necrosis factor α-blocking agents in patients with rheumatoid arthritis. Arthritis Rheum. 56, 448–452.

Kim, M., Townsend, K.R., Wood, I.G., Boukedes, S., Guleria, I., Gabardi, S., El-Chemaly, S., Camp, P.C., Chandraker, A.K., Milford, E.L., 2014. Impact of pretransplant anti-HLA antibodies on outcomes in lung transplant candidates. Am. J. Respir. Crit. Care Med. 189, 1234–1239.

Klein, J., 1986. Seeds of time: fifty years ago Peter A. Gorer discovered the H-2 complex. Immunogenetics 24, 331–338.

Koczan, D., Drynda, S., Hecker, M., Drynda, A., Guthke, R., Kekow, J., Thiesen, H.J., 2008. Molecular discrimination of responders and nonresponders to anti-TNFalpha therapy in rheumatoid arthritis by etanercept. Arthritis Res. Ther. 10, R50.

Kuner, R., Brase, J.C., Sültmann, H., Wuttig, D., 2013. microRNA biomarkers in body fluids of prostate cancer patients. Methods 59, 132–137.

Larsen, M.L., Hørder, M., Mogensen, E.F., 1990. Effect of long-term monitoring of glycosylated hemoglobin levels in insulin-dependent diabetes mellitus. N. Engl. J. Med. 323, 1021–1025.

Lauwerys, B.R., Hachulla, E., Spertini, F., Lazaro, E., Jorgensen, C., Mariette, X., Haelterman, E., Grouard-Vogel, G., Fanget, B., Dhellin, O., 2013. Down-regulation of interferon signature in systemic lupus erythematosus patients by active immunization with interferon α-kinoid. Arthritis Rheum. 65, 447–456.

Lawson, C.A., Brown, A.K., Bejarano, V., Douglas, S.H., Burgoyne, C.H., Greenstein, A.S., Boylston, A.W., Emery, P., Ponchel, F., Isaacs, J.D., 2006. Early rheumatoid arthritis is associated with a deficit in the CD4 (+)CD25(high) regulatory T cell population in peripheral blood. Rheumatology 45, 1210–1217.

Legendre, C., 2014. Antibody-mediated vascular rejection of kidney allograft: characterization of different kidney allograft rejection phenotypes via histology, C4d deposition and donor-specific antibodies. Clin. Exp. Immunol. 178, 59–60.

Lembo, A., Neri, B., Tolley, J., Barken, D., Carroll, S., Pan, H., 2009. Use of serum biomarkers in a diagnostic test for irritable bowel syndrome. Aliment. Pharmacol. Ther. 29, 834–842.

Lequerré, T., Gauthier-Jauneau, A.C., Bansard, C., Derambure, C., Hiron, M., Vittecoq, O., Daveau, M., Mejjad, O., Daragon, A., Tron, F., 2006. Gene profiling in white blood cells predicts infliximab responsiveness in rheumatoid arthritis. Arthritis Res. Ther. 8, R105.

Lindberg, J., Af Klint, E., Catrina, A.I., Nilsson, P., Klareskog, L., Ulfgren, A.K., Lundeberg, J., 2006. Effect of infliximab on mRNA expression profiles in synovial tissue of rheumatoid arthritis patients. Arthritis Res. Ther. 8, R179.

Lindberg, J., Wijbrandts, C.A., Van Baarsen, L.G., Nader, G., Klareskog, L., Catrina, A., Thurlings, R., Vervoordeldonk, M., Lundeberg, J., Tak, P.P., 2010. The gene expression profile in the synovium as a predictor of the clinical response to infliximab treatment in rheumatoid arthritis. PLoS One 5. e11310.

Linder, M.W., Looney, S., Adams Iii, J.E., Johnson, N., Antonino-Green, D., Lacefield, N., Bukaveckas, B.L., Valdes Jr., R., 2002. Warfarin dose adjustments based on CYP2C9 genetic polymorphisms. J. Thromb. Thrombolysis 14, 227–232.

Liu, W., Putnam, A.L., Xu-yu, Z., Szot, G.L., Lee, M., 2006. CD127 expression inversely correlates with FoxP3 and suppressive function of human CD4+ T reg cells. J. Exp. Med. 203, 1701–1711.

Lübbers, J., Brink, M., Van De Stadt, L.A., Vosslamber, S., Wesseling, J.G., Van Schaardenburg, D., Rantapää-Dahlqvist, S., Verweij, C.L., 2013. The type I IFN signature as a biomarker of preclinical rheumatoid arthritis. Ann. Rheum. Dis. 72, 776–780.

Lynch, T.J., Bell, D.W., Sordella, R., Gurubhagavatula, S., Okimoto, R.A., Brannigan, B.W., Harris, P.L., Haserlat, S.M., Supko, J.G., Haluska, F.G., 2004. Activating mutations in the epidermal growth factor receptor underlying responsiveness of non–small-cell lung cancer to gefitinib. N. Engl. J. Med. 350, 2129–2139.

Maillard-Lefebvre, H., Boulanger, E., Daroux, M., Gaxatte, C., Hudson, B.I., Lambert, M., 2009. Soluble receptor for advanced glycation end products: a new biomarker in diagnosis and prognosis of chronic inflammatory diseases. Rheumatology 48, 1190–1196.

Marino, K., Saldova, R., Adamczyk, B., Rudd, P.M., Rauter, A., 2011. Changes in serum N-glycosylation profiles: functional significance and potential for diagnostics. Carbohydr. Chem. 37, 57–86.

Marotte, H., Maslinski, W., Miossec, P., 2005. Circulating tumour necrosis factor-alpha bioactivity in rheumatoid arthritis patients treated with infliximab: link to clinical response. Arthritis Res. Ther. 7, R149–R155.

Marotte, H., Pallot-Prades, B., Grange, L., Tebib, J., Gaudin, P., Alexandre, C., Blond, J., Cazalis, M., Mougin, B., Miossec, P., 2006. The shared epitope is a marker of severity associated with selection for, but not with response to, infliximab in a large rheumatoid arthritis population. Ann. Rheum. Dis. 65, 342–347.

Martinez, A., Salido, M., Bonilla, G., Pascual-Salcedo, D., Fernandez-Arquero, M., De Miguel, S., Balsa, A., De La Concha, E.G., Fernandez-Gutierrez, B., 2004. Association of the major histocompatibility complex with response to infliximab therapy in rheumatoid arthritis patients. Arthritis Rheum. 50, 1077–1082.

Martins, T.B., 2002. Development of internal controls for the Luminex instrument as part of a multiplex seven-analyte viral respiratory antibody profile. Clin. Diagn. Lab. Immunol. 9, 41–45.

Mavragani, C.P., Crow, M.K., 2010. Activation of the type I interferon pathway in primary Sjogren's syndrome. J. Autoimmun. 35, 225–231.

Mellors, J.W., Rinaldo, C.R., Gupta, P., White, R.M., Todd, J.A., Kingsley, L.A., 1996. Prognosis in HIV-1 infection predicted by the quantity of virus in plasma. Science 272, 1167–1170.

Miceli-Richard, C., Comets, E., Verstuyft, C., Tamouza, R., Loiseau, P., Ravaud, P., Kupper, H., Becquemont, L., Charron, D., Mariette, X., 2008. A single tumour necrosis factor haplotype influences the response to adalimumab in rheumatoid arthritis. Ann. Rheum. Dis. 67, 478–484.

Moorman, A.J., Mozaffarian, D., Wilkinson, C.W., Lawler, R.L., Mcdonald, G.B., Crane, B.A., Spertus, J.A., Russo, J.E., Stempien-Otero, A.S., Sullivan, M.D., 2007. In patients with heart failure elevated soluble TNF-receptor 1 is associated with higher risk of depression. J. Card. Fail. 13, 738–743.

Mu, H., Chen, J.J., Jiang, Y., King, M.C., Thomson, G., Criswell, L.A., 1999. Tumor necrosis factor a microsatellite polymorphism is associated with rheumatoid arthritis severity through an interaction with the HLA-DRB1 shared epitope. Arthritis Rheum. 42, 438–442.

Murata, K., Yoshitomi, H., Tanida, S., Ishikawa, M., Nishitani, K., Ito, H., Nakamura, T., 2010. Plasma and synovial fluid microRNAs as potential biomarkers of rheumatoid arthritis and osteoarthritis. Arthritis Res. Ther. 2010 (12), R86.

Mustila, A., Korpela, M., Haapala, A., Kautiainen, H., Laasonen, L., Möttönen, T., Leirisalo-Repo, M., Ilonen, J., Järvenpää, S., Luukkainen, R., 2010. Anti-citrullinated peptide antibodies and the progression of radiographic joint erosions in patients with early rheumatoid arthritis treated with FIN-RACo combination and single disease-modifying antirheumatic drug strategies. Clin. Exp. Rheumatol. 29, 500–505.

Nahm, M.H., Hoffmann, J.W., 1990. Heteroantibody—phantom of the immunoassay. Clin. Chem. 36, 829.

Neumaier, M., 2005. Ethics and quality assessment in genetic testing. J. Int. Federation Clin. Chem. Lab. Med. 16., Available from, http://www.ifcc.org/ejifcc/vol16no2/.

Niewold, T.B., 2014. Type I interferon in human autoimmunity. Front. Immunol. 5, 306.

Niewold, T.B., Harrison, M.J., Paget, S.A., 2007. Anti-CCP antibody testing as a diagnostic and prognostic tool in rheumatoid arthritis. QJM 100, 193–201.

Obermoser, G., Pascual, V., 2010. The interferon-α signature of systemic lupus erythematosus. Lupus 19, 1012–1019.

Othman, E.E.-D.R., Hornung, D., Salem, H.T., Khalifa, E.A., El-Metwally, T.H., Al-Hendy, A., 2008. Serum cytokines as biomarkers for nonsurgical prediction of endometriosis. Eur. J. Obstet. Gynecol. Reprod. Biol. 137, 240–246.

Paczesny, S., Krijanovski, O.I., Braun, T.M., Choi, S.W., Clouthier, S.G., Kuick, R., Misek, D.E., Cooke, K.R., Kitko, C.L., Weyand, A., 2009. A biomarker panel for acute graft-versus-host disease. Blood 113, 273–278.

Parsons, P.E., Matthay, M.A., Ware, L.B., Eisner, M.D., 2005. Elevated plasma levels of soluble TNF receptors are associated with morbidity and mortality in patients with acute lung injury. Am. J. Physiol. Lung Cell. Mol. Physiol. 288, L426–L431.

Pauley, K.M., Satoh, M., Chan, A.L., Bubb, M.R., Reeves, W.H., Chan, E.K., 2008. Upregulated miR-146a expression in peripheral blood mononuclear cells from rheumatoid arthritis patients. Arthritis Res. Ther. 10, R101.

Polman, C.H., Bertolotto, A., Deisenhammer, F., Giovannoni, G., Hartung, H.-P., Hemmer, B., Killestein, J., Mcfarland, H.F., Oger, J., Pachner, A.R., 2010. Recommendations for clinical use of data on neutralising antibodies to interferon-beta therapy in multiple sclerosis. Lancet Neurol. 9, 740–750.

Ponchel, F., Morgan, A.W., Bingham, S.J., Quinn, M., Buch, M., Verburg, R.J., Henwood, J., Douglas, S.H., Masurel, A., Conaghan, P., Gesinde, M., Taylor, J., Markham, A.F., Emery, P., Van Laar, J.M., Isaacs, J.D., 2002. Dysregulated lymphocyte proliferation and differentiation in patients with rheumatoid arthritis. Blood 100, 4550–4556.

Ponchel, F., Verburg, R., Bingham, S., Brown, A., Moore, J., Protheroe, A., Lawson, C., Buch, M., Morgan, A., Douglas, S., Masurel, A., Mcgonagle, D., Markham, A., Ma, D., Van Laar, J., Emery, P., Papadaki, H., Isaacs, J., 2005. IL-7 deficiency and therapy-induced lymphopenia in Rheumatoid Arthritis. Arthritis Res. Ther. 7, 80–92.

Ponchel, F., Goëb, V., Parmar, R., El-Sherbiny, Y., Boissinot, M., El Jawhari, J., Burska, A., Vital, E.M., Harrison, S., Conaghan, P.G., 2014. An immunological biomarker to predict MTX response in early RA. Ann. Rheum. Dis. 73, 2047–2053.

Potter, C., Hyrich, K.L., Tracey, A., Lunt, M., Plant, D., Symmons, D.P.M., Thomson, W., Worthington, J., Emery, P., Morgan, A.W., Wilson, A.G., Isaacs, J., Barton, A., BRAGGSS, 2009. Association of rheumatoid factor and anti-cyclic citrullinated peptide positivity, but not carriage of shared epitope or PTPN22 susceptibility variants, with anti-tumour necrosis factor response in rheumatoid arthritis. Ann. Rheum. Dis. 68, 69–74.

Prince, H.E., 2005. Biomarkers for diagnosing and monitoring autoimmune diseases. Biomarkers 10, 44–49.

Prince, A.M., Jass, D., Brotman, B., Ikram, H., 1973. Specificity of direct solid-phase radioimmunoassay for detection of hepatitis-b antigen. Lancet 1, 1346–1350.

Radstake, T.R., Svenson, M., Eijsbouts, A.M., Van Den Hoogen, F.H., Enevold, C., Van Riel, P.L., Bendtzen, K., 2009. Formation of antibodies against infliximab and adalimumab strongly correlates with functional drug levels and clinical responses in rheumatoid arthritis. Ann. Rheum. Dis. 68, 1739–1745.

Rajkumar, S.V., 2014. Multiple myeloma: 2014 update on diagnosis, risk-stratification, and management. Am. J. Hematol. 89, 998–1009.

Rakieh, C., Nam, J., Hunt, L., Hensor, E., Das, S., Bissell, L., Villeneuve, E., Mcgonagle, D., Hodgson, R., Grainger, A., 2014. Predicting the development of clinical arthritis in anti-CCP positive individuals with non-specific musculoskeletal symptoms: a prospective observational cohort study. Ann. Rheum. Dis. http://dx.doi.org/10.1136/annrheumdis-2014-205227.

Reynier, F., Pachot, A., Paye, M., Xu, Q., Turrel-Davin, F., Petit, F., Hot, A., Auffray, C., Bendelac, N., Nicolino, M., Mougin, B., Thivolet, C., 2010. Specific gene expression signature associated with development of autoimmune type-I diabetes using whole-blood microarray analysis. Genes Immun. 11, 269–278.

Rhodus, N.L., Cheng, B., Myers, S., Bowles, W., Ho, V., Ondrey, F., 2005. A comparison of the pro-inflammatory, NF-κB-dependent cytokines: TNF-alpha, IL-1-alpha, IL-6, and IL-8 in different oral fluids from oral lichen planus patients. Clin. Immunol. 114, 278–283.

Rieder, M.J., Reiner, A.P., Gage, B.F., Nickerson, D.A., Eby, C.S., Mcleod, H.L., Blough, D.K., Thummel, K.E., Veenstra, D.L., Rettie, A.E., 2005. Effect of VKORC1 haplotypes on transcriptional regulation and warfarin dose. N. Engl. J. Med. 352, 2285–2293.

Roelofs, M.F., Wenink, M.H., Brentano, F., Abdollahi-Roodsaz, S., Oppers-Walgreen, B., Barrera, P., Van Riel, P.L.C.M., Joosten, L.A.B., Kyburz, D., Van Den Berg, W.B., Radstake, T.R.D.J., 2009. Type I interferons might form the link between Toll-like receptor (TLR) 3/7 and TLR4-mediated synovial inflammation in rheumatoid arthritis (RA). Ann. Rheum. Dis. 68, 1486–1493.

Rönnblom, L., Eloranta, M.-L., 2013. The interferon signature in autoimmune diseases. Curr. Opin. Rheumatol. 25, 248–253.

Rudd, P., Butler, M., Wilson, I., Jaeken, J., Dwek, R., 2001a. Roles for glycosylation in the immune system. Glycobiology 11, 865.

Rudd, P.M., Elliott, T., Cresswell, P., Wilson, I.A., Dwek, R.A., 2001b. Glycosylation and the immune system. Science 291, 2370–2376.

Saag, M.S., Holodniy, M., Kuritzkes, D., O'brien, W., Coombs, R., Poscher, M., Jacobsen, D., Shaw, G., Richman, D., Volberding, P., 1996. HIV viral load markers in clinical practice. Nat. Med. 2, 625–629.

Saleem, B., Keen, H., Goeb, V., Parmar, R., Nizam, S., Hensor, E.M., Churchman, S.M., Quinn, M., Wakefield, R., Conaghan, P.G., Ponchel, F., Emery, P., 2010. Patients with RA in remission on TNF blockers: when and in whom can TNF blocker therapy be stopped? Ann. Rheum. Dis. 69, 1636–1642.

Satoh, M., Iida, S., Shitara, K., 2006. Non-fucosylated therapeutic antibodies as next-generation therapeutic antibodies. Expert. Opin. Biol. Ther. 6, 1161–1173.

Schilsky, R.L., 2010. Personalized medicine in oncology: the future is now. Nat. Rev. Drug Discov. 9, 363–366.

Schroth, W., Antoniadou, L., Fritz, P., Schwab, M., Muerdter, T., Zanger, U.M., Simon, W., Eichelbaum, M., Brauch, H., 2007. Breast cancer treatment outcome with adjuvant tamoxifen relative to patient CYP2D6 and CYP2C19 genotypes. J. Clin. Oncol. 25, 5187–5193.

Seddiki, N., Santner-Nanan, B., Martinson, J., Zaunders, J., Sasson, S., Landay, A., Solomon, M., Selby, W., Alexander, S.I., Nanan, R., Kelleher, A., Fazekas de St Groth, B., 2006. Expression of interleukin (IL)-2 and IL-7 receptors discriminates between human regulatory and activated T cells. J. Exp. Med. 10, 1693–1700.

Selth, L.A., Roberts, M.J., Chow, C.W., Marshall, V.R., Doi, S.A., Vincent, A.D., Butler, L.M., Lavin, M.F., Tilley, W.D., Gardiner, F., 2014. Human seminal fluid as a source of prostate cancer specific microRNA biomarkers. Endocr. Relat. Cancer 21, L17–L21.

Skapenko, A., Sinisi, S., Redden, L., 2010. Response of early rheumatoid arthritis to treatment with adalimumab plus methotrexate vs methotrexate alone: predicting clinical response by genetic marker analysis. Ann. Rheum. Dis. 69, 158.

Smith, M., Slavotinek, J., Au, V., Weedon, H., Parker, A., Coleman, M., Roberts-Thomson, P., Ahern, M., 2001. Successful treatment of rheumatoid arthritis is associated with a reduction in synovial membrane cytokines and cell adhesion molecule expression. Rheumatology 40, 965–977.

Smith, J., Ibrahim, M., Newell, H., Danskine, A., Soresi, S., Burke, M., Rose, M., Carby, M., 2014. Pre-transplant donor HLA specific antibodies: characteristics causing detrimental effects on survival after lung transplantation. J. Heart Lung Transplant. 33, 1074–1082.

Sorensen, P.S., Ross, C., Clemmesen, K.M., Bendtzen, K., Frederiksen, J.L., Jensen, K., Kristensen, O., Petersen, T., Rasmussen, S., Ravnborg, M., 2003. Clinical importance of neutralising antibodies against interferon beta in patients with relapsing-remitting multiple sclerosis. Lancet 362, 1184–1191.

Sotiriou, C., Piccart, M.J., 2007. Taking gene-expression profiling to the clinic: when will molecular signatures become relevant to patient care? Nat. Rev. Cancer 7, 545–553.

Stuhlmüller, B., Häupl, T., Tandon, N., Hernandez, M., Hultschig, C., Kuban, R., Salfeld, J., Burmester, G., 2005. Microarray analysis for molecular characterization of disease activity and measuring outcomes of anti-tumour necrosis factor therapy in rheumatoid arthritis. Arthritis Res. Ther. 7, 1.

Talpaz, M., Shah, N.P., Kantarjian, H., Donato, N., Nicoll, J., Paquette, R., Cortes, J., O'brien, S., Nicaise, C., Bleickardt, E., Blackwood-Chirchir, M.A., Iyer, V., Chen, T.-T., Huang, F., Decillis, A.P., Sawyers, C.L., 2006. Dasatinib in imatinib-resistant Philadelphia chromosome-positive leukemias. N. Engl. J. Med. 354, 2531–2541.

Terasaki, P.I., Cai, J.C., 2005. Humoral theory of transplantation: further evidence. Curr. Opin. Immunol. 17, 541–545.

Terasaki, P.I., Ozawa, M., 2005. Predictive value of HLA antibodies and serum creatinine in chronic rejection: results of a 2-year prospective trial. Transplantation 80, 1194–1197.

Terasaki, P.I., Kreisler, M., Mickey, R.M., 1971. Presensitization and kidney transplant failures. Postgrad. Med. J. 47, 89–100.

Thurlings, R.M., Boumans, M., Tekstra, J., Van Roon, J.A., Vos, K., Van Westing, D.M., Van Baarsen, L.G., Bos, C., Kirou, K.A., Gerlag, D.M., 2010. Relationship between the type I interferon signature and the response to rituximab in rheumatoid arthritis patients. Arthritis Rheum. 62, 3607–3614.

Tonelli, M., Sacks, F., Pfeffer, M., Jhangri, G.S., Curhan, G., 2005. Biomarkers of inflammation and progression of chronic kidney disease. Kidney Int. 68, 237–245.

Tutuncu, Z., Kavanaugh, A., Zvaifler, N., Corr, M., Deutsch, R., Boyle, D., 2005. Fcγ receptor type IIIA polymorphisms influence treatment outcomes in patients with inflammatory arthritis treated with tumor necrosis factor α-blocking agents. Arthritis Rheum. 52, 2693–2696.

Van Amelsfort, J.M.R., Jacobs, K.M.G., Bijlsma, J.W.J., Lafeber, F., Taams, L.S., 2004. CD4+CD25+ regulatory T cells in rheumatoid arthritis—differences in the presence, phenotype, and function between peripheral blood and synovial fluid. Arthritis Rheum. 50, 2775–2785.

Van Baarsen, L.G., Bos, C.L., Van Der Pouw Kraan, T.C., Verweij, C.L., 2009. Transcription profiling of rheumatic diseases. Arthritis Res. Ther. 11, 207.

Van Baarsen, L.G., Bos, W.H., Rustenburg, F., Van Der Pouw Kraan, T.C., Wolbink, G.J.J., Dijkmans, B.A., Van Schaardenburg, D., Verweij, C.L., 2010a. Gene expression profiling in autoantibody-positive patients with arthralgia predicts development of arthritis. Arthritis Rheum. 62, 694–704.

Van Baarsen, L.G., Wijbrandts, C.A., Rustenburg, F., Cantaert, T., Van Der Pouw, T.C., 2010b. Regulation of IFN respon se gene activity during infliximab treatment in rheumatoid arthritis is associated with clinical response to treatment. Arthritis Res. Ther. 12, R11.

Van Der Pouw Kraan, T.C., Wijbrandts, C.A., Van Baarsen, L.G., Rustenburg, F., Baggen, J.M., Verweij, C.L., Tak, P.P., 2008. Responsiveness to anti-tumour necrosis factor α therapy is related to pre-treatment tissue inflammation levels in rheumatoid arthritis patients. Ann. Rheum. Dis. 67, 563–566.

Van Der Woude, D., Syversen, S.W., Van Der Voort, E.I., Verpoort, K.N., Goll, G.L., Van Der Linden, M.P., Van Der Helm-Van, A.H., Van Der Heijde, D.M., Huizinga, T.W., Kvien, T.K., 2010. The ACPA isotype profile reflects long-term radiographic progression in rheumatoid arthritis. Ann. Rheum. Dis. 69, 1110–1116.

Van Gaalen, F.A., Van Aken, J., Huizinga, T.W., Schreuder, G.M.T., Breedveld, F.C., Zanelli, E., Van Venrooij, W.J., Verweij, C.L., Toes, R.E., De Vries, R.R., 2004. Association between HLA class II genes and autoantibodies to cyclic citrullinated peptides (CCPs) influences the severity of rheumatoid arthritis. Arthritis Rheum. 50, 2113–2121.

Van Holten, J., Smeets, T., Blankert, P., Tak, P., 2005. Expression of interferon β in synovial tissue from patients with rheumatoid arthritis: comparison with patients with osteoarthritis and reactive arthritis. Ann. Rheum. Dis. 64, 1780–1782.

Van Schouwenburg, P.A., Van De Stadt, L.A., De Jong, R.N., Van Buren, E.E., Kruithof, S., De Groot, E., Hart, M., Van Ham, S.M., Rispens, T., Aarden, L., 2012. Adalimumab elicits a restricted anti-idiotypic antibody response in autoimmune patients resulting in functional neutralisation. Ann. Rheum. Dis. 72, 104–109.

Verburg, R., Flierman, R., Sont, J., Ponchel, F., Van Dreunen, L., Levahrt, N., Welling, M., Toes, R., Isaacs, J., Van Laar, J.M., 2005. The outcome of intensive immunosuppression and autologous stemcell transplantation in patients with severe rheumatoid arthritis is associated with the composition of synovial T cell infiltration. Ann. Rheum. Dis. 64, 1397–1405.

Verweij, C.L., Vosslamber, S., 2013. Relevance of the Type I interferon signature in multiple sclerosis towards a personalized medicine approach for interferon-beta therapy. Discov. Med. 15, 51–60.

Vieira, C.A., Agarwal, A., Book, B.K., Sidner, R.A., Bearden, C.M., Gebel, H.M., Roggero, A.L., Fineberg, N.S., Taber, T., Kraus, M.A., 2004. Rituximab for reduction of anti-HLA antibodies in patients awaiting renal transplantation: 1. safety, pharmacodynamics, and pharmacokinetics. Transplantation 77, 542–548.

Vincent, C., Serre, G., Lapeyre, F., Fournié, B., Ayrolles, C., Fournié, A., Soleilhavoup, J., 1989. High diagnostic value in rheumatoid arthritis of antibodies to the stratum corneum of rat oesophagus epithelium, so-called' antikeratin antibodies. Ann. Rheum. Dis. 48, 712–722.

Vis, M., Bos, W.H., Wolbink, G., Voskuyl, A.E., Twisk, J.W., Van De Stadt, R., Hamann, D., Dijkmans, B.A., Lems, W.F., 2008. IgM-rheumatoid factor, anti-cyclic citrullinated peptide, and anti-citrullinated human fibrinogen antibodies decrease during treatment with the tumor necrosis factor blocker infliximab in patients with rheumatoid arthritis. J. Rheumatol. 35, 425–428.

Vital, E., Israelsson, L., Nogueira, L., Malmstrom, V., El-Sherbiny, Y., Rawstron, A., Serre, G., Klareskog, L., Ponchel, F., Emery, P., 2014. ACPA fine specificity is associated with increased plasmablast numbers and worse clinical response to rituximab in rheumatoid arthritis. Ann. Rheum. Dis. 73, A14–A15, 450.

Weinberg, E.O., Shimpo, M., Hurwitz, S., Tominaga, S.-I., Rouleau, J.-L., Lee, R.T., 2003. Identification of serum soluble ST2 receptor as a novel heart failure biomarker. Circulation 107, 721–726.

Wijbrandts, C.A., Dijkgraaf, M.G.W., Kraan, M.C., Vinkenoog, M., Smeets, T.J., Dinant, H., Vos, K., Lems, W.F., Wolbink, G.J., Sijpkens, D., Dijkmans, B.a.C, Tak, P.P., 2008. The clinical response to infliximab in rheumatoid arthritis is in part dependent on pretreatment tumour necrosis factor α expression in the synovium. Ann. Rheum. Dis. 67, 1139–1144.

Wright, H.L., Bucknall, R.C., Moots, R.J., Edwards, S.W., 2012. Analysis of SF and plasma cytokines provides insights into the mechanisms of inflammatory arthritis and may predict response to therapy. Rheumatology 51, 451–459.

Yao, Y., Richman, L., Morehouse, C., De Los Reyes, M., Higgs, B.W., Boutrin, A., White, B., Coyle, A., Krueger, J., Kiener, P.A., 2008. Type I interferon: potential therapeutic target for psoriasis? PLoS One 3. e2737.

Yao, Y., Higgs, B.W., Morehouse, C., De Los Reyes, M., Trigona, W., Brohawn, P., White, W., Zhang, J., White, B., Coyle, A.J., Kiener, P.A., Jallal, B., 2009a. Development of potential pharmacodynamic and diagnostic markers for anti-IFN-alpha monoclonal antibody trials in systemic lupus erythematosus. Hum. Genomics Proteomics 2009, 374312.

Yao, Y., Richman, L., Higgs, B.W., Morehouse, C.A., De Los Reyes, M., Brohawn, P., Zhang, J., White, B., Coyle, A.J., Kiener, P.A., Jallal, B., 2009b. Neutralization of interferon-alpha/beta-inducible genes and downstream effect in a phase I trial of an anti-interferon-alpha monoclonal antibody in systemic lupus erythematosus. Arthritis Rheum. 60, 1785–1796.

Yong, P.L., Russo, P., Sullivan, K.E., 2008. Use of sirolimus in IPEX and IPEX-like children. J. Clin. Immunol. 28, 581–587.

Zivojinovic, S.M., Pejnovic, N.N., Sefik-Bukilica, M.N., Kovacevic, L.V., Soldatovic, I.I., Damjanov, N.S., 2012. Tumor necrosis factor blockade differentially affects innate inflammatory and Th17 Cytokines in Rheumatoid Arthritis. J. Rheumatol. 39, 18–21.

Zweig, M.H., Csako, G., Benson, C.C., Weintraub, B.D., Kahn, B.B., 1987. Interference by anti-immunoglobulin-g antibodies in immunoradiometric assays of thyrotropin involving mouse monoclonal-antibodies. Clin. Chem. 33, 840–844.

INDEX

Note: Page numbers followed by *f* indicate figures and *t* indicate tables.

J

K

L

M

S

Kolibri 360 GmbH
Ferdinand-Jühlke-Straße 7
99095 Erfurt, Deutschland
produktsicherheit@kolibri360.de